Atlas and Text of Aspiration Biopsy Cytology

The First Century 1890-1990 SANS TACHE

Atlas and Text of Aspiration Biopsy Cytology

Kenneth C. Suen, M.D., F.R.C.P.(C)

Pathologist
Vancouver General Hospital

Consulting Pathologist
Cancer Control Agency of British Columbia

Clinical Professor of Pathology
University of British Columbia
Vancouver, British Columbia, Canada

WILLIAMS & WILKINS
Baltimore • Hong Kong • London • Sydney

Editor: Timothy S. Satterfield
Associate Editor: Linda Napora
Project Editor: Klementyna L. Bryte
Designer: Wilma Rosenberger
Illustration Planner: Ray Lowman
Production Coordinator: Charles E. Zeller

Cover Illustrations: Aspirate smear showing pleomorphic adenoma of the parotid gland *(left)* and histologic section of the resected pleomorphic adenoma *(right).*

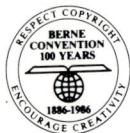

Library of Congress Cataloging-in-Publication Data
Suen, Kenneth C.
    Atlas and text of aspiration biopsy cytology / Kenneth C. Suen.
        p.   cm.
    Includes index.
    ISBN 0-683-08024-5
    1. Biopsy, Needle—Atlases.   2. Diagnosis, Cytologic—Atlases.
  I. Title.
    [DNLM: 1. Biopsy, Needle—methods—atlases.   WB 17 S944a]
  RB43.S84   1990
  616.07'58—dc20
  DNLM/DLC
  for Library of Congress   89-5722
                                                                    CIP

                                        89 90 91 92 93
                                    1 2 3 4 5 6 7 8 9 10

Foreword

To many, aspiration biopsy is a rather opaque subject or an arcane science practiced by a few superspecialists. This, of course, is no longer the situation, as it has moved from being a topic of interest for a small number to being the order of the day in modern major pathology programs. Dr. Kenneth Suen is one individual who showed keen interest in aspiration biopsy early in his career, when in the early 1970s he was a Fellow in Surgical Pathology at Memorial Sloan-Kettering Cancer Center. By the late 1970s he was responsible for setting up a highly regarded aspiration biopsy system at the Vancouver General Hospital. He has been involved in applying this technique and teaching it to other pathologists and residents over the past decade. Dr. Suen is truly a hands-on pathologist, who sees patients, performs the biopsy aspirations by himself, and interprets them with his colleagues. His expert opinions are highly valued, as reflected by the large number of cases sent to him in consultations by pathologists throughout Canada and beyond.

It gives me great pleasure to see that Dr. Suen's considerable expertise, now translated into print, can be shared by all pathologists. This book is not simply an atlas with brief legends accompanying the illustrations. It contains comprehensive text with consideration of all common entities that constitute the "bread and butter" of aspiration biopsy, with the exception of the central nervous system lesions, which are traditionally in the domain of the neuropathologists. The book also includes many uncommon entities that are beyond the experience of any one laboratory, the inclusion of which was possible because of the vast amount of material available to the author from both on-site and consultation cases. To condense so much information into a single-volume monograph is a formidable undertaking. It takes someone like Dr. Suen, who not only understands the subject thoroughly but also writes clearly and succinctly, to accomplish this feat. Dr. Suen uses hematoxylin and eosin (H & E) staining for his aspirates. Since the comparison of aspiration cytology with histology is very important, histopathologists who interpret aspiration cytology will find diagnostic similarities between the cells in the smears stained with H & E and those in the histologic sections. In interpreting cytologic smears, the author emphasizes not only cell morphology but also pattern recognition, thus achieving a high diagnostic accuracy. This combined approach reflects his wide experience and knowledge in surgical pathology. The opening chapter and the chapters on thyroid, liver, breast, and soft tissue, in my opinion, provide many practical solutions to especially difficult problems.

I heartily recommend this book of fine needle aspiration cytology, written by an acknowledged leader in the field, to all those engaged in the daily practice of this very useful diagnostic procedure.

David F. Hardwick, M.D., F.R.C.P.(C)
Professor and Head
Department of Pathology
University of British Columbia

Preface

The widespread use of fine needle aspiration biopsy (FNAB) in clinical medicine has created a need for an up-to-date text with explanatory illustrations to aid pathologists, residents, and cytotechnologists in interpreting FNAB. It is my hope that this book will meet that need and serve as a practical guide. The volume has been kept to a usable size, and yet includes virtually all of the common as well as many not-so-common lesions of the human body. For all of the important pathologic entities, the characteristic cell morphology, cellular pattern, histologic correlation, differential diagnosis, and interpretative pitfalls are presented.

The style and content of this book have been influenced by the four convictions I developed from my involvement with teaching residents about FNAB. First, in order to be a competent cytopathologist one must be a competent histopathologist because the cytologic changes in FNAB mirror the histologic changes. To master FNAB, the pathologist must be knowledgeable in the normal and pathologic conditions of the organs involved. For this reason, throughout the book the cytologic photomicrographs are matched, whenever feasible, with the corresponding histologic sections. Second, the "pattern recognition" approach is an integral part of FNAB interpretation and will be emphasized. The pathologist is doing the technique an injustice and the patient a disservice if he or she just examines the morphology of the individual cells without paying close attention to the cellular pattern. Third, as diagnosticians, we should no longer be satisfied with the cytologic diagnosis of cells as merely benign or malignant. Whenever possible, an attempt should be made to classify the tumors according to their histogenesis. Together with the pattern recognition approach, immunocytochemistry and electron microscopy facilitate accurate typing of many forms of cancer and are fully applicable to aspirated material. Fourth, many times clinical data help to clarify an otherwise insoluble differential diagnostic problem. The pathologist engaging in FNAB must work closely with the clinician and radiologist; this team approach will provide the optimal milieu for a correct diagnosis.

Acknowledgments

Many pathologists helped me in different ways in the production of this book. In particular, Dr. Jean LeRiche of the Cancer Control Agency of British Columbia and Drs. Nazma Jetha and Edward Jones of the Shaughnessy Hospital, Vancouver, generously allowed me to review their cases. I would like to thank Dr. David F. Hardwick, Head, Department of Pathology, University of British Columbia, and Dr. Noel F. Quenville, Head, Division of Anatomical Pathology, Vancouver General Hospital, without whose support this book would probably have taken twice as long to finish. I also appreciate the fine needle aspiration cytotechnologists, Cori-Ann Greene and Charlene Martin, for their unabating devotion in this technique and their meticulous preparation of the specimens.

Last, but not least, I thank my wife, Peggy, and my children, Meredith and Kevin, for their forbearance toward a husband and parent whose mind was constantly preoccupied.

Explanatory Notes

Figure Legends

    To avoid repetitions and save space in the figure legends, we have adopted the following format:

    The routine stain used for needle aspirates is either the Papanicolaou or hematoxylin and eosin stain. Because there are no significant tinctorial differences in black and white photomicrographs, the type of routine stain used is not specified in the legends. However, other stains used are identified.

Abbreviations

ABC	aspiration biopsy cytology
CT	computed tomography
FNAB	fine needle aspiration biopsy
H & E	hematoxylin and eosin
MGG	May-Grünwald Giemsa
N/C ratio	nuclear/cytoplasmic ratio
Pap stain	Papanicolaou stain

Contents

1

Introduction and General Considerations

Fine needle aspiration biopsy (FNAB) is simple, speedy, safe, cost-effective, and accurate. Three major factors have contributed to its increasing popularity. First, we are now witnessing a gradual shift from inpatient hospital care to outpatient care due to demand for medical cost containment.[1-3] In numerous instances, surgical biopsy necessitating anesthetic and surgical expertise is now being replaced by FNAB, which can be readily performed in the outpatient department. Second, contemporary advances in cross-sectional imaging techniques enable accurate localization of mass lesions. Anatomic sites that were formerly inaccessible by exfoliative cytology can now be investigated by aspiration cytology, procured under ultrasound or computed tomography (CT) guidance. Third, modern refinements in cytologic diagnosis including use of immunocytochemistry, electron microscopy, flow cytometry, and image analysis have acclerated the acceptability of FNAB.

The simplicity of the aspiration technique, however, does not mean interpretation is less demanding than that of surgical biopsy specimens. In fact, at the present time a major factor that limits the optimal use of this procedure is the shortage of properly trained cytotechnologists and pathologists. **Table 1.1** lists the advantages and disadvantages of fine needle aspiration biopsy.

Table 1.1. Fine Needle Aspiration Biopsy

Advantages
1. The technique is an economical, outpatient procedure.
2. It has wide patient acceptance because it is less traumatic than the conventional tissue biopsy.
3. It is rapid. Results can be available in 20–30 minutes.
4. It can be repeated as often as necessary.
5. It is highly accurate in experienced hands.
6. Even when the diagnosis is not definite, a less-than-certain diagnosis will often provide useful information to guide the clinician to choose future investigations.
7. Other uses:
    a. Aspirate material is suited for bacteriologic, electron microscopic, immunocytochemical, and other studies.
    b. The technique can be used intraoperatively in lieu of frozen sections, particularly in carcinoma of the pancreas.

Disadvantages
1. The technique is not suitable for investigation of many nonneoplastic conditions where detailed examination of tissue architecture is necessary for diagnosis.
2. Considerable training and experience are required before the results become reliable.
3. The procedure may produce complications, e.g., bleeding, infection, and seeding of tumor cells. Complications, however, are far less than those of conventional biopsy.

SOURCES OF MATERIAL

The volume of material available to the author for study is considerable. There are approximately 25,000 cases of FNAB accumulated in our files since 1978. These cases are derived from two large medical centers where I am a pathologist. Vancouver General Hospital is an acute care general hospital with 1000 beds (it had 1700 beds a few years ago), where FNAB is used as an initial investigation rather than at the end of a long sequence of diagnostic procedures. About 1200 aspiration biopsies are performed each year. The Cancer Control Agency of British Columbia is a cancer treatment and research center with a mandate to provide optimal care to all cancer patients in the province. About 1800 aspiration biopsies are preformed annually for tumor recurrence, staging, and follow-up in patients who already have a diagnosis of cancer before referral. All types of malignancies are encountered, diagnoses and follow-up data are computerized, and opportunities for cytohistologic correlation are superb. In addition, there are about 1000 FNABs (mainly breast aspirates) sent to us annually by individual clinicians who perform the procedure at their offices.

ASPIRATION TECHNIQUE

At our institutions, superficial masses are aspirated by clinicians and pathologists. The needles used are 21–23 gauge, 25 or 38 mm (1 or 1.5 inches) long **(Fig. 1.1)**. The needle is connected to a 12–ml air-tight plastic syringe, which is fitted snugly in a syringe holder **(Fig. 1.2)**. The latter is purchased from Precision Dynamics Corporation, Burbank, CA. This unit requires only one hand to achieve strong, repetitive suction so that the other hand is free to immobilize the mass.

For aspiration of superficial masses, local anesthesia is not necessary. The skin overlying the mass is cleansed with an antiseptic. After the needle has entered the mass, the plunger is retracted to create a vacuum in the syringe. The needle is moved back and forth several times in the lesion as material is being sucked into the needle by the negative pressure. Most of the time the cell sample remains in the needle and is not visible in the syringe barrel. Before withdrawing the needle from the lesion, suction must be released to avoid aspiration of the material into the syringe barrel. To expel the sample onto the glass slides, the needle is quickly detached from the syringe and the plunger is retracted to allow air to fill the syringe. The needle is then reattached and the content is ejected forcefully onto the slides by pushing down the plunger. Usually an average of three smears can be made per puncture. If a smear is too thick, it can be spread out evenly with the tip of the needle or with another glass slide. If the aspirated material is scanty, it should be expressed directly onto the slide without further manipulation. After slide prep-

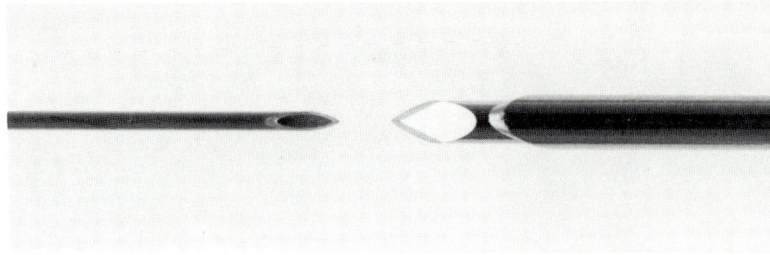

Figure 1.1.   A 22-gauge fine needle for aspiration biopsy *(left)*. A Tru-cut needle *(right)* for histologic biopsy is shown for comparison.

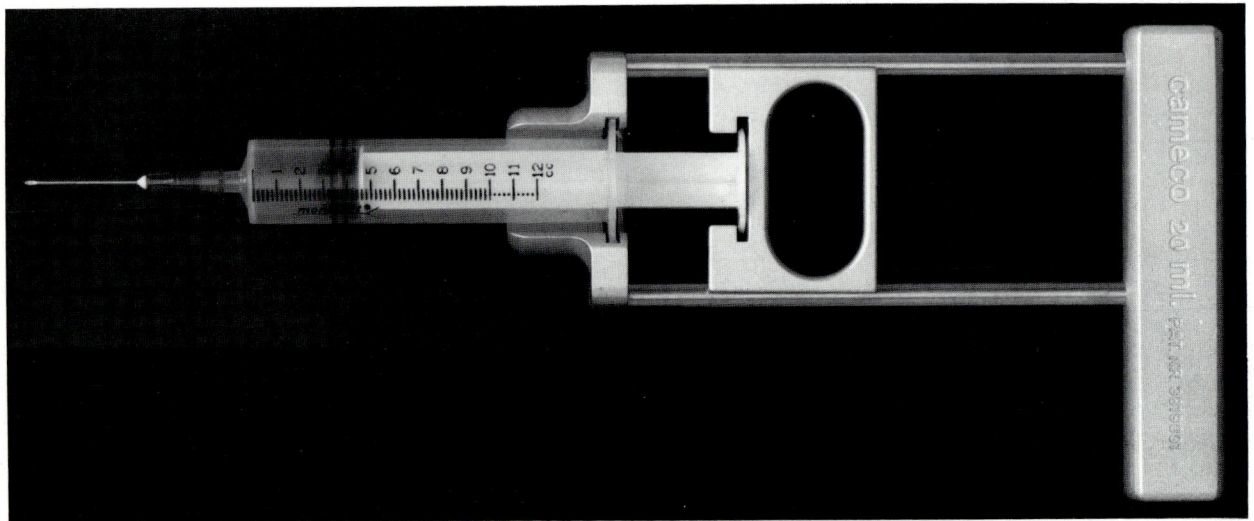

Figure 1.2.   A single grip syringe holder fitted with a 12-ml plastic syringe.

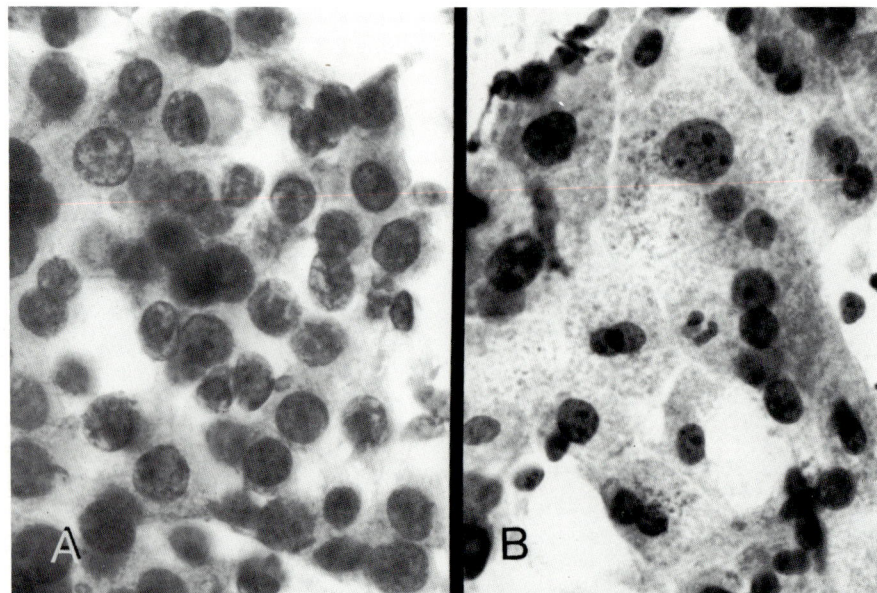

Figure 1.3.   A, Hepatocellular carcinoma, ABC. Note morphologic purity. × 500. **B**, Cirrhosis, ABC. Note spectrum of morphologic changes, ranging from normality to marked atypia. × 500.

Table 1.2. Rapid Hematoxylin and Eosin Stain for Fine Needle Aspirates

After the smears are prepared and before the slightest trace of drying occurs, fix them in 95% ethanol or Clarke's fixative for at least 2 minutes. Then pass the slides through the following sequence:

1. Tap water	10 dips
2. Carazzi's hematoxylin[a]	¾ minute
3. Tap water	10 dips
4. Lithium carbonate (bluing solution)	10 dips
5. Tap water	10 dips
6. Eosin	20 seconds
7. 95% ethyl alcohol	10 dips
8. 95% ethyl alcohol	10 dips
9. 100% ethyl alcohol	10 dips
10. 100% ethyl alcohol	10 dips
11. Xylene	10 dips
12. Xylene	10 dips
13. Mount with mounting medium and coverslip	

[a] *Preparation of Carazzi's hematoxylin*

This double-strength modification of Carazzi's original formula is intended to be used as a progressive stain. It works well on cytologic and frozen section materials.

Hematoxylin	2 gm
Glycerol	200 ml
Potassium alum	50 gm
Distilled water	800 ml
Potassium iodate	0.4 gm
	(1000 ml)

1. Dissolve the hematoxylin in the glycerol.
2. Dissolve the alum in 700 ml of water.
3. Allow to stand overnight.
4. Add the alum solution to the hematoxylin solution, mixing thoroughly.
5. Dissolve the iodate in the remaining 100 ml of water. Avoid heating if possible.
6. Add the iodate solution to the hematoxylin mixture, mixing constantly.
7. Filter into Coplin jar for use. Solution is ready for use immediately. It has reliable storage life of 6 months at room temperature, and it will remain usable for longer if stored at 4°C.

aration, the syringe with the needle is then thoroughly rinsed with a balanced salt solution and is used for Cytospin preparation (Cytospin II, Shandon Instruments, Sewickley, PA). Any visible tissue fragments in the rinse should be gently removed with a pair of forceps and transferred to formalin or Bouin's fixative for cell block preparation as needed. We recommend quick staining of the smears, followed by immediate reading to assess the adequacy of the aspirated material. If the specimen is considered inadequate or if more material is needed for special procedures, such as special stains, electron microscopy, and bacteriologic culture, the puncture can be repeated many times provided the patient's general condition permits.

For nonpalpable or deep-seated masses, such as pulmonary, intraabdominal, and retroperitoneal lesions, aspiration may be performed with a 90–200 mm long, fine needle. Fluoroscopy, ultrasound, and computed tomography (CT) may be used to guide and monitor the placement of the needle, which is usually aimed at right angle to the body wall and tumor. These biopsies require local anesthesia but do not require hospitalization. To obtain the best results, an experienced radiologist should perform or supervise the procedure and the appropriate radiologic facility be used. Discussions of the imaging techniques are available in radiologic publications.[4–7] It is our policy that a cytotechnologist is on site to assist the radiologist.

The former will prepare, stain, and assess the adequacy of the aspirated material. This not only ensures optimal specimen fixation and preparation, it also enables the cytotechnologist to make certain that the requisition form contains all the relevant information necessary for interpretation of the biopsy.

In order to enable more physicians to do aspiration biopsy, some workers have advocated collection of the aspirated samples in a preservative.[8–10] The aspiration is performed in the usual manner. The aspirated material is then ejected directly into a container filled with 30–50 ml of Saccomanno's Carbowax solution or 50% ethanol, and the syringe also is flushed thoroughly. This circumvents the necessity of having a cytotechnologist present at the time of the aspiration and permits transportation of the specimen, at the convenience of the aspirator, to a laboratory, where proper smears can be prepared by trained personnel.

FIXATION AND STAINS

If the Papanicolaou or hematoxylin and eosin staining method is to be used, immediate fixation of slides in a recommended fixative for 2–3 minutes is crucial. Delay in fixation results in cellular distortion and in poor preservation of nuclear detail. Paper clips are placed on one end of the slides to separate them in the fixative bottle and allow adequate fixation. The routine fixative we use is 95% ethyl alcohol or Clarke's fixative. Clarke's fixative consists of 3 parts of 100% alcohol and 1 part of glacial acetic acid. The latter lyses the red blood cells, thus providing a cleaner background in case of a bloody aspirate. If sufficient material is aspirated, it is recommended that at least one or two slides be left air-dried in case a Romanovsky stain is needed.

There are many different routine staining methods used for aspiration specimens and each has its proponents. Regardless of the opinions expressed in this book, the choice of routine stain will surely continue to generate heated debates. We recommend the use of hematoxylin and eosin (H & E) or Papanicolaou's technique, which is outlined in **Tables 1.2** and **1.3**, respectively. We use Carazzi's hematoxylin because the conventional Harris' or Gill's hematoxylin tends to overstain the nuclei. The Carazzi's hematoxylin gives ex-

Table 1.3. Rapid Papanicolaou's Stain for Fine Needle Aspirates

After the smears are prepared and before the slightest trace of drying occurs, fix them in 95% ethanol or Clarke's fixative for at least 2 minutes. Then pass the slides through the following sequence:

1. Tap water	10 dips
2. Carazzi's hematoxylin	¾ minute
3. Tap water	10 dips
4. Lithium carbonate (bluing solution)	10 dips
5. Tap water	10 dips
6. 95% alcohol	10 dips
7. 95% alcohol	10 dips
8. Orange-G 6	¾ minute
9. 95% alcohol	10 dips
10. 95% alcohol	10 dips
11. Eosin azure-65	¾ minute
12. 95% alcohol	10 dips
13. 95% alcohol	10 dips
14. 100% alcohol	10 dips
15. 100% alcohol	10 dips
16. Xylene	10 dips
17. Xylene	10 dips
18. Mount with mounting medium and coverslip	

cellent and crisp nuclear detail when used as a double strength solution with a shortened staining time (some variations in staining time by trial and error are sometimes necessary to obtain optimal staining).

While H & E and Papanicolaou's techniques are popular among cytopathologists in North America,[11–13] the Romanovsky staining technique, e.g., May-Grünwald Giemsa (MGG), performed on air-dried smears, is widely used in Europe. **Table 1.4** compares the H & E technique and the May-Grünwald Giemsa technique. If one aims at an overall diagnostic accuracy of 90–95%, then air-dried, Romanovsky stained smears are totally adequate. But if one wishes to do better than that, I personally believe that meticulously prepared, wet-fixed smears are indispensable. The alcohol-fixed, Papanicolaou or H & E stained smears are crucial for examination of nuclear detail. On the other hand, in aspirations of palpable breast masses it does not matter to us what stain one uses or whether the smears are wet-fixed or air-dried, because we are aiming at diagnosing unequivocally only 80–85% of the breast cancers. The diagnosis of the remainder requires confirmatory frozen section examination or surgical biopsy (see Chapter 6).

PREREQUISITES TO ACCURATE INTERPRETATION

Steps necessary to ensure optimal results of FNAB are listed below:

1. The puncture is performed by someone familiar with the technique and interpreted by a pathologist interested in FNAB. An unskillful aspirator and a disinterested pathologist will render the technique totally useless. A negative biopsy is less significant if the aspirator is uncertain of the precise location of the needle relative to the lesion than if he or she is certain that the nodule was entered and adequately sampled. The best result is obtained when the individual who interprets the aspirate also performs the puncture.[14]
2. Multiple punctures from different sites of the lesion ensure adequate, representative samples.
3. A devoted, conscientious cytotechnical staff ensures optimal preparation, fixation, and staining of the specimens.
4. Immediate staining and reading of the direct smears ensures adequacy of the specimen. If the specimen is considered inadequate, aspiration is immediately repeated, patient's condition permitting.
5. The aspirate is processed by a number of methods, including direct smearing, cytocentrifuge (or filter) preparation, and cell block.
6. Other specialized diagnostic techniques are readily available to the FNAB service, e.g., special stains,[15] immunocytochemistry,[16–18] and electron microscopy.[19–21]
7. All relevant clinical and radiologic data are communicated to the pathologist (team approach).
8. A good quality assurance program ensures a high-quality practice. Every effort should be made to follow up all cases. In modern computerized laboratories, a monthly print-out listing all surgical tissue diagnoses that have preceding FNAB diagnoses should be available to cytopathologists and cytotechnologists for quality control purposes. Review of the cytologic diagnoses in light of the histologic diagnoses helps the cytopathologist to formulate new, and to improve on existing, cytologic criteria.[22]

HOW TO EVALUATE A SMEAR

One should always examine the smear first with low-power magnification (×4 objective). This enables the observer to scan the smear thoroughly and rapidly, to identify tissue fragments and architectural pattern, to evaluate the background, and to select noteworthy areas for further examination under high magnification. Attention should always be paid to the edges of the smear because quite often the cells are concentrated there. Finally, when examining the nuclear detail, one should not hesitate to use the oil immersion objective.

When examining a smear, the cytopathologist should routinely go through a mental check list that includes the following points:

1. The number of cells present (cellularity);
2. The cellular composition of the smear;
3. The morphology of the individual cells;
4. The arrangement of cells (cell pattern);
5. The background in which the cells are found (extracellular material).

Cellularity of the Smear

In general, aspirates from malignant tumors show the highest cellularity due to the loss of cellular cohesion of the malignant cells. Benign tumors, in contrast, usually show hypocellularity in the smears. Inevitably, exceptions occur. Hypocellularity can be seen in a malignant aspirate because of inadequate suction by an inexperienced aspirator, or because sample is from a desmoplastic tumor in which the tumor cells are bound down by fibrous tissue. Conversely, some benign tumors (e.g., fibroadenoma of the breast) can be very cellular.

Table 1.4.   Comparison of H & E (or Papanicolaou) Stained Smears and May-Grünwald Giemsa Stained Smears

Hematoxylin and Eosin Stain	May-Grünwald Giemsa Stain
Fixation	
95% ethanol (prompt fixation crucial; if smear is thin, it may dry out before it can be fixed)	Air drying (convenient for clinicians who perform the procedure)
Nuclear detail	
Excellent and crisp	Poorly preserved; chromatin and nucleolar features are often obscured by heavy staining
Cytoplasmic detail	
Poor; cytoplasmic granules and secretory products less well visualized	Good; cytoplasmic granules and secretory products better visualized
Cytoplasmic outline	
Well defined; original cell shape better preserved	Less well defined; air drying effect
Cell groups (cytologic patterns)	
Easy to visualize due to lighter staining of cytoplasm	Heavy staining renders study of large cell groups difficult
Extracellular material	
Poor staining of extracellular material	Highlights extracellular material (fibromyxoid matrix, basement membrane material, etc.)
Keratin staining	
Excellent	Poor
Lymphoproliferative disorders	
Nuclear membrane irregularities (cleaved nuclei) and nucleoli better appreciated	Good differential staining of lymphoid cells
Stain familiar to pathologists and permits comparison with histologic sections	Stain familiar to hematologists, but does not permit comparison with histologic sections

Cellular Composition of the Smear

The presence of a highly atypical or even cytologically malignant cell in a smear does not necessarily denote malignancy. Its significance must be interpreted in the context of other cells present. When examining a smear, one should always attempt to answer the following questions: Is the smear composed of one cell type? If so, are the cellular alternations in each cell more or less similar to each other (morphologic uniformity) or is there a continuous spectrum of cytologic changes, varying from normality to marked atypia? If the smear is composed of more than one cell type, what are they? Are they derived from the same tissue of origin or from different sources? Do they all appear malignant or is there a mixture of malignant and benign cells?

To illustrate the diagnostic importance of cellular composition, there are no better examples than hepatocellular carcinoma (HCC) and cirrhotic liver aspirates. The former typically shows a monomorphic population of liver cells with uniformity of malignant changes, whereas the latter reveals a spectrum of changes from normality to severe atypia in the liver cells (**Fig. 1.3**). Moreover, other cell types, including bile ductular cells and fibroblasts, are present in the cirrhotic liver but absent in HCC (see Chapter 9 for detailed discussion). In general, aspirates consisting of a monomorphic population of cells are likely derived from neoplasms. Nevertheless, not all neoplasms show morphologic purity. Kline et al.[23] have recognized three morphologic types of tumor cells in aspirates of melanomas, i.e., small, medium, and large cells, and together they constitute a recognizable diagnostic pattern (**Fig. 1.4**). We have described the characteristic polymorphous cellular composition of pheochromocytomas, i.e., polygonal cells, bizarre giant cells, and spindle cells (**Fig. 1.5**).[24] Novice pathologists who try to interpret the giant cells and spindle cells without paying attention to the surrounding uniform polygonal cells are likely to think that the aspirate is derived from a giant cell carcinoma or sarcoma. In certain tumors, the aspiration biopsy cytology (ABC) typically shows a bimorphic cell population, e.g., synovial sarcoma (**Fig. 1.6**), mixed müllerian tumor, epithelioid leiomyoblastoma, thymoma, Warthin's tumor, and pleomorphic adenoma of the salivary gland. In still other tumors, the aspirates frequently comprise neoplastic as well as nonneoplastic cells. This is best exemplified by prostatic adenocarcinoma. Unlike HCC, which usually grows as a large mass, prostatic carcinoma has the tendency to infiltrate and admix with the normal prostatic glands. Hence, both malignant and benign prostatic glands can be seen side by side in the smear (**Fig. 1.7**). A unique opportunity is therefore present to compare and contrast the cytologic changes of the malignant cells and the normal cells, thereby rendering the diagnosis relatively easy.

The above remarks serve as a brief introduction only, and many other examples are to be found later in the book. It is important to stress that one should not study cytologic changes in isolation. They will make more sense when viewed in relation to one another.

Cell Morphology

In conventional exfoliative cytology, one depends heavily on nuclear alternations in determining whether a cell is malignant or benign. Long-established nuclear features that are generally regarded as indication of malignancy are outlined in **Table 1.5**.

In ABC, on the other hand, the general criteria for malignancy are not necessarily applicable to every case. The cytologic criteria of malignancy in many cases are organ-specific rather than general, and the mere knowledge of the general features of a cancer cell is

not sufficient. Even strict adherence to the nuclear criteria uncommonly may result in a false-positive diagnosis; conversely, some malignant lesions may lack the nuclear criteria of malignancy. For example, large bizarre cells can be seen in pleomorphic lipoma, atypical fibroxanthoma, degenerated schwannoma, and pheochromocytoma; the presence of these cells does not mean that the tumors are malignant (see discussions later in this book under individual tumors). On the other hand, cells from some thyroid carcinomas, bronchioloalveolar carcinoma of the lung, colloid carcinoma of the breast, and pseudomyxoma peritonei may appear deceptively bland. Before the final diagnosis is made, one must consider features other than cell morphology, such as cell pattern, smear composition, and background.

While nuclear characteristics provide the most information as to whether the cell is malignant or benign, cytoplasmic texture and staining reaction aid in establishing the functional characteristic and hence the cell type. Dense refractile eosinophilic cytoplasm would suggest keratinized squamous cells, whereas vacuolated cytoplasm may be due to mucin vacuoles (in glandular cells), lipids (in lipoblasts and histiocytes), or fat and glycogen (in renal cell carcinoma). Eosinophilic granular cytoplasm would be consistent with oncocytes and other cell types such as hepatocytes and renal tubular cells. Cyanophilic granular cytoplasm may be seen in carcinoid and other neuroendocrine tumors, acinic cell tumors, and melanomas. In every aspirate, an accurate assessment of cytoplasmic size, shape, border, texture, and cytoplasmic inclusions should be made. **Table 1.6** tabulates and **Figures 1.8–1.17** illustrate the appearance of the various common cell types encountered in FNAB, recognition of which aids in correct differential diagnosis.

Concept of Cytologic Pattern

Traditional teaching of exfoliative cytology stresses individual cell morphology. Needle aspiration biopsy has the added advantage of providing specimens of a type bordering on surgical biopsy. As our experience with FNAB is increasing, lesions that exhibit characteristic cellular patterns are continually encountered. By architectural pattern, I refer to the arrangement of cells seen in an aspirate specimen. Hence, careful analysis of the interrelationship of the cells in cell groups, which may be cohesive or noncohesive, is central to our appreciation of cytologic patterns. For pathologists who are not familiar with FNAB, it often comes as a surprise when it is pointed out to them that some patterns are so characteristic that the correct diagnosis can be made instantaneously (**Fig. 1.18**), e.g., the papillary pattern in papillary thyroid carcinoma, trabecular pattern in hepatocellular carcinoma, and cribriform pattern in adenoid cystic carcinoma. A word of caution is necessary here: as in histopathology, the more anaplastic tumors in each category of the tumors may not have a sufficiently developed pattern to be recognizable.

The cellular patterns that can be identified with confidence in FNAB are listed in **Table 1.7** and illustrated in **Figures 1.19–1.29**.

Table 1.5.   **General Nuclear Criteria of Malignancy**

Increased nuclear size resulting in an increase in nucleocytoplasmic ratio
Nuclear membrane irregularities
Irregular chromatin distribution
Hyper- or hypochromasia with good preservation
Extreme variation of nuclear size and shape
Macronucleoli
Abnormal mitoses

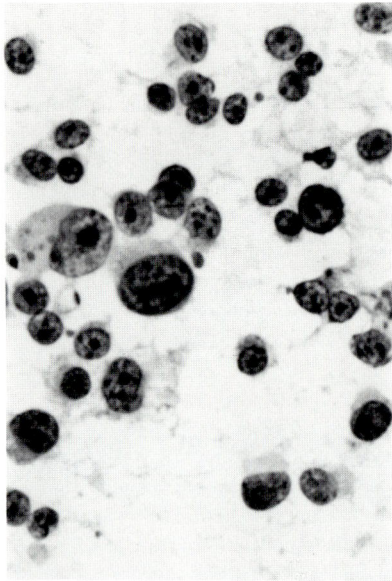

Figure 1.4. Malignant melanoma, ABC. Note characteristic triphasic cell population of small, medium, and large tumor cells. ×500.

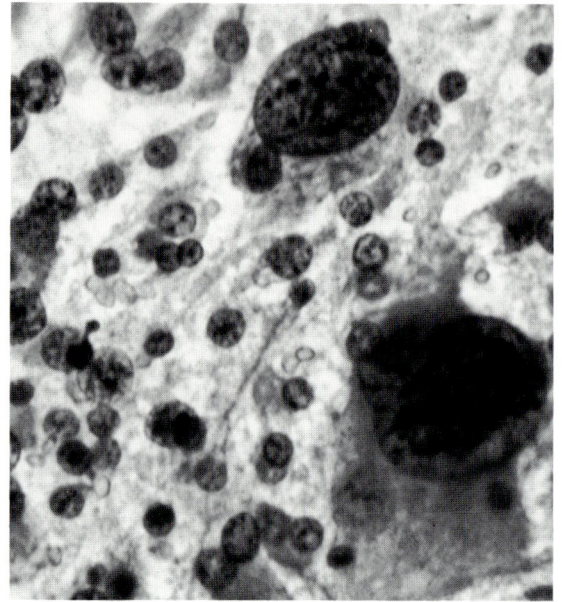

Figure 1.5. Pheochromocytoma, ABC. Note polymorphous cell population. ×500.

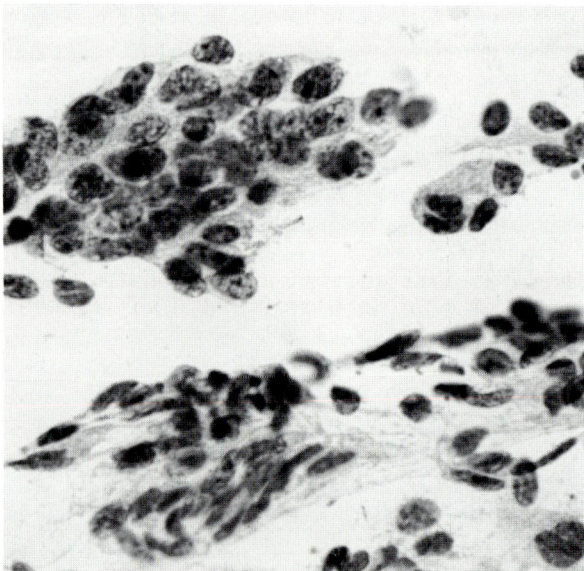

Figure 1.6. Synovial sarcoma, ABC. Note biphasic cell population of epithelial cells and spindle cells. ×500.

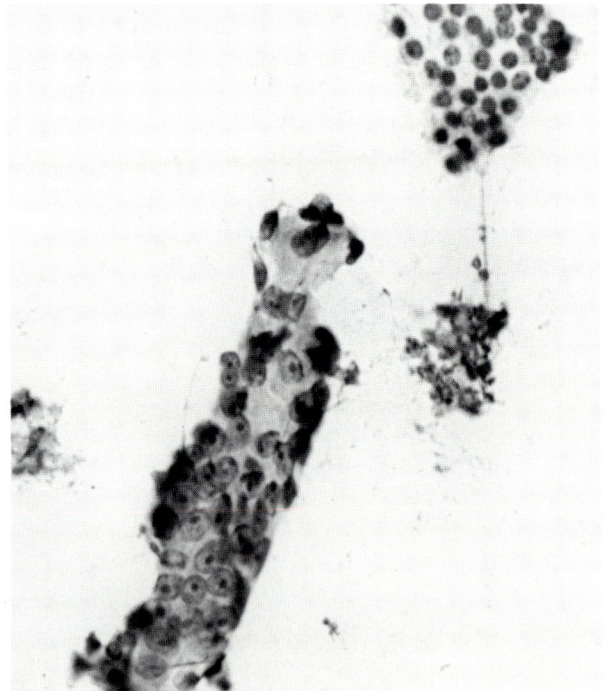

Figure 1.7. Prostatic adenocarcinoma, ABC. Note malignant and benign prostatic glands lying side by side. ×500.

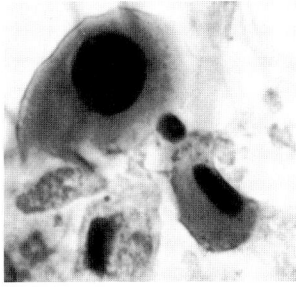

Figure 1.8. Malignant keratinizing squamous cells with refractile eosinophilic cytoplasm and sharp edges, ABC. × 500.

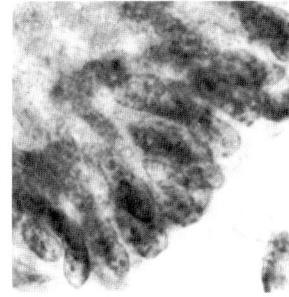

Figure 1.9. Malignant columnar cells from adenocarcinoma of colon, ABC. × 500.

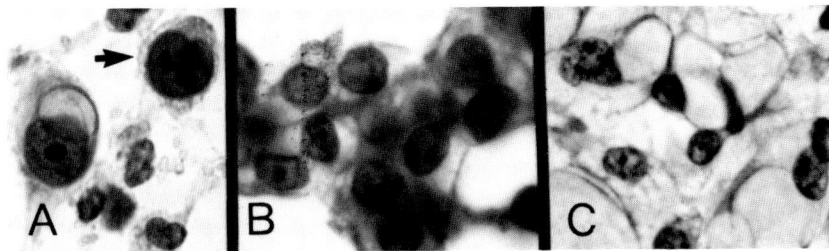

Figure 1.10. Vacuolated cells without compressed nuclei, ABC. **A**, Adenocarcinoma. *Arrow* indicates multiple small vacuoles. × 500. **B**, Renal cell carcinoma. × 500. **C**, Chordoma. × 500.

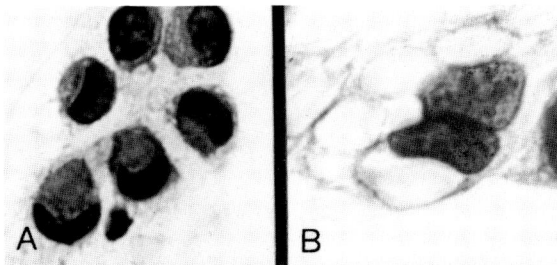

Figure 1.11. Vacuolated cells with compressed nuclei, ABC. **A**, Signet-ring cell adenocarcinoma. × 500. **B**, Liposarcoma. × 1000.

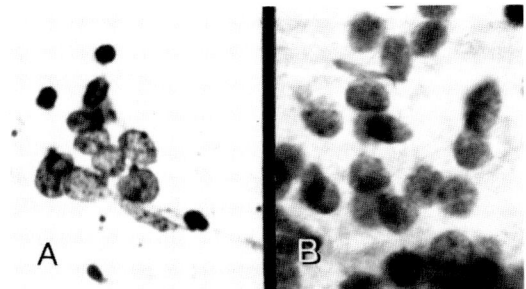

Figure 1.12. Small round cells, ABC. **A**, Oat cell carcinoma. Note nuclear crowding and molding. × 500. **B**, Neuroblastoma. Note rosette arrangement. × 500.

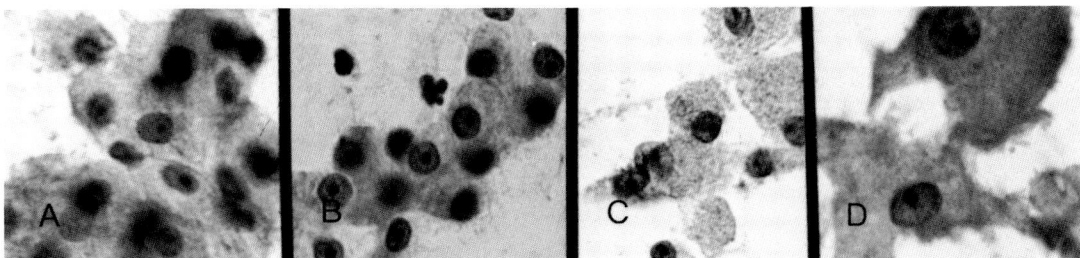

Figure 1.13. Polygonal cells with abundant granular cytoplasm, ABC. **A**, Oncocytoma of thyroid. × 500. **B**, Hepatocellular carcinoma. × 500. **C**, Granular cell myoblastoma. × 500. **D**, Alveolar soft part sarcoma. × 500.

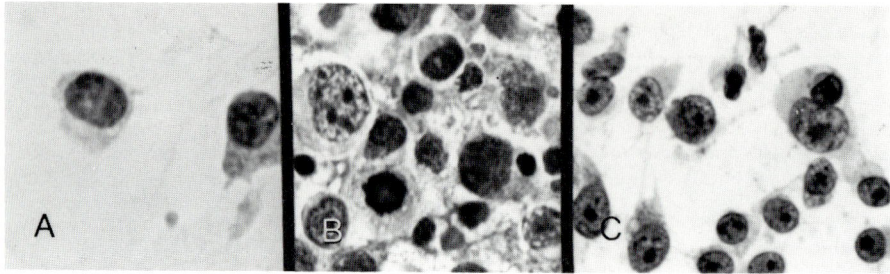

Figure 1.14.   Plasmacytoid cells with eccentric nuclei, ABC. **A,**   Multiple myeloma. ×1000. **B,** B-cell immunoblastic lymphoma. ×500. **C,** malignant melanoma. ×500.

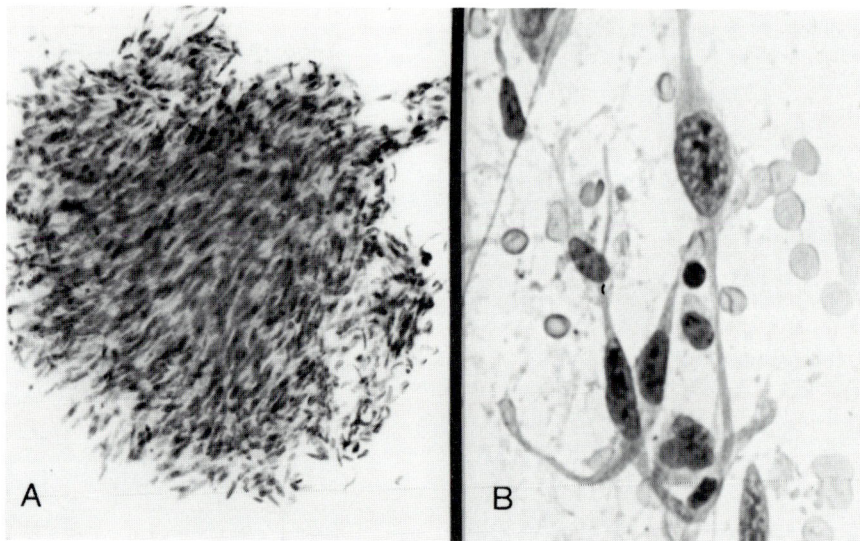

Figure 1.15.   Spindle cells, ABC. **A,** Sarcoma. Aspirate from a leiomyosarcoma. Note spindle cells with a fascicular pattern. ×125. **B,** Carcinoma. Aspirate from a lymph node with metastatic squamous cell carcinoma of the esophagus. ×500.

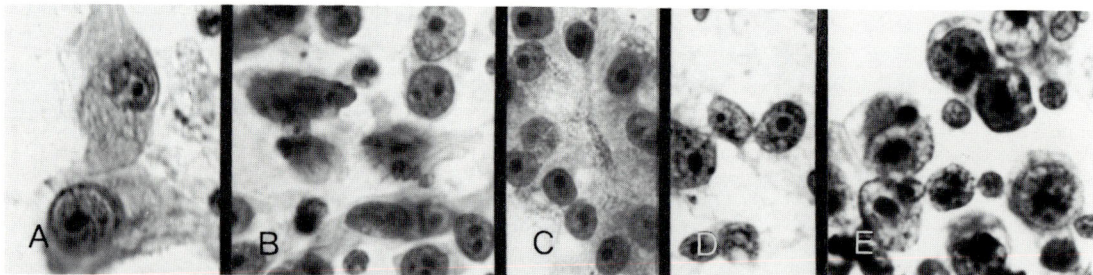

Figure 1.16.   Cells with macronucleoli, ABC. **A,** Reactive cells in postchemotherapy lung aspirate. **B,** Adenocarcinoma of stomach. **C,** Hepatocellular carcinoma. **D,** Malignant melanoma. **E,** Germ cell tumor; seminomatous component. All ×500.

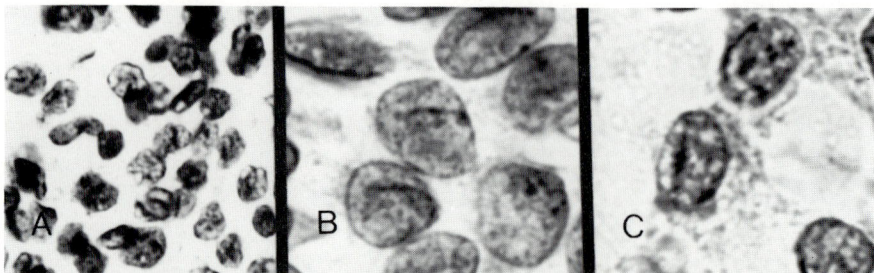

Figure 1.17.   Cells with grooved nuclei, ABC. **A,** Cleaved cell lymphoma. ×500. **B,** Papillary carcinoma of thyroid. ×1000. **C,** Granulosa cell tumor. ×1000.

Table 1.6. Cell Types Recognizable in Needle Aspirates

1. Malignant keratinizing cells **(Fig. 1.8)**
   Squamous cell carcinoma
   Caution: Degenerated cells of any type may show cytoplasmic eosinophilia and pyknotic nuclei, mimicking malignant squamous cells.
2. Malignant columnar cells **(Fig. 1.9)**
   Adenocarcinoma, particularly from gastrointestinal tract
3. Vacuolated cells without compressed nuclei **(Fig. 1.10)**
   Adenocarcinoma
   Clear cell carcinoma, particularly from kidney and ovary
   Adrenocortical tumor
   Chordoma
   Caution: Degenerated cells of any type may develop cytoplasmic vacuolation. Also rule out histiocytes.
4. Vacuolated cells with compressed nuclei **(Fig. 1.11)**
   Adenocarcinoma, particularly the signet-ring variant
   Liposarcoma
5. Small round cells **(Fig. 1.12)**
   Small cell anaplastic (oat cell) carcinoma
   Lymphoma
   Neuroblastoma
   Embryonal rhabdomyosarcoma
   Ewing's tumor
   Wilms' tumor
   Carcinoid tumor
6. Polygonal cells with abundant granular eosinophilic cytoplasm and central nuclei **(Fig. 1.13)**
   Oncocytoma
   Hepatocytic tumor
   Renal cell carcinoma (granular cell type)
   Adrenocortical tumor
   Granular cell myoblastoma
   Alevolar soft part sarcoma
7. Plasmacytoid cells **(Fig. 1.14)**
   Multiple myeloma
   Immunoblastic lymhoma
   Melanoma
   Medullary thyroid carcinoma
   Transitional cell carcinoma
8. Spindle cells **(Fig. 1.15)**
   Mesenchymal neoplasms
   Spindle cell carcinomas (squamous carcinoma, renal cell carcinoma)
   Spindle cell melanoma
   Spindle cell thymoma
   Neuroendocrine tumors
   Mesothelioma
9. Bizarre giant cells
   Any anaplastic neoplasms may contain bizarre giant cells, but giant cells are a constant feature in the following tumors **(Figs. 5.19; 7.19; 14.22)**
   Giant cell anaplastic carcinoma
   Pleomorphic sarcomas
   Choriocarcinoma
   Hodgkin's disease
   Some benign tumors (pleomorphic lipoma, atypical fibroxanthoma, and pheochromocytoma)
10. Cells with macronucleoli **(Fig. 1.16)**
    In addition to poorly differentiated carcinomas and sarcomas, the following neoplasms characteristically show macronucleoli
    Adenocarcinoma
    Hepatocellular carcinoma
    Malignant melanoma
    Germ cell tumors
    Caution: Tissue repair, chronic inflammation, radiation and postchemotherapy can induce macronucleoli in benign reactive cells.
11. Cells with grooved nuclei **(Fig. 1.17)**
    Cleaved cell lymphocytic lymphoma
    Papillary carcinoma of the thyroid
    Granulosa cell tumor
12. Cells with pigment granules **(Fig. 4.24)**
    Malignant melanoma (melanin pigment)
    Hepatocellular carcinoma (bile pigment)
    Caution: rule out histiocytes
13. Cells with cytoplasmic eosinophilic globules **(Figs. 9.7 and 14.21)**
    Hepatocellular carcinoma
    Yolk sac tumor
    Some sarcomas
    Plasmacytoma

Table 1.7. Some Common Cytologic Patterns Recognizable in Needle Aspirates

1. Dispersed (single) cell pattern **(Fig. 1.19)**
   Well-differentiated squamous cell carcinoma
   Malignant lymphoma
   Many anaplastic tumors
2. Glandular tissue fragments with large lumina **(Fig. 1.20)**
   Adenocarcinomas, particularly those from the gastrointestinal tract, lung, uterus, and ovary
3. Tissue fragments with demarcated curved borders **(Figs. 1.20 and 1.21)**
   Adenocarcinoma
   Papillary carcinoma
4. Papillary pattern **(Figs. 1.21 and 1.22)**
   Carcinomas of the thyroid, ovary, gastrointestinal tract, and lung
5. Cell balls **(Fig. 1.23)**
   Bronchioloalveolar carcinoma
   Mesothelioma
6. Cell balls with uniform round fenestrations **(Fig. 1.24)**
   Adenoid cystic carcinoma
   Follicular thyroid neoplasms
7. Acinar pattern **(Fig. 1.25)**
   The distinction between acinar and glandular pattern is necessarily arbitrary. The former has tiny lumina.
   Carcinoid tumor or other neuroendocrine tumors
   Prostatic carcinoma
   Breast carcinoma
   Acinic cell tumor
8. Rosette pattern **(Fig. 1.26)**
   This pattern differs from acinar pattern in that the central area is not occupied by a lumen, but contains granular material or fibrils.
   Neuroblastoma
   Ewing's sacoma
   Granulosa cell tumor (Call-Exner bodies)
9. Thick trabecular pattern **(Fig. 1.27)**
   Hepatocellular carcinoma
10. Thin trabecular (ribbon) pattern **(Fig. 1.28)**
    Carcinoid tumor and other neuroendocrine tumors
    Thyroid adenoma
    Breast carcinoma
    Hepatocellular adenoma and hepatoblastoma
11. Fascicular pattern **(Figs. 1.15A and 1.29)**
    Soft tissue tumors and sarcomas
    Spindle cell carcinoma
12. Mixed cellular pattern **(Fig. 1.6)**
    a. Mixture of spindle and epithelial cells e.g., synovial sarcoma, mesothelioma, Wilms' tumor, malignant mixed mesodermal tumor, pleomorphic adenoma of salivary gland, leiomyoblastoma, etc.
    b. Mixture of squamous and glandular cells e.g., mucoepidermoid carcinoma, adenosquamous carcinoma
    c. Mixture of epithelial cells and lymphocytes e.g., thymoma, seminoma, medullary breast carcinoma, Warthin's tumor, branchial cleft cyst, and Hashimoto's thyroiditis

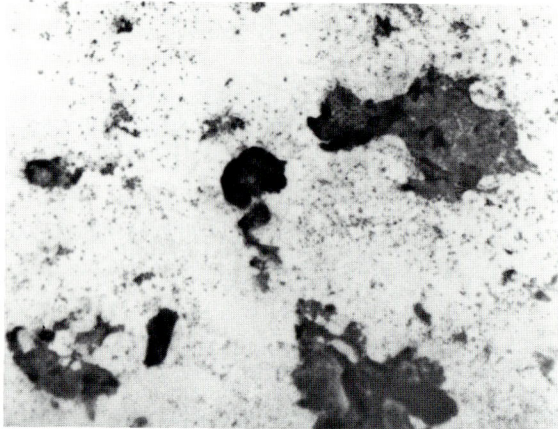

Figure 1.18.

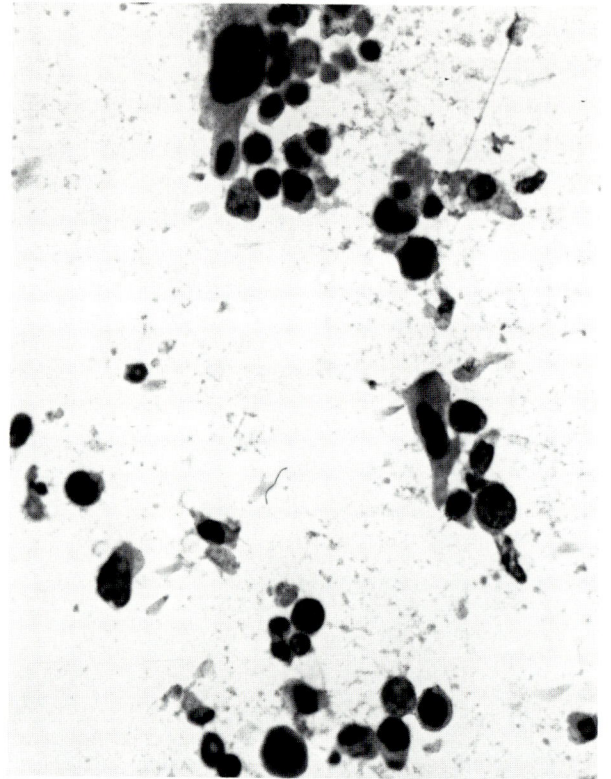

Figure 1.19.

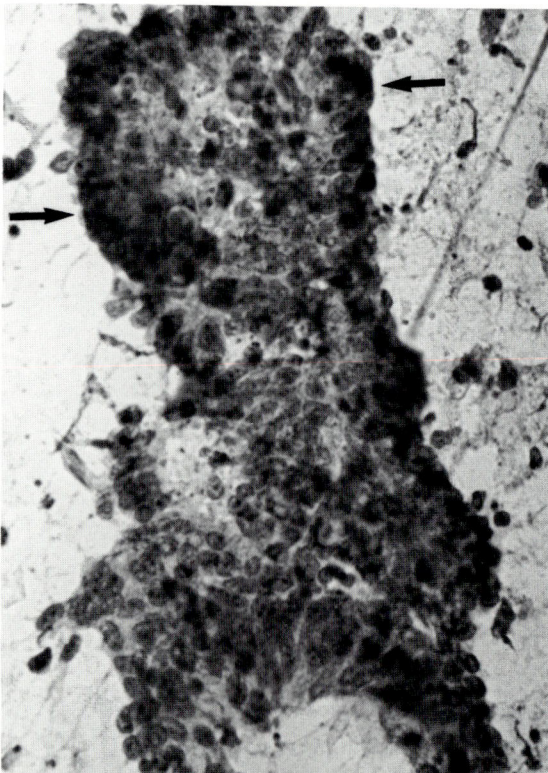

Figure 1.18.   Low-power view of an aspirate obtained from a thyroid nodule. There are numerous small and large tissue fragments as well as single cells. To an experienced cytopathologist, this cytologic appearance is characteristic of papillary thyroid carcinoma. ×60.

Figure 1.19.   Dispersed cell pattern in well-differentiated squamous carcinoma, ABC. ×310.

Figure 1.20.   Glandular fragments in adenocarcinoma of colon, ABC. Note smooth curved borders *(arrows)* and central lumina. ×310.

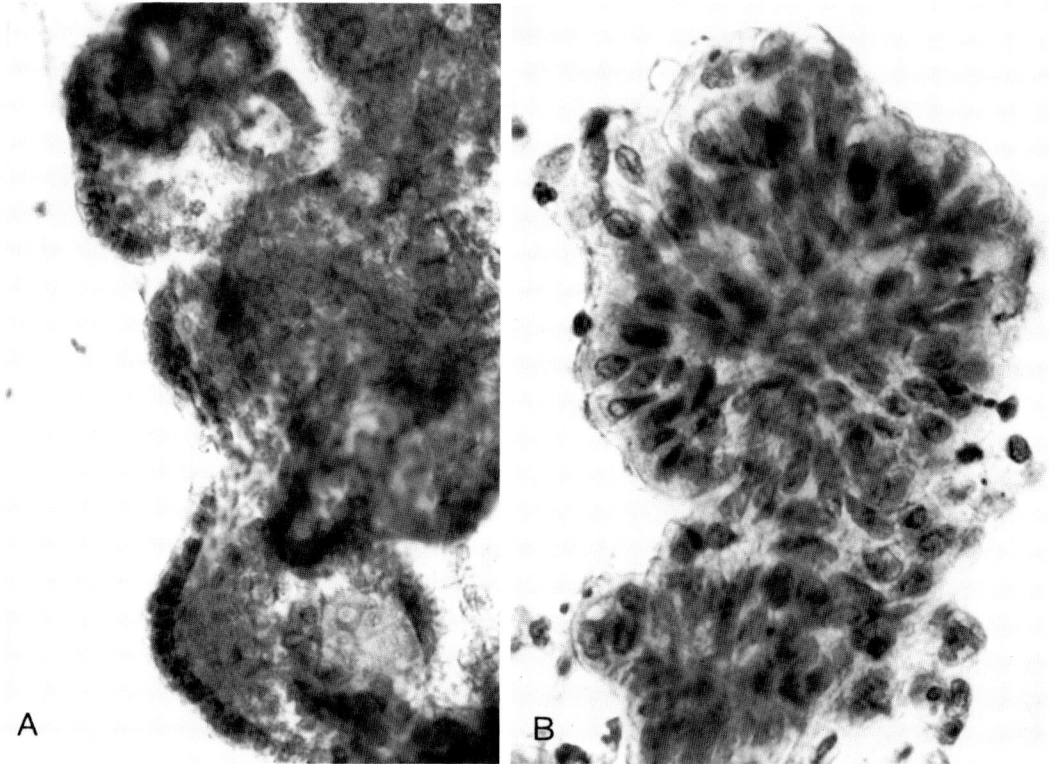

Figure 1.21. Tissue fragments in papillary adenocarcinoma, ABC. **A** and **B**, Note well-defined curved borders. **A,** ×200; **B,** ×500.

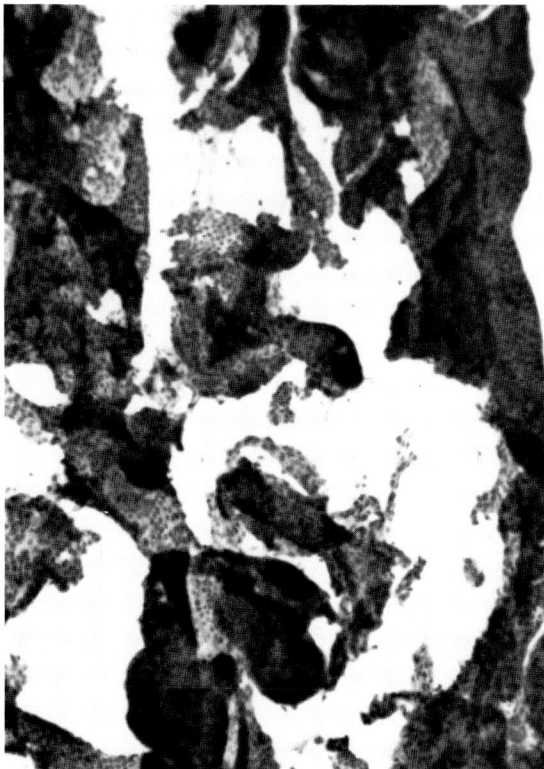

Figure 1.22. Three-dimensional, anastomosing papillary fronds in papillary thyroid carcinoma, ABC. ×125.

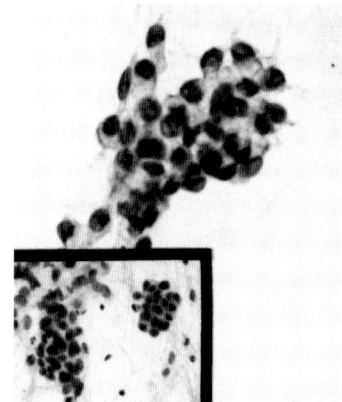

Figure 1.23. Cell balls in bronchioloalveolar carcinoma, ABC. × 500; *inset*, ×125.

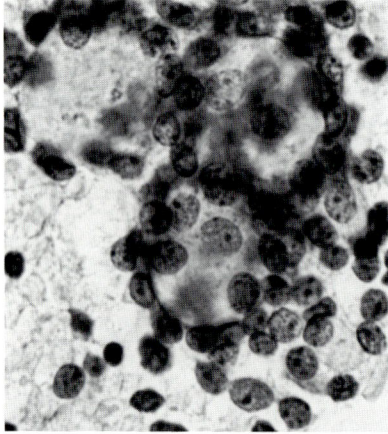

Figure 1.24. Cell balls in adenoid cystic carcinoma, ABC. Note three-dimensional ball-like masses of stromal substance enclosed by tumor cells. ×500.

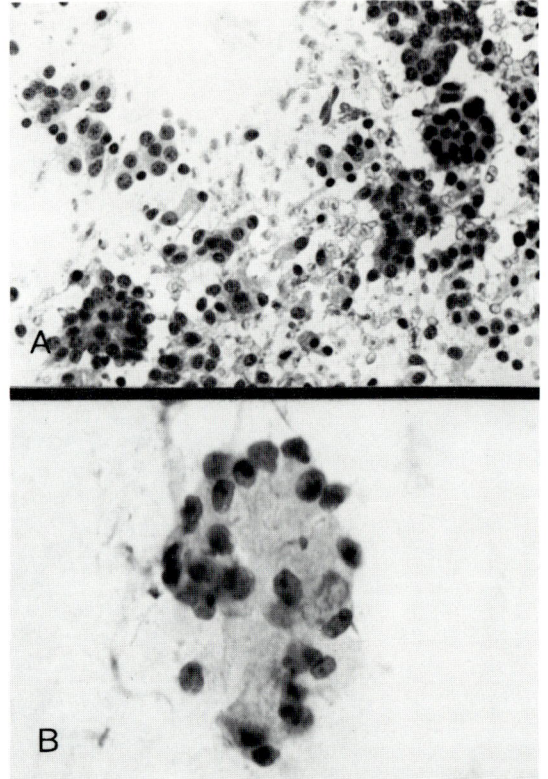

Figure 1.25. Acini, ABC. **A,** Carcinoid tumor. Note relatively uniform cells. ×180. **B,** Prostatic adenocarcinoma. Note atypical cells with prominent nucleoli. ×500.

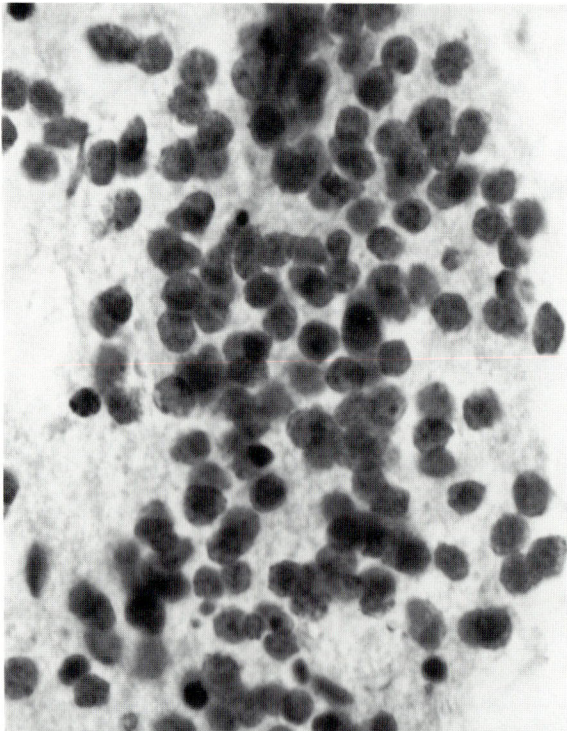

Figure 1.26. Rosette pattern in neuroblastoma, ABC. Note granular-fibrillary background. ×500.

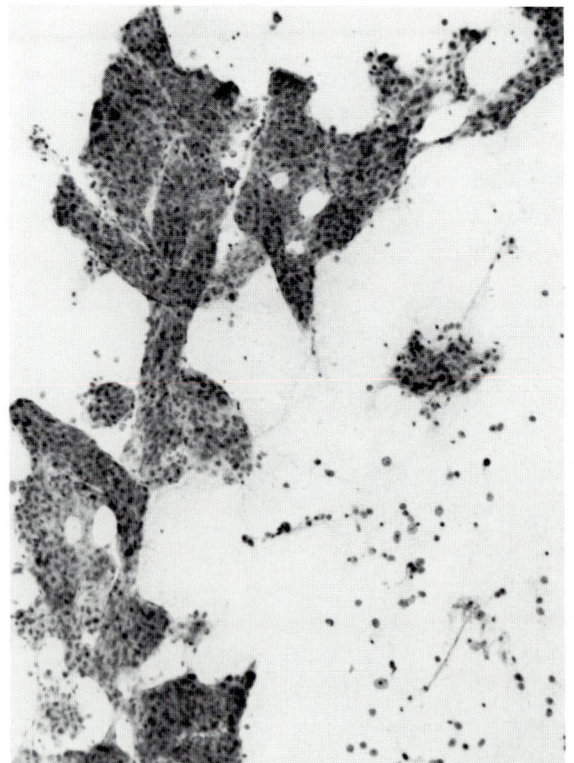

Figure 1.27. Thick trabecular pattern in hepatocellular carcinoma, ABC. ×125.

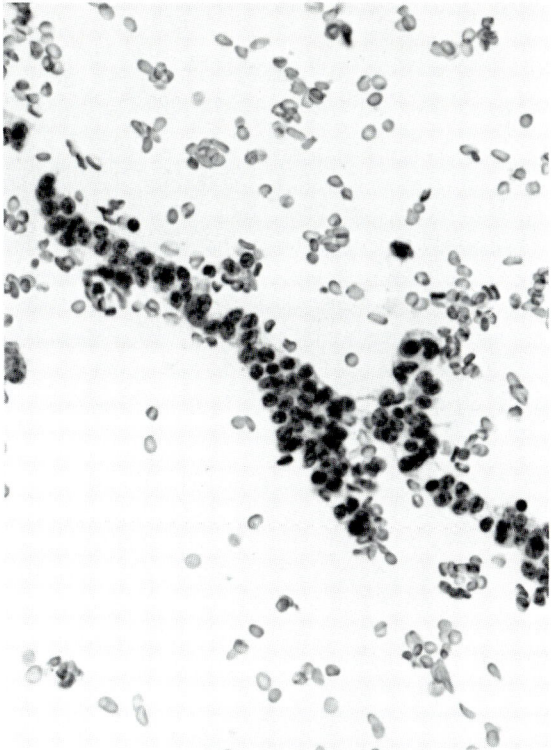

Figure 1.28.

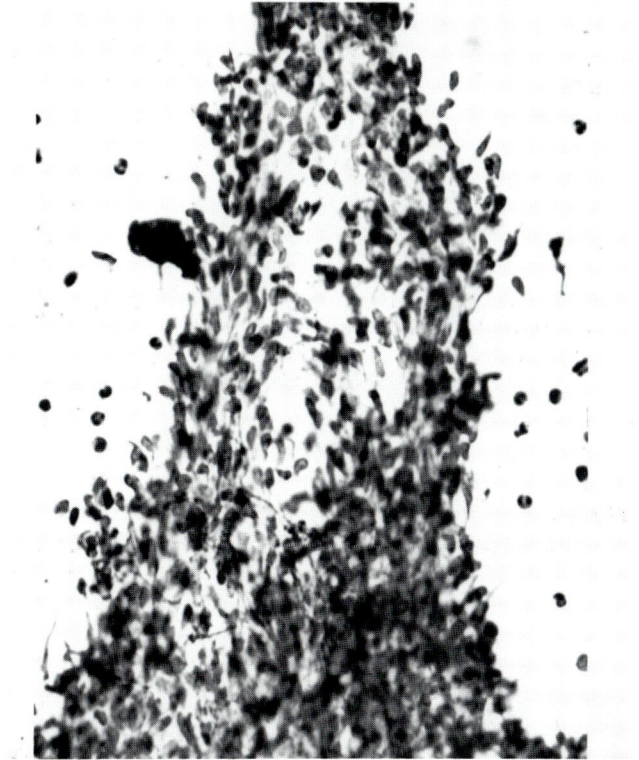

Figure 1.29.

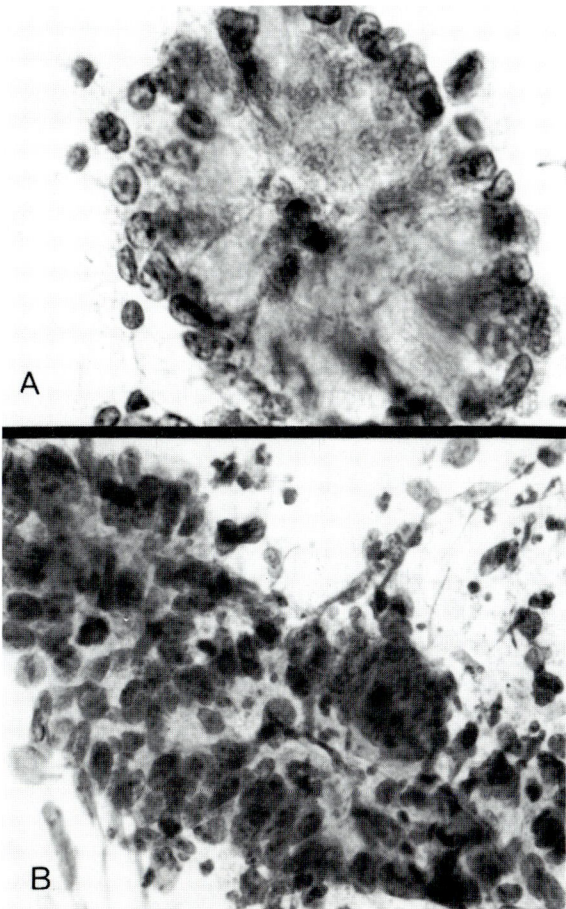

Figure 1.30.

Figure 1.28.   Thin cords or ribbons in carcinoid tumor, ABC. ×180.

Figure 1.29.   Fascicular pattern in leiomyosarcoma, ABC. ×180.

Figure 1.30.   Contrasting benign and malignant glandular patterns, ABC. A, Benign gland. Note cohesive uniform cells with basal nuclei. ×500. B, Malignant gland. Note cell crowding and nuclear stratification. ×500.

Table 1.8.   Cellular Patterns Suggestive of Malignancy

1. Disoriented cellular arrangement, e.g., nuclear crowding and molding, loss of nuclear polarity.
2. Loss of cell cohesion within cell groups and increased number of isolated cells.
3. Presence of a cytologic pattern that is not seen normally in the organ from which the aspiration material is obtained, e.g., trabeculae, rosettes, cell balls.

Table 1.9.   Reasons for False-negative Results in FNAB

1. **Technical Problems**
   Sampling error/ geographic miss
   Inadequate suction
   Improper processing
2. **Nature of the Lesion**
   Densely fibrotic masses
   Necrosis or cystic changes
   Extremely well-differentiated tumors
   Organ-specific limitations (e.g., thyroid)
3. **Pathologist's Misinterpretation**
   Inexperience

Table 1.10.   Reasons for False-positive Results in FNAB

Failure to recognize reactive, degenerative, or metaplastic changes
Failure to recognize postradiation or chemotherapy changes
Diagnosis based on few cells
Diagnosis based on poorly preserved cells
Clinical misinformation

The way the cells are arranged in the smears may provide information not only on their histogenesis but also on whether the lesion is malignant or benign (**Table 1.8** and **Fig. 1.30**).

Smear Background

The background of a smear may provide valuable diagnostic information. Amyloid material may be observed in medullary carcinoma, psammoma bodies in papillary carcinoma, and eosinophilic fibrillary material in neuroblastoma. A large amount of mucin in the background should raise the possibility of mucinous tumors. Fibromyxoid background is often seen in pleomorphic adenoma of the salivary gland and some soft tissue tumors. Evaluating the amount of colloid material aids in differentiating a benign follicular thyroid lesion from a follicular carcinoma, which generally has scanty colloid.

CLINICO-CYTOLOGIC CORRELATION

Adequate clinico-cytologic correlation implies a close working relationship among the clinician, the radiologist, and the cytopathologist (team approach). A good history, pertinent physical and radiologic findings, the age and sex of the patient, and the site and nature of the lesion, whether solid or cystic, must be communicated to the pathologist. Most cystic lesions in the body are benign (breast cysts, renal cysts), yet the epithelial lining may occasionally be so atypical as to mimic cancer. If the patient has a documented cancer, the previous slides should be reviewed and compared with the current cytologic smears whenever feasible. Previous treatment of cancer with chemotherapy or radiation may lead to bizarre cytologic atypia, which may cause confusion with malignancy. This information should always be indicated on the requisition to prevent a potential false-positive diagnosis. The pathologist on his or her part must be familiar with the situations in which false-negative and false-positive cytologic diagnoses may occur (**Tables 1.9** and **1.10**). This knowledge can then be correlated with the clinical situation.

In addition, the pathologist must fully understand the clinical implication of his or her diagnosis. A cytologic diagnosis of poorly differentiated carcinoma can be readily accepted in an elderly patient who has an abdominal mass and a previous colon cancer. In a young patient, potentially curable cancers, such as lymphoma and germ cell tumor, must enter into the differential diagnosis whenever a "poorly differentiated carcinoma" is considered.[25]

Undoubtedly, ready availability of clinical data is important, but the cytopathologist should not be biased by the clinical information, the primary function of which is to safeguard an inappropriate cytologic diagnosis. Because there is a danger of reading the expected into the cytologic picture if the pathologist knows beforehand the clinician's diagnosis, the pathologist should look at the cytology before seeing the clinical data. This initial unbiased opinion may have to be subsequently modified when the clinical and radiological findings are made known, but this approach at least has the merit of giving each case a totally fresh appraisal.[26] When all the cytologic data are accumulated, they must fit the clinical and radiologic findings.

REPORTING

In many instances, fine needle aspiration cytology represents the definitive diagnosis on which treatment will be based; it is obvious the numerical system, class I-V, traditionally used in gynecologic smears does not transmit sufficient information to the clinicians. Reports of FNAB not only provide data (or facts) but also information. The latter is interpretive reporting based on sound knowledge.[27] Information directs physicians to take actions if necessary, such as seeking further knowledge, confirming or excluding a diagnosis, or choosing a particular mode of treatment. Hence, nomenclature comparable to that in surgical pathology should be used whenever feasible. If a definitive interpretation is not possible, statements indicating the differential diagnostic possibilities and their relative likelihood should be included. If a cytologic diagnosis requires histologic confirmation, this request should be included in the cytologic report. A negative report issued by the pathologist should be clearly stated as to the effect that the biopsy is negative because there are only normal cells intrinsic to the site of aspiration or because the aspirate is strongly suggestive of a benign lesion. In the former instance, the finding might well be the result of a sampling error. By repeating the biopsy from different areas of the lesion, the operator may enhance the significance of a negative finding. In the case in which the diagnosis suggests a benign lesion, an evaluation of the entire clinical situation would determine the next course of action.

References

1. Japko L. New federal regulations and the future practice of cytology. Diagn Cytopathol 1985;1:263–266.

2. Lambird P. New payment systems: A brillant opportunity for cytology. Diagn Cytopathol 1985;1:261–262.

3. Kaminsky DB. Aspiration biopsy in the context of the new Medicare fiscal policy. Acta Cytol 1984;28:333–336.

4. Zornoza J. Percutaneous needle biopsy. Baltimore: Williams & Wilkins, 1981.

5. Grant EG, Richardson JD, Smirniotopoulos JG, Jacobs NM. Fine needle biopsy directed by real-time sonography: Technique and accuracy. AJR 1983;141:29–34.

6. Letourneau J, Elyaderani MK, Castaneda-Zuniga WR. Percutaneous biopsy, aspiration and drainage. Chicago: Year Book Medical Publishers, 1987.

7. Cooperberg PL, Rowley VA. Abdominal imaging techniques. In: Suen KC. Guides to clinical aspiration biopsy. Retroperitoneum and intestine. New York: Igaku Shoin, 1987:13–21.

8. Young GP. Enabling more physicians to do aspiration biopsy. Diagn Cytopathol 1986;2:229–230.

9. Atkinson BF. Carbowax fixation of needle aspirates. Diagn Cytopathol 1986;2:231–232.

10. Olson NJ, Gogel HK, Williams WL, Mettler FA, Jr. Processing of aspiration cytology samples. An alternative method. Acta Cytol 1985;29:943

11. Pak HY, Yokota SB, Teplitz RL. Rapid staining techniques employed in fine needle aspirations. Acta Cytol 1983;27:81–82.

12. Gublin N. Hematoxylin-and-eosin staining of fine needle aspirate smears. Acta Cytol 1984;28:648.

13. Koss LG. The thin needle aspiration: An important diagnostic tool. Einstein Q J Biol Med 1984;2:73–85.

14. Japko L. Aspiration biopsy: The pathologist as hands-on consultant. Diagn Cytopathol 1986;2:233–235.

15. Sachdeva R, Kline TS. Aspiration biopsy cytology and special stains. Acta Cytol 1981;25:678–683.

16. Nadji M. The potential value of immunoperoxidase techniques in diagnostic cytology. Acta Cytol 1980;24:442–447.

17. Osborn M, Weber K. Tumor diagnosis by intermediate filament typing: A novel tool for surgical pathology. Lab Invest 1983;48:372–394.

18. Domagala W, Lubinski J, Weber K, Osborn M. Intermediate filament typing of tumor cells in fine needle aspirates by means of monoclonal antibodies. Acta Cytol 1986;30:214–224.

19. Kindblom LG, Walaas L, Widehn S. Ultrastructural studies in the preoperative cytologic diagnosis of soft tissue tumors. Semin Diagn Pathol 1986;3:317–344.

20. Wills EJ, Carr S, Philips J. Electron microscopy in the diagnosis of percutaneous fine needle aspiration specimens. Ultrastruct Pathol 1987;11:361–387.

21. Mackay B, Fanning T, Brunner JM, Steglich MC. Diagnostic electron microscopy using fine needle aspiration biopsies. Ultrastruct Pathol 1987;11:659–672.

22. Hyman MP. Programs in cytopathology: How do you evaluate performance and how can you improve? Pathologist 1985;39:19–21.

23. Kline TS, Kannan V. Aspiration biopsy cytology of melanoma. Am J Clin Pathol 1982;77:597–601.

24. Suen KC. Adrenal. In Guides to clinical aspiration biopsy. Retroperitoneum and intestine. New York: Igaku Shoin, 1987:165–189.

25. Ledermann JA, Crawford SM, Philip PA, Bagshawe KD. Curable metastatic cancer in young women. Br Med J 1987;295:432–433.

26. Underwood JCE. Introduction to biopsy interpretation and surgical pathology, 2nd ed. Berlin: Springer-Verlag, 1987:79.

27. Speicher CE, Smith JW. Interpretive reporting. Clin Lab Med 1984;4:41–60.

2

Thyroid

Thyroid nodules are common, but only a small proportion of them are malignant. The incidence of thyroid cancers is 30–60 new cases per 1 million population per year, or 0.003–0.006%.[1] Differentiation between benign and malignant nodules by conventional means, such as thyroid function tests, radioisotope scan, thyroid suppression test and ultrasonography, results in a low yield of cancer in surgically excised specimens. Many investigators[2,3] have shown that fine needle aspiration biopsy (FNAB) is the single most sensitive, specific, and cost-effective method in the investigation of the solitary "cold" thyroid nodule.

The role of FNAB is to aid in the selection for surgery of nodules that have a high probability of malignancy.[4] Used in this manner, FNAB is primarily a screening rather than a diagnostic procedure, and a conclusive cytologic diagnosis is not always required. Any "suspicious" cytologic report should lead to further investigation that would clarify the issue and in most instances this would mean surgical exploration. At our institution, the prevalence of malignancy in the excised nodules was 14% prior to the FNAB era and 47% after the advent of FNAB.[4] Other workers have reported similar experience. Silver and associates[5] reported that the percentage of malignant thyroid tumors in their surgical patients has doubled from 16 to 35% since the advent of FNAB. Hawkins et al.[6] showed that the percentage of patients who underwent surgery decreased from 61% the 1st year to 14% the 5th year after introduction of FNAB, and the diagnosis of thyroid cancer in surgical specimens increased from 8.3% the 1st year to 37.3% the 5th year. Not only has the preoperative use of FNAB reduced the number of unnecessary thyroidectomies, but it has also uncovered many clinically unsuspected cancers that would otherwise have been followed medically.[7] **Figure 2.1** outlines the role of FNAB in the sequential approach to the apparently solitary thyroid nodule.

NONNEOPLASTIC LESIONS
Nodular Goiter

Nodular goiter is a common condition, which affects all age groups, and it is four to nine times as frequent in women as in men. The diseased gland is enlarged and distorted by multiple nodules. Although some nodular goiters may appear to be solitary on clinical and ultrasonic examinations, microscopic examination of the resected specimens will generally reveal multinodularity. Histologically, the essential pathologic process is one of hyperplasia and involution. The nodules contain an endless variety of differently shaped follicles **(Fig. 2.2)**. At one end of the spectrum, there are crowded follicles formed by tall hyperplastic epithelial cells, leaving only a small follicular cavity. At the other end, as a result of involutional

changes, the follicles are enlarged and distended by large amounts of colloid; the follicular epithelial cells are flattened and cuboidal. Degenerative changes are common, such as hemorrhage, fibrosis, calcification, and cyst formation.

Aspiration Cytology

Cytologic Pattern. Aspirates obtained from nodular goiters are generally hypocellular **(Fig. 2.3)**, although the less commonly encountered hyperplastic nodules can yield cell-rich specimens. The follicular cells are orderly spaced in a circular manner to form small follicles **(Fig. 2.3 *inset*)** or are arranged in small monolayered sheets **(Fig. 2.4)**. Hyperplastic nodules yield much larger tissue fragments composed of numerous follicle units **(Fig. 2.5)** or monolayered tissue fragments that have a regular, honeycomb appearance **(Fig. 2.6)**.

The smear background shows a variable, but usually abundant, amount of colloid. The colloid is present either as discrete clumps or as a diffuse pale amorphous sheet dominating the background **(Fig. 2.3)**; it stains eosinophilic with H & E and variably pink to green with Papanicolaou stain. Also in the background may be seen variable numbers of macrophages, with or without hemosiderin pigment in the cytoplasm **(Fig. 2.4)**.

Cell Morphology. The follicular epithelial cells **(Figs. 2.3–2.6)** are cuboidal or low columnar, small and uniform, and have a moderate amount of somewhat ill-defined, pale, eosinophilic cytoplasm. The nuclei are perfectly round and slightly larger than small lymphocytes. The chromatin is compact, granular, and uniformly stained. Nucleoli are rarely seen. Occasionally, the follicular cells may be stripped of cytoplasm and appear as bare nuclei, which may be mistaken for lymphocytes by the unwary.

Diagnostic Pitfalls and Discussion. Although aspirates from most of the nodular goiters are hypocellular, hypocellularity is by no means monopolized by nodular goiters. A thyroid neoplasm also may give rise to a hypocellular specimen if suction by the aspirator is inadequate or if the neoplasm is desmoplastic. The latter situation occurs more often in anaplastic thyroid carcinoma than in well-differentiated carcinoma (see "Anaplastic Carcinoma"). Attention to clinical data, such as rapid growth, hardness, and fixation of the mass, is helpful in arriving at the correct diagnosis of anaplastic carcinoma. Nodular goiter is diagnosed when hypocellularity is seen in an appropriate cellular milieu (abundant colloid in the background and/or scattered histiocytes) and in an appropriate clinical setting (multinodularity and/or cystic changes on ultrasonography). The question as to what constitutes a satisfactory specimen is often raised. The answer given by Kline for breast aspiration applies equally well to thyroid aspiration: "an adequate sample is one that is competently and vigorously taken."[8] Each thyroid sample should contain at least

16

four to six groups of follicular epithelial cells; however, we still consider a biopsy sufficient for the diagnosis of colloid goiter even though few follicular cells are seen, provided there is a large amount of colloid present along with the assurance by an experienced aspirator that the aspirate is taken from the lesion. On the other hand, a hypocellular specimen is "unsatisfactory" if it is awkwardly retrieved by an inexperienced physician.[8]

Aspirates obtained from hypercellular nodular goiters may be confused with those obtained from thyroid neoplasms.[9] For example, the cytologic features depicted in **Figure 2.5** may be mistaken for follicular adenoma, and the many tissue fragments in **Figure 2.6** may suggest papillary carcinoma (see **Figure 2.31** and "Papillary Carcinoma"). It is important to remember that although hyperplastic goiters yield cellular aspirates, examination of the tissue fragments under high magnification will reveal regular, well-spaced cells and the familiar honeycomb pattern.

Occasional atypical follicular cells with enlarged and hyperchromatic nuclei, probably representing a regressive change, may be seen in aspirates of nodular goiters and should not be mistaken for malignancy. Unlike malignant tumors, the atypical cells in nodular goiters are few in number and admixed with benign-appearing follicular cells.

Thyroid Cysts

Benign cysts of the thyroid are common. They result from cystic degeneration of nodular goiters or hemorrhage into preexisting nodules. Cystic papillary carcinoma also occurs but is uncommon and discussed under "Papillary Carcinoma."

Aspiration Cytology

The amount of fluid aspirated may range from a few drops to as much as 30 or 40 ml; it may be clear or turbid, yellow or dark brown. The aspirates **(Fig. 2.7)** are hypocellular and the predominant cell type is the histiocyte. The histiocytes may contain hemosiderin pigment in the cytoplasm, indicative of previous hemorrhage into the cyst. Follicular epithelial cells are small and few in number, occurring in small groups, like those seen in nodular goiters. The nuclei of some follicular cells may show pyknosis, a feature of degeneration. A variable amount of colloid may be seen in the background.

Diagnostic Pitfalls. Most of the cystic lesions of the thyroid are benign. Following a single aspiration, two-thirds of the cysts in Frable's series did not recur.[10] On the other hand, it is important to remember that about 4% of the papillary carcinomas are cystic, and dilution of the neoplastic cells by cystic fluid may result in a false-negative diagnosis. Walfish et al.[11] cautioned that pathologists should always suspect a cystic cancer when the cyst is larger than 4 cm in diameter or when there is prompt reaccumulation of hemorrhagic fluid after repeated aspirations.

Chronic Lymphocytic (Hashimoto's) Thyroiditis

Chronic lymphocytic, or Hashimoto's, thyroiditis is the most common form of thyroiditis.[12] It is an autoimmune disease; microsomal and thyroglobulin antibodies are frequently found in the blood of these patients. Therefore, serologic tests for these antibodies are diagnostically useful. Clinically, both lobes of the thyroid are diffusely enlarged. In about 5–10% of the cases, however, the disease presents as a localized nodule, mimicking a neoplasm. The classic histologic picture **(Fig. 2.8)** is a diffuse process, consisting of lymphocytic infiltrate, follicular cells undergoing Hürthle cell transformation (see below), and fibrosis.

Aspiration Cytology

Cytologic Pattern. The aspirates are cellular, unless there is exuberant fibrosis. Two distinct populations of cells—the follicular epithelial cells and the lymphocytes—are present in variable proportion **(Fig. 2.9)**. The follicular cells are arranged in small follicles or loose sheets, while the lymphocytes are characteristically noncohesive and scattered singly in the background.

Cell Morphology. The epithelial cell component consists of regular follicular cells as well as follicular cells that show Hürthle cell transformation. Hürthle cells **(Figs. 2.9 and 2.10)** are large polygonal cells that have abundant granular cytoplasm, which is eosinophilic with H & E stain or cyanophilic with Papanicolaou stain. Nucleoli may be prominent. The inflammatory component consists of predominantly lymphocytes in varying stages of maturation, and occasional plasma cells and tingible body macrophages can sometimes be seen.

Diagnostic Pitfalls. Cytologic diagnosis of chronic lymphocytic thyroiditis is easily made when ABC exhibits the classic pattern of dual cell population.[13] However, the condition has been known to be one of the principal sources of confusion with carcinoma, particularly Hürthle cell tumors **(Fig. 2.11)**,[9,14–15] but mistakes are likely to disappear after reasonable experience.[15] Most problems occur in the interpretation of Hürthle cells in the absence of, or in the presence of only a scanty number of, lymphocytes. Needle aspirates from different areas of the lesion should be obtained to ensure more representative samples. As a rule, if lymphocytes are seen in the background or admixed with the Hürthle cells, caution is needed to make the diagnosis of Hürthle cell neoplasm. In **Table 2.1** are compared the clinical and cytologic features of chronic lymphocytic thyroiditis and Hürthle cell tumor (see also "Hürthle Cell Tumors").

Chronic lymphocytic thyroiditis may coexist with papillary or follicular carcinoma, and the neoplastic cells may be mistaken for benign reactive cells and vice versa. Familiarity with the appearances of the papillary and follicular neoplastic groups (discussed later) aids in separating neoplastic cells from reactive follicular cells.

Chronic lymphocytic thyroiditis may be confused with malignant lymphoma. However, lymphomas of the thyroid gland are usually rapidly growing and clinically malignant tumors. Cytologically, the lymphocytes in chronic lymphocytic thyroiditis are benign-appearing, show various degrees of maturation, and are admixed with plasma cells; whereas in malignant lymphoma, the lymphocyte population is generally monomorphic and shows nuclear atypia.[16]

Table 2.1. Comparison of Chronic Lymphocytic Thyroiditis and Hürthle Cell Neoplasm

Chronic Lymphocytic Thyroiditis	Hürthle Cell Neoplasm
Clinical Examination	
Generally diffuse enlargement	Solitary nodule
Antithyroid Antibodies	
Elevated	Not elevated
FNAB Findings	
Hürthle Cells	
Mixture of benign-appearing and atypical Hürthle cells	Monomorphic population of atypical Hürthle cells
Normal Follicular Cells	
Generally present	Scant or absent
Lymphocytes and Plasma Cells	
Present	Absent

Thyroid nodule
|
Radioiodine scan

"Hot" or "warm"
nodule indicates
neoplasia unlikely

"Cold" or "cool"
nodule
|
Ultrasound

Cystic
|
FNAB

Solid
|
FNAB

Benign
cytology

Suspicious
cytology

Suspicious
cytology

Benign
cytology

Follow-up
(± thyroxine therapy)

Surgery

Follow-up
(± thyroxine therapy)

Reevaluation
after 6 months
(or sooner if
clinically indicated)

Reevaluation
after 6 months
(or sooner if
clinically indicated)

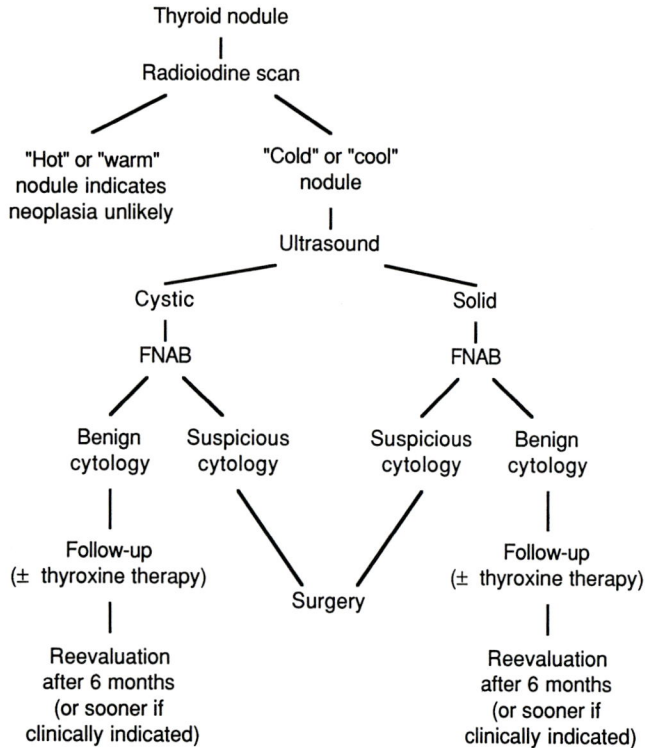

Figure 2.1. Role of fine needle aspiration biopsy (FNAB) in the sequential approach to the cold thyroid nodule.

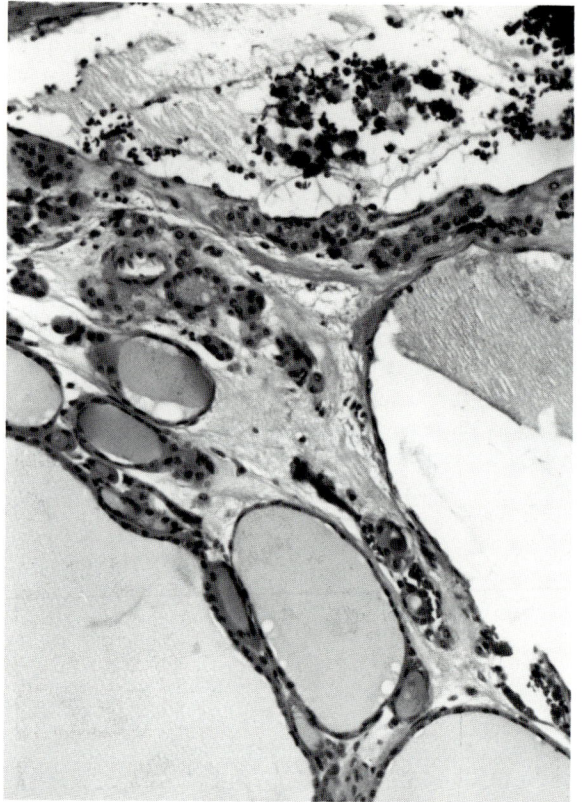

Figure 2.2. Histologic features of nodular goiter. Note varying-sized follicles, lined by low cuboidal epithelium and distended with colloid. Also note collection of macrophages in an area of cystic degeneration *(top)*. ×125.

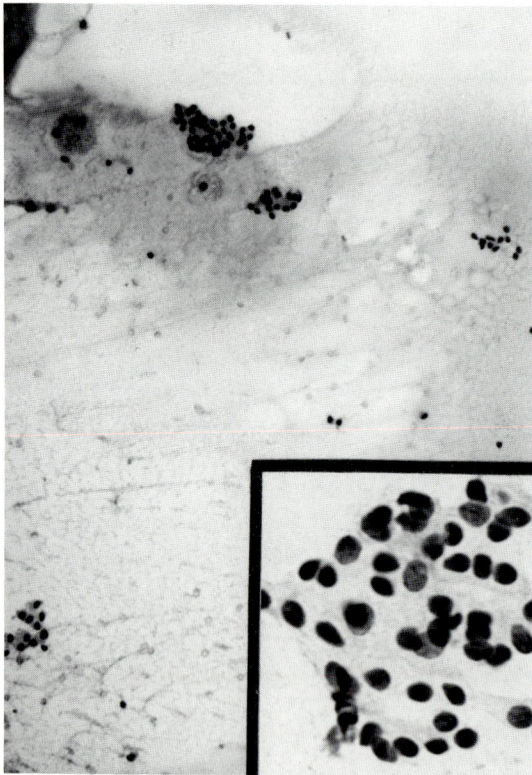

Figure 2.3. Nodular goiter, ABC. The smear is hypocellular, with scattered, small groups of follicular epithelial cells. Note diffuse thin layer of colloid covering part of the background. *Inset* shows high magnification view of the follicles. ×125; inset, ×500.

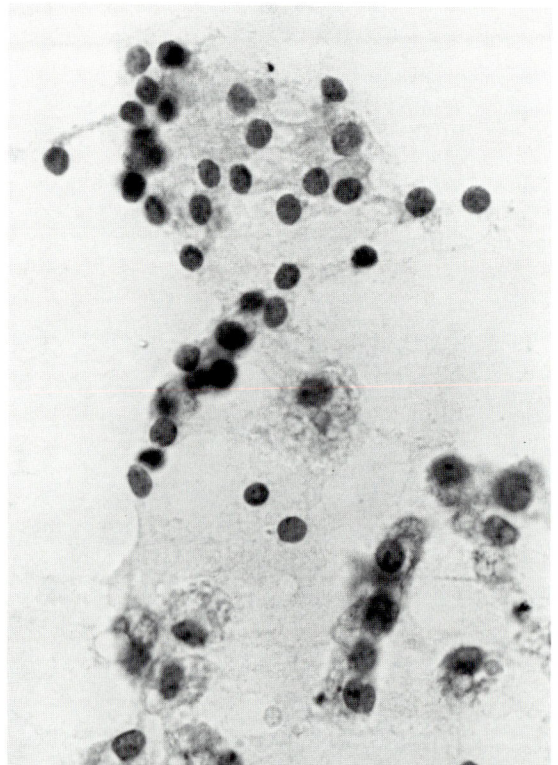

Figure 2.4. Nodular goiter, ABC. Note small monolayer of uniform follicular cells with bland nuclei. The larger cells with foamy cytoplasm are histiocytes *(lower half* of figure). ×500.

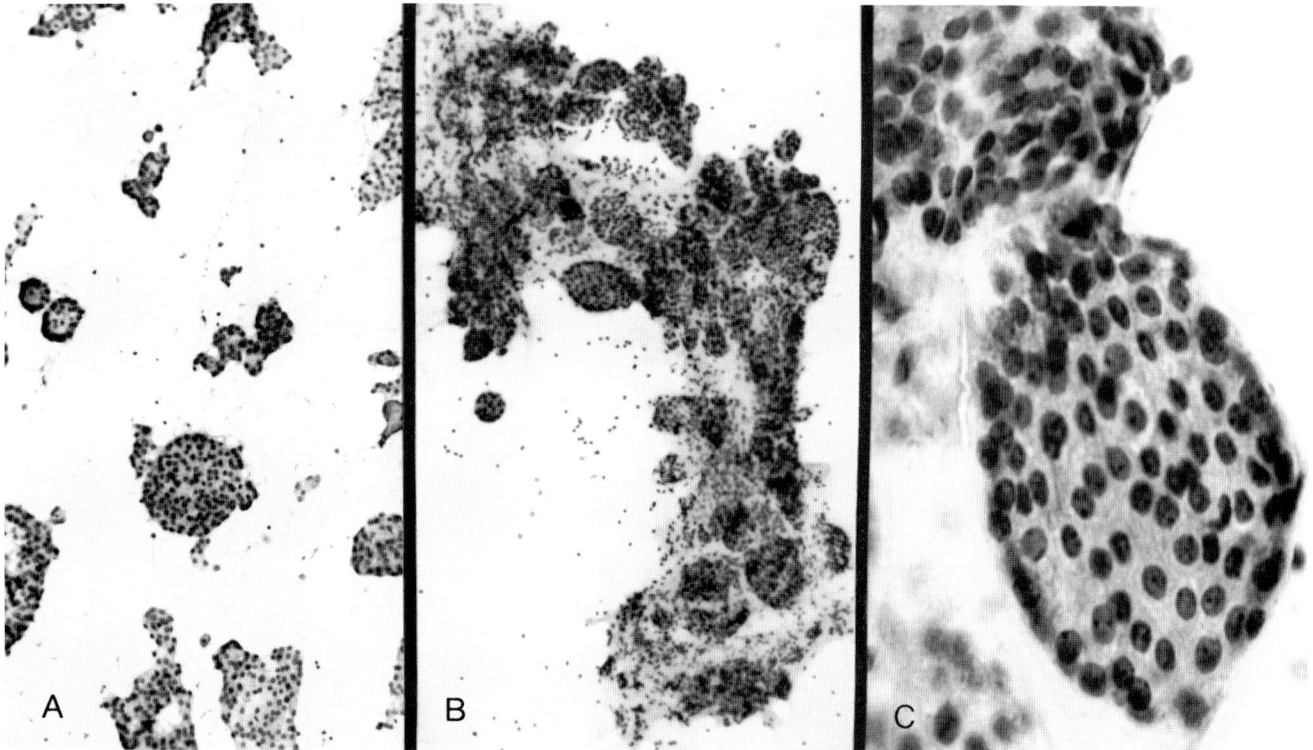

Figure 2.5. Hyperplastic nodular goiter, ABC. **A**, The smear is hypercellular, showing many small and large cell balls with a follicular pattern. ×125. **B**, Large tissue fragment composed of numerous well-developed follicles. ×75. **C**, High magnification view of a follicular cell ball. Note cellular uniformity and retention of nuclear polarity. ×500.

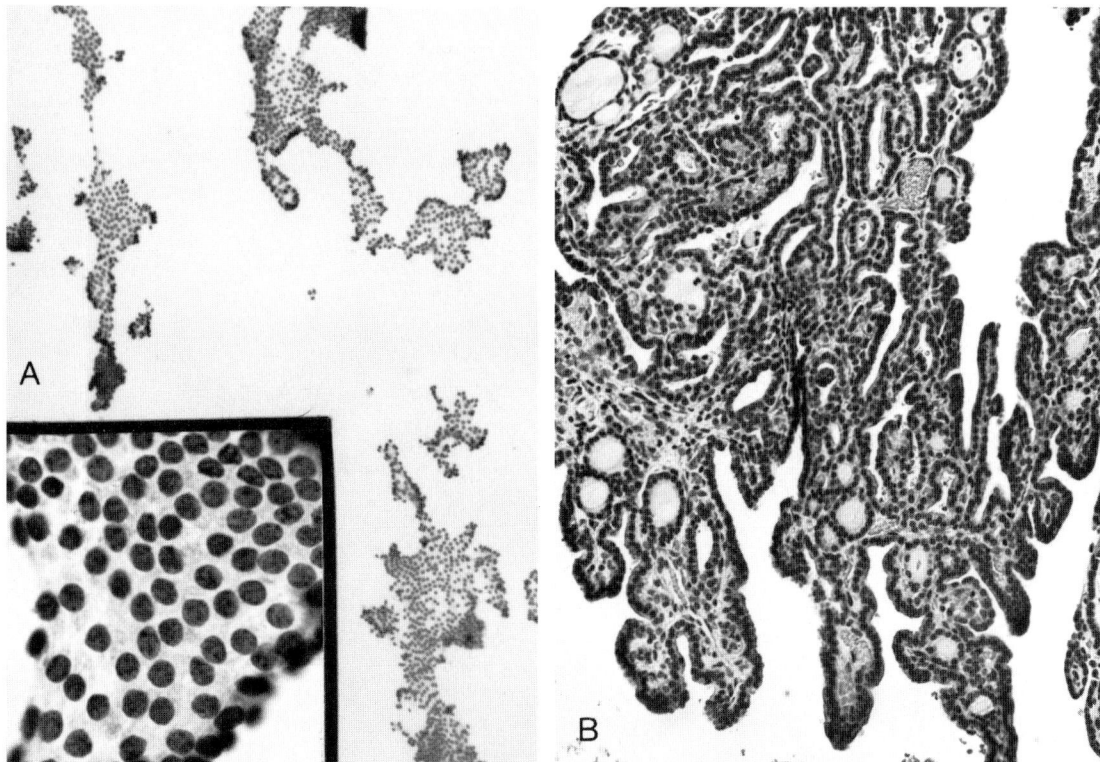

Figure 2.6. Hyperplastic nodular goiter. **A**, ABC. The smear shows many large monolayered tissue fragments, superficially resembling the monolayered tissue fragments seen in papillary carcinoma. Compare this with **Figure 2.31.** *Inset* shows follicular cells at higher magnification. Note honeycombing. ×75; *inset*, ×310. **B**, Histologic section of the hyperplastic nodular goiter showing pseudopapillae, covered by benign cuboidal follicular cells and containing many small secondary follicles in the stalks. ×125.

19

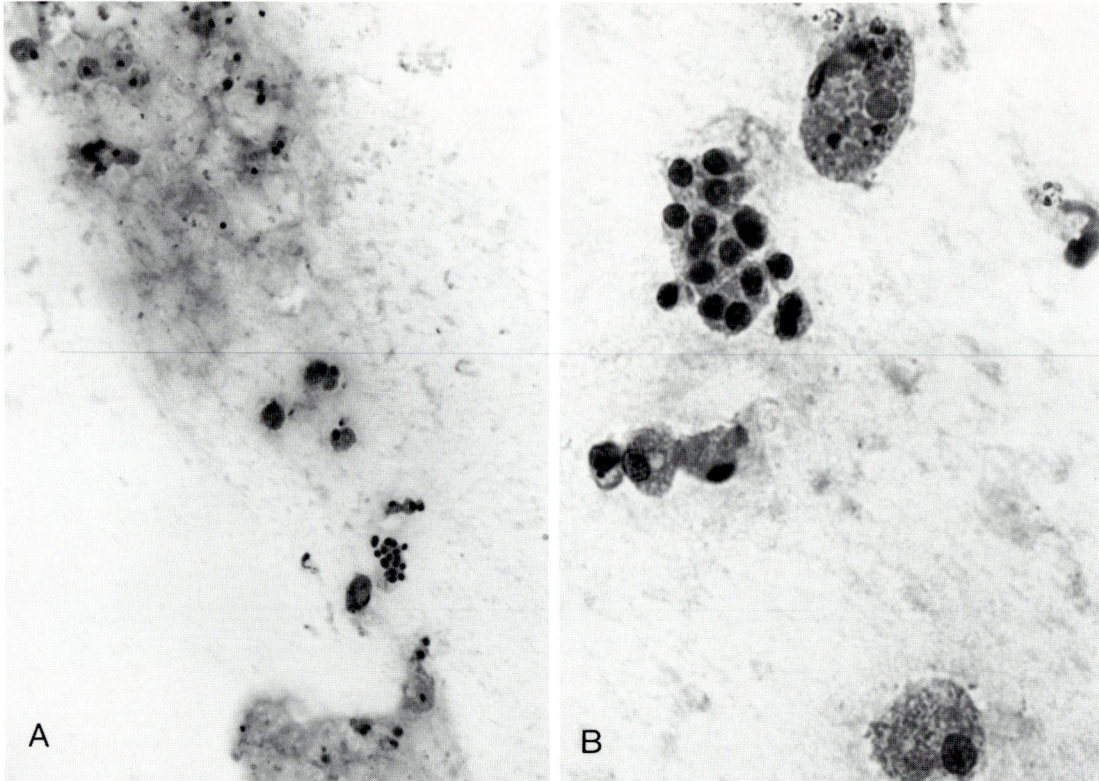

Figure 2.7.

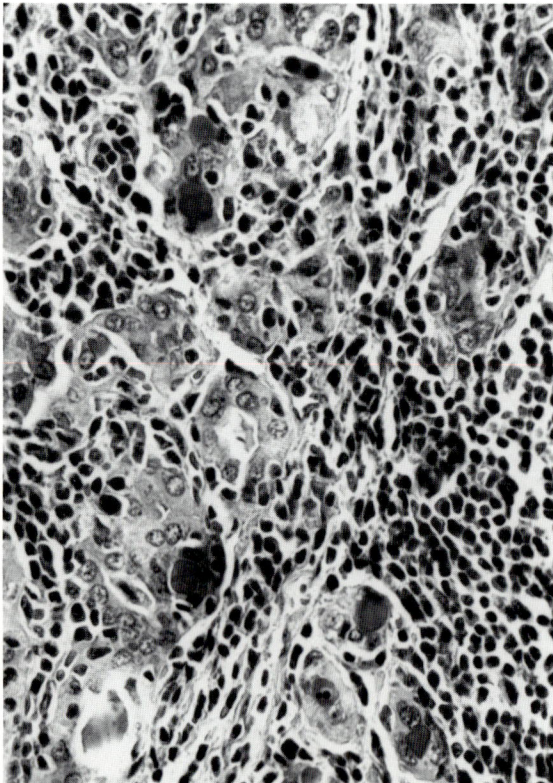

Figure 2.7. Thyroid cyst, ABC. **A,** Low-power view showing paucity of cells and a cystic background. ×75. **B,** Higher power view showing a cluster of small follicular cells and several hemosiderin-laden histiocytes. ×500.

Figure 2.8. Chronic lymphocytic thyroiditis, histologic section. Note lymphocytic infiltrate and follicular cells with Hürthle cell change. ×310.

Figure 2.8.

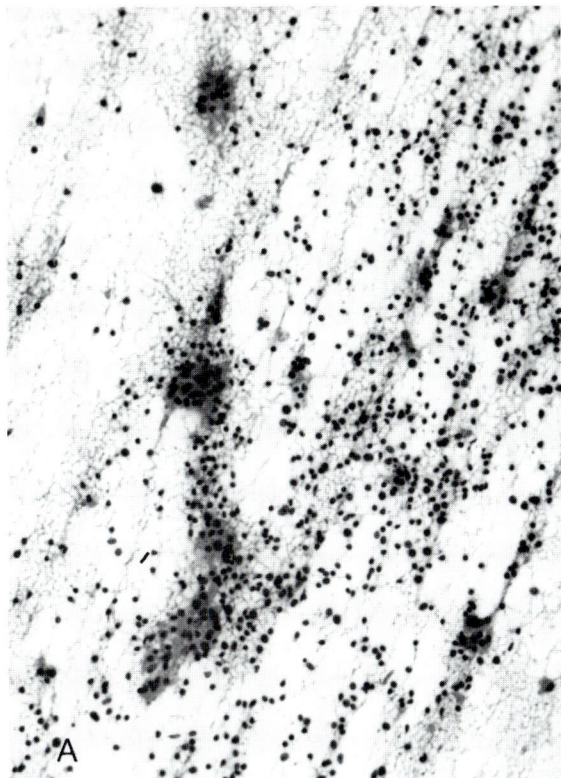

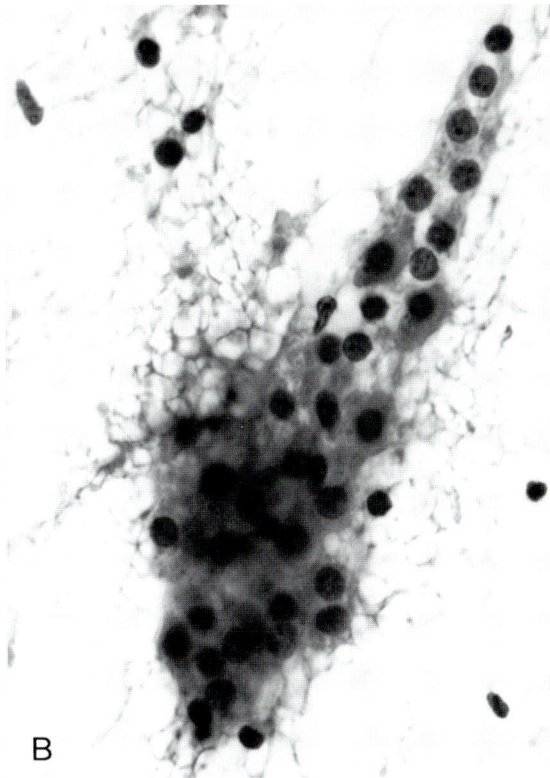

Figure 2.9. Chronic lymphocytic thyroiditis, ABC. **A**, Note small, cohesive groups of Hürthle cells, admixed with dispersed lymphocytes. ×125. **B**, A close-up view of a group of Hürthle cells. The nuclei are modestly enlarged. The cytoplasm is granular and eosinophilic. ×500.

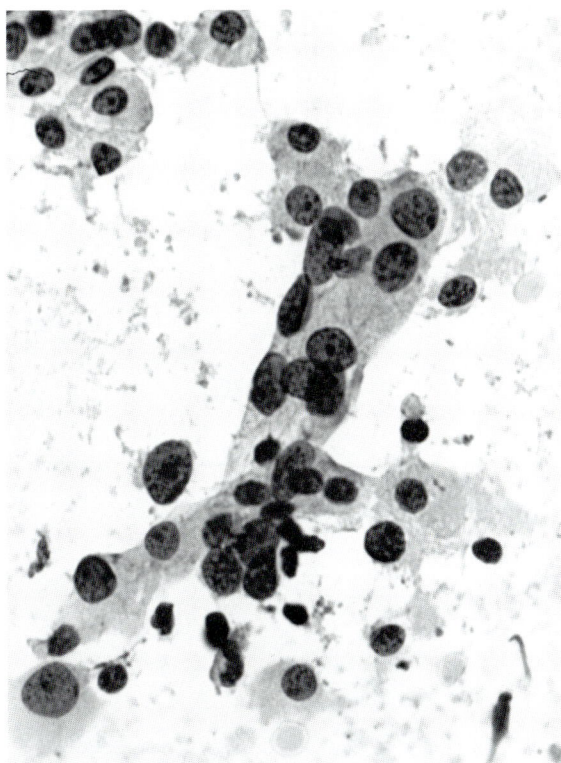

Figure 2.10. Chronic lymphocytic thyroiditis, ABC. Note atypical, enlarged Hürthle cells, admixed with some "regular," smaller Hürthle cells. This spectrum of changes from regular to large pleomorphic Hürthle cells is characteristic of the disease. ×500.

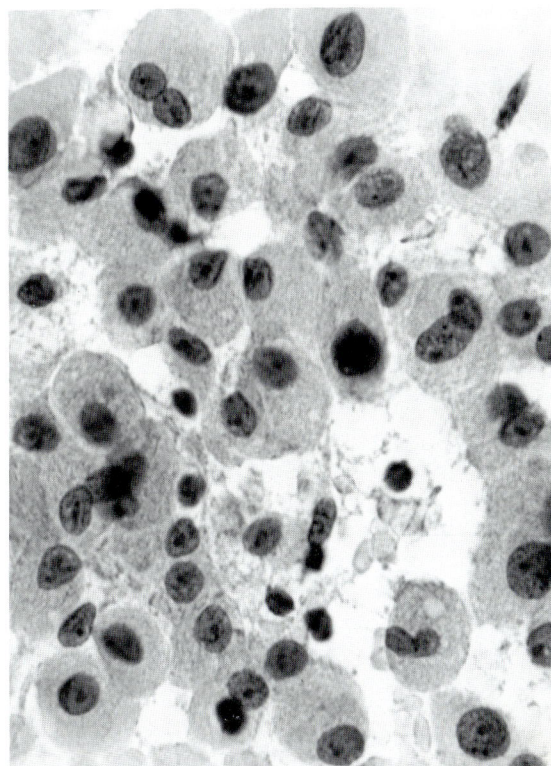

Figure 2.11. Chronic lymphocytic thyroiditis, diagnostic trap. ABC shows a monomorphic population of Hürthle cells with prominent nuclei and almost no lymphocytes. Unless another area of the smear shows more classic changes of chronic lymphocytic thyroiditis, the morphologic purity seen here may cause confusion with Hürthle cell neoplasm. ×500.

Subacute (Granulomatous) Thyroiditis

Subacute thyroiditis is a spontaneously remitting inflammatory condition that may last for a few weeks or several months.[12] The thyroid gland is tender and diffusely enlarged, but it also may be asymmetrical with predominant involvement of one lobe. Histologically, one sees a mixture of subacute, chronic, and granulomatous inflammatory changes, along with parenchymal destruction and fibrosis. The histologic hallmark is the granuloma, composed of multinucleated giant cells clustered about foci of ruptured or degenerating follicles (Fig. 2.12).

Aspiration Cytology

The ABC (Fig. 2.13) shows admixture of lymphocytes, plasma cells, and polymorphonuclear leukocytes, accompanied by epithelioid histiocytes and multinucleated foreign-body-type giant cells, some of which may be enormous in size.[17] A few small groups of follicular epithelial cells are usually present, but Hürthle cells are not seen.

Diagnostic Pitfalls.   In some instances of subacute thyroiditis, a heavy lymphocytic infiltrate along with paucity of multinucleated giant cells may lead to the erroneous diagnosis of chronic lymphocytic (Hashimoto's) thyroiditis.

Papillary carcinoma may enter into the differential diagnosis because multinucleated giant cells are encountered in both subacute thyroiditis and papillary carcinoma.

NEOPLASTIC LESIONS
Follicular Adenoma

Thyroid adenoma is a benign neoplasm, with a predominance in females as much as 6:1. In contrast to nodular goiters, adenomas are encapsulated and generally solitary. Six histologic types are recognized: simple, colloid (macrofollicular), microfollicular, trabecular, Hürthle cell, and atypical.[18,19] Except for being solitary and encapsulated, the simple and the colloid adenoma (Fig. 2.14) are histologically indistinguishable from nodular goiters. All these lesions are basically composed of large colloid-filled follicles, lined by flat or cuboidal epithelium, an observation that has led some authorities to question whether these adenomas are indeed true neoplasms or dominant nodules of nodular goiters.[19] On the other hand, the microfollicular and the trabecular adenoma (Figs. 2.15 and 2.16) are truly cellular neoplasms, with a histologic pattern differing from that of the surrounding tissue. The microfollicular adenoma is composed of small closely packed follicles, with only a small amount of colloid; whereas trabecular adenoma resembles embryonal thyroid tissue and has a trabecular pattern, devoid of colloid. Not uncommonly, a mixed pattern may be found within the same tumor. Atypical adenomas (Fig. 2.17) show cellular atypia, but lack evidence of capsular or vascular invasion. Despite morphologic variations, all adenomas have a benign behavior as long as there is no capsular or vascular invasion demonstrated. Hürthle cell adenoma will be discussed separately later in this chapter.

Aspiration Cytology

Cytologic Pattern.   Smear cellularity is variable, depending on the type of adenoma. In simple and colloid adenomas, the smears are moderately cellular, whereas in microfollicular, trabecular, and atypical adenomas the smears are usually hypercellular. The tumor cells occur singly, but more often they are arranged in follicular units or in large tissue fragments with a follicular pattern. In simple and colloid adenomas, the cytologic appearance resembles that of

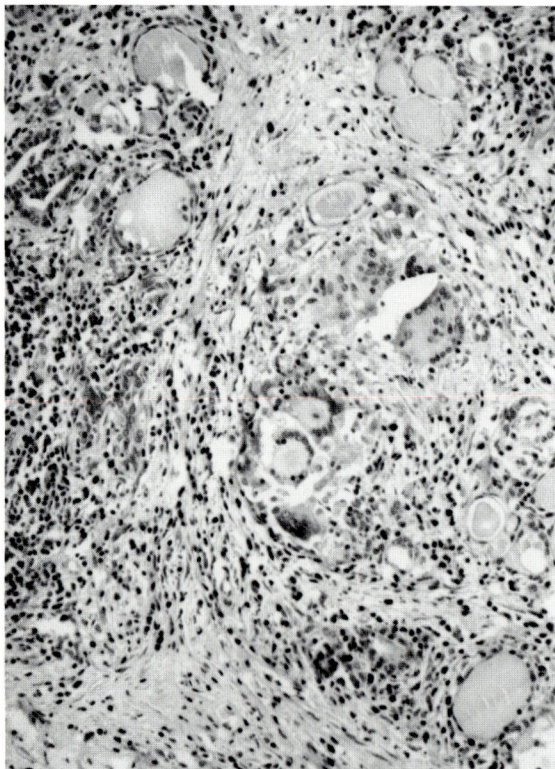

Figure 2.12.   Histology of subacute thyroiditis showing chronic granulomatous inflammation, along with fibrosis and destruction of follicles. ×125.

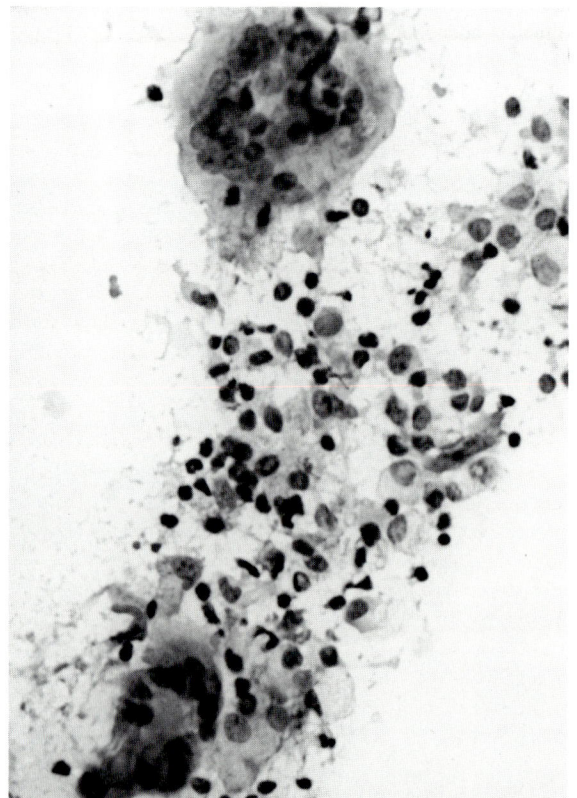

Figure 2.13.   Subacute thyroiditis, ABC. Note admixture of histiocytes, lymphocytes, and multinucleated giant cells. ×500.

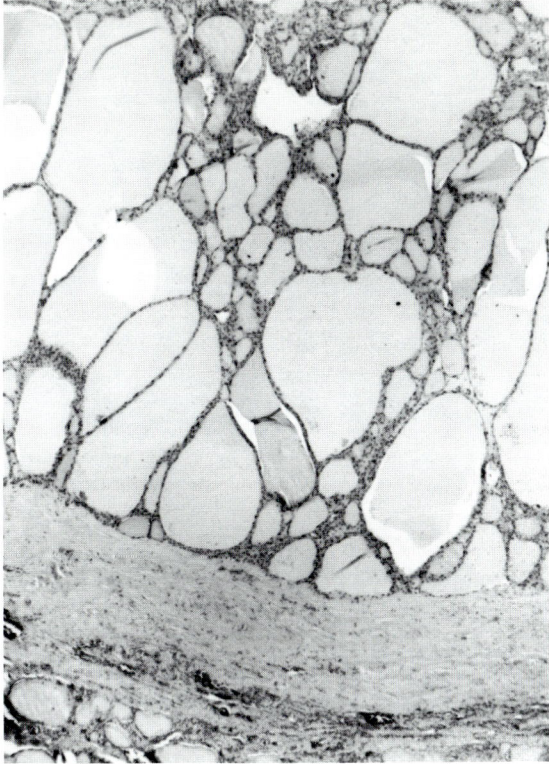

Figure 2.14. Histologic section of colloid (macrofollicular) adenoma. Note large follicles filled with colloid. ×75.

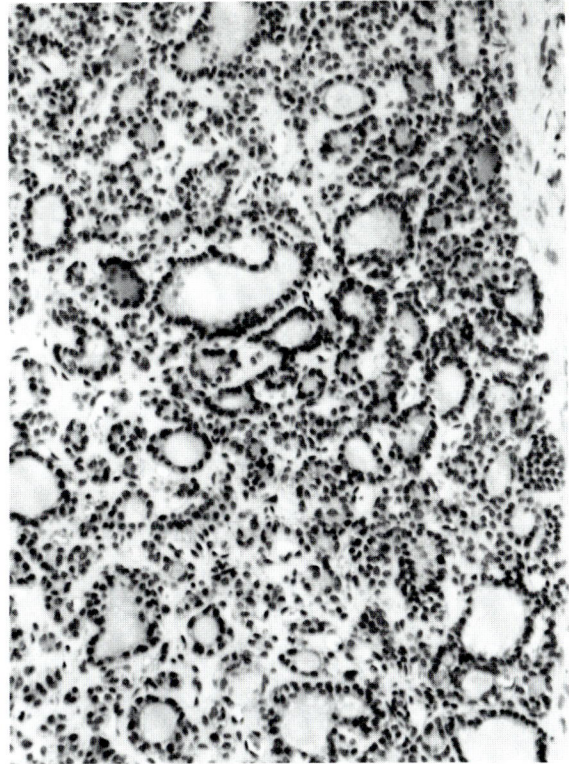

Figure 2.15. Histologic section of microfollicular adenoma. The tumor is cellular and composed of numerous, crowded small follicules with a small amount of colloid only. ×125.

hyperplastic goiter; the uniform follicles are composed of regularly spaced cells and have smooth external contours (**Fig. 2.18**). In microfollicular adenomas, the follicular units are irregular and composed of more crowded and disorganized cells (**Figs. 2.19** and **2.20**). In trabecular adenomas, a trabecular pattern is evident (**Fig. 2.21**). A variable amount of colloid is seen in simple and colloid adenomas, and scant or absent colloid is the norm in microfollicular, trabecular, and atypical adenomas.

Cell Morphology. The follicular cells (**Figs. 2.18–2.21**) vary from normal to slightly enlarged. The nuclei are round or oval. The chromatin is finely granular and evenly distributed. The nuclear membranes are thin and smooth. The nucleoli, if present, are small.

In atypical adenomas (**Fig. 2.22**), the cells show various degrees of nuclear atypia, with nuclear enlargement, prominent nucleoli, and uneven distribution of chromatin.

Well-differentiated Follicular Carcinoma

Follicular carcinomas account for about a quarter of all thyroid cancers and are second to papillary carcinomas in frequency. Although the histologic spectrum of follicular carcinomas is very broad, ranging from regular follicular growth at one end to solid anaplastic growth with a few follicles at the other end, the majority are well-differentiated. The histology of many well-differentiated encapsulated carcinomas may closely resemble cellular follicular adenoma. The diagnosis of carcinoma in such instances rests on the histologic demonstration of capsular invasion or angioinvasion. Unfortunately, these findings are not observed in FNA specimens.

Aspiration Cytology

The smear pattern is hypercellular. The cells are arranged in disorganized follicular units, unstructured cell sheets, or single cells.

Although well-differentiated follicular carcinoma may cytologically closely resemble adenoma (**Fig. 2.23**), with experience, one would be able to appreciate the subtle nuclear and architectural abnormalites in many, but not all, of the cases (**Fig. 2.24**). The diagnostic criteria published in the literature[20–24] are summarized below:

1. Smear hypercellularity with an increase in number of dissociated cells.
2. Cell group hypercellularity with cellular disarray. Within the cell groups, there is disorganization and crowding of the component cells.
3. Increase in nuclear size. Many carcinomas tend to have larger nuclei than adenomas. The nuclear enlargement, if present, should affect practically all tumor cells. A few cells with enlarged hyperchromatic nuclei can be seen in nodular goiters or adenomas and should not be interpreted as malignant.
4. Prominent nucleoli. We have found this criterion very useful, provided it is present in all or most nuclei. However, the absence of prominent nucleoli does not necessarily mean that the lesion is not carcinoma. Nucleolar prominence is best appreciated in technically optimal, ethanol-fixed smears stained with the Papanicolaou or H & E technique and examined with a ×100 oil immersion lens. This criterion, however, does not apply to Hürthle cells, which tend to show prominent nucleoli even when they are benign.
5. Chromatin clumping and parachromatin clearing.
6. Scant or absent colloid in the background.

Most of the criteria described above are subtle changes that require experience for interpretation, and they are relative rather than absolute. For instance, the nucleoli seen in follicular carcinomas will not be judged prominent at all when compared with those seen in conventional adenocarcinomas. The architectural arrangement may

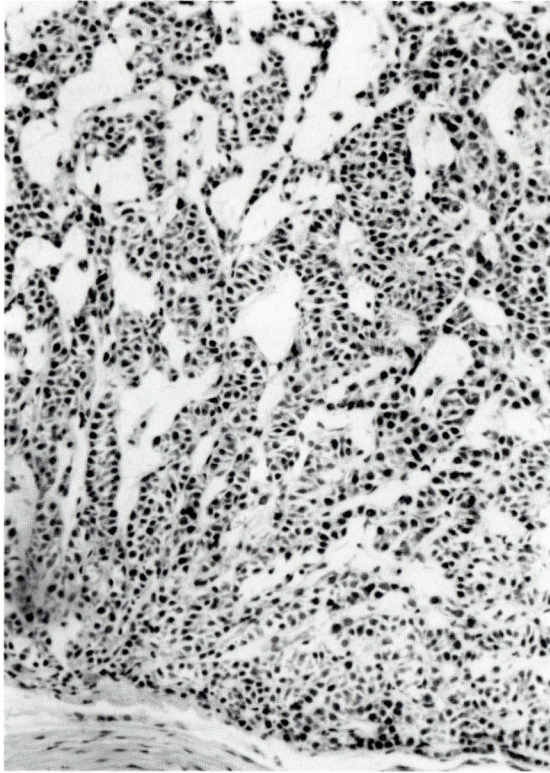

Figure 2.16. Histologic section of trabecular adenoma showing tumor cells arranged in trabeculae. ×125.

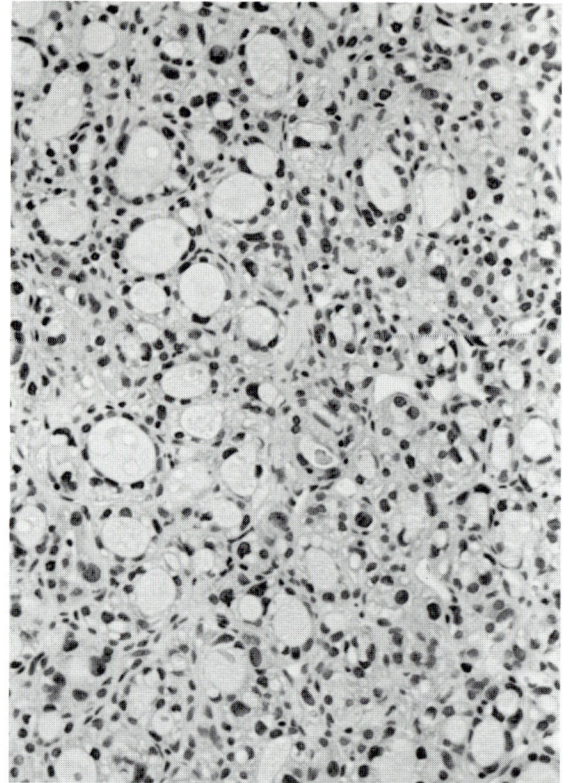

Figure 2.17. Histologic section of atypical adenoma. Note cellular atypia. ×160.

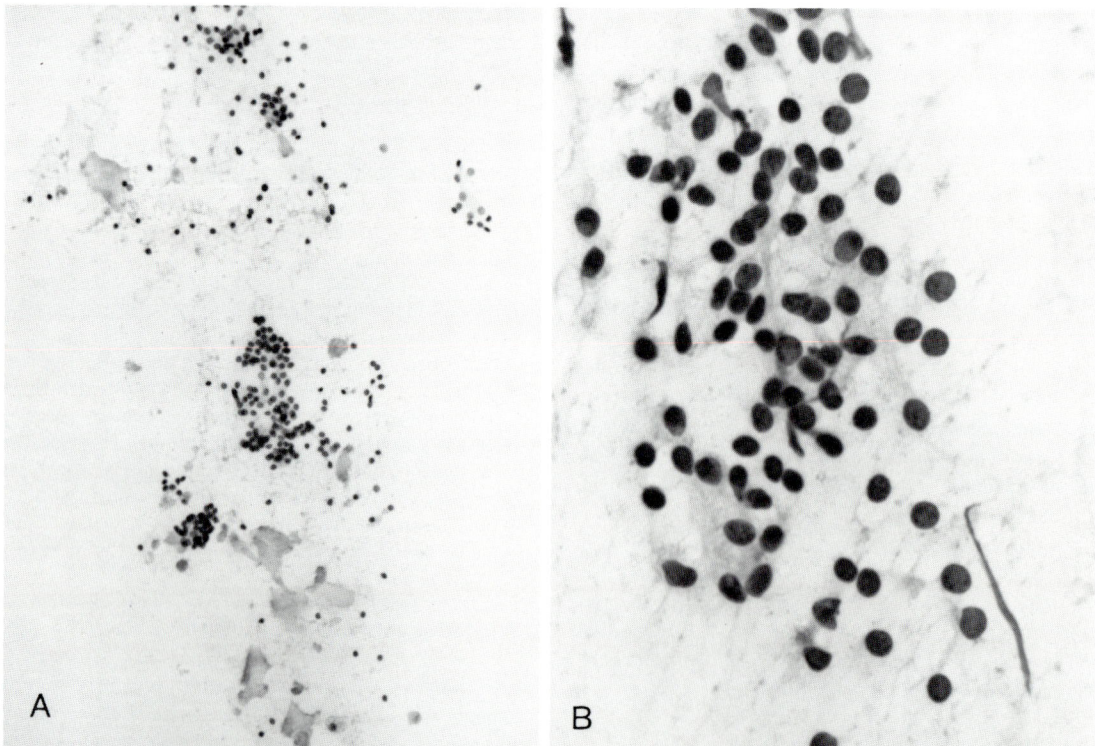

Figure 2.18. Colloid (macrofollicular) adenoma, ABC. **A,** Note follicular cell groups and large clumps of colloid. ×75. **B,** Higher magnification view of the follicular cells. Note perfectly round, evenly staining nuclei and minimal crowding. ×500.

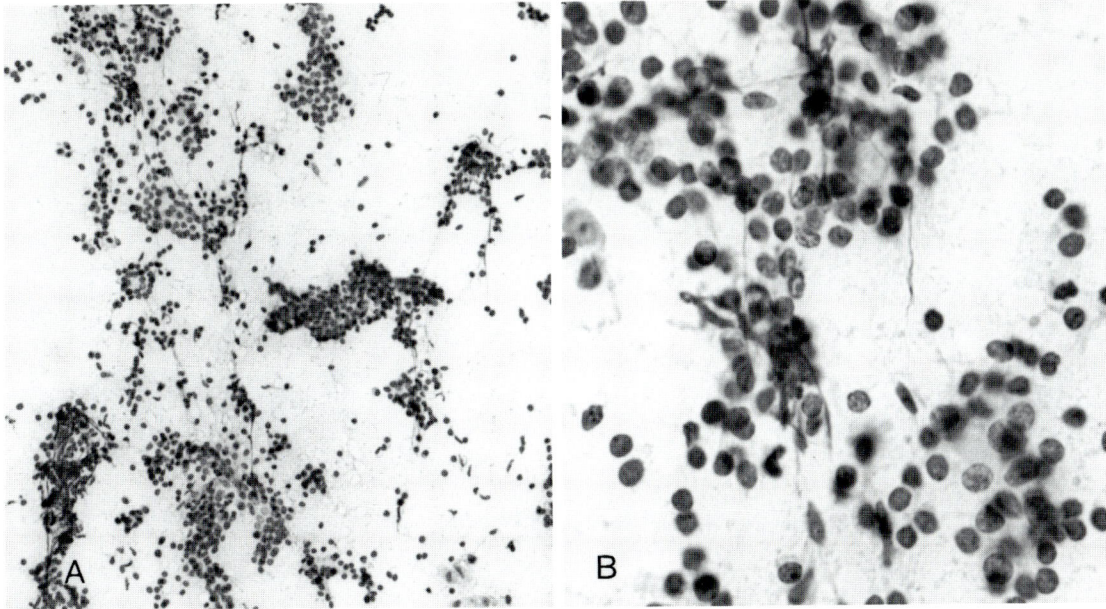

Figure 2.19.

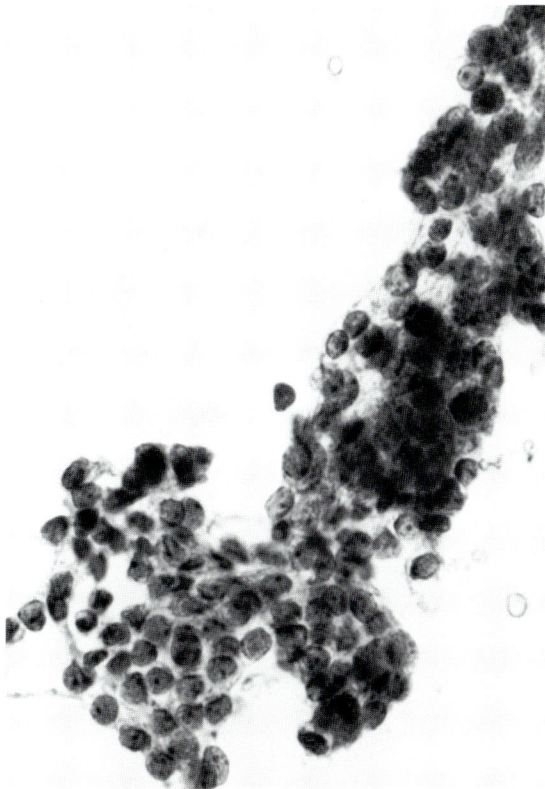

Figure 2.19. Microfollicular adenoma, ABC. **A,** Note hypercellularity, consisting of numerous tissue fragments as well as single cells. ×75. **B,** Note cell crowding and microfollicular arrangement. ×500.

Figure 2.20. Microfollicular adenoma, ABC. Note large hypercellular tissue fragment. The background is devoid of colloid. ×500.

Figure 2.20.

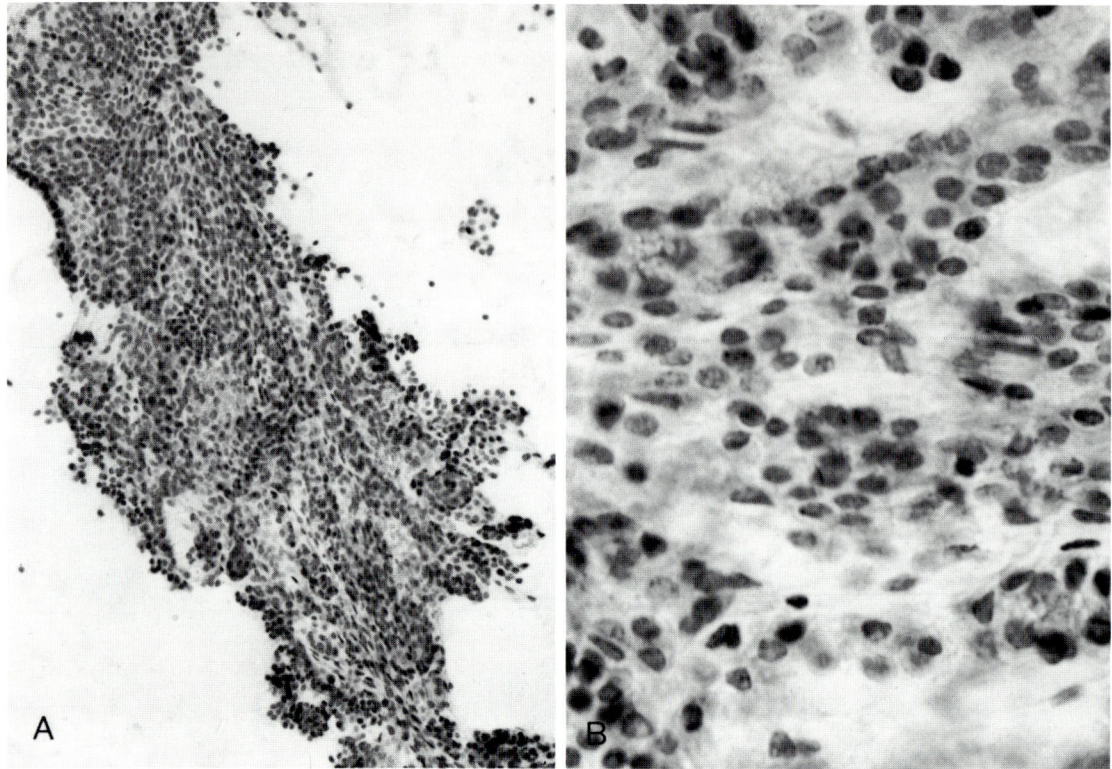

Figure 2.21.

Figure 2.21. Trabecular adenoma, ABC. **A,** Large tissue fragment composed of follicular cells in trabecular arrangement. ×75. **B,** Neoplastic trabeculae at higher magnification. ×500.

Figure 2.22. Atypical adenoma, ABC. Note hypercellularity, follicular pattern, and individual cells with nuclear atypia. ×125.

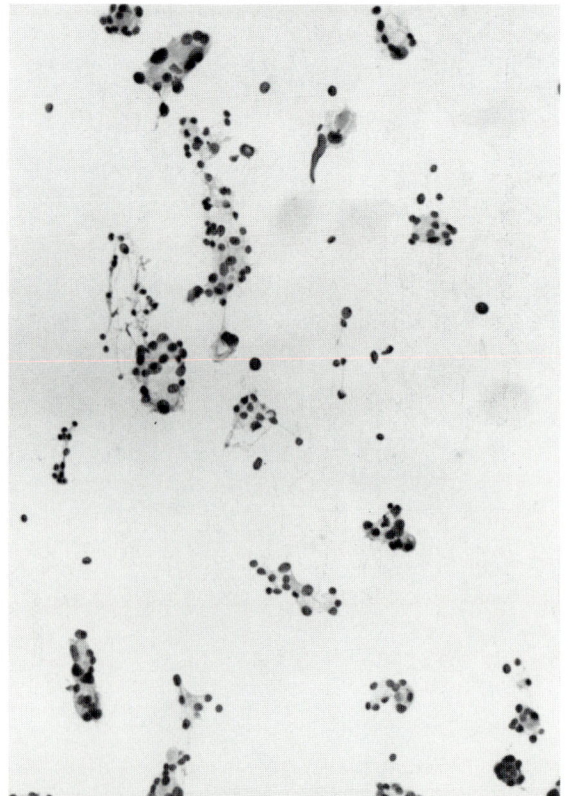

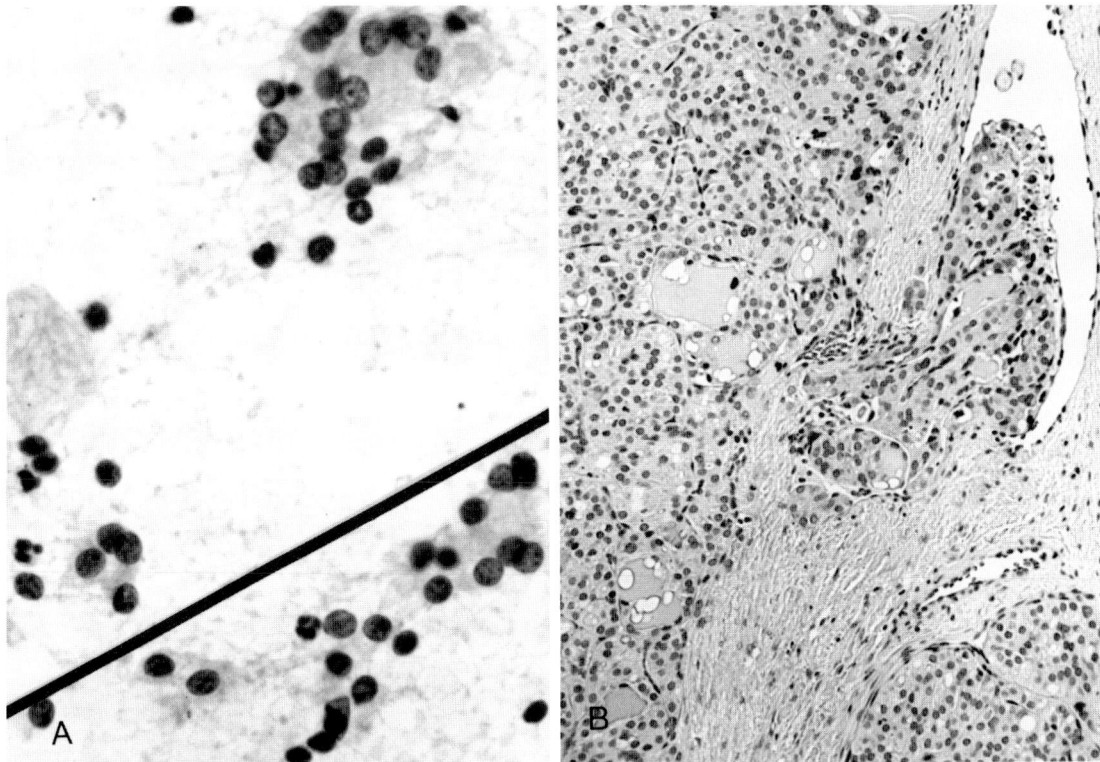

Figure 2.23. Well-differentiated follicular carcinoma. **A**, Aspirate. The tumor cells closely resemble those of follicular adenoma in appearance. Nevertheless, tumor cells are slightly larger and some show subtle chromatin clumping, parachromatin clearing, and nucleoli. ×500. **B**, Histology. Note hypercellular, microfollicullar pattern and vascular invasion by tumor. ×125.

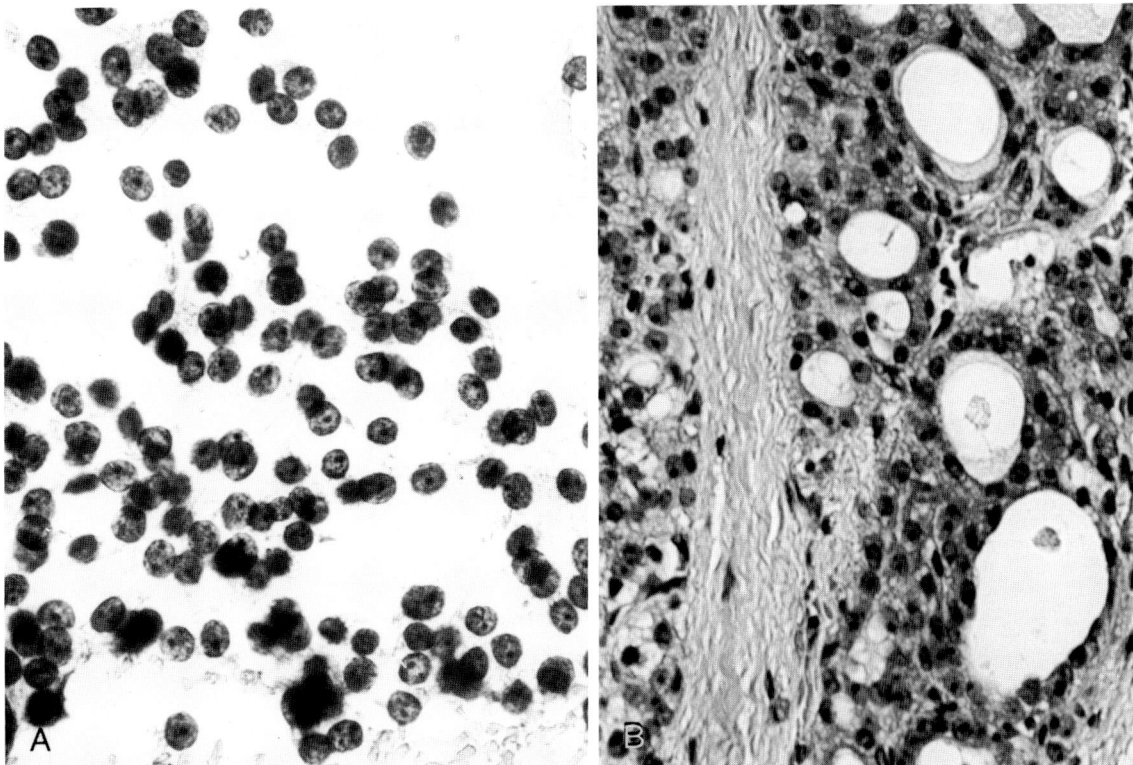

Figure 2.24. Well-differentiated follicular carcinoma. **A**, Aspirate with a hypercellular smear pattern. The cell nuclei are enlarged and each shows a prominent nucleolus. Also note clumped chromatin and uneven condensation of chromatin material at the nuclear membranes. ×500. **B**, Histology of the well-differentiated follicular carcinoma. Note prominent nucleoli. ×310.

not be regarded disorganized by the conventional cytologic standard, but it becomes apparent when compared with the uniform arrangements seen in goiters and some adenomas. According to Kini et al.,[24] increased nuclear size and architectural disarray are the two most useful criteria that help differentiate malignant from benign follicular lesions.

Approach to Cytologic Interpretation of Well-differentiated, Cellular Follicular Lesions

In the past, smear hypercellularity was often taken to mean neoplasia and many hyperplastic nodular goiters were excised unnecessarily. This approach has been challenged recently.[9,20,24] Well-differentiated, cellular follicular lesions of the thyroid gland embrace a broad spectrum of pathologic conditions. Conceptually and in practice, it is helpful to divide these follicular lesions into three cytologic categories: groups I, II, and III, according to their probability of malignancy (Table 2.2).[20] The cytologic features of each of these three groups are recapitulated in Table 2.3. It is important to remember that all these criteria must be interpreted together in making the diagnosis. Each cytologic group is not sharply defined, and a cytologic feature in one group may overlap with that in another group. Follicular carcinomas rarely masquerade as group I lesions; hence, lesions in this group can be treated medically with thyroxine suppression and reevaluated in 6 months. Lesions in groups II and III, on the other hand, are to be treated by surgery.

Kini and associates[24] estimated that about 70% of well-differentiated follicular carcinomas were correctly diagnosed or suspected cytologically. The majority of the remaining cases were interpreted as cellular adenoma (our group II) and were excised. About 1–2% were underdiagnosed as nodular goiter. Thyroid cancers that are missed by FNAB are generally well-differentiated and slow-growing. Admittedly, identification of all thyroid cancers is possible only if all nodules are routinely excised. This is, of course, impractical. Judicious follow-up with repeat aspiration would eventually identify these missed cases and is preferable to routine surgery of all solitary cold nodules.[25]

Papillary Carcinoma

This is the most common type of thyroid carcinoma, accounting for two-thirds of all thyroid malignancy. The tumors are low-grade, and many patients survive 10–20 years after surgery. The typical histology consists of papillary fronds covered by epithelium of neoplastic cells with overlapping, "ground-glass" nuclei (Figs. 2.25 and 2.26). Many cases show a mixture of neoplastic follicles and papillae. When a tumor shows entirely a follicular pattern and yet the nuclei retain the characteristics of papillary carcinoma (discussed below), it is referred to as the "follicullar variant" of papil-

Table 2.2.   Cytologic Categories of Cellular, Well-differentiated Follicular Lesions of the Thyroid[a]

Group I	Group II	Group III
Hyperplastic nodular goiter	Microfollicular adenoma	Follicular carcinoma
Simple adenoma	Trabecular adenoma	Atypical adenoma
Colloid adenoma	Some follicular carcinomas	Some microfollicular and trabecular adenomas

[a] From Suen KC. How does one separate follicular lesions of the thyroid by fine-needle aspiration biopsy? Diagn Cytopathol 1988;4:78–81.

Table 2.3.   Cytologic Features of the Various Cellular Well-differentiated Follicular Lesions of the Thyroid[a]

	Group I	Group II	Group III
Cellularity of smear	Low to high	Generally high	Generally high
Cellularity within cell groups	Low to moderate	Moderate	Moderate to high
Follicular units[b]	Well-formed with smooth contour	Moderately well-formed	Moderately to poorly formed
Cell arrangement in cell groups[b]	Well spaced (honeycomb appearance)	Some crowding	Crowded and disorganized
Colloid	Variable	Scant	Scant
Cell morphology			
Nuclear size	Small	Moderate	Moderate to large
Nuclear outline	Smooth and round	Smooth and round	Slightly irregular
Nucleoli[b]	Absent	Small	Often prominent in virtually all cells
Chromatin[b]	Uniformly distributed	Uniformly distributed	Slightly irregularly distributed

[a] From Suen KC. How does one separate follicular lesions of the thyroid by fine-needle aspiration biopsy? Diagn Cytopathol 1988;4:78–81.
[b] Features that have more discriminatory value.

lary carcinoma (Fig. 2.27). Biologically, both the mixed and the follicular variant behave like pure papillary carcinoma.[26,27]

Aspiration Cytology

Cytologic Pattern.   Aspirates are highly cellular. Tumor cells are typically arranged in tissue fragments of various sizes (see Fig. 1.18). Single cells are also present but are not prominent. Kini and associates[28] have described in detail three types of tissue fragments: papillary, monolayered, and multilayered. Figures 2.28 and 2.29 show papillary tissue fragments with a characteristic stereoscopic and branching configuration. The three-dimensional configuration is best appreciated if one moves the plane of focus of the microscope up and down. At higher magnification, cell crowding and nuclear overlapping are evident, and the peripheral cells are arranged in a palisade, forming smooth external borders (Fig. 2.30).

The second type of tissue fragments is the monolayered cell sheet (Figs. 2.31–2.33). The component cells within the cell sheets are slightly larger and more pleomorphic than those seen in the papillary tissue fragments and frequently exhibit a squamoid appearance.

The third type of tissue fragments is multilayered and unstructured (Fig. 2.34). There is considerable crowding and overlapping of the component cells, with loss of cell polarity. The external borders of these tissue fragments are jagged. The multilayered tissue fragment is a nonspecific finding and can be seen in aspirations of any highly cellular tumors.

In the follicular variant of papillary carcinoma (Fig. 2.35), tumor cells are arranged to form disorganized follicular units or unstructured cell groups. Typical papillary tissue fragments are sparse or absent.

Cell Morphology.   The neoplastic cells are larger than the

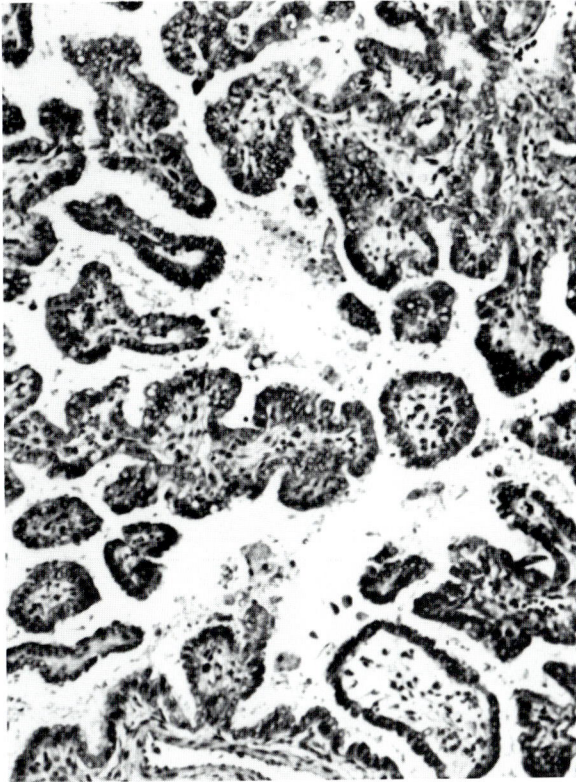

Figure 2.25. Typical histology of papillary carcinoma. Note numerous papillary fronds. ×75.

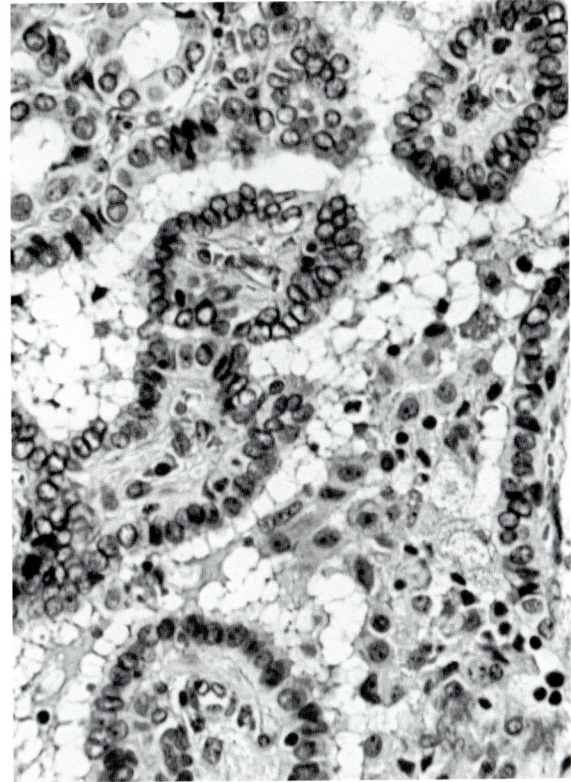

Figure 2.26. Histology of papillary carcinoma at higher magnification showing the characteristic overlapping, ground-glass nuclei. ×310.

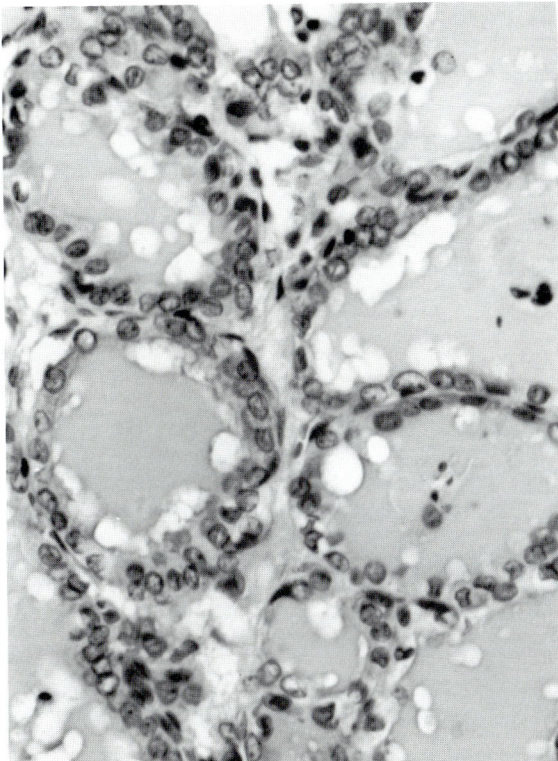

Figure 2.27. Follicular variant of papillary carcinoma, histologic section. Note follicular formation and the ground-glass appearance of nuclei. ×310.

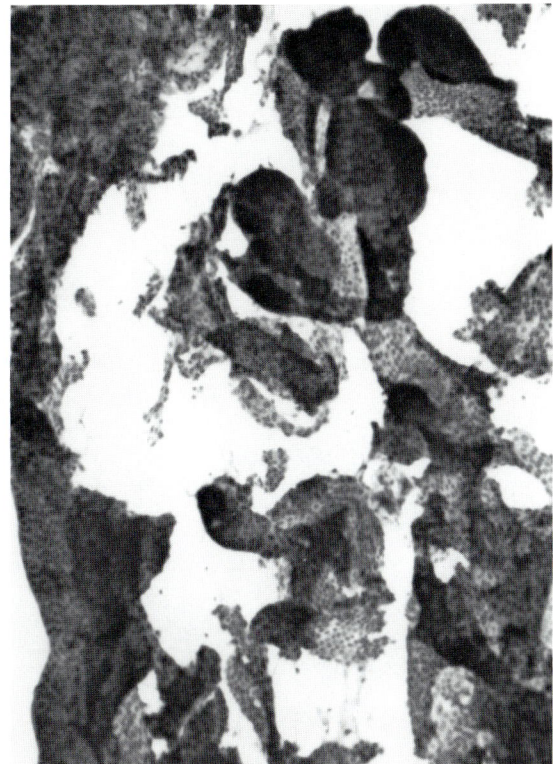

Figure 2.28. Papillary carcinoma, ABC. Typical low-power view showing irregular, branching papillary tissue fragments. ×125.

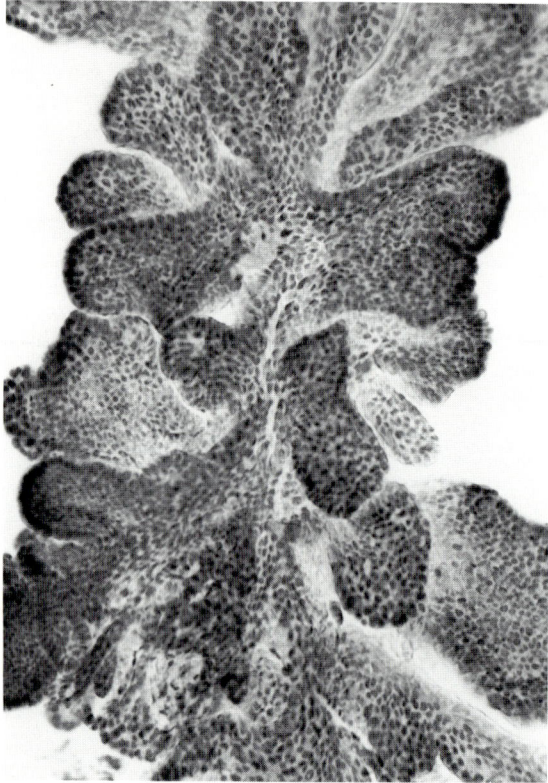

Figure 2.29.

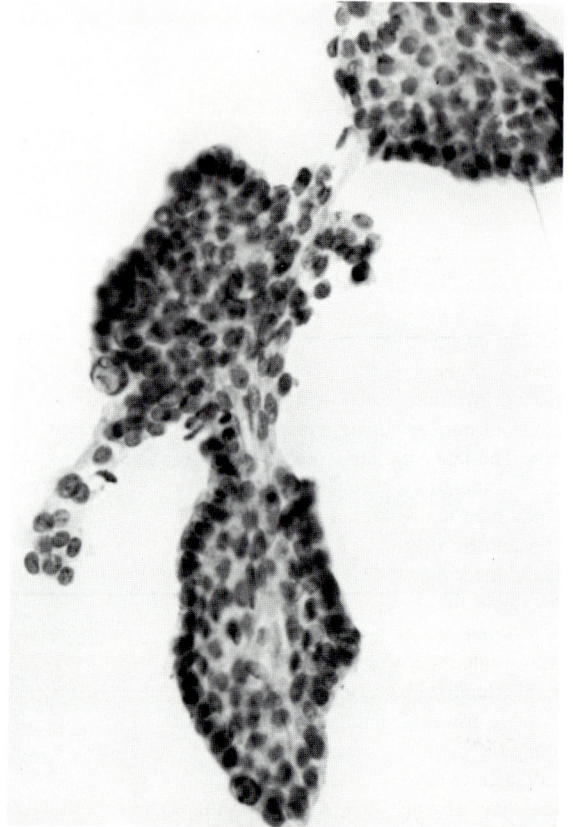

Figure 2.30.

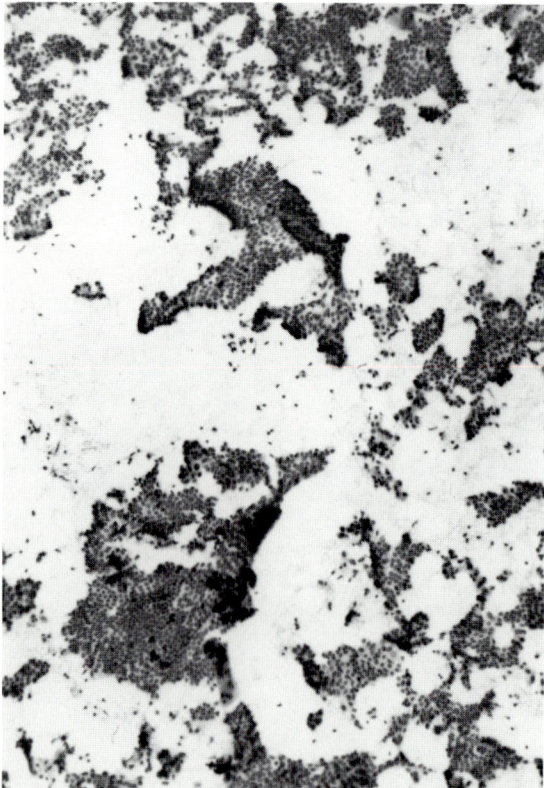

Figure 2.31.

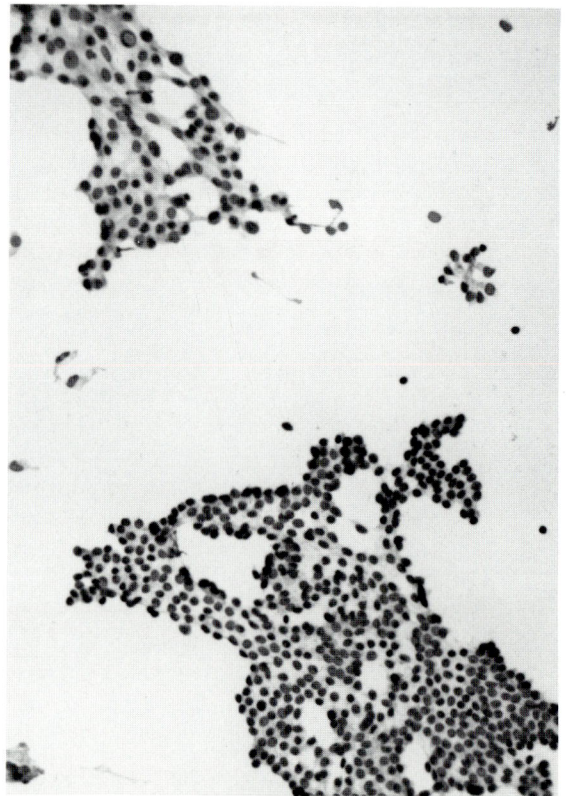

Figure 2.32.

normal follicular cells. The nuclear/cytoplasmic ratio is high. The nuclei are vesicular and pale staining, with a central micronucleus. The chromatin is often so powdery that the nuclei may have a ground-glass appearance (**Figs. 2.34** and **2.35**). The nuclear membranes are irregular, and some nuclei show grooves and notches (**Fig. 2.36**).[29] In our experience, both ground-glass nuclei and nuclear grooves are more readily seen in paraffin-embedded tissue sections than in needle aspirates.

Another cytologic characteristic is the presence in some nuclei of well-defined ''holes,'' or pseudoinclusions (**Fig. 2.33**). These nuclear holes, which can be seen in up to 60% of our cases, represent cytoplasmic invaginations.[30,31]

Smear Background.   There is very little or no colloid in the background. Multinucleated giant histiocytes (**Fig. 2.37**) are seen in about 20% of our cases, and psammoma bodies (**Fig. 2.38**) in about 15–20%. The latter are laminated calcific spherules, 30–100 μm in diameter, scattered singly or in groups, surrounded by cancer cells or incorporated within papillary fragments.

Diagnostic Pitfalls.   The diagnosis of papillary carcinoma can usually be made with great accuracy by FNAB. However, the following diagnostic pitfalls can occur.

1. About 4% of our cases of papillary carcinoma are cystic, and the aspirated tumor cells may be so diluted by the fluid that they may be overlooked, leading to a diagnosis of benign cyst. Generally, the cytologic criteria for diagnosing these cases are the same as those for noncystic papillary carcinoma. The main differences are that papillary cell groups may be very sparse or absent, degenerative changes may obscure cell detail, and a cytologic diagnosis of suggestive of papillary carcinoma may have to be made on scanty evidence.[32,33] It is important that, after evacuation of the cystic content, any residual solid area, if present, should be aspirated. Prompt reaccumulation of fluid is also an indication for repeat biopsy or excision of the lesion.

2. The follicular variant of papillary carcinoma (**Fig. 2.35**) may be mistaken for follicular adenoma. The identification of ground-glass nuclei, nuclear grooves, and intranuclear pseudoinclusions aids in correct diagnosis. A diligent search of the smears may disclose diagnostic papillary tissue fragments, even though the latter may not show up on histology examination.

3. Concomitant chronic lymphocytic thyroiditis and thyroid neoplasm can occur in the same patient. In such cases, tumor cells may be misinterpreted as reactive epithelium or masked completely by the florid changes of thyroiditis, resulting in a false-negative diagnosis.

4. The large monolayered tissue fragments obtained from hyperplastic nodular goiters may be confused with the monolayered tissue fragments of papillary carcinoma. Despite hypercellularity, ABC of the former (**Fig. 2.6**) shows uniform cells in honeycomb arrangement while the latter (**Figs. 2.31–2.33**) shows disturbed nuclear polarity, large nuclei with nuclear holes and grooves, and a powdery chromatin pattern.

5. Both psammoma bodies and multinucleated giant histiocytes are extremely helpful, but by no means specific, in diagnosing papillary carcinoma. Calcific material similar to psammoma body can be found occasionally in degenerated areas of nodular goiter and in chronic lymphocytic thyroiditis,[34] and multinucleated histiocytes are a constant feature of subacute thyroiditis.

Hürthle (Oxyphilic) Cell Tumors

Of all the thyroid neoplasms, Hürthle cell tumors are most controversial regarding their classification and behavior. It is not clear whether Hürthle cell tumor is a definite histopathologic entity or whether Hürthle cell change is just a secondary event that can take place in follicular and papillary tumors. To compound the problem further, some authorities regard all Hürthle cell neoplasms as potentially malignant,[35] while others do not subscribe to this extreme view.[19,36]

Histologically, Hürthle cell tumor (**Fig. 2.39**) is composed of large polygonal cells, with abundant granular eosinophilic (oxyphilic) cytoplasm. Nuclei are large and have prominent nucleoli. It is usually difficult to differentiate between Hürthle cell adenoma and carcinoma based on cell morphology. Rosai[19] has indicated that most Hürthle cell lesions lacking obvious morphologic signs of malignancy behave in a benign fashion. Criteria similar to those used for follicular carcinoma—capsular and vascular invasion—also apply with these tumors.[36]

Aspiration Cytology

Aspirates from Hürthle cell tumors (**Fig. 2.40**) are cellular and have scant or no colloid in the background. The cells occur singly, in monolayers, or in tissue fragments with follicle-like arrangement. Characteristic Hürthle cells are large, polygonal cells with abundant eosinophilic granular cytoplasm. The nuclei are also enlarged, round to oval, and have fine chromatin and relatively large nucleoli. In Hürthle cell carcinoma (**Fig. 2.41**), there is more nuclear atypia and nucleoli are more prominent. Nevertheless, there is considerable overlap in the cytologic features of Hürthle cell adenoma and Hürthle cell carcinoma.[37] Hence, the noncommittal term Hürthle cell tumor

Figure 2.29.   Papillary carcinoma, ABC. This huge papillary tissue fragment is composed of many well-developed, three-dimensional papillary fronds with smooth, sharply demarcated external borders. The component cells are tightly packed and superimposed. Also note palisade orientation of the peripheral cells. ×125.

Figure 2.30.   Papillae at higher magnification, ABC. Note smooth borders and three-dimensional configuration, which is best appreciated by moving the plane of focus of the microscope up and down. ×310.

Figure 2.31.   Papillary carcinoma, ABC. Variably sized monolayered tissue fragments. ×75.

Figure 2.32.   Monolayered tissue fragments in papillary carcinoma, ABC. ×125.

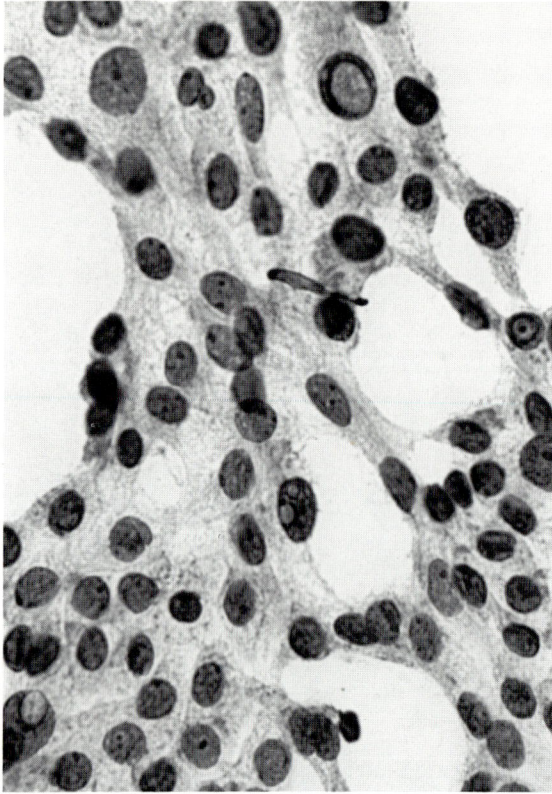

Figure 2.33.

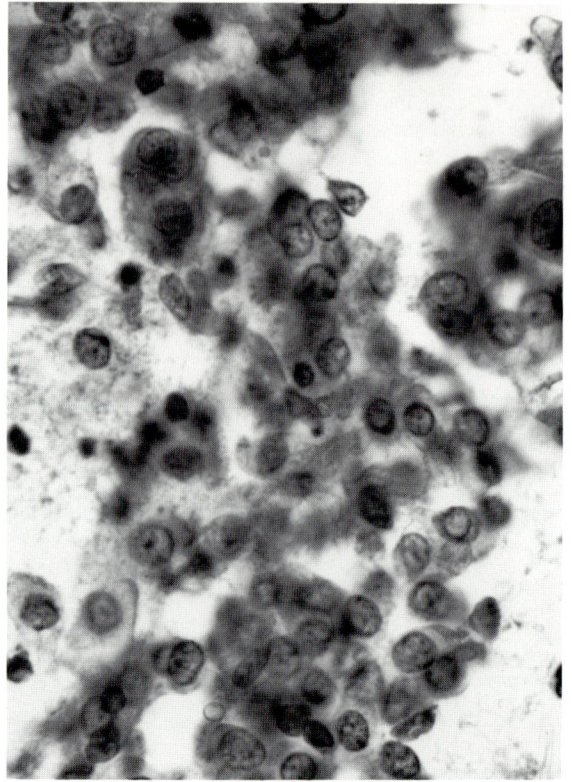

Figure 2.34.

Figure 2.33. High magnification view of monolayered tissue fragment (same case as **Figure 3.32**). The tumor cells are large, with loss of polarity and modest degree of nuclear pleomorphism. Note intranuclear cytoplasmic pseudoinclusions, often referred to as nuclear holes. ×500.

Figure 2.34. Multilayered tissue fragment from papillary carcinoma, ABC. Note overlapping, disorganized cells with ground-glass nuclei. ×500.

Figure 2.35. Follicular variant of papillary carcinoma, ABC. Note abortive follicles formed by neoplastic cells having pale, powdery chromatin, and micronucleoli. Intranuclear cytoplasmic pseudoinclusions are also seen. ×455.

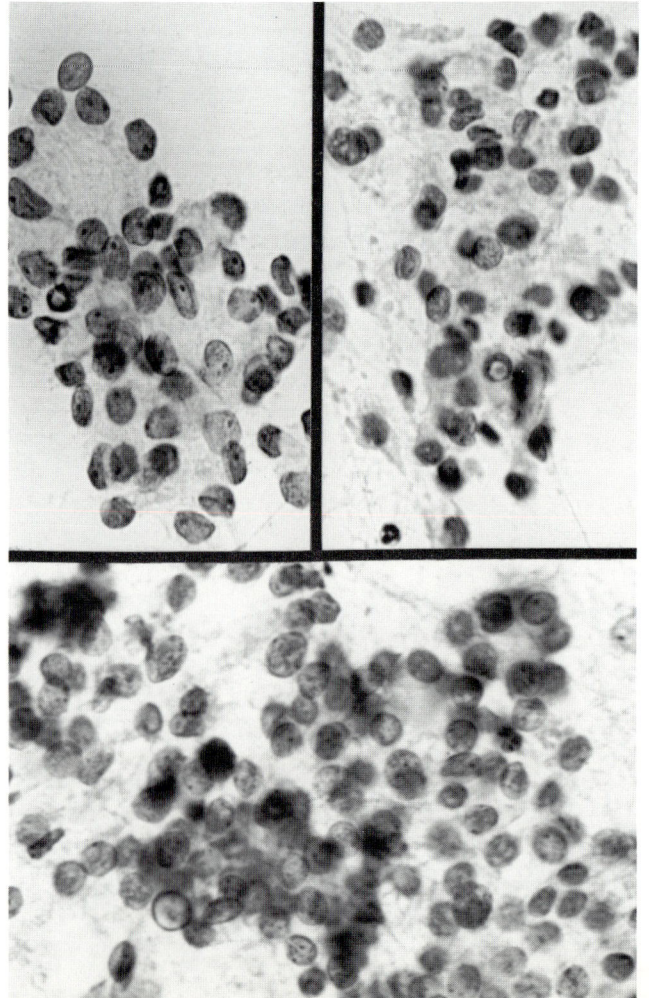

Figure 2.35.

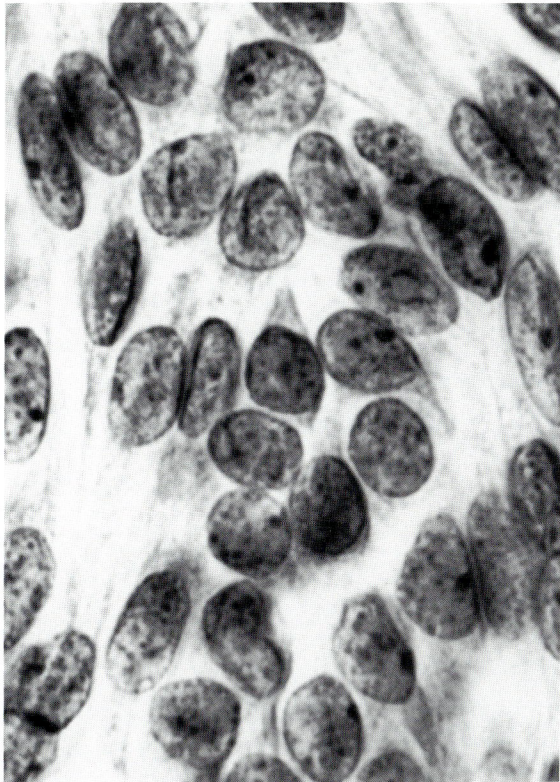

Figure 2.36. Papillary carcinoma, ABC. Close-up view to show nuclear detail. Note atypical nuclei with grooves, notches, and micronucleoli. ×1200.

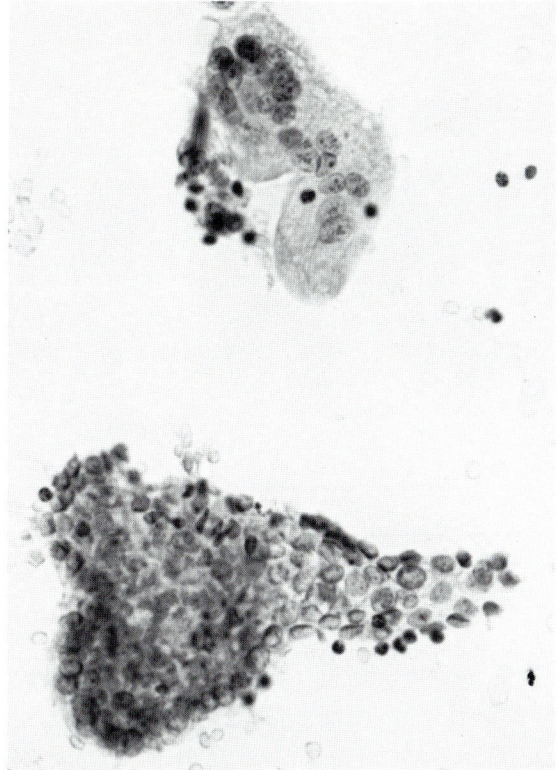

Figure 2.37. Papillary carcinoma, ABC. Note a multinucleated histiocytic giant cell and an adjacent papillary tissue fragment showing overlapping, ground-glass nuclei. ×310.

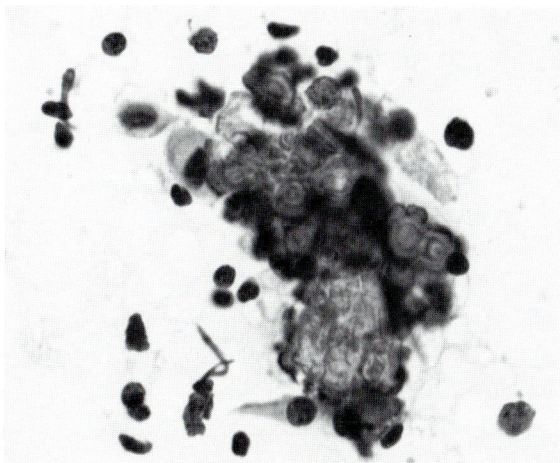

Figure 2.38. Papillary carcinoma, ABC. A group of psammoma bodies, characterized by laminated calcific spherules, surrounded by tumor cells. ×500.

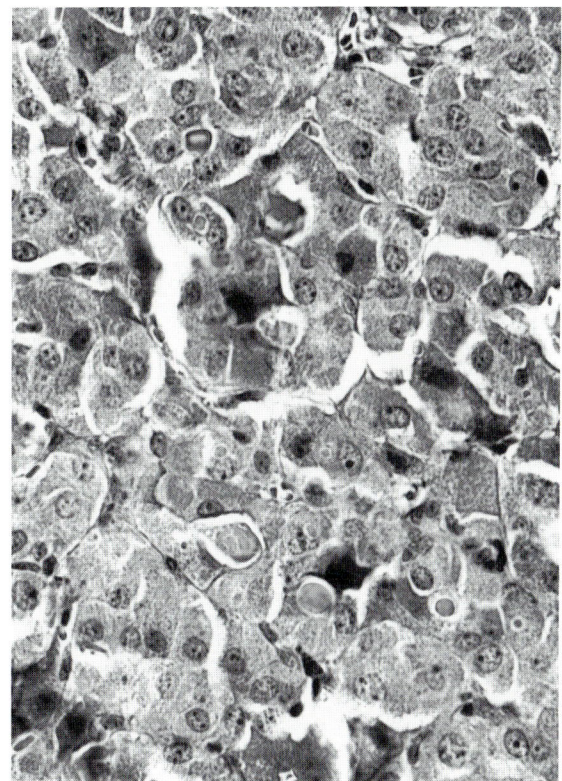

Figure 2.39. Histology of Hürthle cell carcinoma. Note large, polygonal cells with granular eosinophilic cytoplasm and prominent nucleoli. The tumor subsequently metastasized to the lungs. ×310.

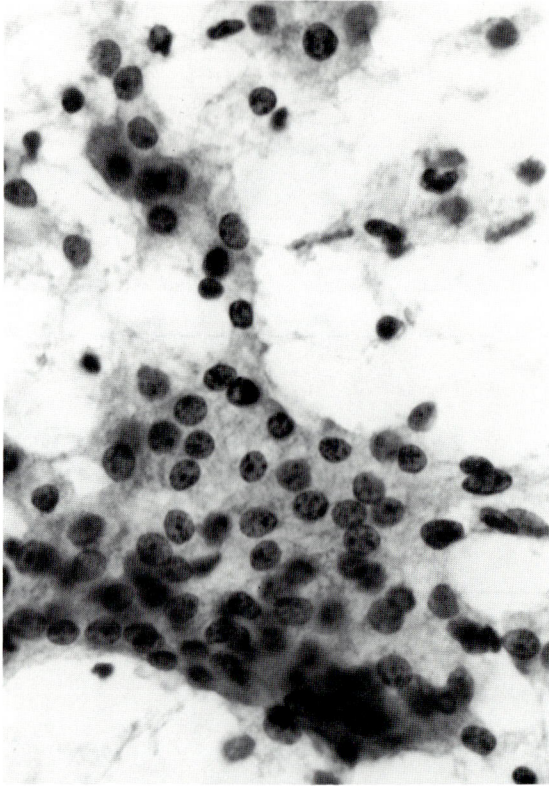

Figure 2.40. Hürthle cell adenoma, ABC. Note monomorphic population of large, polygonal cells with abundant granular cytoplasm. The tumor cells are cytologically benign-appearing. ×500.

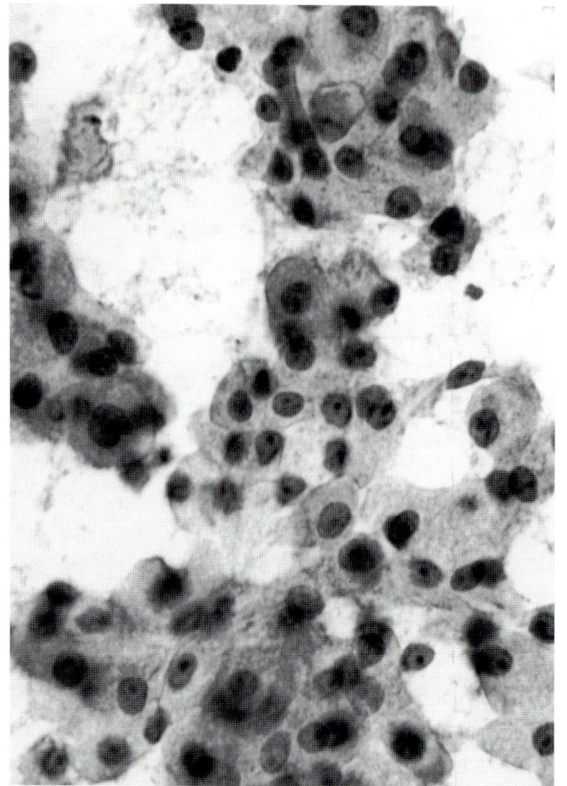

Figure 2.41. Hürthle cell carcinoma, aspirate from the case shown in **Figure 2.39.** Note nucleolar prominence and nuclear membrane irregularity. ×500.

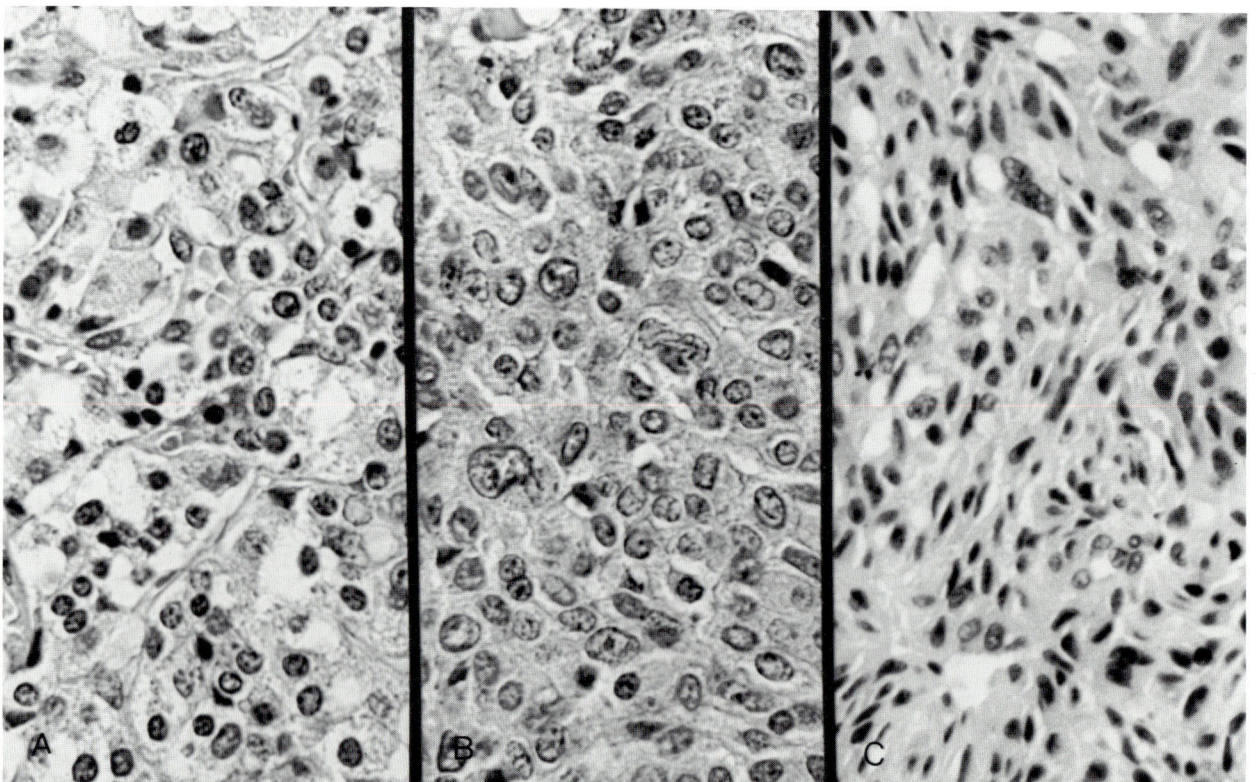

Figure 2.42. Histologic spectrum of medullary carcinoma. **A,** Uniform polygonal cells with round nuclei, granular chromatin, and cyanophilic granulated cytoplasm. These cells resemble those from carcinoid tumors. ×500. **B,** Larger cells showing nuclear pleomorphism and nucleoli. ×500. **C,** Spindle and giant cells. X310.

should be used in FNAB diangosis and all such tumors should be excised.

Diagnostic Pitfalls. Hürthle cell neoplasms must be distinguished from nonneoplastic conditions, such as Hashimoto's thyroiditis and nodular goiters that contain metaplastic Hürthle cell nodules. Aspirates from Hürthle cell neoplasms usually show a single population of neoplastic Hürthle cells. By contrast, the atypical Hürthle cells in these nonneoplastic conditions are frequently admixed with some "normal" Hürthle cells that have regular and smaller nuclei.[38] Other features, such as lymphocytes in chronic lymphocytic thyroiditis, and colloid and histocytes in nodular goiter, should be carefully searched for in order to arrive at the correct diagnosis. When clinical and laboratory data support a diagnosis of Hashimoto's thyroiditis, caution is advised before making a cytologic diagnosis of Hürthle cell tumor.

Medullary Carcinoma

Medullary thyroid carcinomas, constituting 2–8% of all thyroid cancers, are derived from the parafollicular cells, or C cells, of the thyroid follicles. These C cells are a distinct category from the follicular cells and are believed to originate embryologically from the neural crest. They secrete calcitonin, which plays a crucial role in the regulation of bone resorption. Most of the medullary thyroid carcinomas occur sporadically, but a genetic predisposition to the neoplasm also exists in about 10–20% of the cases, which may be associated with neoplasms of other endocrine glands, like pheochromocytoma and parathyroid hyperplasia or adenoma.

Histologically, medullary carcinoma manifests a varied appearance **(Fig. 2.42)**. The majority of the tumors consist of medium-sized polygonal cells having an organoid or carcinoid-like growth pattern, but spindle cells and pleomorphic giant cells may be seen focally or extensively.[39,40] Another characteristic feature is the presence of amyloid in the tumor stroma.

Aspiration Cytology

Cytologic Pattern. The smear pattern is generally cellular, showing predominantly dissociated cells **(Fig. 2.43)**. Some tumor cells may form sheets or clusters, but papillary and follicular configurations are not seen.

Cell Morphology. The prototypic cells **(Fig. 2.43B)**, resembling those seen in carcinoid tumors, are characterized by polygonal shape, central or eccentric oval nuclei, and coarse uniformly distributed chromatin. Binucleation is common. Nucleoli are generally not prominent. The eccentric nuclei impart a plasmacytoid appearance. The amphophilic cytoplasm displays fine granulation in a few or sometimes in all cells. Some of the polygonal cells may show a greater degree of nuclear pleomorphism. These cells tend to have a coarser chromatin pattern, with an irregular nuclear membrane and single or multiple nucleoli **(Fig. 2.44)**. The second cell type is the spindle cells, which are observed in only one-third of the cases. These cells have elongated nuclei; the cytoplasm is finely granulated. The cells may show a whorled, or sometimes a streaming, pattern **(Fig. 2.45)**. The third cell type is the giant cells, which are least common. The nuclei of these giant cells can be extremely hyperchromatic and enormous in size **(Figs. 2.43 and 2.44)**.[39] When an aspirate specimen contains all three cell types, a polymorphous, disconcerting cellular picture is observed.

If medullary carcinoma is suspected, the cytopathologist should look carefully for amyloid deposits **(Fig. 2.46)**. These are amorphous pink deposits that may be confused with colloid. The former, however, can be demonstrated by Congo-red stain.[41]

Diagnostic Pitfalls. Kini and coworkers[42] reported that accurate diagnosis of medullary carcinoma was relatively simple when there was a combination of spindle cells and rounded cells, whereas one cell type alone led to diagnostic error.

The cytopathologist may have difficulties in separating medullary carcinoma from follicular carcinoma and adenoma. It is important to remember that when cell clusters are seen in medullary carcinoma, they show considerable disorganization, unlike the usual follicular pattern seen in follicular tumors. There also are more dissociated cells in aspirates of medullary carcinoma. The cytoplasm of the cells is finely granulated, and an immunoperoxidase stain will demonstrate calcitonin in the cytoplasm **(Fig. 2.47)**.

The spindle and giant cells seen in medullary carcinoma may be confused with those derived from anaplastic thyroid carcinoma. The identification of the prototypic polygonal cells that resemble carcinoid tumor cells among the spindle and giant cells aids in separating medullary carcinoma from the pleomorphic cells of anaplastic carcinoma.

Poorly Differentiated ("Insular") Carcinoma

Poorly differentiated thyroid carcinoma, a relatively uncommon entity recently described in detail by Rosai et al.,[43] is a much more aggressive tumor than the well-differentiated (papillary and follicular) carcinomas, but it is less aggressive than the anaplastic thyroid carcinoma. Microscopically, the neoplastic cells are small and round, with scanty cytoplasm **(Fig. 2.48A)**. Tumor necrosis, extensive capsular invasion, and blood vessel invasion by tumor are common. The growth pattern is reminiscent of that seen in the insular type of carcinoid tumor; the tumor cells form large solid nests or islands containing a variable number of poorly developed, small follicles.

Aspiration Cytology

Cell Morphology. The neoplastic cells are small, round, and relatively uniform, with little variation from cell to cell **(Fig. 2.48B)**. Although superficially there appears to be little nuclear pleomorphism, careful examination reveals unevenness of nuclear membranes. The chromatin, although finely granular, is irregularly distributed. Nucleoli may be prominent or inconspicuous.

Cytologic Pattern. The tumor cells are arranged into varying-sized groups, with no obvious polarity. Because cytoplasm is scanty, the cells are closely packed, resulting in nuclear crowding.

Diagnostic Pitfalls. The monotonous appearance of the small uniform tumor cells is characteristic,[44] but it may at the same time mislead the unwary pathologist to believe that he or she is dealing with an adenoma. One should always keep the possibility of poorly differentiated insular carcinoma in mind when one encounters the following cytologic features in the smears: tightly grouped small cells with scant cytoplasm, overlapping nuclei, loss of nuclear polarity within the cell groups, and a necrotic background.

Occasionally, malignant lymphoma also enters into the differential diagnosis. Again the characteristic cell grouping is a feature of epithelial neoplasm and not of lymphoma.

Anaplastic Carcinoma

This is a highly malignant tumor, occurring in older patients usually 65 years old and over.[45] Clinically, it is a rapidly growing tumor with a hard consistency, and frequently extends throughout the gland and into adjacent soft tissues. The tumor consists of spindle cells, giant cells, and squamoid cells in various proportions. In about one-third of cases, adequate sampling will reveal a better differentiated (follicular or papillary) component in the tumor. Tumor necrosis and mitoses are common findings.

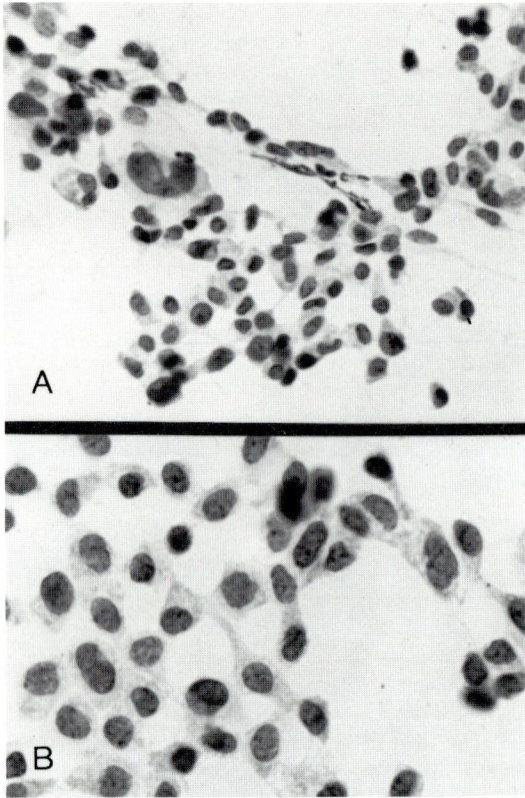

Figure 2.43.

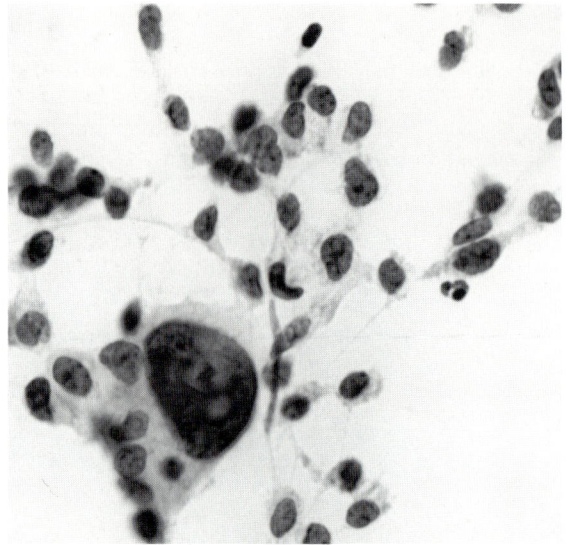

Figure 2.44.

Figure 2.43.   Medullary carcinoma, ABC. **A**, Note the characteristic polymorphous cellular pattern, composed of uniform small polygonal cells, pleomorphic giant cells, and spindle cells. ×310. **B**, High magnification to show the uniform, polygonal cells with granulated cytoplasm, resembling carcinoid tumor cells ×500.

Figure 2.44.   Medullary carcinoma, ABC. Note polygonal tumor cells, which are slightly more pleomorphic than those shown in **Figure 43B**, and a bizarre, hyperchromatic giant cell. ×500.

Figure 2.45.   Medullary carcinoma, ABC. Note spindle cells in whorled pattern. ×500.

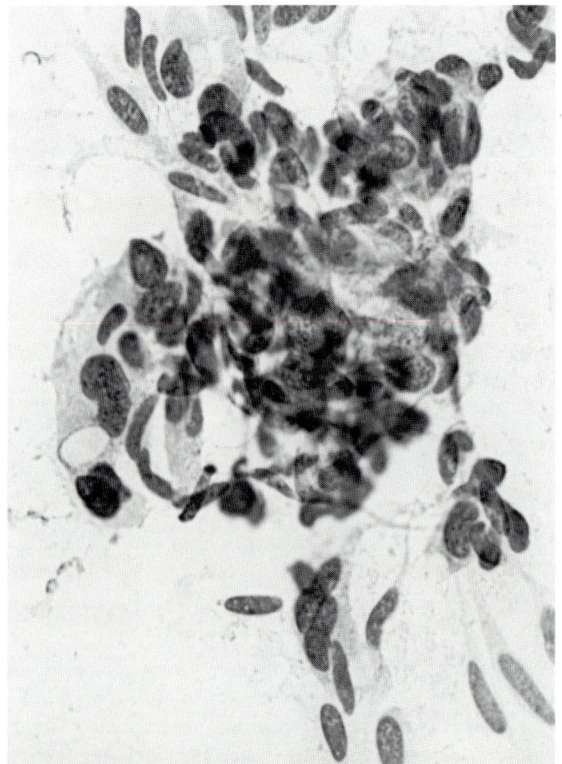

Figure 2.45.

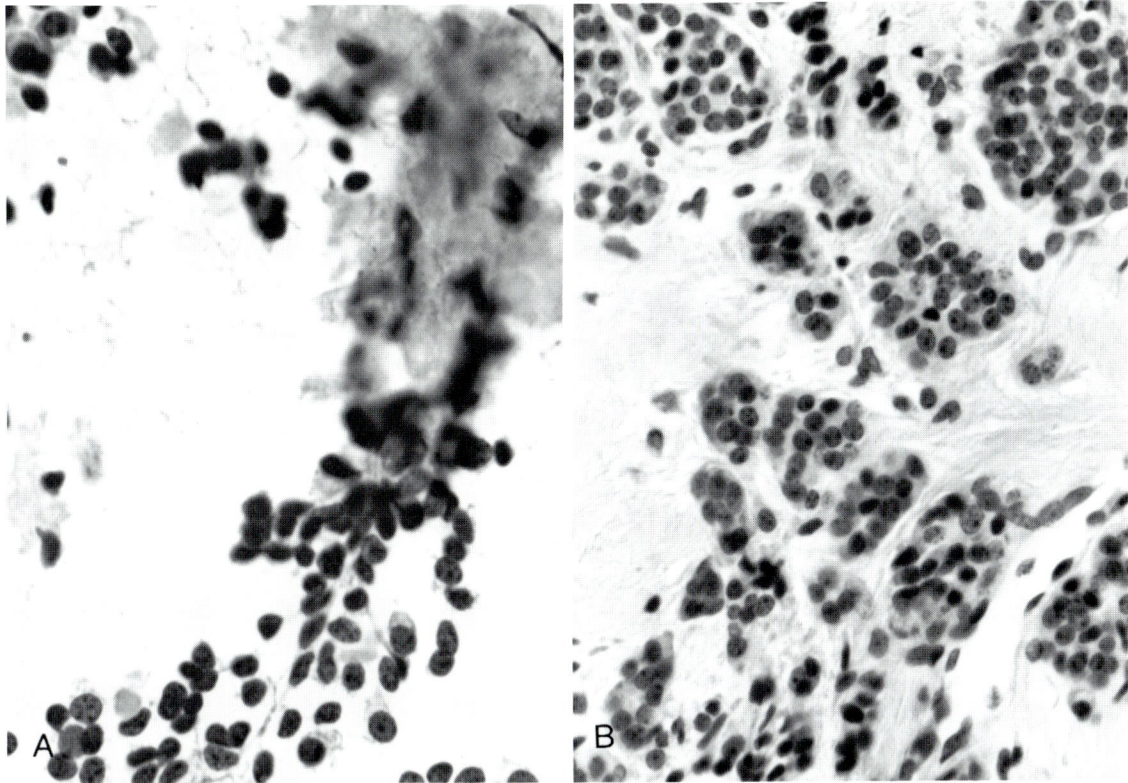

Figure 2.46.

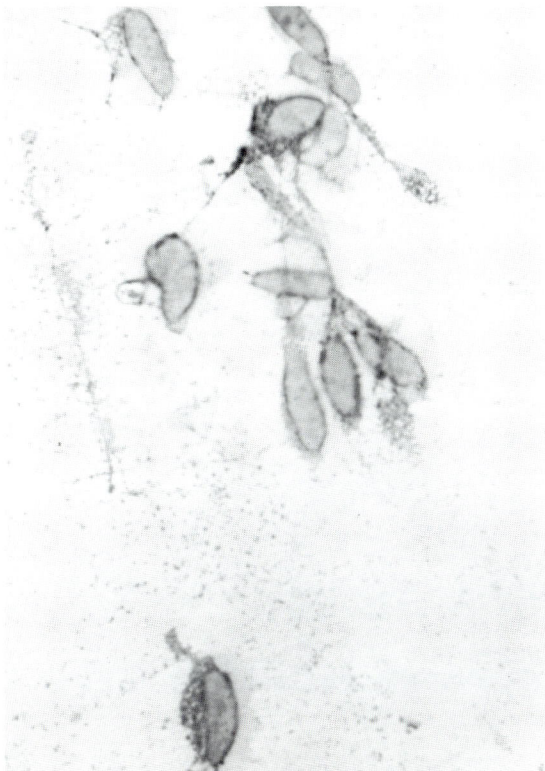

Figure 2.46. Medullary carcinoma. **A,** ABC. Note extracellular, eosinophilic, amorphous material representing amyloid. ×500. **B,** Histologic section of medullary carcinoma with an amyloid stroma. ×310.

Figure 2.47. Medullary carcinoma, ABC. Neoplastic spindle cells showing positive immunoreactivity for calcitonin. Immunoperoxidase preparation. ×500.

Figure 2.47.

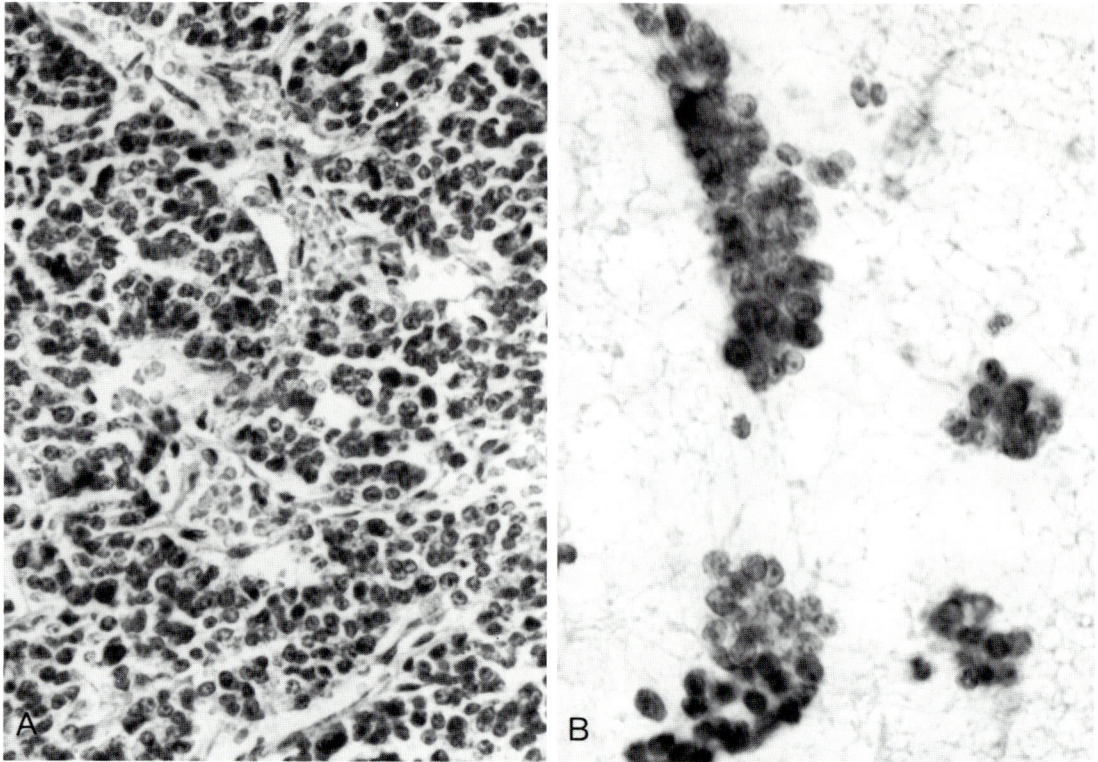

Figure 2.48.   Poorly differentiated (insular) carcinoma. **A,** Typical histology showing small, round cells growing in nests. ×310. **B,** ABC. Note small, round cell with granular chromatin, micronucleoli, and scant cytoplasm. Because there is little or no cytoplasm, the cells are closely packed. ×500.

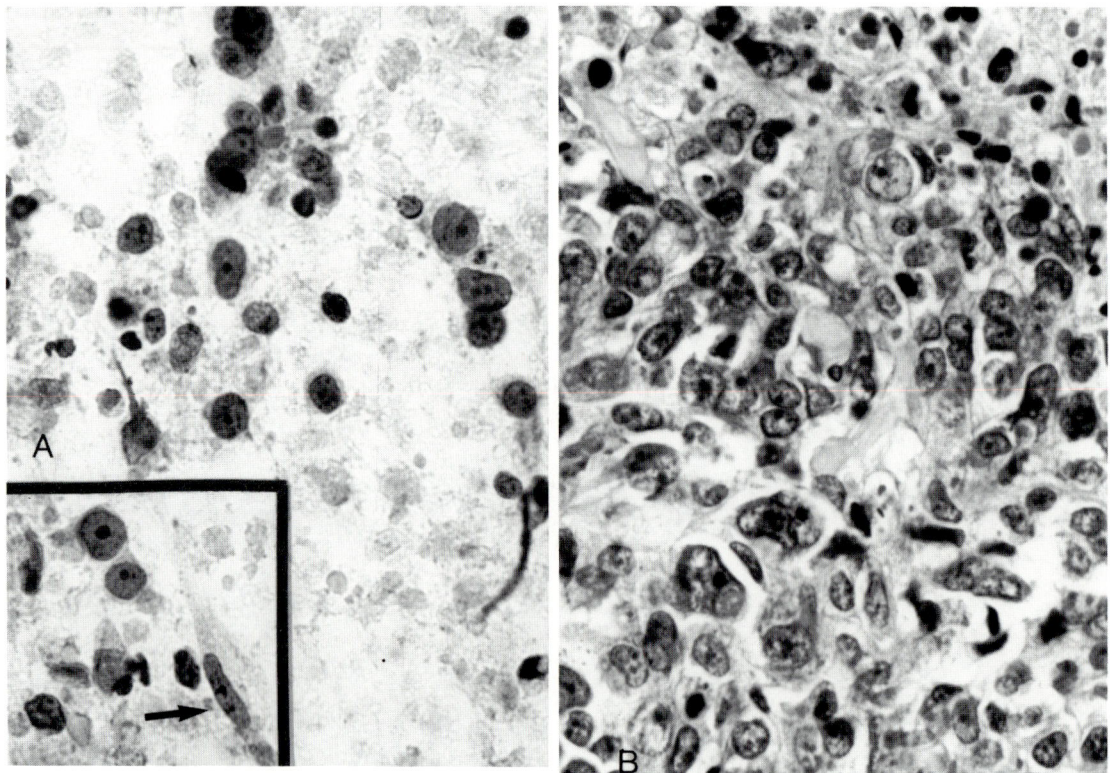

Figure 2.49.   Anaplastic carcinoma. **A,** ABC. Note tumor cells with large nuclei, prominent nucleoli, coarse chromatin, and irregular nuclear outline. *Arrow* indicates a spindle cell. Necrotic debris is seen in the background. ×500. **B,** Histology. Note morphologic similarities between histology and cytology of the tumor. ×500.

In the past, the so-called small cell thyroid carcinoma was regarded as a subtype of anaplastic carcinoma. Rosai et al.[43] have pointed out that tumors so designated in the past were in fact poorly differentiated (insular) carcinomas, medullary carcinomas (see **Fig. 2.46**), or malignant lymphomas.

Aspiration Cytology

Provided the sample is adequate (see "Diagnostic Pitfalls"), the cytologic diagnosis of anaplastic carcinomas usually presents no problem, because cytologic criteria of malignancy are quite obvious in these cases.[46]

Cell Morphology. The tumor cell nuclei, varying considerably in size and shape, are hyperchromatic with irregular, clumped chromatin, and many have prominent nucleoli. Malignant spindle and giant cells are not infrequent (**Figs. 2.49** and **2.50**). Osteoclast-like giant cells are also observed in some of our material. Cell necrosis is a very common finding.

Cytologic Pattern. The aspirates consist of both single cells and disorganized cell groups. Papillary or follicular pattern is generally not discernible, unless a better differentiated area is aspirated. A necrotic background with ghost tumor cells and inflammatory cells is common.

Diagnostic Pitfalls. Unlike well-differentiated thyroid cancers, some of the anaplastic carcinomas are desmoplastic. Aspirations from these tumors may yield poorly cellular specimens, which are a source of false-negatives. Similarly, if a necrotic area of the tumor is aspirated, the smears may consist of entirely necrotic material or inflammatory cells, resulting in a false-negative diagnosis (**Fig. 2.51**). It is important to remember that anaplastic carcinomas are clinically malignant and occur typically in older patients (>65 year of age); hence a negative or unsatisfactory aspiration diagnosis should always be viewed in light of the clinical findings.

Table 2.4. Comparison of the Cytologic Features of Anaplastic Carcinoma and Medullary Carcinoma

	Anaplastic Carcinoma	Medullary Carcinoma
Prototype cells	Anaplastic cells with obvious malignant features	Relatively uniform polygonal cells with granular cytoplasm
Bizarre giant cells	Common	Not uncommon
Osteoclastic-like giant cells	May be present	Not present
Spindle cells	Common	Not uncommon
Necrosis	Common	Uncommon
Amyloid background	Absent	May be present
Immunostaining for calcitonin	Negative	Positive

Pleomorphic giant cells can be seen in anaplastic carcinoma as well as in medullary carcinoma. **Table 2.4** compares the cytologic features of these two tumors. Finally, when an anaplastic carcinoma is composed predominantly or exclusively of spindle cells it can simulate a sarcoma. Immunoperoxidase staining and electron microscopic studies aid in correct classification of the tumor.

Malignant Lymphoma

Malignant lymphomas, representing less than 5% of primary thyroid neoplasms, appear as rapidly enlarging masses. Histologically most are of the diffuse large cell type (formerly classified as histiocytic lymphomas). The frequent concomitant occurrence of chronic lymphocytic thyroiditis has led to the suggestion that malignant lymphoma might evolve from preexisting thyroiditis.[47]

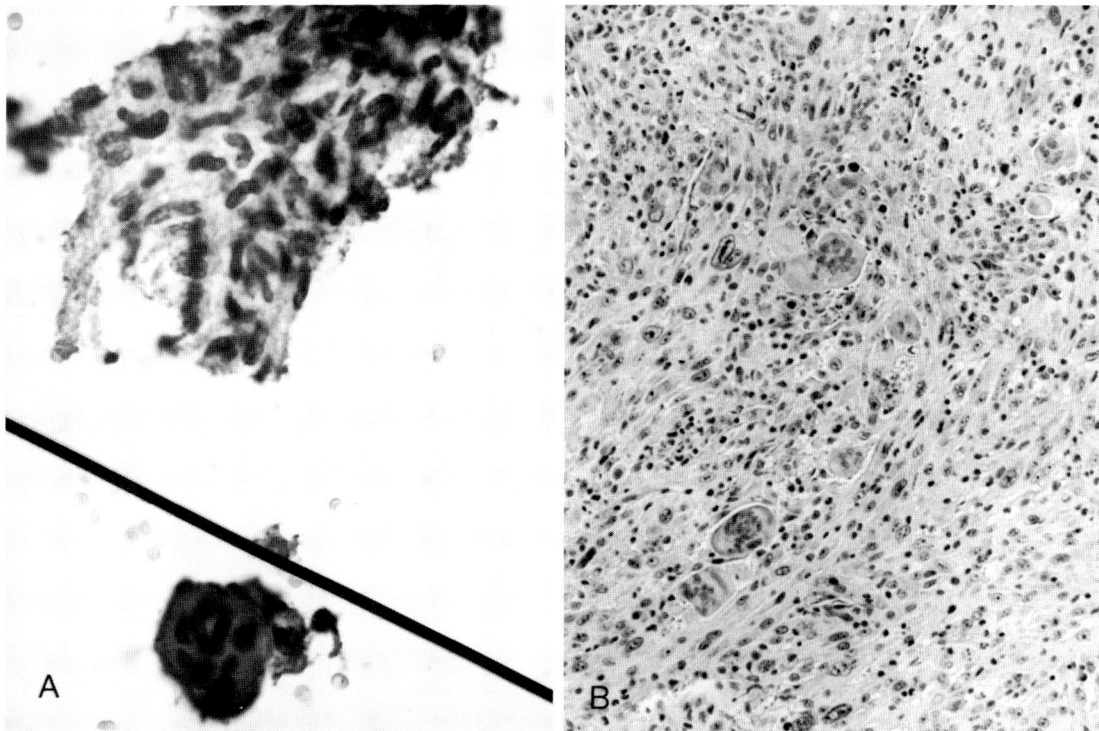

Figure 2.50. Anaplastic spindle and giant cell carcinoma. **A,** ABC. Note tissue fragment composed of spindle cells. There is also an osteoclast-like giant cell (inset). × 310. **B,** Histologic section. Note admixture of malignant spindle cells and giant cells. Also present are a few osteoclast-like multinucleated cells. × 120.

Figure 2.51. Necrotic anaplastic carcinoma (potential false-negative diagnosis). The aspirate shows only scattered acute inflammatory cells. This cytologic picture would have been misinterpreted as acute thyroiditis or abscess if the pathologist were not given the clinical data. ×310.

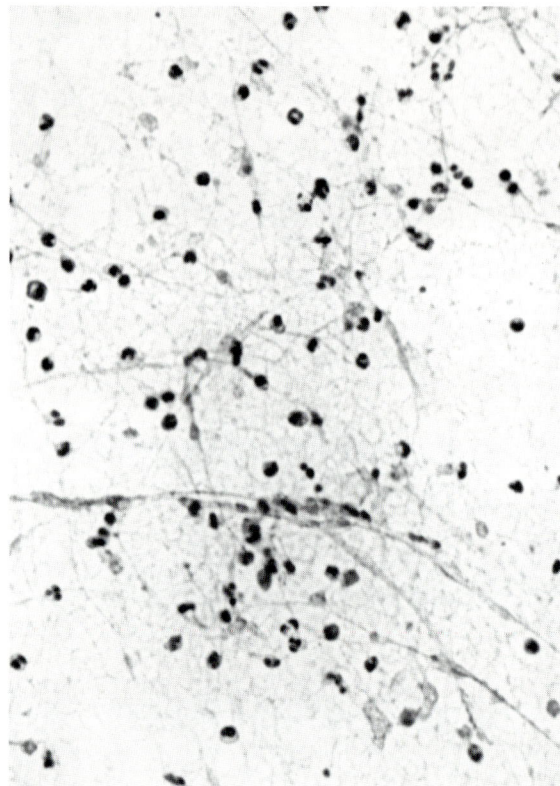

The cytologic features of malignant lymphoma is described in Chapter 4. Chronic lymphocytic thyroiditis is the main differential diagnosis.[16] Features that are diagnostic of chronic lymphocytic thyroiditis include small lymphocytes, admixed with other types of inflammatory cells, and Hürthle cells. A clinical presentation of a rapidly enlarging mass along with an aspirate showing monomorphic population of atypical lymphocytes would favor malignant lymphoma.

Metastatic Tumors

The occurrence of a nodule in the thyroid gland of a patient with a history of cancer at another site presents a diagnostic prob- lem, which can be readily resolved by FNAB. Such a lesion could be a benign thyroid goiter, a metastasis from the original cancer, or an independent primary thyroid cancer. Review of the histologic slides of the previous cancer and knowledge of the common types of cancer metastatic to the thyroid gland should facilitate FNAB interpretation. Shimaoka and coworkers[48] found metastatic disease in the thyroid gland upon autopsy in 9.5% of 1980 patients who had malignant tumors. The most common tumors were malignant melanoma (39%), and carcinoma of the breast (21%), kidney (12%), and lung (11%). Moreover, laryngeal carcinoma frequently invades the thyroid by direct extension.

References

1. DeGroot LJ, Larsen PR, Refetoff S, Stanbury JB. The thyroid and its diseases, 5th ed. New York: John Wiley & Sons, 1984:756–831.
2. Van Herle AJ, Rich P, Ljung BME, et al. The thyroid nodule. Ann Intern Med 1982;96:221–232.
3. Silverman JF, West RE, EW Larkin, Park HM, Finley JL, Swanson MS, Fore WW. The role of fine needle aspiration biopsy in the rapid diagnosis and management of thyroid neoplasm. Cancer 1986;57:1164–1170.
4. Suen KC, Quenville NF. Fine needle aspiration biopsy of the thyroid gland: A study of 304 cases. J Clin Pathol 1983;36:1036–1045.
5. Silver CE, Brauer RJ, Schreiber K. Cytologic evaluation of thyroid nodules. New criteria for surgery. N Y State J Med 1984;84:109–112
6. Hawkins F, Bellido D, Bernal C, et al. Fine needle aspiration biopsy in the diagnosis of thyroid cancer and thyroid disease. Cancer 1987;59:1206–1209.
7. Stavric GD, Karanfilski BT, Kalamaras AK, Serafimov NZ, Georgiev- ska BS, Korubin VH. Early diagnosis and detection of clinically non-suspected thyroid neoplasia by the cytologic method. Cancer 1980;45:340–344.
8. Kline TS. Handbook of fine needle aspiration biopsy cytology, 2nd ed. New York: Churchill Livingstone, 1988:204.
9. Atkinson B, Ernst CS, LiVolsi VA. Cytologic diagnosis of follicular tumors of the thyroid. Diagn Cytopathol 1986;2:1–3.
10. Frable WJ. Aspiration biopsy of the thyroid. Head & Neck Cancer 1985;1:238–244.
11. Walfish PG, Hazani E, Strawbridge HTG, Miskin M, Rosen IB. Combined ultrasound and needle aspiration cytology in the assessment and management of hypofunctioning thyroid nodule. Ann Intern Med 1977;87:270–274.
12. Volpé R. The pathology of thyroiditis. Hum Pathol 1978;9:429–438
13. Friedman M, Shimaoka K, Rao U, Tsukada Y, Cavigan M, Tamura K. Diagnosis of chronic lymphocytic thyroiditis (nodular presentation) by needle aspiration. Acta Cytol 1981;25:513–522.

14. Guarda LA, Baskin HJ. Inflammatory and lymphoid lesions of the thyroid gland: Cytopathology by fine-needle aspiration. Am J Clin Pathol 1987;87:14–22.

15. Kini SR, Miller JM, Hamburger JI. Problems in the cytologic diagnosis of the "cold" thyroid nodule in patients with lymphocytic thyroiditis. Acta Cytol 1981;25:506–512.

16. Matsuda M, Sone H, Koyama H, Ishiguro S. Fine needle aspiration cytology of malignant lymphoma of the thyroid. Diagn Cytopathol 1987;3:244–249.

17. Persson PS. Cytodiagnosis of thyroiditis. A comparative study of cytological, histological, immunological, and clinical findings in thyroiditis. Acta Med Scand Suppl 1968;483:7–100.

18. Meissner WA, Warren S. Tumors of the thyroid gland. Atlas of tumor pathology. 2nd Series, Fascicle 4. Washington D.C.: Armed Forces Institute of Pathology, 1968:45–46.

19. Rosai J. Ackerman's surgical pathology, 6th ed. St. Louis: CV Mosby, 1981:330–378.

20. Suen KC. How does one separate cellular follicular lesions of the thyroid by fine-needle aspiration biopsy? Diagn Cytopathol 1988;4:78–81.

21. Miller JM, Kini SR, Hamburger JI. Needle biopsy of the thyroid. New York: Praeger, 1983:22–167.

22. Lang W, Atay Z, Georgii A: The cytological classification of follicular tumors in the thyroid gland. Virchows Archiv A (Pathol Anat Histopathol) 1978;378:199–211.

23. Boon ME, Lowhagen T, Willems JS. Planimetric studies on fine needle aspirates from follicular adenoma and follicular carcinoma of the thyroid. Acta Cytol 1980;24:145–148.

24. Kini SR, Miller JM, Hamburger JI, Smith-Purslow MJ. Cytopathology of follicular lesions of the thyroid gland. Diagn Cytopathol 1985;1:123–132.

25. Hamburger JI. Consistency of sequential needle biopsy findings for thyroid nodules: Management implications. Arch Intern Med 1987;147:97–99.

26. Vickery AL. Thyroid papillary carcinoma. Pathological and philosophical controversies. Am J Surg Pathol 1983;7:797–807.

27. Rosai J, Zampi G, Carcangiu ML. Papillary carcinoma of the thyroid. A discussion of its several morphologic expressions, with particular emphasis on the follicular variant. Am J Surg Pathol 1983;7:809–817.

28. Kini SR, Miller JM, Hamburger JI, Smith MJ. Cytopathology of papillary carcinoma of the thyroid by fine needle aspiration. Acta Cytol 1980;24:511–521.

29. Chan JCK, Saw D. The grooved nucleus. A useful diagnostic criterion of papillary carcinoma of the thyroid. Am J Surg Pathol 1986;10:672–679.

30. Gray A, Doniach I. Morphology of the nuclei of papillary carcinoma of the thyroid. Br J Cancer 1969;23:49–51.

31. Christ ML, Haja J. Intranuclear cytoplasmic inclusions (invaginations) in thyroid aspirations. Frequency and specificity. Acta Cytol 1919;23:327–331.

32. Goellner JR, Johnson DA. Cytology of cystic papillary carcinoma of the thyroid. Acta Cytol 1982;26:797–799.

33. Ruiz-Velasco R, Waisman J, Van Herle AJ. Cystic papillary carcinoma of the thyroid gland. Acta Cytol 1978;22:38–42.

34. Dugan JM, Atkinson BF, Avitabile A, Schimmel M, Livolsi VA. Psammoma bodies in fine needle aspirate of the thyroid in lymphocytic thyroiditis. Acta Cytol 1987;31:330–334.

35. Thompson NW, Dunn EL, Batsakis JG, Nishiyama RH. Hürthle cell lesions of the thyroid gland. Surg Gynecol Obstet 1974;139:555–560.

36. Rosai J, Carcangiu ML: Pathology of thyroid tumors: Some recent and old questions. Hum Pathol 1984;15:1008–1012.

37. Kini SR, Miller JM, Hamburger JI. Cytopathology of Hürthle cell lesions of the thyroid gland by fine needle aspiration. Acta Cytol 1981;25:647–652.

38. Nilsson G. Nuclear size classes in the follicular epithelium of lymphoid thyroiditis. Acta Pathol Microbiol Scand Sect A Pathol 1976;84:165–171.

39. Kadudo K, Miyauchi A, Ogihara T, Takai SI, et al. Medullary carcinoma of the thyroid. Giant cell type. Arch Pathol Lab Med 1978;102:445–447.

40. Mendelsohn G, Bigner SH, Eggleston JC, Baylin SN4B, Wells SA, Jr. Anaplastic variants of medullary carcinoma. Am J Surg Pathol 1980;4:333–341.

41. Geddie WR, Bedard YC, Strawbridge HTG: Medullary carcinoma of the thyroid in fine needle aspiration biopsies. Am J Clin Pathol 1984;82:552–558.

42. Kini SR, Miller JM, Hamburger JI, Smith MJ. Cytopathologic features of medullary carcinoma of the thyroid. Arch Pathol Lab Med 1984;108:156–159.

43. Rosai J, Saxen EA, Woolner L: Undifferentiated and poorly differentiated carcinoma. Semin Diagn Pathol 1985;2:123–136.

44. Limbert E, Soares J, Botelho L, Sobrinho-Simoes M. "Insular" thyroid carcinoma—clinicopathological study of 12 cases. In Jaffiol C, Milhaud G. Thyroid cancer. Amsterdam: Excerpta Medica, 1985:317–319.

45. Carcangiu ML, Steeper T, Zampi G, Rosai J. Anaplastic thyroid carcinoma: A study of 70 cases. Am J Clin Pathol 1985;83:135–158.

46. Schneider V, Frable WJ. Spindle and giant cell carcinoma of the thyroid. Cytologic diagnosis by fine needle aspiration. Acta Cytol 1980;24:184–189.

47. Burke JS, Butler JJ, Fuller LM: Malignant lymphomas of the thyroid. Cancer 1977;39:1587–1602.

48. Shimaoka K, Sokal JE, Pickren JW. Metastatic neoplasms in the thyroid gland. Cancer 1962;15:557–565.

3

Salivary Glands

The easily accessible major salivary glands are optimal targets for fine needle aspiration biopsy, and even intraoral minor salivary gland swellings can be readily aspirated via a direct transoral route.[1] The standard technique of FNAB used for superficial lesions as described in Chapter 1 is applicable. FNAB should be used frequently since increasing experience will improve diagnostic accuracy.[2–10]

In addition to diagnosing intrinsic salivary gland lesions, FNAB is useful for differentiating salivary gland from nonsalivary gland masses. For instance, based on clinical examination it is sometimes difficult to differentiate between tumors of the parotid gland and high cervical swellings, such as upper jugular chain lymph nodes and branchial cleft cyst. Similar difficulty is experienced in separating tumors of the submandibular gland from submandibular lymph nodes. FNAB should become part of the pretreatment evaluation of all salivary gland masses. A preoperative diagnosis enables the clinician to promptly institute the appropriate management.[11–13]

Pragmatic Considerations

In general, FNAB diagnosis of the common salivary gland neoplasms, i.e., pleomorphic adenoma and Warthin's tumor, are fairly easy. On the other hand, diagnosis of many of the malignant salivary gland neoplasms (acinic cell carcinoma, low-grade mucoepidermoid carcinoma, and adenoid cystic carcinoma) is more difficult because they are histologically well-differentiated. Therefore, they may be confused with benign neoplasms on FNAB and vice versa. Layfield and associates[9] have suggested that in difficult situations it is wise to simply diagnose the tumor as salivary gland neoplasm, type not specified. Such a diagnosis encourages the surgeon to perform a limited resection with frozen-section examination before doing a radical procedure.

Diagnostic Accuracy

Conflicting reports exist in the literature regarding the accuracy of needle biopsy interpretation of salivary glands. The discrepancy is likely a reflection of the experience of the workers involved. Byers et al.[14] reviewed eight cases of needle biopsy of the submaxillary gland and found that only one was correctly diagnosed. The other seven cases revealed insufficient material in three, false-negative diagnosis in two, and malignancy of the incorrect cell type in two. Frable and Frable,[3,15] presenting their own FNAB experience along with a summary of that of several others, reported that the technique is accurate, with a significant increase in accuracy since its introduction in early years. In Frable's series,[15] the sensitivity for the presence of a benign or malignant neoplasm was 93% and the specificity was 99%. More recently, Qizilbash et al.[16] studied 146 cases and reported an overall accuracy of 98% and sensitivity of

87.5%. There were three false-negative diagnoses and no false-positive diagnosis. O'Dwyer et al.[11] reported an overall diagnostic accuracy of 90%, a sensitivity of 73% for diagnosing malignant tumors, and a specificity of 94% for benign tumors. Our results at Vancouver General Hospital and the Cancer Control Agency of British Columbia are recorded in **Table 3.1.**

Two recent studies[9,10] showed that frozen section and FNAB diagnoses of salivary lesions had similar sensitivity, specificity, and accuracy rate, and these workers concluded that FNAB was as good a method of diagnosing salivary gland tumors as frozen section.

Table 3.1. Results of FNAB of 279 Cases of Primary Salivary Gland Lesions (VGH-CCABC, 1981–1985)[a]

Type (no.)	Correct Cytologic Diagnosis	False-positive	False-negative[b]
Mucoepidermoid carcinoma[c] (12)	9		3
Adenoid cystic carcinoma[c] (14)	12		2
Acinic cell carcinoma[c] (6)	4		2
Malignant mixed tumors (2)	2		
Lymphoma[d] (4)	4		
Pleomorphic and monomorphic adenomas[c] (178)	168	1[e]	9
Warthin's tumor (34)	32		2
Benign lymphoepithelial lesion (2)	2		
Sialadenitis (27)	25	2[f]	

Overall diagnostic accuracy of FNAB = 92.5%
Sensitivity for detecting malignant tumors = 81%
Sensitivity for detecting benign lesions = 95%

[a]VGH, Vancouver General Hospital. CCABC, Cancer Control Agency of British Columbia.
Due to the referral pattern at these institutions, the distribution of the salivary gland lesions shown in this table does not necessarily reflect their true incidence in the general population.
[b]A negative cytologic report should not be considered final. Clinico-cytologic correlation or further investigation is required.
[c]A cytologic report "consistent with salivary gland neoplasm" is counted as a correct diagnosis.
[d]A cytologic report "suspicious for lymphoma" is counted as a correct diagnosis.
[e]Mistaken for squamous cell carcinoma.
[f]Mistaken for pleomorphic adenoma in one case and "neoplasm, type not specified" in the other case.

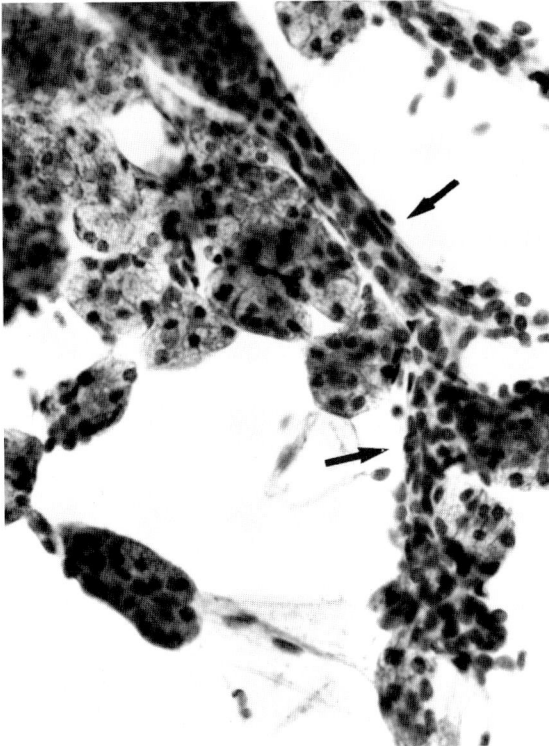

Figure 3.1. Normal salivary gland, ABC. A ductal-acinar complex, composed of branching intercalated ducts (arrows) surrounded by acini. Note finely granulated cytoplasm of the acinic cells. ×310.

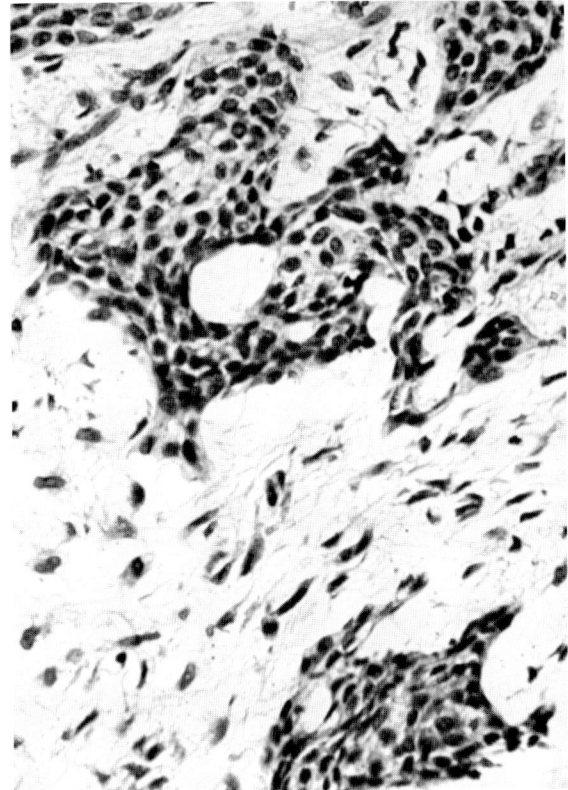

Figure 3.2. Pleomorphic adenoma, histologic section. Note irregular islands of epithelial cells, isolated spindle myoepithelial cells and typical myxoid stroma. ×310.

Normal Aspiration Cytology

The ABC of normal salivary gland tissue shows sparse groups of cells derived from acini and intralobular ducts. Single acinar and ductal cells are seldom seen. The acinar units are formed by low columnar or cuboidal cells having a small, bland, basally located nucleus and ample finely granulated or vacuolated basophilic cytoplasm. The acini are often seen to be in continuity with the intercalated ducts, forming a ductal-acinar complex (Fig. 3.1). The ductal cells are smaller, cuboidal or columnar, and arranged in small tubules. The nuclei are small and round, and the cytoplasm is eosinophilic. The N/C ratio is higher than that of the acinar cells. Other normal ABC findings include occasional adipose tissue and other connective tissue elements.

BENIGN NEOPLASMS

When tumors arising in both major and minor salivary glands are included, about 75–80% of salivary gland neoplasms are benign. Pleomorphic adenomas (benign mixed tumors) comprise 85% of the benign salivary gland tumors; Warthin's tumors comprise about 10% and the remaining 5% are monomorphic adenomas.[17–22]

Pleomorphic Adenoma (Mixed Tumor)

Pleomorphic adenoma is most often found in the parotid gland, and constitutes about 70% of all neoplasms found in this gland.[19,21,22] Clinically these tumors usually present as slowly growing, painless masses. The term "mixed tumor" was originally introduced to draw attention to the variegated histologic appearance, showing admixture of epithelial and mesenchymal elements (Fig. 3.2). The current consensus is that these tumors probably arise from the epithelial and myoepithelial cells of the intercalated ducts and that the "mesenchy-

mal" components are a product of the myoepithelial cells.[21] Approximately 36% of pleomorphic adenomas show equal proportions of epithelial and mesenchymal elements; 22% are predominantly epithelial, with another 12% being extremely cellular.[19]

Aspiration Cytology

The aspirates are cellular and consist of three components: ductal epithelial cells, myoepithelial cells, and stroma (Fig. 3.3A). The proportion of each of these elements in any one tumor is highly variable.

The ductal epithelial cells (Fig. 3.3, B and C) are round, oval, or low columnar, with monotonous nuclei and moderate amounts of pale cytoplasm. The nuclei may be central or eccentric, with fine chromatin pattern and smooth nuclear membranes. Some epithelial cells occur singly; most are arranged in well-demarcated flat sheets, multilayered tissue fragments, or in ductal or acinar arrangement. Not uncommonly, haphazard branching of the clusters may give rise to a low-power impression of deer antlers.[24]

The myoepithelial cells (Fig. 3.3D) are spindle or stellate-shaped, with bland nuclei. These cells occur in loose cell groups or, more often, occur singly within the stromal tissue fragments. Transitional forms between the epithelial cells and the spindle cells may be discernible.

The stromal tissue fragments (Fig. 3.3D) may be amorphous, mucoid, or have a finely fibrillar structure, and stain pink or blue with the hematoxylin and eosin stain and grey to green with the Papanicolaou method. In areas in which the matrix is more deeply stained, the background resembles chondroid tissue (Fig. 3.3E).

Diagnostic Pitfalls. The cytologic diagnosis of pleomorphic adenomas generally poses no problems. Zajicek[23] reported that, prior

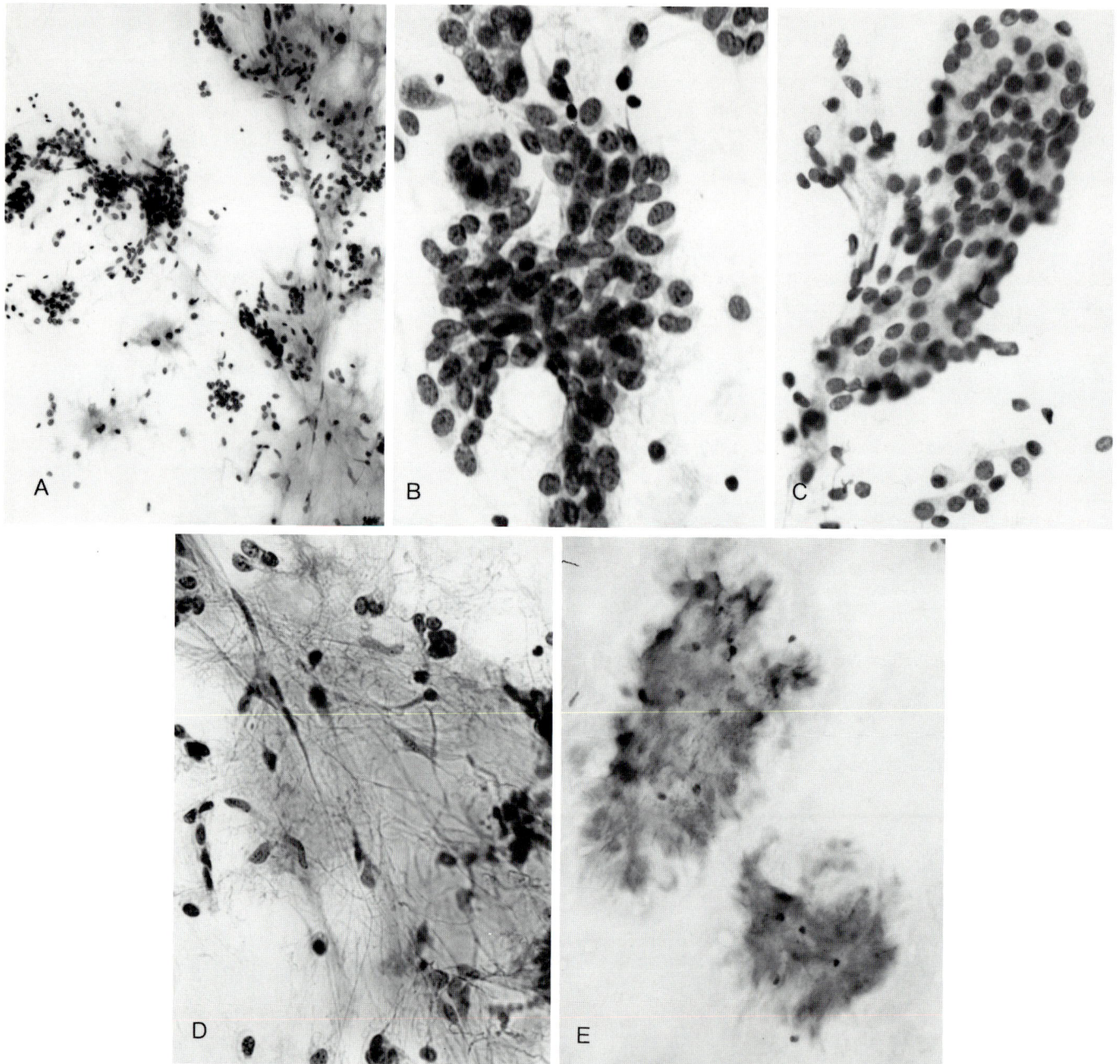

Figure 3.3. Pleomorphic adenoma, composite ABC. **A,** Note numerous epithelial cells lying singly and in cohesive clusters. There is abundant myxoid stromal tissue with enmeshed spindle cells. ×100. **B,** A cellular tissue fragment composed of benign ductal epithelial cells. ×420. **C,** Benign epithelial cells in acinar arrangement. ×260. **D,** Admixture of epithelial cells, myoepithelial cells, and myxofibrillary stroma. Note a gradual transition of ovoid or cuboidal epithelial cells to spindle cells. ×260. **E,** Two fragments of deeply basophilic chondroid stroma. ×260.

to 1966, 92.5% of all cases were recognizable from FNAB and, at present, virtually all of these tumors are recognizable. The following diagnostic pitfalls, however, must be kept in mind. Epithelial hypercellularity in pleomorphic adenomas may lead to the mistaken diagnosis of adenoid cystic carcinoma, especially when the hyperplastic epithelial cells are arranged in three-dimensional crowded cell clusters.[25,26] In this setting, careful evaluation of the scattered single cells helps distinguish pleomorphic adenoma from adenoid cystic carcinoma, since the single cells in the latter generally diplay cytologic atypia.[24] (See ''Adenoid Cystic Carcinoma.'')

Intracellular mucin may be seen occasionally in pleomorphic adenomas and, together with the abundant extracellular myxoid or mucoid matrix, confusion with a mucoepidemoid carcinoma or adenocarcinoma may arise.[9]

Kline[1] and Frable[15] cautioned that benign pleomorphic adenoma can sometimes show epithelial atypia, and Zajicek[23] reported cytologic atypia in patients who had received prior radiotherapy. One should remember that epithelial atypia in an otherwise typical pleomorphic adenoma does not usually mean that the lesion is malignant. Malignant pleomorphic adenomas are extremely uncommon (see below).

To reduce the likelihood of confusion with other tumors, multiple samples from different areas of the lesion may have to be taken. When doubt exists as to the malignant nature of a salivary gland tumor, it is better to classify the lesion as salivary gland neoplasms, not otherwise specified.[9]

Monomorphic Adenoma

Monomorphic adenomas are benign salivary neoplasms that are generally considered to be distinct from pleomorphic adenoma.[19] From the viewpoint of cytodiagnosis, we consider the tumor to be a variant of pleomorphic adenoma that lacks the stromal or mesenchymal component.

Aspiration Cytology

The ABC is cellular. The ductal epithelial cells resemble those seen in pleomorphic adenomas. They are present in clusters, trabeculae and acini, and as isolated cells. The uniform epithelial cells have a round or oval nucleus with a moderate amount of pale cytoplasm. Cellular pleomorphism is not found. The stroma, if present, is scanty and composed of loose fibrous tissue. The myxoid or chondroid tissues, so often seen in pleomorphic adenomas, are not seen in monomorphic adenomas.

Diagnostic Pitfalls. This author has recently reviewed a case of monomorphic adenoma (**Fig. 3.4**) of the submandibular gland that was misinterpreted on FNAB as metastatic squamous cell carcinoma in a patient who had a concurrent squamous cell carcinoma of the buccal mucosa. Review of the aspirate showed, in addition to the group of poorly preserved atypical cells that were mistaken for malignant cells (**Fig. 3.4A**), many benign epithelial cells (**Fig. 3.4B**). Novice pathologists often make the mistake of making a malignant diagnosis based on one or two groups of questionable atypical cells. If due consideration had been given to the overall composition of the smears, i.e., a group of atypical cells amidst many benign-appearing cells, an erroneous diagnosis of carcinoma could have been avoided.

In general, the benign cytologic appearances of the cells of monomorphic adenomas are easily recognized on FNAB.[27] However, like pleomorphic adenoma, monomorphic adnenoma may be confused with adenoid cystic carcinoma.[28,29] (See ''Adenoid Cystic Carcinoma.'')

Warthin's Tumor

Warthin's tumor (papillary cystadenoma lymphomatosum) is a benign tumor involving predominantly the parotid gland and only occasionally arises in other salivary glands. Clinically the tumor is well-defined and soft in consistency. Histologically it shows columnar or cuboidal oncocytic epithelial cells lining cystic spaces with a lymphocytic infiltrate in the supporting stroma (**Fig. 3.5**).

Aspiration Cytology

Warthin's tumor is suspected if the aspirate contains a few drops of brownish liquid material (thus, indicative of a cystic lesion). The ABC (**Fig. 3.6**) consists of varying proportions of two populations of cells: oncocytic cells and lymphocytes. The oncocytes are large polygonal or columnar cells, with a bland basal nucleus and abundant brightly eosinophilic cytoplasm. They may occur singly or as irregular flat sheets. The lymphocytes, exhibiting a dispersed cellular pattern, are mainly of the small type, but larger germinal center cells and plasma cells may also be present. Amorphous and granular debris with oncocytic ''ghost'' cells are present in the background.

Diagnostic Pitfalls. Cytologic diagnosis of Warthin's tumor, in our experience, is relatively easy. Some workers have warned of the occasional difficulties in obtaining representative material from fluid samples that dilute the cellular components, resulting in false-negative reports.[30] On the other hand, a false-positive diagnosis may occur when the oncocytes are degenerated and appear atypical, mimicking the squamous cells of mucoepidermoid carcinomas.[26] As a rule, however, in mucoepidermoid carcinomas polymorphonuclear leukocytes rather than lymphocytes are seen in the background (see below).

Interpretation of the lymphocytes may occasionally cause problems. One should be aware that an exuberant lymphoid component is not an exclusive feature of Warthin's tumors. Like others,[31] we have observed similar lymphocytic infiltrate, albeit uncommon, in acinic cell carcinomas. Branchial cleft cysts also yield numerous lymphocytes on FNAB, but the epithelial lining cells are usually of the mature squamous type (**Fig. 3.7**). When the lining epithelium undergoes oncocytic metaplasia, then the branchial cleft cyst mimics a Warthin's tumor.

MALIGNANT NEOPLASMS

Malignant neoplasms constitute about 20% of all salivary gland tumors. The incidence of malignant tumors is higher in the minor than in the major salivary glands: 56% of all tumors in the minor salivary glands of the palate are malignant, versus 32% in the submandibular gland and 13% in the parotid gland.[32]

Mucoepidermoid Carcinoma

Mucoepidermoid carcinoma, constituting between 3 and 9% of all salivary gland tumors, is the most common malignant tumor to arise in the major salivary glands.[18,22] Histogenetically, these tumors probably originate from the epithelium of the large salivary ducts.[33] Microscopic examination shows multiple, irregular cell nests that contain cystic spaces as well as solid areas. The solid areas are composed of predominantly squamous, or epidermoid, cells, some of which have also become hydropic. Cystic spaces filled with mucin and lined mainly by mucous cells are commonly seen, particularly in well-differentiated tumors (**Fig. 3.8**).

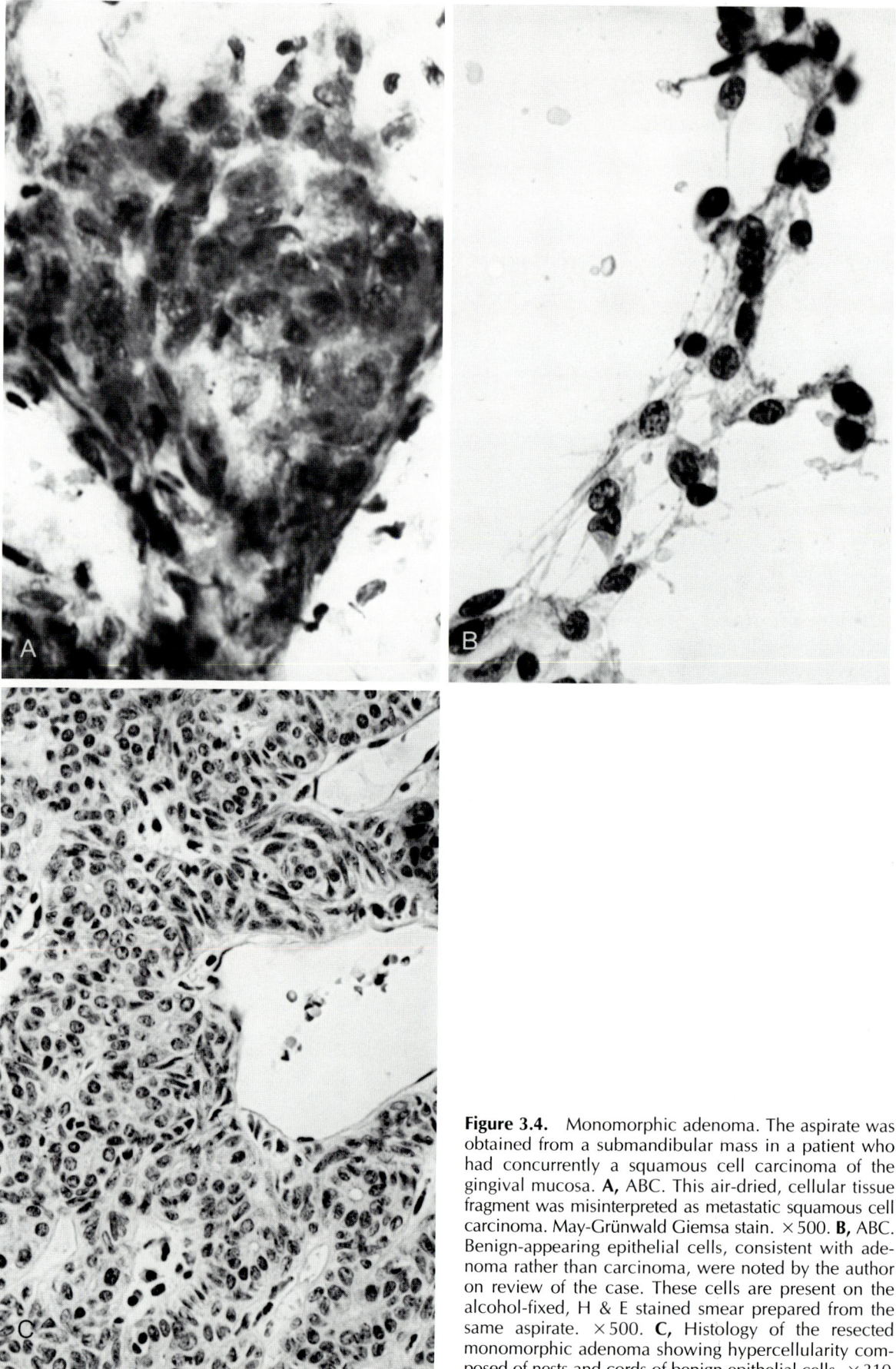

Figure 3.4. Monomorphic adenoma. The aspirate was obtained from a submandibular mass in a patient who had concurrently a squamous cell carcinoma of the gingival mucosa. **A,** ABC. This air-dried, cellular tissue fragment was misinterpreted as metastatic squamous cell carcinoma. May-Grünwald Giemsa stain. ×500. **B,** ABC. Benign-appearing epithelial cells, consistent with adenoma rather than carcinoma, were noted by the author on review of the case. These cells are present on the alcohol-fixed, H & E stained smear prepared from the same aspirate. ×500. **C,** Histology of the resected monomorphic adenoma showing hypercellularity composed of nests and cords of benign epithelial cells. ×310.

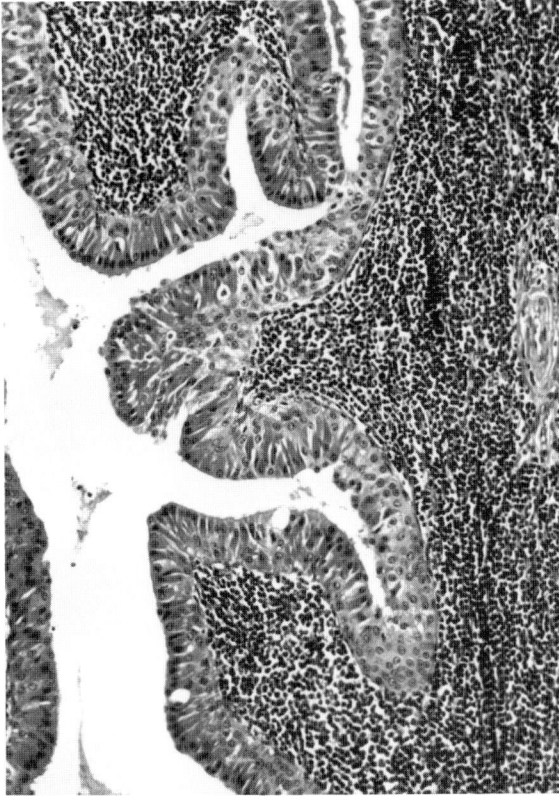

Figure 3.5.

Figure 3.5. Warthin's tumor, histologic section. Note cystic space lined by oncocytic epithelium and stroma infiltrated by numerous lymphocytes. ×310.

Figure 3.6. Warthin's tumor, ABC. **A,** Note columnar-shaped oncocytes with abundant eosinophilic cytoplasm, scattered lymphocytes, and granular debris consisting of anucleated cell remnants (ghost cells). ×125. **B,** Note admixture of oncocytes and lymphocytes in a cystic background. The oncocytes with brightly eosinophilic cytoplasm and dark pyknotic nuclei may be mistaken for malignant squamous cells by the unwary. ×500.

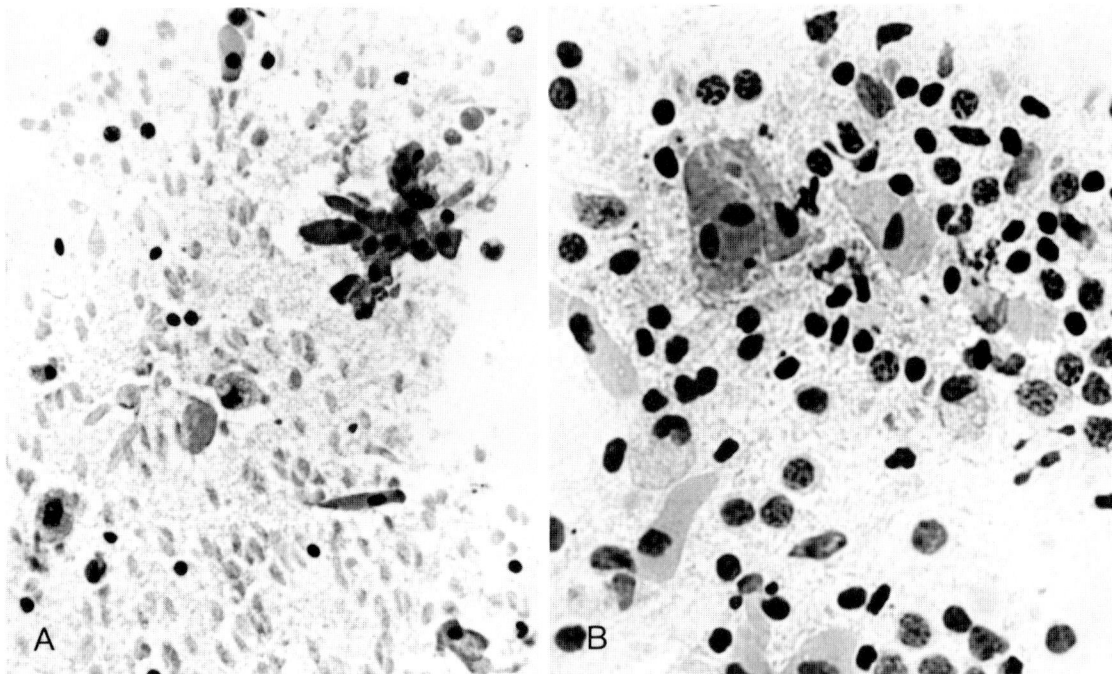

Figure 3.6.

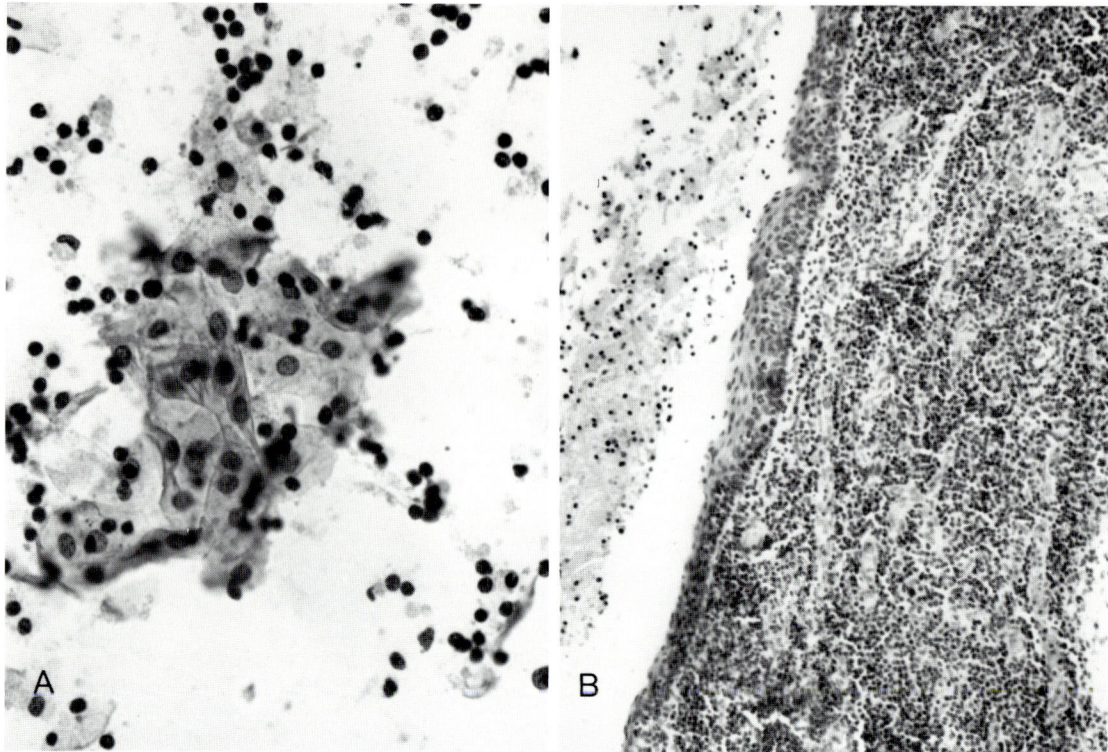

Figure 3.7.

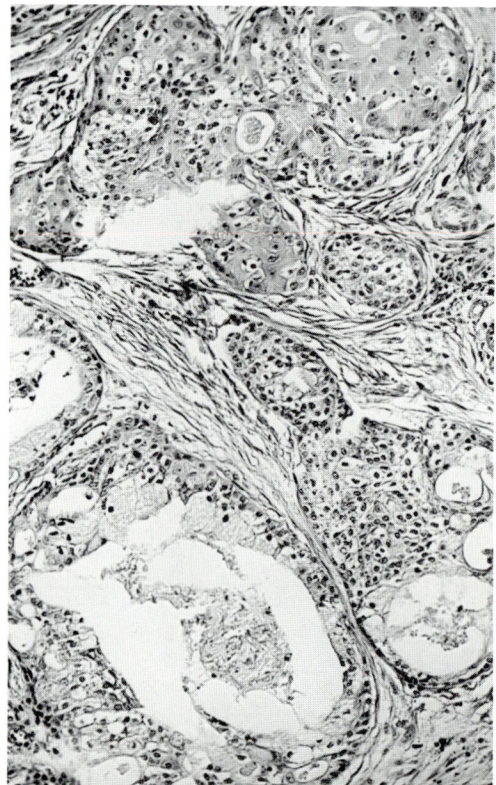

Figure 3.7. Branchial cleft cyst. **A,** Note numerous lymphocytes and benign mature squamous cells. ×310. **B,** Histology of branchial cleft cyst showing benign squamous mucosa and lymphoid infiltrate in the wall. ×125.

Figure 3.8. Low-grade mucoepidermoid carcinoma, histologic section. Note solid and cystic areas with epidermoid and mucous cells. ×110.

Figure 3.8.

Aspiration Cytology

Cell Type.   Varying proportions of squamous cells and mucous cells are seen in mucoepidermoid carcinomas. The squamous cells are usually of the intermediate type, resembling the malpighian layer of the squamous epithelium **(Fig. 3.9A)**.[16,24] Squamous cells have a central, rather uniform nucleus and a scant to moderate amount of eosinophilic cytoplasm. Some of the intermediate squamous cells have mucin-positive perinuclear vacuoles.[25] More mature squamous cells **(Fig. 3.9B)** with overt cytoplasmic keratinization can be seen but they are uncommon. The mucous cells **(Fig. 3.9A)** are large, columnar, and sometimes swollen or balloon-shaped, with distinct cell boundaries. The nuclei are small, bland, eccentrically situated, and frequently displaced by intracytoplasmic vacuoles. The cytoplasm is pale, foamy, or vacuolated and may show a positive reaction for mucicarmine and periodic acid-Schiff (PAS) stains. When isolated, the mucous cells may resemble histiocytes.[24,25]

In a small number of cases, the mucoepidermoid carcinoma is poorly differentiated, and shows a greater degree of cellular anaplasia and cytologic pleomorphism. In these cases, tissue fragments of poorly differentiated intermediate squamous cells usually predominate **(Fig. 3.10)**, with a proportional decrease in mucous cells. Keratinizing squamous cells are rarely found.

Cellular Pattern.   The cellularity of the smears depends very much on the area of the lesion aspirated. From solid areas, the aspirates are cellular. The cells appear in small irregular sheets or clusters. A mixture of both squamous and mucous cells can be seen within the same cluster; this is especially obvious in the well-differentiated tumors **(Fig. 3.9)**.

The aspirates obtained from cystic areas are hypocellular. The background consists of amorphous, eosinophilic debris or mucous material with entrapped polymorphonuclear leukocytes.

Diagnostic Pitfalls.   Interpretation of FNAB of mucoepidermoid carcinomas is difficult if the observer is not familiar with the cytologic features of these tumors. Most of the errors are false-negative results, which occur in the following circumstances.[1,9,23,26] *(a)* Aspirations from the cystic areas of the tumor may yield few cells. Hence, multiple aspirations from solid areas of the lesion are imperative to obtain representative material. *(b)* Inflammatory cells and debris may be prominent and obscure the neoplastic cells. *(c)* In some well-differentiated mucoepidermoid carcinomas, the neoplastic cells may appear so bland that they may be misinterpreted as benign cells.

False-positive diagnoses also occur. Benign mixed tumors with extracellular mucoid material, chronic sialadenitis with atypical squamous cells, and Warthin's tumors with degenerated oncocytes have all been mistaken for well-differentiated mucoepidermoid carcinoma.[9,23]

In poorly differentiated mucoepidermoid carcinomas, cytologic diagnosis of malignancy generally poses no problems because the cells are cytologically malignant, but correct classification may not be possible if only anaplastic cells are present.[23,33]

Adenoid Cystic Carcinoma

Any salivary gland tissue can be the site of an adenoid cystic carcinoma, but there is a much higher incidence within the minor salivary glands, where this lesion is the most commonly diagnosed malignancy. Adenoid cystic carcinoma accounts for less than 4% of all neoplasms in the parotid gland, 10% in the submandibular gland, and 60–70% in the minor salivary glands.[20,32,34] The typical histology **(Fig. 3.11)** consists of many nests and columns of cells arranged concentrically around gland-like spaces, giving rise to a cribriform pattern. The majority of these ''cystic spaces'' are pseudocysts filled with replicated basement membrane material, although small true glandular lumina can also be formed.[20]

Aspiration Cytology

In most cases, adenoid cystic carcinoma is easily recognized because of the typical arrangement of the cells and the presence of amorphous hyaline globules (corresponding to the basement membrane-like material in the pseudocysts seen in histologic sections).[35–38] FNAB is especially useful in detecting recurrence.

Cellular Pattern.   The two-dimensional cribriform pattern seen in histologic sections is represented in the smears by three-dimensional cell balls, filled with globules of amorphous hyaline material **(Fig. 3.12)**. The neoplastic cells characteristically encircle the hyaline globules, which stain colorless or light blue with the Papanicolaou technique, pink with hematoxylin and eosin, and bright red to purple with the May-Grünwald Giemsa stain. In addition to the numerous cell balls, dissociated cells and irregular cell sheets with haphazardly arranged cells are seen.

Cell Morphology.   The neoplastic cells are reminiscent of ''basaloid'' cells, which are rather small and uniform, having round nuclei and little cytoplasm. Small nucleoli can be seen **(Fig. 3.12B)**. Since the individual cells are only minimally atypical, the appropriate pattern of cellular arrangement should be looked for before a confident diagnosis of adenoid cystic carcinoma is rendered.

Diagnostic Pitfalls.   Adenoid cystic carcinoma can be diagnosed by FNAB with a fair degree of certainty, provided their distinctive features are present and recognized.[35–38] Cellular pleomorphic adenomas have been confused with adenoid cystic carcinoma.[24–26] In general, cells from adenoid cystic carcinomas tend to show minimally greater nuclear atypia and nucleoli (compare **Figs. 3.3C** and **3.12B**). Another point to remember is that if there is any suggestion of myxoid or chondroid tissue in a smear, caution should be exercised in diagnosing adenoid cystic carcinoma.

The ABC of monomorphic adenomas may also simulate adenoid cystic carcinoma.[28,29] Hood et al.[28] have emphasized the architectural arrangements of the cells and the tinctural properties of the hyaline material in separating these two tumors. According to these authors, the smears obtained from monomorphic adenomas have a greater tendency to show irregular branching bands and clumps of epithelial cells, whereas in adenoid cystic carcinomas one finds three-dimensional cell balls with a typical sieve-like pattern, with long axes of the cells oriented parallel to the borders of the cell balls. The hyaline globules, when present in monomorphic adenomas, are small and few, and stain more eosinophilic with hematoxylin and eosin than those in adenoid cystic carcinomas.

Acinic Cell Carcinoma

Acinic cell carcinoma occurs primarily in the parotid glands, accounting for 2.5–4% of all parotid gland tumors.[33] It is much less frequently found in other salivary glands. The tumor is slow growing and is often mistaken for a pleomorphic adenoma on clinical examination.

Aspiration Cytology

Cellular Pattern.   The aspirates generally show high cellularity. There are many large and small cell sheets, variable numbers of isolated cells, and bare nuclei. The diagnostic cell sheets contain numerous acinar units and cystic spaces **(Fig. 3.13)**. No ductal epithelium are seen among the acinic tumor cells.

Cell Morphology.   The monomorphic, round or polygonal acinic cells have central or basal nuclei with a regular chromatin

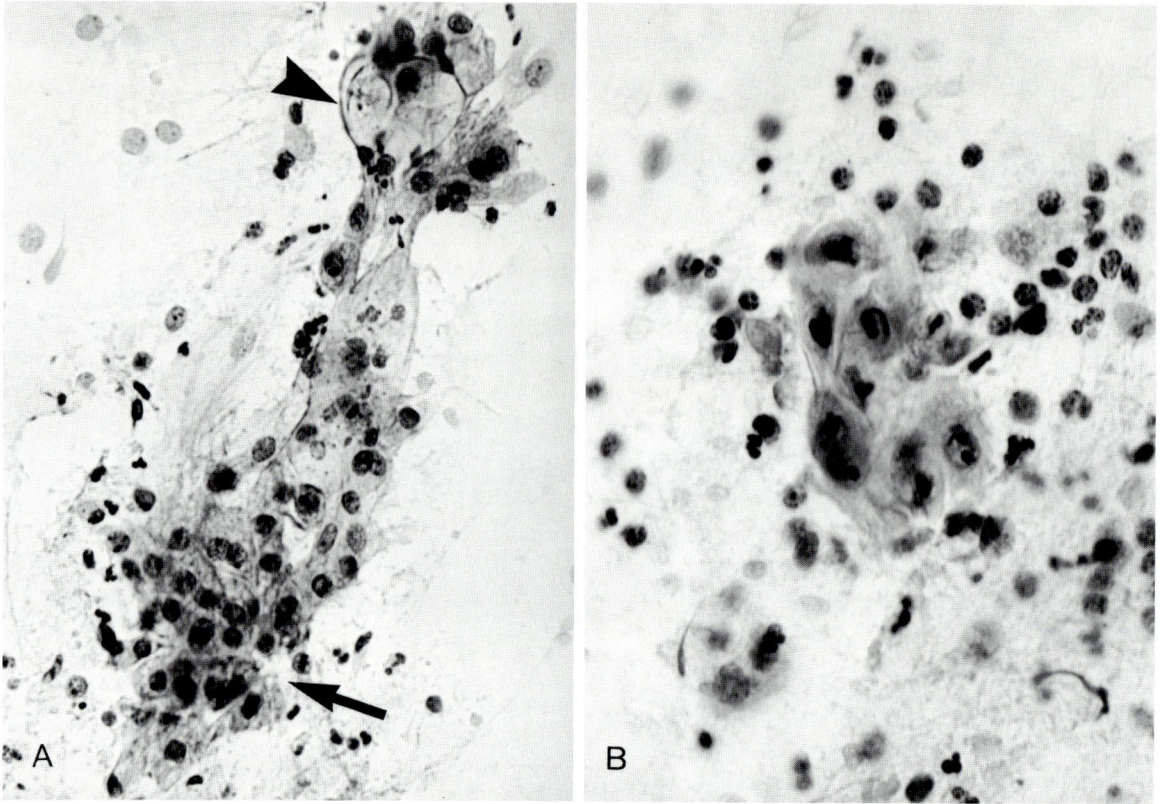

Figure 3.9.

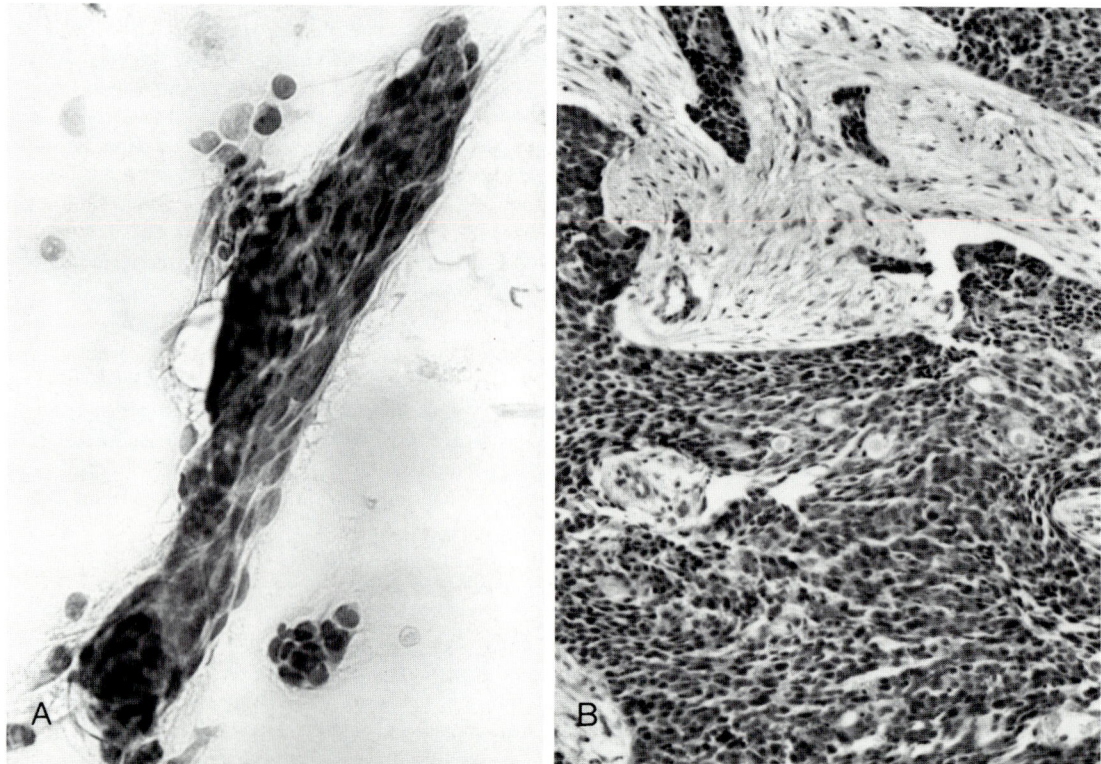

Figure 3.10.

pattern and inconspicuous nucleoli. The cytoplasm is basophilic and finely granulated, reticulated or vacuolated **(Fig. 3.13)**. The cytoplasmic granules are positive for the periodic acid-Schiff reaction after diastase digestion.

In a small percentage of cases, the tumor cells are less differentiated and show a greater degree of anisonucleosis, nuclear atypia, and prominent macronucleoli **(Fig. 3.14)**.

Diagnostic Pitfalls. FNAB of acinic cell carcinoma has often yielded low sensitivity because many of these tumors are cytologically well-differentiated. Review of the literature shows an overall false-negative rate of 35%.[3] In Zajicek's series,[23] 26 of the 34 acinic cell carcinomas did not show any nuclear atypia or nuclear polymorphism. In such cases, the cytopathologist must differentiate between acinic cell carcinoma and normal acinic tissue. The former is characterized by abundance of acinic cells with formation of irregular acini (as oppposed to the regular cohesive acini in normal ABC; see **Fig. 3.1**), the absence of relationship with ductal epithelium, and the presence of many isolated cells and bare nuclei.[31]

In poorly differentiated acinic cell carcinomas, recognition of malignancy is not difficult, but correct typing of the tumor may not be feasible. In general, acinic cell carcinoma can be distinguished from other salivary gland tumors by the presence of cytoplasmic granules that are PAS-positive after diastase digestion.

Malignant Mixed Tumor

The term *malignant mixed tumor* encompasses three morphologic entities.[19,21] The first group consists of tumors in which the epithelial cells have undergone malignant change (usually an adenocarcinoma) and remnants of a mixed tumor matrix can still be identified. The term *carcinoma ex pleomorphic adenoma* is used to refer to this group of tumors. The second group consists of tumors in which both the epithelial and stromal components are morphologically malignant. The tumors in the third group show a histology not much different from that of benign mixed tumor and yet the tumor metastasizes to distant organs—the so-called metastasizing benign mixed tumor.

The first group of tumors is relatively more common and may account for as much as 2% of all mixed tumors. We have encountered two such cases on FNAB. In each case, the malignant cells were considered to be adenocarcinoma and remnants of mixed tumor stroma were seen **(Fig. 3.15)**. Tumors in the second group are essentially carcinosarcomas. The smears show both malignant epithelial cells as well as fibrosarcoma-like cells. Tumors in the third group are indistinguishable from benign mixed tumor on FNAB. Histologically, the observation of an infiltrative growth pattern, i.e., tumor invasion outside the capsule, is suggestive of metastatic potential in what otherwise appears to be a benign mixed tumor.

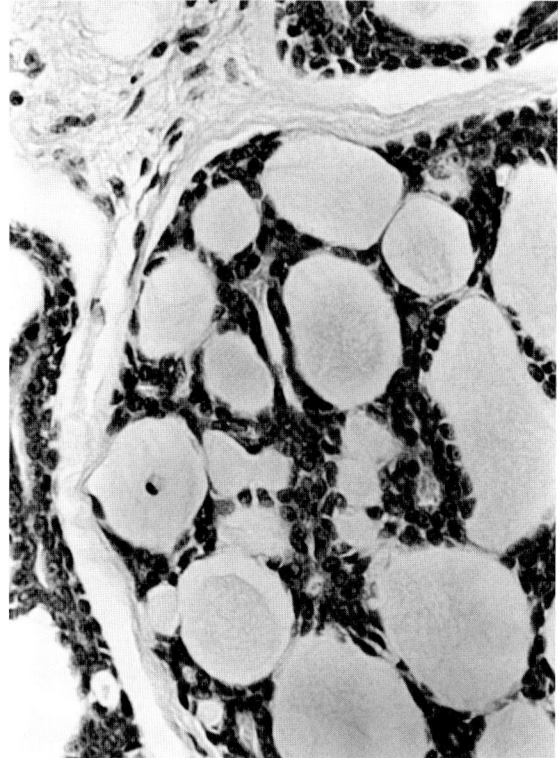

Figure 3.11. Adenoid cystic carcinoma, histologic section. Note cribriform pattern formed by tumor cells surrounding round spaces, filled with basement membrane-like material. ×310.

Other Carcinomas

Adenocarcinomas and undifferentiated carcinomas of the salivary glands are malignant epithelial neoplasms that cannot be classified into the specific types of carcinoma described above. Most of the adenocarcinomas of the salivary glands arise from larger intralobular ducts or excretory ducts and histologically do not differ from adenocarcinoma of other organs. The tumor may be papillary or nonpapillary. The former is the predominant form, and on FNAB it resembles papillary carcinoma of the breast.

Undifferentiated carcinoma occur rarely. The tumor usually grows in a solid pattern. The small cell variant resembles oat cell carcinoma of the lung. It is the most lethal of all salivary gland tumors.

Lymphoma

Lymphoid tissue and lymph nodes are normally present in and around the salivary glands and may be the site of a malignant lym-

Figure 3.9. Low-grade mucoepidermoid carcinoma, ABC. **A,** Note cell sheet composed of mucinous goblet cells *(arrowhead)* and smaller compact intermediate squamous cells *(arrow)*. Note also polymorphonuclear leukocytes in the background. ×500. **B,** Note cluster of more mature squamous cells with dense keratinized cytoplasm and sharp cell borders. Also note inflammatory diathesis. ×500.

Figure 3.10. High-grade mucoepidermoid carcinoma. **A,** ABC. Note cellular tissue fragment composed of poorly differentiated epidermoid cells with a high N/C ratio. ×500. **B,** Histology. Note predominance of nonkeratinizing squamous cells with occasional interspersed mucinous cells. ×310.

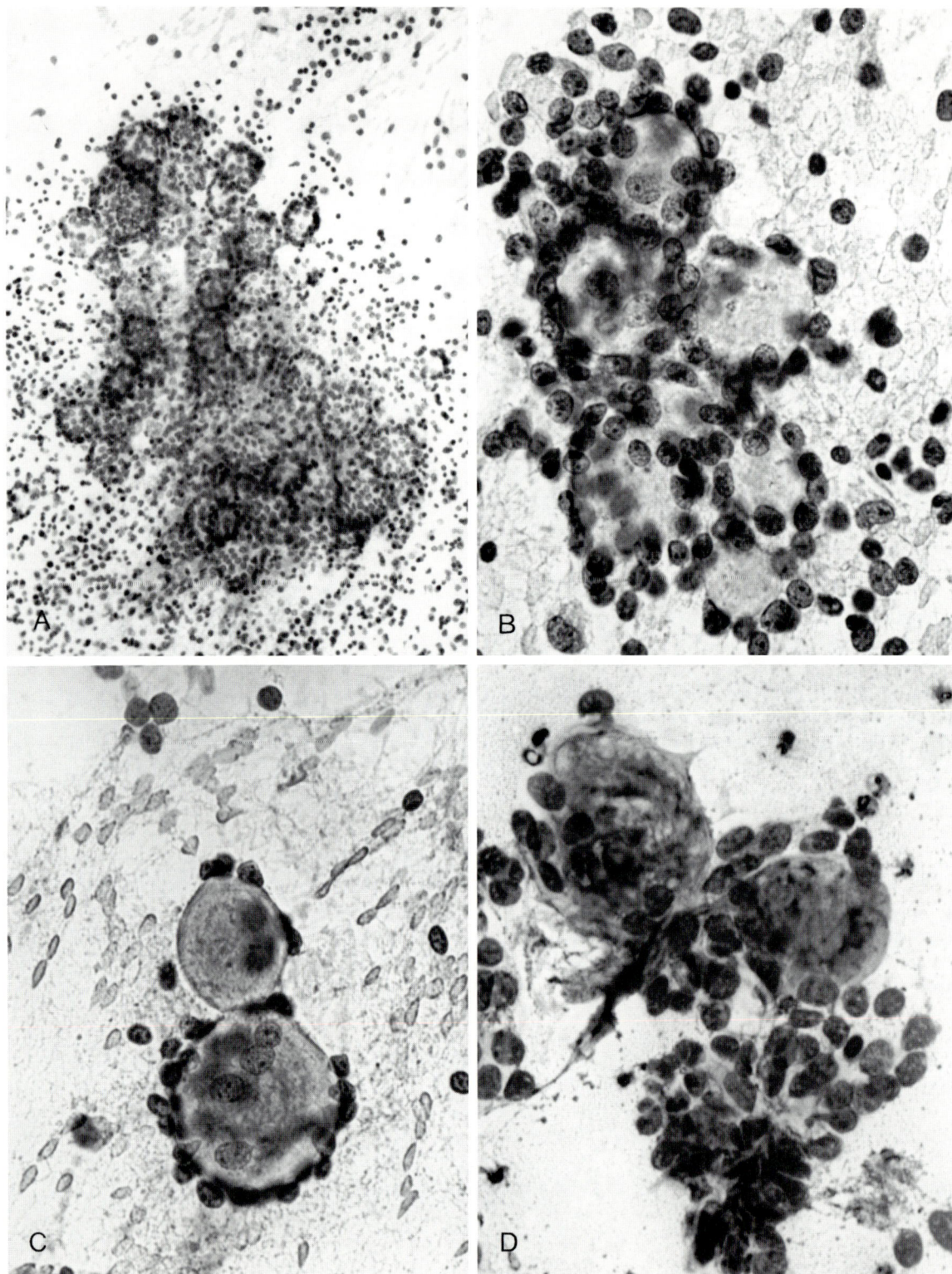

Figure 3.12. Adenoid cystic carcinoma, ABC. **A** and **B,** Tissue fragments showing cribriform or cell-ball pattern created by circular arrangement of tumor cells around hyaline globules. **A,** ×125; **B,** ×500. **C,** Note eosinophilic hyaline globules rimmed by tumor cells. ×500. **D,** MGG stained smear for comparison. Note deeply metachromatic globules. May-Grünwald Giemsa stain. ×500.

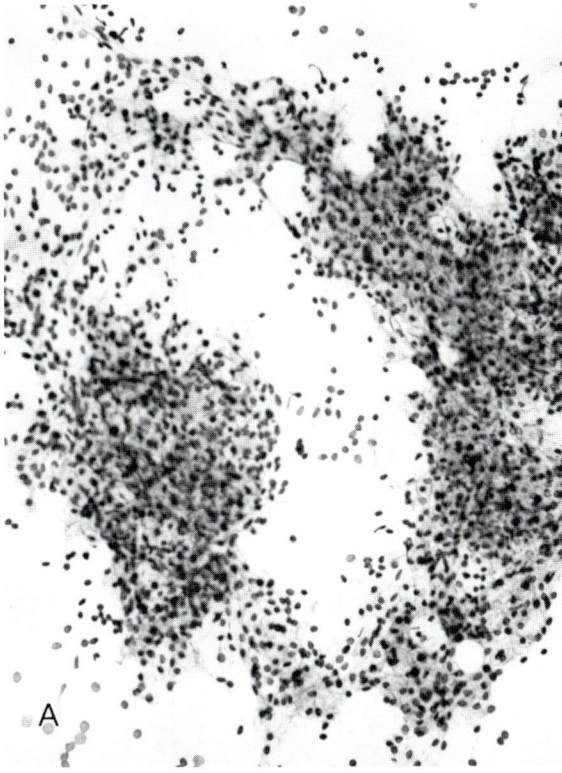

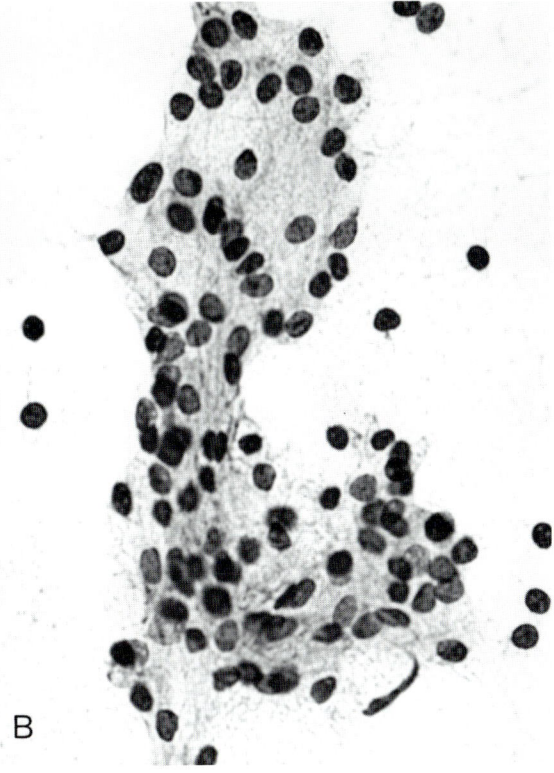

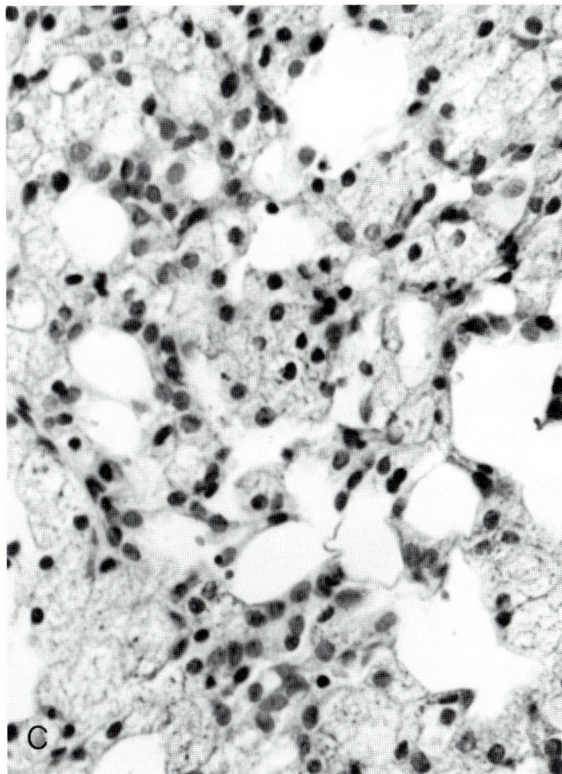

Figure 3.13. Acinic cell carcinoma. **A,** ABC. Note hypercellularity and tumor cells arranged in acinar pattern. ×125. **B,** ABC. Higher magnification to show the acinar units. Note cellular uniformity and ample basophilic granular cytoplasm. ×500. **C,** Histology. Note morphologic similarities of tumor cells in aspirate and tissue section. ×310.

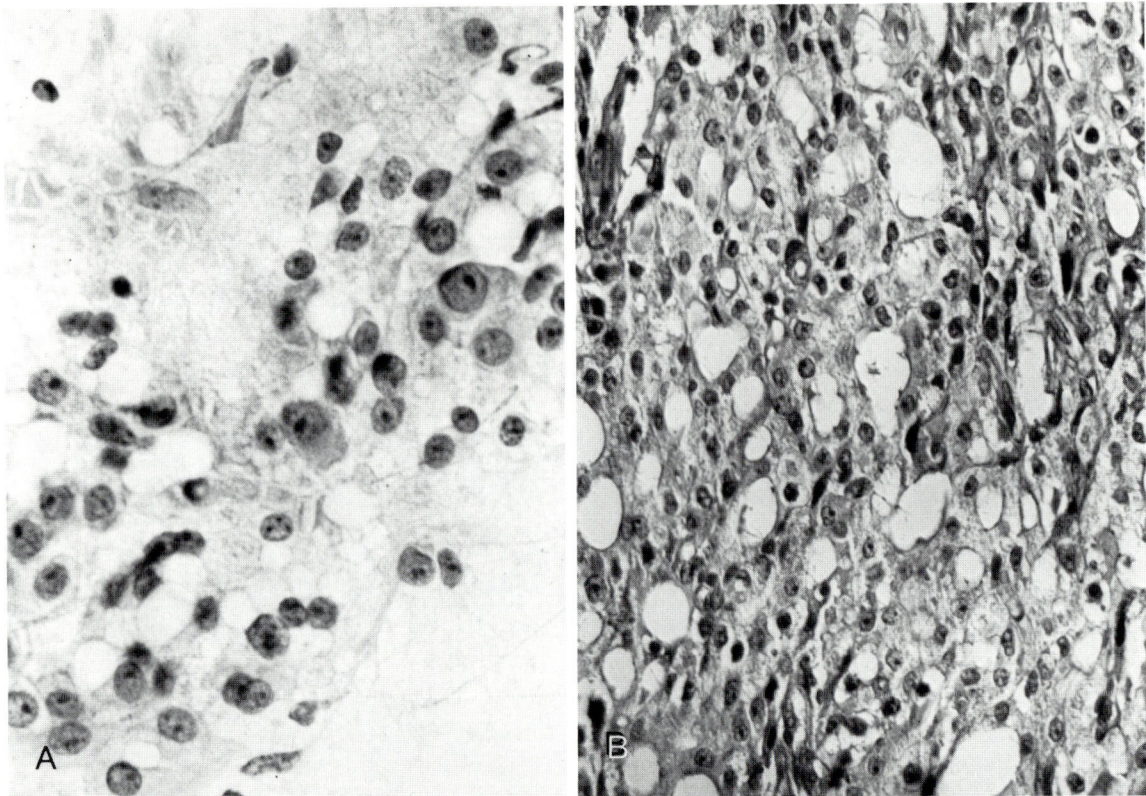

Figure 3.14. Acinic cell carcinoma. **A,** ABC. The neoplastic cells in this case are more anaplastic than those shown in **Fig. 3.13.** Note prominent nucleoli and irregularly thickened nu- clear membranes. The cytoplasm is finely granular or almost clear. ×500. **B,** Histology of the resected acinic cell carcinoma. ×310.

phoma. In fact, lymphoma of the salivary glands is more common than has been previously recognized.[39] The entire spectrum of non-Hodgkin's lymphomas (see Chapter 4) seen at other sites can be seen in the salivary glands; on the other hand, Hodgkin's disease of the salivary glands is uncommon. Distinction by FNAB between small cell lymphocytic lymphoma and the benign lymphoepithelial lesion (BLL) may be difficult. The problem is further compounded by the recent recognition that patients with BLL have a greater risk of developing a malignant lymphoma.[39–41]

Metastatic Tumors

Tumors may metastasize to the lymph nodes in and around the salivary glands, particularly the parotid, and secondarily involve the gland tissue. In one series, metastatic tumor accounted for 13% of 68 malignant salivary gland tumors.[42] The predominant histologic types of metastases are melanomas and squamous cell carcinomas, generally from the ipsilateral skin and mucosal surfaces of the head and neck region. Metastases from distant sites are encountered much less frequently and are primarily carcinomas of the kidney, lung, and breast.

INFLAMMATORY AND TUMOR-LIKE LESIONS
Benign Lymphoepithelial Lesion

Benign lymphoepithelial lesion is enlargement of salivary glands characterized microscopically by (a) diffuse lymphocytic infiltration, (b) atrophy of the acinar parenchyma, and (c) replacement of the intralobular ducts by islands of epithelial and myoepithelial cells, forming the so-called epithelial islands **(Fig. 3.16).** Immunologic

factors probably play a crucial role in its pathogenesis. One-third to one-half of the patients afflicted with Sjögren's syndrome have BLL in the salivary glands. Recently, BLL has also been observed in the salivary glands of intravenous drug users.[43] In some patients, BLL is a forerunner of malignant lymphoma or carcinoma.[39–41]

Aspiration Cytology

The ABC shows two distinct populations of cells, namely the lymphoid cells and the epithelial cells **(Fig. 3.17).** The former usually predominate and are scattered small mature and larger activated lymphocytes. Occasional plasma cells and plasmacytoid lymphocytes are also present. The epithelial cells are polygonal in shape, with vesicular nuclei, uniform chromatin structure, and frequently conspicuous nucleoli. They occur in irregular cohesive clusters or sheets, surrounded by lymphoid cells.

Diagnostic Pitfalls. The principal differential diagnosis is malignant lymphoma. The notion that the epithelial islands are pathognomonic of BLL has been challenged. Epithelial islands were observed in 14 of the 59 histologically studied cases of malignant lymphomas.[39] As a rule, malignant lymphomatous infiltrates are monomorphic, whereas BLL is polymorphic. However, the distinction between BLL and small cell lymphocytic lymphoma can be extremely difficult. Immunocytochemistry is helpful: if the cells can be shown to be polyclonal, as evidenced by staining for κ and λ light chains, the process is likely reactive. A monoclonal lymphoid infiltrate generally means that the lesion is a lymphoma. Other criteria, such as bone marrow and lymph node involvement and serum monoclonal gammopathy, are also useful in making a correct diagnosis.

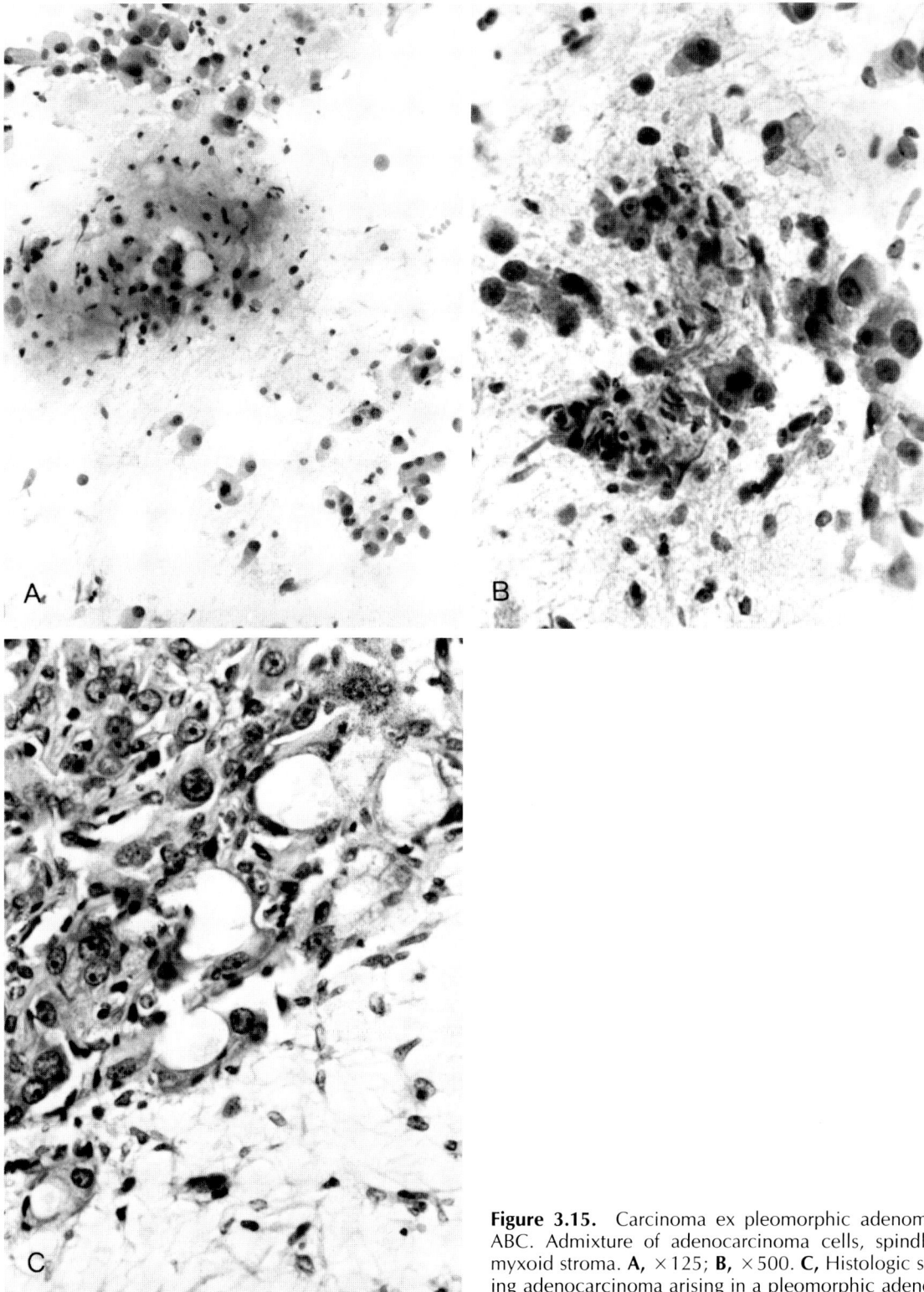

Figure 3.15. Carcinoma ex pleomorphic adenoma. **A** and **B,** ABC. Admixture of adenocarcinoma cells, spindle cells, and myxoid stroma. **A,** ×125; **B,** ×500. **C,** Histologic section showing adenocarcinoma arising in a pleomorphic adenoma. ×310.

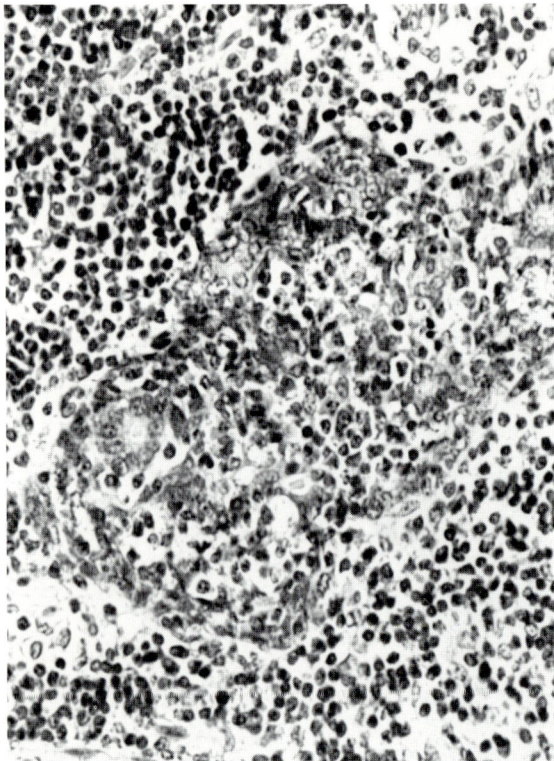

Figure 3.16. Benign lymphoepithelial lesion, histology. Note diffuse lymphocytic infiltrate and an epithelial island. ×125.

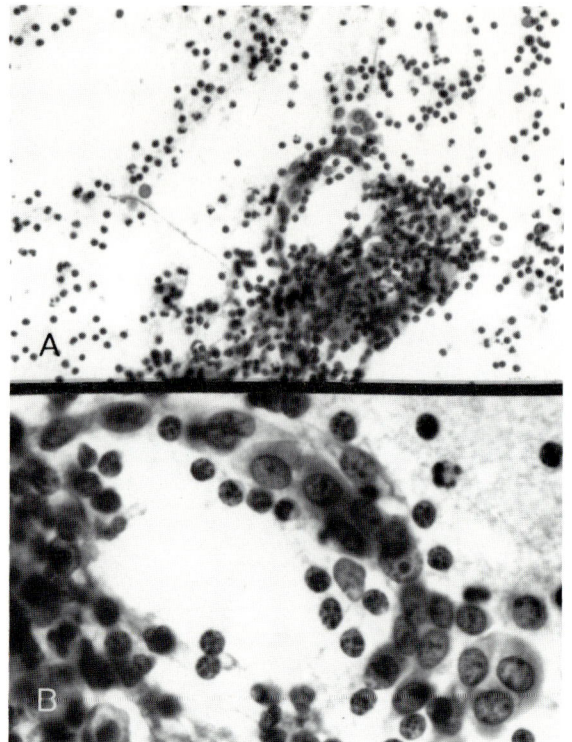

Figure 3.17. Benign lymphoepithelial lesion, ABC. **A** and **B,** Note scattered benign lymphocytes admixed with clusters of epithelial cells having small distinct nucleoli and moderate amount of eosinophilic cytoplasm. **A,** ×125; **B,** ×500.

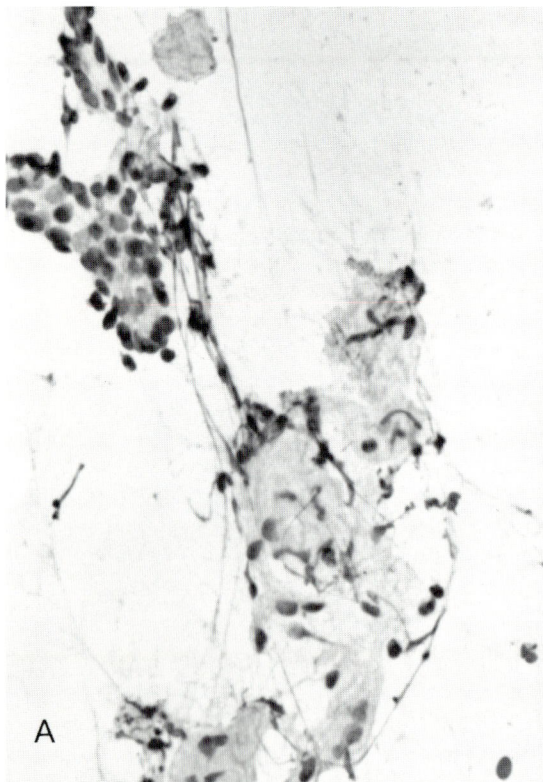

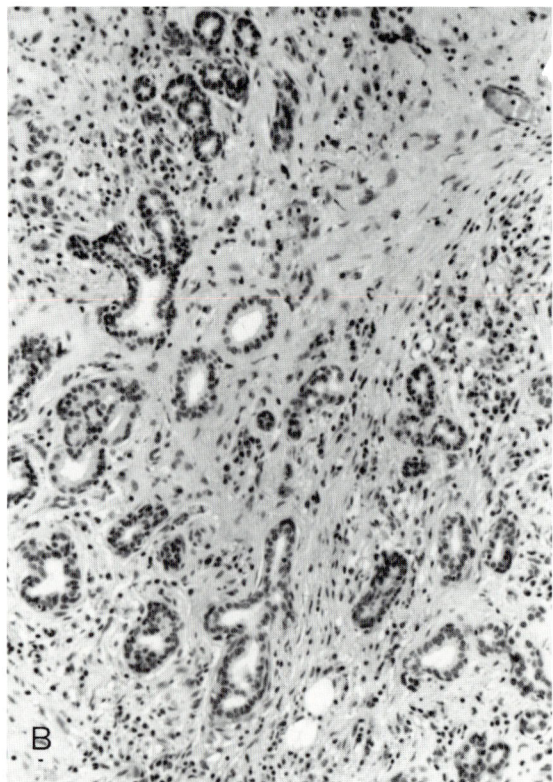

Figure 3.18. Chronic sialadenitis mistaken for pleomorphic adenoma. **A,** ABC. Note epithelial cells in acinar arrangement and a fragment of exuberant fibrous connective tissue. ×310. **B,** His-tology of the chronic sialadenitis showing reactive and regenerative ductal epithelium and fibrosis. ×125.

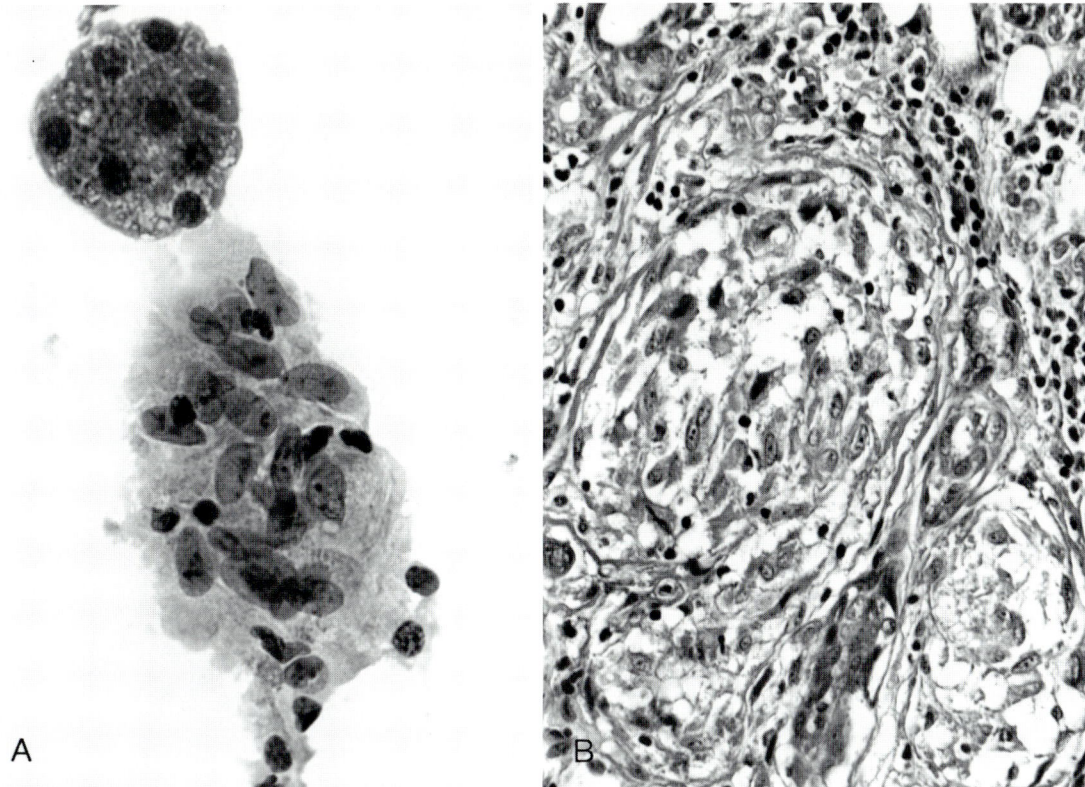

Figure 3.19. Sarcoidosis involving the parotid gland. **A,** ABC. Note cluster of epithelioid cells intermingled with a few lymphocytes. A normal acinus is also seen. ×500. **B,** Histology of sarcoidosis (not the same case). Note noncaseating epithelioid granulomas. ×310.

Sialadenitis

Acute sialadenitis can be of bacterial or viral (e.g., mumps) origin. The onset of the disease is sudden and the salivary gland swelling is tender. Since diagnosis is usually made on clinical features, FNAB is superfluous.

Chronic sialadenitis can present as a localized painless swelling that may mimic a neoplasm. Depending on the area aspirated, FNAB may show normal salivary gland components or may show lymphocytes, plasma cells, histiocytes, and variable amounts of ductal, acinar, and fibrous tissues. We have encountered a case of chronic sialadenitis of the submandibular gland, which was misinterpreted as pleomorphic adenoma on FNAB. The aspirate was cellular, with a large amount of ductal epithelium and fibrous stromal tissue **(Fig. 3.18)**. The histologic examination of the excised specimen showed atrophy of the acinar tissue and a preponderance of residual reactive ductal elements that had given rise to the numerous epithelial tissue fragments seen on the aspirate. Moreover, the reactive fibrous stroma seen in the chronic sialadenitis simulated the fibromyxoid stroma of a mixed tumor.

Granulomatous Diseases

Tuberculosis, sarcoidosis, and cat scratch disease cause salivary gland enlargements that may clinically simulate neoplasms. FNAB is diagnostically valuable. In the two cases in our file of sarcoidosis of parotid gland, the smears revealed small rounded masses of epithelioid cells **(Fig. 3.19)**. The epithelioid cells are plump, elongated cells, with reniform vesicular nuclei, single or multiple small nucleoli, and ample, lightly eosinophilic cytoplasm. The cytoplasmic membranes are generally ill-defined. There was a sprinkling of mature lymphocytes on the background; the absence of necrotic debris rendered the possibility of tuberculosis unlikely. The diagnosis of sarcoidosis is often suggested by radiologic evidence of hilar lymphadenopathy, a positive Kveim test, and a negative tuberculin skin test. Frable and Frable[44] reported the successful use of FNAB to confirm the clinical diagnosis of six cases of sarcoidosis with palpable disease in the head and neck area. They noted that typical sarcoid granulomas were easily identified in all cases.

For a description of the cytologic features of tuberculosis and cat scratch disease, readers are referred to Chapter 4, under "Benign Lymphadenopathies."

References

1. Kline TS. Handbook of fine needle aspiration cytology, 2nd ed. New York: Churchill Livingstone, 1988:121–152.
2. Nahum AM. The needle biopsy comes of age [Editorial]. Head Neck Surg 1981;3:437.
3. Frable WJ, Frable M. Thin-needle aspiration biopsy in the diagnosis of head and neck tumors. Laryngoscope 1974;84:1069–1076.
4. Strong MS. Aspiration cytology in the management of head and neck neoplasms. In Evans PHR, Robin PE, Fielding JWL. Head and neck cancer. New York: Alan R Liss, 1983:97–101.
5. Eneroth CM, Zajicek J. Aspiration biopsy of salivary gland tumors. II. Morphologic studies on smears and histologic sections from oncocytic tumors. Acta Cytol 1965;9:355–361.

6. Eneroth CM, Zajicek J. Aspiration biopsy of salivary gland tumors. III. Morphologic studies on smears and histologic sections from 368 mixed tumors. Acta Cytol 1966;10:440–454.

7. Eneroth CM, Jakobsson P, Zajicek J. Aspiration biopsy of salivary gland tumors. V. Morphologic investigations on smears and histologic sections of acinic cell carcinoma. Acta Radiol Suppl 1971;310:85–93.

8. Zajicek J, Eneroth CM, Jakobsson P. Aspiration biopsy of salivary gland tumors. VI. Morphologic studies on smears and histologic sections from mucoepidermoid carcinoma. Acta Cytol 1976;20:35–41.

9. Layfield LJ, Tan P, Glasgow BJ. Fine needle aspiration of salivary gland lesions. Arch Pathol Lab Med 1987;111:346–353.

10. Cohen MB, Ljung BME, Boles R. Salivary gland tumors: Fine needle aspiration vs. frozen section diagnosis. Arch Otolaryngol Head Neck Surg 1986;112:867–869.

11. O'Dwyer P, Farrar WB, James AG, Finkelmeier W, McCabe DP. Needle aspiration biopsy of major salivary gland tumor. Its value. Cancer 1986;57:554–557.

12. Fechner RE. Diagnosis of salivary gland neoplasms. In Chretien PB, Johns ME, Shedd DP, Strong EW, Ward PH. Head and neck cancer, Vol. 1. Philadelphia: BC Decker, 1984:219–222.

13. Bedrossian CWM, Martinez F, Silverberg AB. Fine needle aspiration. In Gnepp DR. Pathology of the head and neck. New York: Churchill Livingstone, 1988:25–99.

14. Byers RM, Jesse RH, Guillamondegui OM, Luna MA. Malignant tumors of the submaxillary gland. Am J Surg 1973;126:450–463.

15. Frable WJ. Thin needle aspiration biopsy. Philadelphia: WB Saunders, 1982.

16. Qizilbash AH, Sianos J, Young JEM, Archibald SD. Fine needle aspiration biopsy cytology of major salivary glands. Acta Cytol 1985;29:503–512.

17. Eneroth CM. Histological and clinical aspects of parotid tumors. Acta Otolaryngol Suppl 1964;191:5–99.

18. Foote FW Jr, Frazell EL. Tumors of the major salivary glands. Atlas of tumor pathology, Section IV, Fascicle 11. Washington D.C.: Armed Forces Institute of Pathology, 1954.

19. Batsakis JG. Tumors of the head and neck. Baltimore: Williams & Wilkins, 1974.

20. Batsakis JG, Regezi JA. The pathology of head and neck tumors: Salivary glands, Part 4. Head Neck Surg 1979;1:340–349.

21. Peel RL, Gnepp DR. Diseases of the salivary glands. In Barnes L. Surgical pathology of the head and neck, Vol. 1. New York: Marcel Dekker, 1985:533–645.

22. Perzin KH. Systemic approach to the pathologic diagnosis of salivary gland tumors. Prog Surg Pathol 1982;4:137–179.

23. Zajicek J. Aspiration biopsy cytology, Part I. Cytology of supradiaphragmatic organs. Basel: S Karger, 1974:30–65.

24. Geisinger KR, Weidner N. Aspiration cytology of salivary glands. Semin Diagn Pathol 1986;3:219–226.

25. Koss LG, Woyke S, Olszewski W. Aspiration biopsy. Cytologic interpretation and histologic bases. New York: Igaku Shoin, 1984:191–222.

26. Lindberg LG, Akerman M. Aspiration cytology of salivary gland tumors: Diagnostic experience from six years of routine laboratory work. Laryngoscope 1976;86:584–594.

27. Hruban RH, Erozan YS, Zinreich SJ, Kashima HK. Fine needle aspiration cytology of monomorphic adenomas. Am J Clin Pathol 1988;90:46–51.

28. Hood IC, Qizilbash AH, Salama SS, Alexopoulou I. Basal cell adenoma of parotid. Difficulty of differentiation from adenoid cystic carcinoma on aspiration biopsy. Acta Cytol 1983;27:515–520.

29. Layfield LJ. Fine needle aspiration cytology of a trabecular adenoma of the parotid gland. Acta Cytol 1985;29:999–1002.

30. Kline TS, Merriam JM, Shapshay SM. Aspiration biopsy of the salivary gland. Am J Clin Pathol 1981;76:263–269.

31. Palma O, Torri AM, de Cristofaro JA, Fiaccavento S. Fine needle aspiration cytology in two cases of well-differentiated acinic-cell carcinoma of the parotid gland. Acta Cytol 1985;29:516–521.

32. Eneroth CM. Salivary gland tumors in the parotid gland, submandibular gland, and the palate region. Cancer 1971;27:1415–1418.

33. Batsakis JG, Chinn E, Reggezi JA, Repola DA. The pathology of head and neck tumors: Salivary glands, Part 2. Head Neck Surg 1978;1:167–180.

34. Perzin KH, Gullane P, Clairmont AC. Adenoid cystic carcinomas arising in salivary glands. Cancer 1978;42:265–282.

35. Lozowski MS, Mishriki Y, Solitare GB. Cytologic features of adenoid cystic carcinoma: Case report and literature review. Acta Cytol 1983;27:317–322.

36. Plafker J, Nosher JL. Fine needle aspiration of liver with metastatic adenoid cystic carcinoma. Acta Cytol 1983;27:323–325.

37. Anderson RJ, Johnston WW, Szpak CA. Fine needle aspiration of adenoid cystic carcinoma metastatic to the lung. Cytologic features and differential diagnosis. Acta Cytol 1985;29:527–532.

38. Smith RC, Amy RW. Adenoid cystic carcinoma metastatic to the lung. Report of a case diagnosed by fine needle aspiration biopsy cytology. Acta Cytol 1985;29:533–534.

39. Colby TV, Dorfman RF. Malignant lymphomas involving the salivary glands. Pathol Annu 1979;14 (Part 2):307–324.

40. Kelly DR, Spiegel JC, Maves M. Benign lymphoepithelial lesion of the salivary glands. Arch Otolaryngol 1975;101:71–75.

41. Causey JQ. The benign lymphoepithelial lesion—a harbinger of neoplasia. South Med J 1976;69:60–63.

42. Grage TB, Lober PH. Malignant tumors of the major salivary glands. Surgery 1962;52:284–294.

43. Smith FB, Rajdeo H, Panesar N, Bhuta K, Stahl R. Benign lymphoepithelial lesion of the parotid gland in intravenous drug users. Arch Pathol Lab Med 1988;112:742–745.

44. Frable MA, Frable WJ. Fine needle aspiration biopsy in the diagnosis of sarcoid of the head and neck. Acta Cytol 1984;28:175–177.

4

Lymph Nodes

Fine needle aspiration is a simple and cost-effective technique that can be routinely used in patients presenting with persistent lymphadenopathy. Within this setting, a cytologic diagnosis of benign hyperplasia, malignant lymphoma, or metastatic cancer is sought.[1] Subsequent investigation and management of the patient will then depend on the cytologic findings and the clinical correlation (**Fig. 4.1**).

Palpable, superficial lymph nodes can be easily aspirated without radiologic guidance.[1–2] Aspirations of abdominal and retroperitoneal lymph nodes necessitate imaging localization and are performed by radiologists.[3,4] When a malignant lymphoma is clinically suspected, the assistance of a cytotechnologist or pathologist is essential so that optimal fixation of the specimen is achieved and additional material is prepared for immunocytochemical and other special studies, if needed.

FNAB of the lymph node is useful in the following situations:

1. In diagnosing metastatic neoplasms;
2. In rendering a primary diagnosis of lymphoma in selected cases (see later discussion);
3. In documenting the evolution of a previously diagnosed low-grade lymphoma to a higher grade lymphoma;
4. In assessing the extent or recurrence of the lymphoma following histologic diagnosis;
5. In the diagnosis of nonspecific lymphadenitis, and sometimes in the diagnosis of a specific inflammatory condition, e.g., tuberculosis, cat scratch disease;
6. In providing material for culture and other special studies.

BENIGN LYMPHADENOPATHIES

Antigenic stimulation of lymph nodes results in nodal enlargement, with germinal center hyperplasia containing a great number of small and large lymphocytes, both cleaved and noncleaved, and many tingible body histiocytes. The expanded interfollicular areas contain plasma cells, neutrophils, immunoblasts, and histiocytes. Hence, in smears obtained from a reactive lymph node, there is a diverse cell population composed of numerous lymphocytes in varying stages of maturation, plasmacytes, immunoblasts, and histiocytes. In contrast to epithelial cells, which tend to form clusters or tissue fragments, lymphoid cells are noncohesive and tend to spread all over the smear as single cells. However, occasional lymphoid aggregates or clumps may also be seen due to cell crowding as opposed to true cellular adherence. The lymphoid aggregates lack an organoid pattern.

Acute Lymphadenitis

Acute lymphadenitis is usually caused by an infection or inflammation in the area the lymph node drains. Common examples are the cervical lymphadenitis associated with acute pharyngitis and the inguinal lymphadenitis in infections about the genitals and in the lower extremities. Clinically, the regional node may be tender and may show localized edema. It is seldom aspirated because the diagnosis is clinically apparent and the disease resolves with antibiotic therapy. ABC may reveal many polymorphonuclear leukocytes among a varied population of lymphocytes. When the bacteria have been carried to the node, they may multiply and produce an abscess, in which case the aspirate contains pus. The latter should then be sent for culture of the organisms.

Chronic Lymphadenitis and Lymphoid Hyperplasia

In chronic lymphadenitis the nodes are painless, and a specific cause is often not apparent. ABC shows a polymorphous cellular picture (**Fig. 4.2**), as opposed to the monomorphic cellular picture seen in non-Hodgkin's lymphomas (see below). Along with a variable number of plasma cells and phagocytic histiocytes, there are numerous lymphocytes in varying stages of maturation, ranging from small lymphocytes, which usually predominate, to medium size lymphocytes to large transformed lymphocytes (immunoblasts).

Dermatopathic lymphadenopathy is merely reactive lymphoid hyperplasia associated with chronic dermatitis. Macrophages containing melanin pigment are seen in the aspirates (**Fig. 4.3**).

Diagnostic Pitfalls. Cytologic interpretation of abnormal lymph nodes may be extremely difficult for the novice cytopathologist because benign lymphoid hyperplasia can mimic malignant lymphoma and vice versa. For example, benign proliferation of large transformed lymphocytes may be misinterpreted to be malignant lymphoma (see "infectious mononucleosis"); conversely, certain low-grade non-Hodgkin's lymphomas may resemble reactive lymphoid hyperplasia on FNAB. To separate benign and malignant lymphoproliferative lesions, one must be thoroughly familiar with the cytopathology of the various forms of malignant lymphomas. (For further discussion on diagnostic pitfalls, see "Malignant Lymphomas.")

Infectious Mononucleosis

Of the viral lymphadenopathies, infectious mononucleosis can be regarded as the prototype. In most instances the clinical diagnosis is readily apparent based on clinical features, peripheral blood picture, and an elevated heterophil antibody titer. Only occasional atypical cases are subjected to FNAB or surgical biopsy.[5] The ABC (**Fig. 4.4**) shows, in addition to the usual features of lymphadenitis as previously described, many large transformed lymphocytes and immunoblasts dominating the smear. The transformed lymphocytes have an intermediate or large vesicular nucleus and one or two distinct nucleoli often situated close to the nuclear membrane. The cytoplasm is basophilic or amphophilic. The immunoblasts are large plas-

(I)
Lymph node clinically benign

FNAB benign   FNAB malignant   FNAB uncertain

Lymphoma   Metastatic tumor

Reassurance and follow-up   Surgical biopsy   Individualized workup and therapy   Follow-up or surgical biopsy

(II)
Lymph node clinically malignant

FNAB benign   FNAB malignant   FNAB uncertain

Lymphoma   Metastatic tumor

Surgical biopsy   Institute therapy in selected cases; otherwise surgical biopsy   Individualized workup and therapy   Surgical biopsy

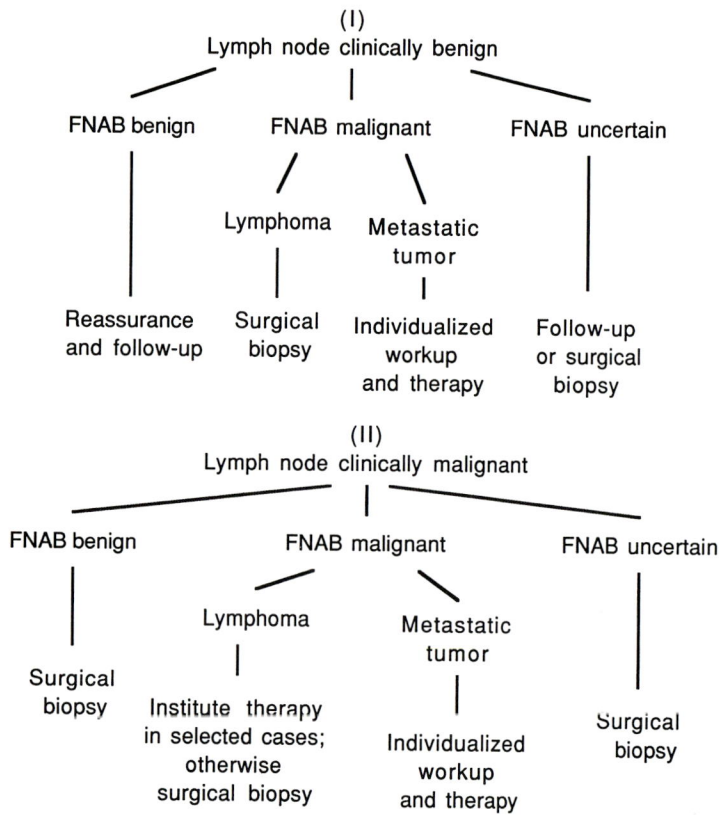

Figure 4.1. Flow diagram for use of fine needle aspiration biopsy of lymph nodes.

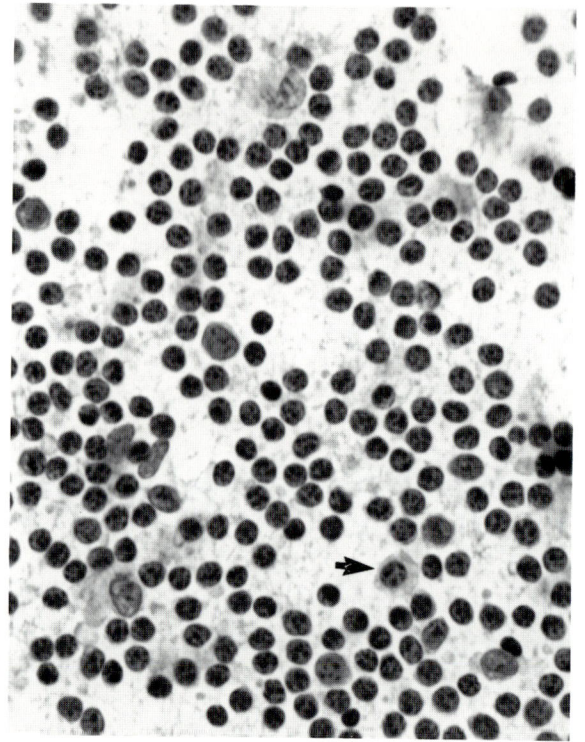

Figure 4.2. Chronic nonspecific lymphadenitis, ABC. Note a polymorphous cell population of small and large lymphocytes and histiocytes. *Arrow* indicates a plasma cell. ×500.

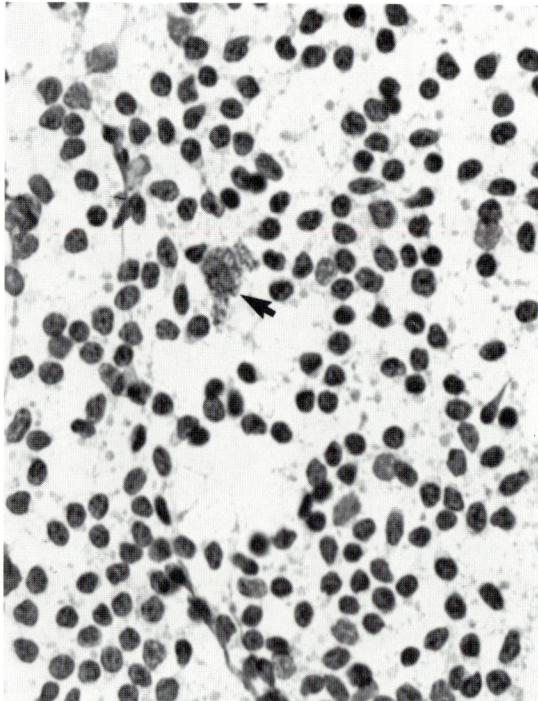

Figure 4.3. Dermatopathic lymphadenitis, ABC. Note many small "mature" lymphocytes, some larger lymphocytes, and a pigment-containing histiocyte *(arrow).* ×500.

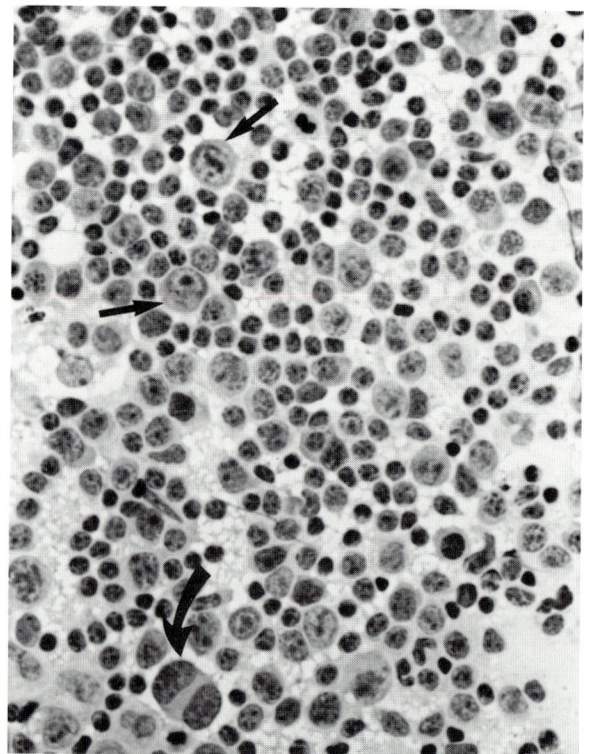

Figure 4.4. Infectious mononucleosis, lymph node aspirate. Note many transformed lymphocytes, large immunoblasts with prominent nucleoli *(arrows)* and a binucleated immunoblast *(curved arrow)* in a background of follicular hyperplasia. ×450.

macytoid cells (20–30 μm in diameter), having a large vesicular nucleus and one prominent amphophilic or basophilic nucleolus. The cytoplasm is abundant and basophilic. Transitional forms of transformed lymphocytes and immunoblasts are frequently seen.

Diagnostic Pitfalls. When binucleated immunoblasts are seen, they must be distinguished from Reed-Sternberg cells (see ''Hodgkin's disease''). When there is an excessive proliferation of immunoblasts, the cytologic picture may mimic immunoblastic non-Hodgkin's lymphoma.

Aspirates from lymph nodes with toxoplasmosis or necrotizing granulomatous inflammation may show cytologic features overlapping with those of infectious mononucleosis.[5] In the former two conditions, although there is a relative high percentage of transformed lymphocytes, granulomatous elements are also apparent (see below).

Granulomatous Lymphadenitis

Necrotizing granulomatous lymphadenitis is a common condition, caused by various organisms including *Mycobacterium tuberculosis*, atypical mycobacteria, *Histoplasma*, and *Coccidioides*, the first two being most frequently encountered in our practice. A cheesy or purulent material is frequently aspirated in cases of tuberculous lymphadenitis.[6] The aspiration cytology of active tuberculosis falls into two groups: ABC in which epithelioid granulomas are present and ABC in which no granulomas are found but large amounts of necrotic debris with variable numbers of leukocytes, histiocytes, and lymphocytes are present.[7] In ABC, necrotizing granulomas are represented by aggregates of epithelioid histiocytes admixed with necrotic debris **(Fig. 4.5)**. The epithelioid histiocyte is a large plump cell with an elongated or reniform vesicular nucleus, a small nucleolus, and an ample amount of pale ill-defined cytoplasm. The indistinct cell borders of the histiocytes give the cell aggregates a syncytial appearance. Another characteristic cell is the Langhans' cell, which is a giant histiocyte with 40–50 nuclei arranged around the periphery of the cell (see Chapter 7). Langhans' giant cells are not always seen in the smears.

When a granulomatous disease is suspected, a Ziehl-Neelsen stain or an auramine-rhodamine fluorescent stain for acid-fast bacilli and stains for fungi can be done either on the direct smears or on cell blocks.[6–8] Aspirated material should also be sent for culture.

Cat scratch disease causes granulomatous lymphadenitis along with formation of multiple suppurative microabscesses. Its cytologic picture is similar to that described for tuberculosis, except that numerous polymorphonuclear leukocytes in lieu of lymphocytes are present in the background **(Fig. 4.6)**. Correct cytologic diagnosis of cat scratch disease is feasible, when a pertinent clinical history is obtained.[9]

Sarcoidosis and toxoplasmosis give rise to noncaseating granulomas composed of epithelioid histiocytes. The granulomas are generally large and confluent in sarcoidosis, whereas in toxoplasmosis the granulomas are small and discrete, occurring in a background of lymphoid hyperplasia.[10] The cytologic features of sarcoidosis are discussed in Chapter 3 (see **Fig. 3.19**).

MALIGNANT LYMPHOMAS

Malignant lymphomas are the primary neoplasms of the lymphoreticular tissues and are divided into two broad categories: non-Hodgkin's lymphoma (NHL) and Hodgkin's disease. Non-Hodgkin's lymphomas account for about 3% of all cancers (excluding skin cancer and carcinoma in situ) and are four times more common than Hodgkin's lymphoma and account for 10 times as many deaths as Hodgkin's lymphoma.[12] Malignant lymphomas occur in all age

groups, with an increased incidence in age in NHL. In Hodgkin's disease, the distribution curve is bimodal, with the first peak between 20 and 30 years of age and the second peak after 50 years of age.[13]

Diagnostic Accuracy

Although the results of diagnosing malignant lymphoma by FNAB are mixed, in experienced hands the accuracy rate is high, being in the range of 85–94%.[14–18a] Orell and Skinner[16] reported full agreement between cytologic and histologic classification in 44 of 53 cases of NHLs, and they were able to correctly assign 48 of 49 cases diagnosed by FNAB to good or bad prognostic groups. When cytologic evaluation is combined with immunocytochemistry, the results were even better. In one series of 111 cases of lymphoma, correct diagnosis and classification was made in 91% of the cases, diagnosis of suspected lymphoma in 4.5%, benign in 1%, and inadequate material in 4.5%.[15]

Analysis of our own experience based on 180 cases at the Cancer Control Agency of British Columbia[19] showed that FNAB had a positive impact on patient management in 170 cases and a negative impact in 10 cases. The positive influence included prompt institution of appropriate therapy (84), rapid solution to the clinical situation (65), improved understanding of the clinical situation (78), and elimination of unnecessary surgical procedure (minor (local anesthetic), 31; intermediate (general anesthetic), 88; major (laparotomy or thoracotomy), 18). The negative effects were, for the most part, temporary; they led to unnecessary investigation (1), delayed therapy (3), incorrect therapy (4), and were a source of confusion (10).

In fairness to fine needle aspiration, one should also note that even histologic evaluation of lymphomas is not infallible. In a review of a large number of cases by the Pathology Panel and Repository Center for Lymphoma Clinical Studies,[20] disagreement between referring and panel pathologists on subclassification of lymphoma occurred in up to 25% of the cases and disagreement on whether or not the resected tissues showed evidence of malignancy in as many as 6% of the cases.

Non-Hodgkin's Lymphoma

A number of NHL classification systems have been in use, based on either morphologic or immunologic features.[21–23] Despite the many different classification systems, all authorities have agreed on two points: the larger the cells the poorer the prognosis, and diffuse growth pattern indicates a poorer prognosis than nodular growth pattern of the same cell type.[24,25]

In 1982, an international group of experts introduced a practical formulation of non-Hodgkin's lymphomas to allow translation between the major classification schemes.[26] Based on morphologic rather than immunologic criteria, the Working Formulation nomenclature is readily applicable to cytologic specimens **(Table 4.1)**.[4,15,19,27]

The lymphocyte population in the majority of NHLs is monomorphic, although a small number of the ubiquitous small histiocytes and small lymphocytes may be present. Although it is generally not feasible to decide by FNAB if the neoplastic lymphocytes are arranged in nodular or diffuse form, identification of small cell and large cell categories and the histologic subtype of lymphoma **(Fig. 4.7)** can be achieved with a high degree of accuracy.

Malignant Lymphoma, Small Lymphocytic

This disease is the nodal counterpart of chronic lymphocytic leukemia. It generally affects patients over 40 years of age and runs an indolent course with a favorable prognosis. The smears consist

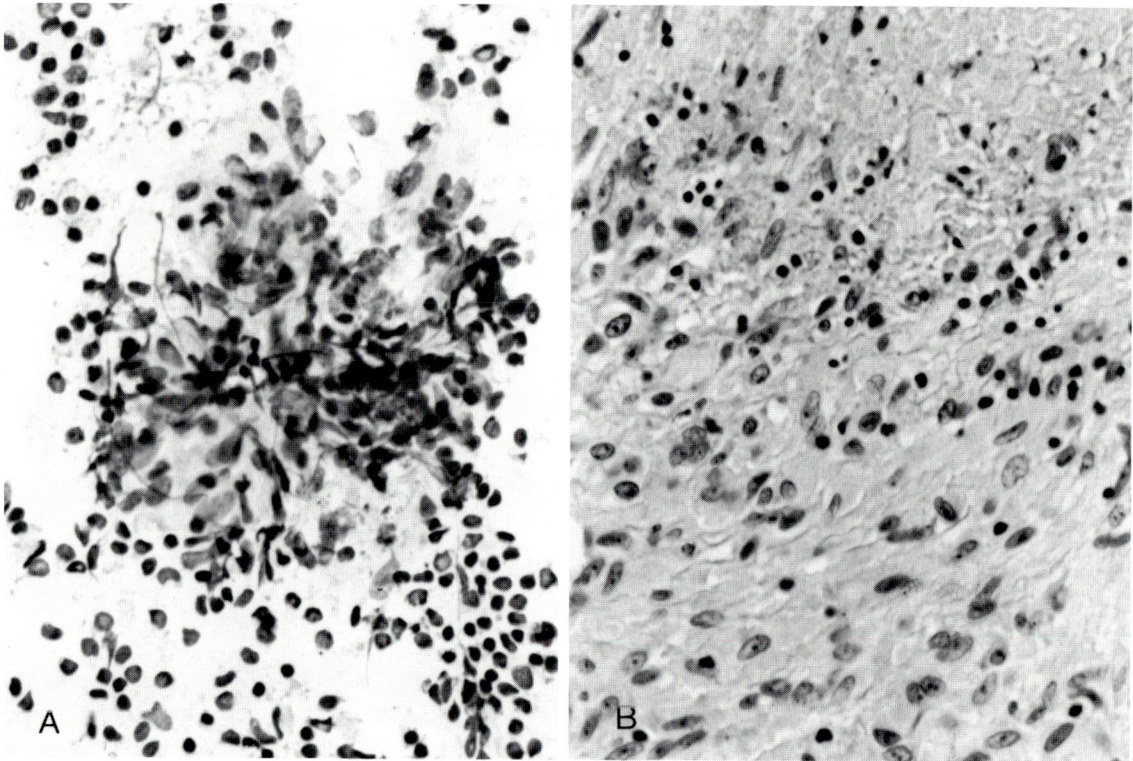

Figure 4.5.

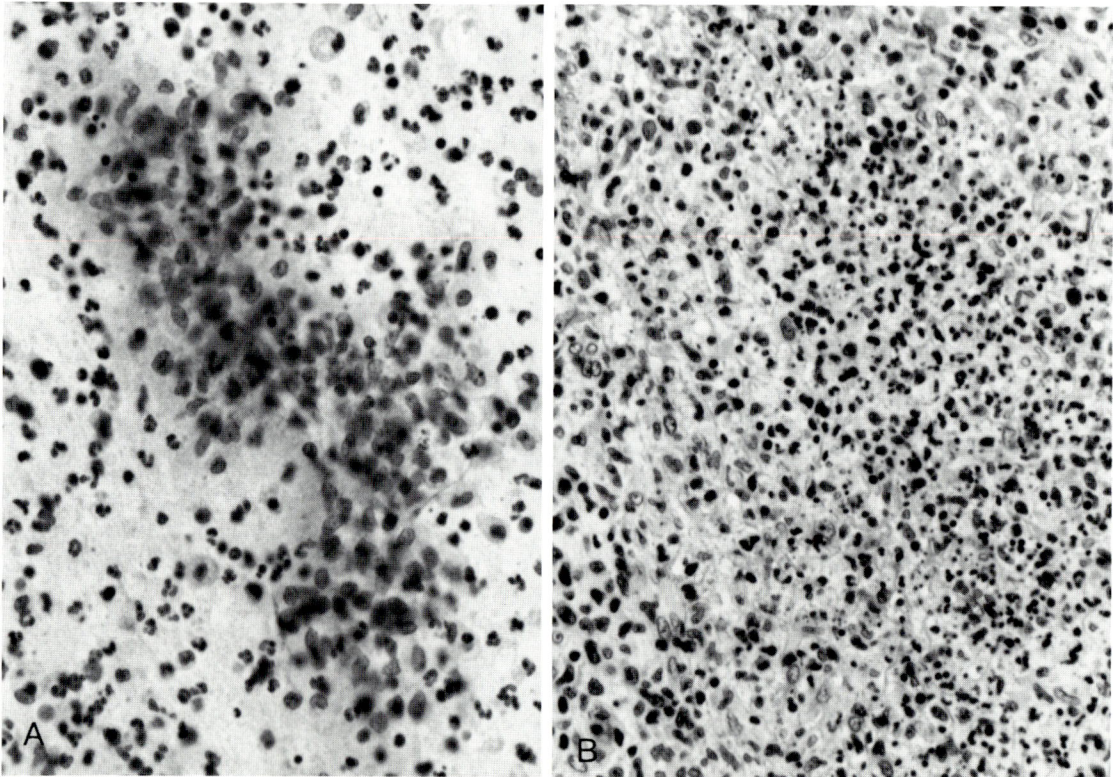

Figure 4.6.

Table 4.1.   Cytologic Classification of Non-Hodgkin's Lymphoma[a]

Low grade	Small lymphocyte
	Small cleaved cell
	Mixed small and large cell
	Large cell
	Cleaved and noncleaved
	Immunoblastic
	Small noncleaved cell
	Burkitt's
	Non-Burkitt's
High grade	Lymphoblastic (convoluted cell)

[a] Terminology is adopted from the Working Formulation.[26] The pattern of growth (follicular or diffuse) is not apparent on FNAB.

entirely of small lymphocytes, which are morphologically indistinguishable from normal lymphocytes. The cells are small (8–9 μm), with a round or oval nucleus. The chromatin is made up of coarse, mosaic-shaped chromocenters, and the nucleoli are either inconspicuous or not evident. The cytoplasm is scanty or invisible (**Fig. 4.8**).

Approximately 15% of patients with small lymphocytic lymphoma have a serum monoclonal gammopathy. The aspirates from these cases show, in addition to the small lymphocytes, variable numbers of plasmacytoid lymphocytes (**Fig. 4.9**) with eccentric nuclei, moderate to abundant amphophilic or basophilic cytoplasm, and occasional cytoplasmic and/or nuclear immunoglobulin (Ig) inclusions. When the lymphoma is accompanied by IgM monoclonal dysproteinemia, the term "Waldenström's macroglobulinemia" is used.

Malignant Lymphoma, Small Cleaved Cell

The aspirates consist of entirely small cleaved lymphocytes or a mixture of small cleaved lymphocytes and a small number of small lymphocytes. The small cleaved cells (**Fig. 4.10**) are slightly larger than a small lymphocyte. The nuclei are cleaved or indented. The chromatin pattern is moderately fine to coarse, and nucleoli are present but usually small. Cytoplasm is scanty.

Malignant Lymphoma, Mixed Small and Large Cell

This category comprises a heterogeneous group of lymphomas of mixed cell population (**Fig. 4.11**). Some of these in which the small lymphocytes show cleaved nuclei are of follicular center cell origin. Others are of T-cell origin, consisting of large and small lymphocytes with irregular but noncleaved nuclei.

Malignant Lymphoma, Large Cell

These neoplasms assume a wide range of microscopic appearance. Two subsets are generally recognized: (a) large cell, cleaved or noncleaved and (b) large cell, immunoblastic.

In the first subset (**Fig. 4.12**), the lymphocytes have large nuclei, which are three to four times as large as those of small lymphocytes and may be cleaved or noncleaved (round). Both cleaved and noncleaved cells may be present or one of the two may be predominant. The chromatin pattern is finely stippled and nucleoli are large. The amount of cytoplasm is variable.

In the second subset, the large cells show immunoblastic features (**Fig. 4.13**). The cells are large (20–30 μm) with abundant basophilic or amphophilic cytoplasm. The nuclei are uniformly round, centrally or eccentrically placed, and have thick nuclear membranes and one or more large, irregular, sharp nucleoli.

Malignant Lymphoma, Small Noncleaved Cell

The small noncleaved cells are larger than small cleaved lymphocytes, but smaller than large cleaved or noncleaved lymphocytes. This group of lymphomas encompasses Burkitt's and non-Burkitt's types. The most striking feature of Burkitt's lymphoma is the uniformity of the tumor cells (**Fig. 4.14**). The regular nuclei are rounded or oval, sometimes slightly notched, and are about the size of macrophage nuclei. They have an evenly distributed but rather coarse chromatin. The nuclear membrane is prominent. Two to five moderately prominent basophilic nucleoli are present in each nucleus. A distinct rim of amphophilic or basophilic cytoplasm is evident. Mitoses are frequent.

Small noncleaved cell lymphomas that show too much nuclear variation and pleomorphism to be classified as Burkitt's lymphoma are called small noncleaved cell lymphoma, non-Burkitt's type. Many of these tumors are difficult to distinguish from large cell lymphoma on purely histologic and cytologic grounds.

Malignant Lymphoma, Lymphoblastic

Lymphoblastic lymphomas are usually composed of lymphocytes with convoluted nuclei. Most cases are of T-cell origin. The lymphocytes are of medium size (15–20 μm), with nuclei that are larger than those of small cleaved lymphocytes but smaller than those of immunoblasts. The nuclei show finely dispersed chromatin and small or inconspicuous nucleoli. The nuclear membranes typically possess deep convolutions, imparting a lobulated or cerebriform appearance (**Fig. 4.15**). It must be noted that there is a wide variation in the percentage of convoluted lymphocytes not only among different cases but among materials from different sites in the same case as well. It has been estimated that on the average about 47% of the cells have convoluted nuclei.[28]

Diagnostic Pitfalls in Non-Hodgkin's Lymphomas

Cytologic atypia is minimal or absent in low-grade NHLs and obvious in high-grade NHLs.[14,27,29,30] In low-grade (well-differentiated) NHLs, 20–36% of the cases cannot be distinguished from benign lymphadenopathy; on the other hand, 90% of the high-grade (poorly differentiated) NHLs can be identified correctly by FNAB.[30]

At the present time, FNAB is not used routinely as the sole

Figure 4.5.   Tuberculous lymphadenitis. A, ABC. Note a group of elongated epithelioid cells with ill-defined pale cytoplasm, admixed with necrotic debris. The cells scattered in the background are lymphocytes. ×310. **B**, Histologic section of a caseating granuloma (not from the same case). Note area of necrosis (upper field) and elongated epithelioid histiocytes (lower field). ×310.

Figure 4.6.   Cat scratch disease. A, Lymph node aspirate. Note a syncytial group of epithelioid cells. Unlike tuberculous inflammation, the background shows numerous polymorphonuclear leukocytes. ×310. **B**, Histologic section (not from the same case) showing a microabscess, source of the polymorphonuclear leukocytes, rimmed by epithelioid histiocytes. ×310.

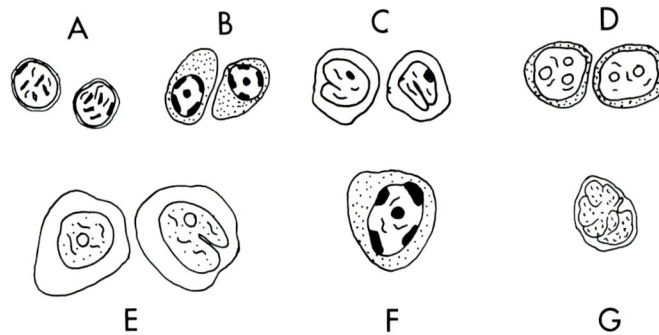

Figure 4.7. Non-Hodgkin's lymphoma cell types. **A**, small lymphocyte; **B**, small plasmacytoid lymphocyte; **C**, small cleaved cell; **D**, small noncleaved cell; **E**, large cell, cleaved and noncleaved; **F**, large cell, immunoblastic; **G**, convoluted cell (lymphoblast).

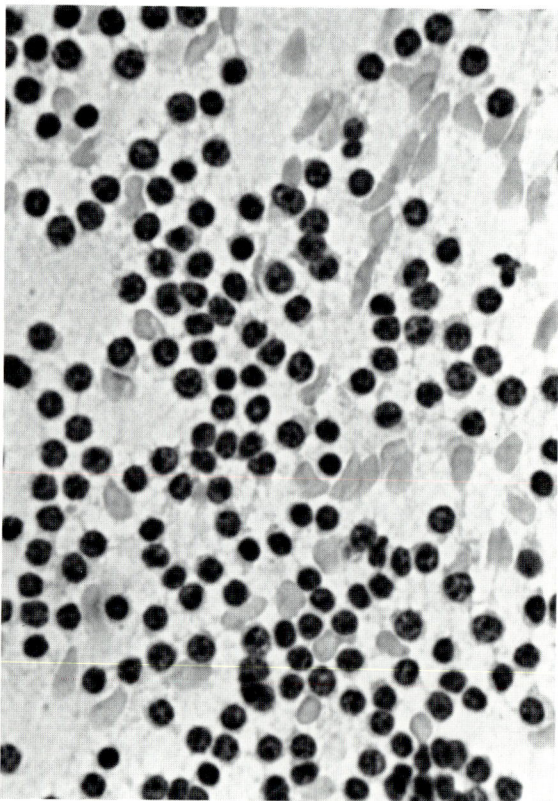

Figure 4.8. Malignant lymphoma, small lymphocytic, ABC. The cells are small with regular round nuclei, indistinguishable from nonneoplastic small lymphocytes. ×500.

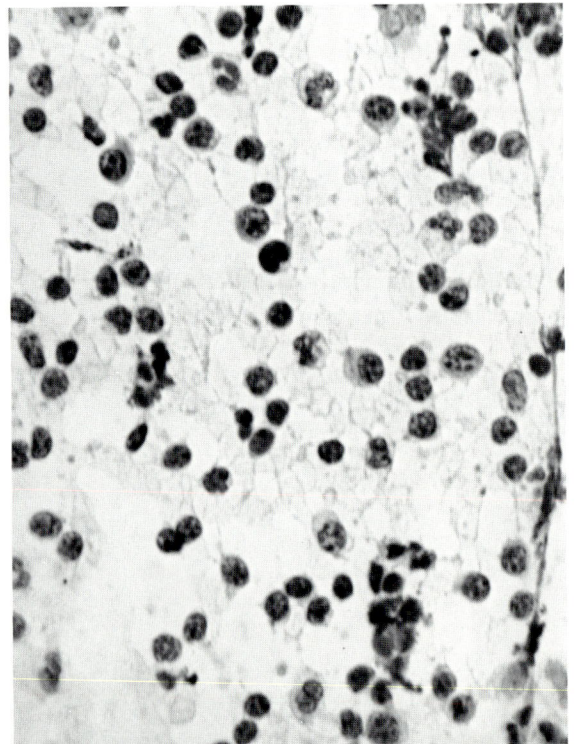

Figure 4.9. Malignant lymphoma, small lymphocytic-plasmacytoid, ABC. Note admixture of small lymphocytes and plasmacytoid lymphocytes. The latter have eccentric nuclei and a fair amount of cytoplasm. The patient subsequently proved to have Waldenström's macroglobulinemia. ×500.

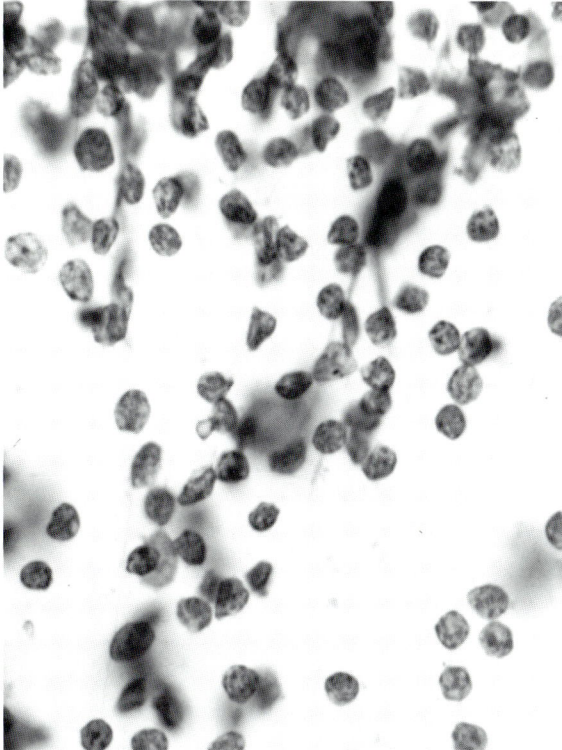

Figure 4.10. Malignant lymphoma, small cleaved cell, ABC. Note irregular nuclei with linear cleavage planes. ×500.

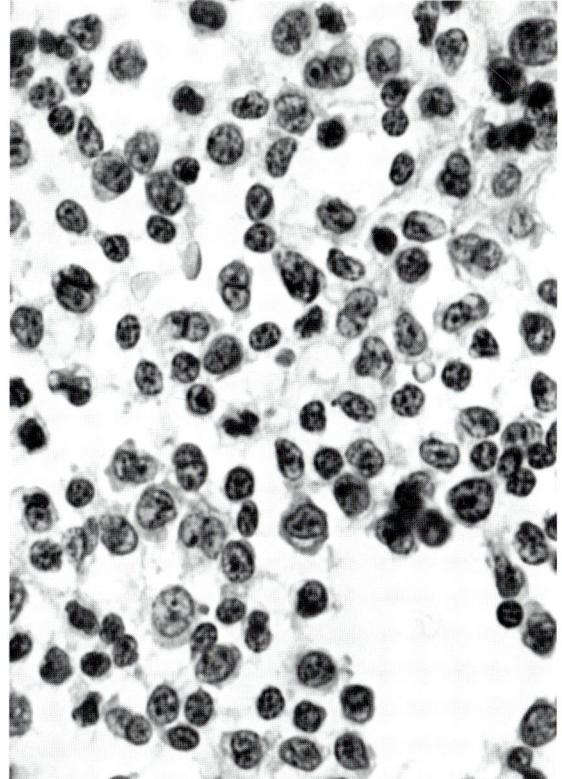

Figure 4.11. Malignant lymphoma, mixed small and large cell, ABC. There is a roughly equal mixture of small and large cells. ×500.

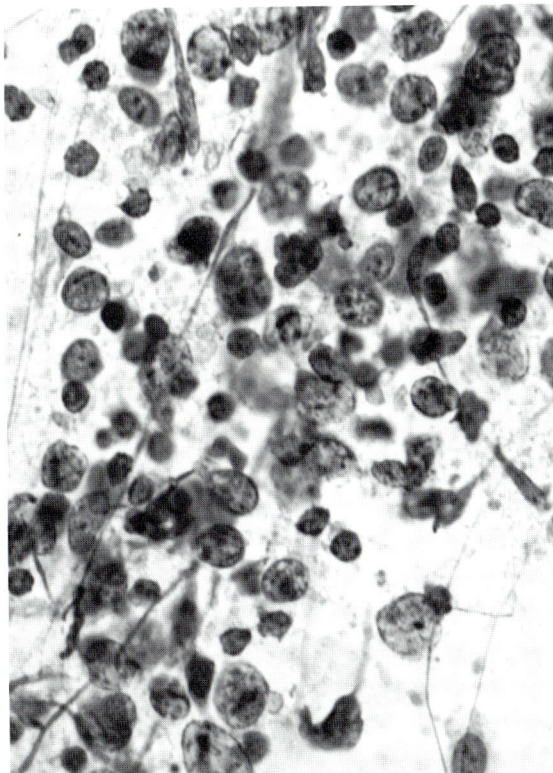

Figure 4.12. Malignant lymphoma, large cell, ABC. Note large atypical lymphocytes, and in this case both cleaved and non-cleaved cells are seen. ×500.

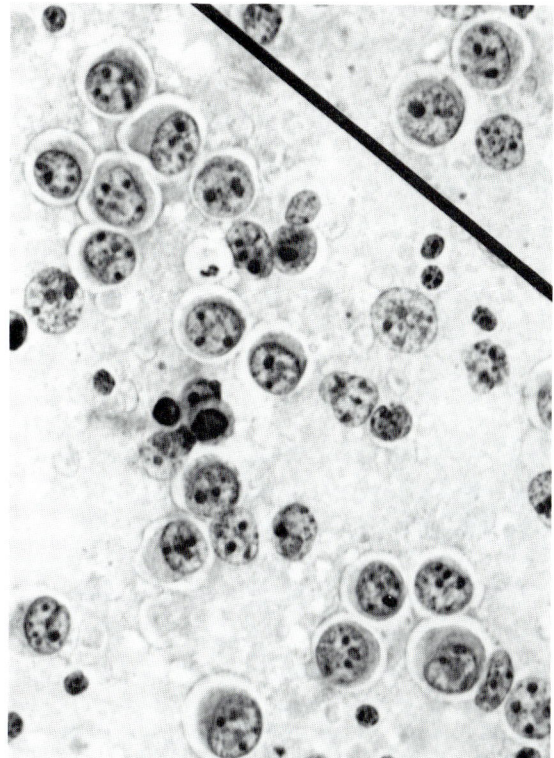

Figure 4.13. Malignant lymphoma, large cell, immunoblastic, ABC. Note large round nuclei with macronucleoli. Many cells demonstrate plasmacytoid differentiation, characterized by nucleus eccentricity and ample basophilic cytoplasm. ×500.

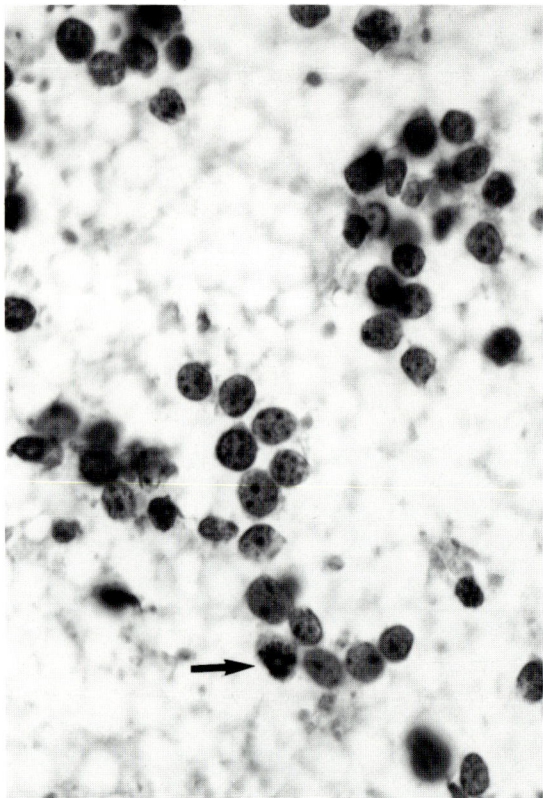

Figure 4.14. Malignant lymphoma, small noncleaved cell (Burkitt's type), ABC. Note uniformity of tumor cells, with rounded nuclei containing coarse chromatin and distinct nucleoli. The tumor cells have a high mitotic rate (*arrow* shows a mitosis). ×500.

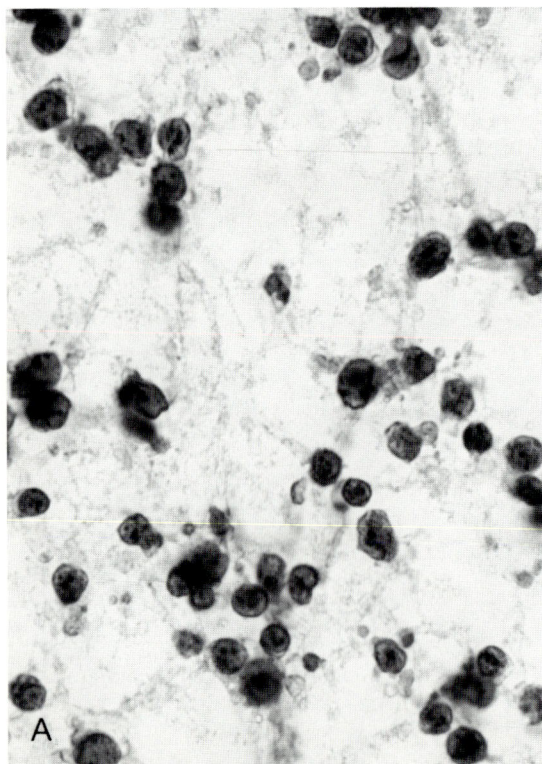

Figure 4.15. Malignant lymphoma, lymphoblastic (convoluted cell type), ABC. **A** and **B**, Note medium-sized lymphocytes with a finely dispersed chromatin pattern, small or inconspicuous nucleoli. Convoluted nuclei are seen in some cells. **A**, ×500; **B**, ×1250.

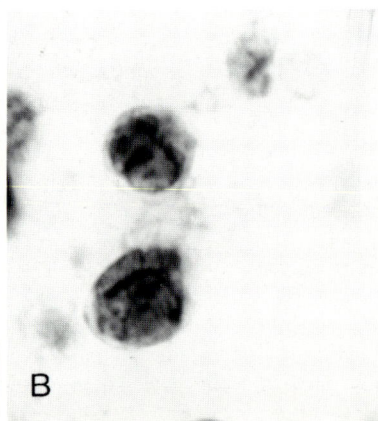

basis for the initial diagnosis of malignant lymphoma, except in selected types of NHL (see below). Confirmatory surgical biopsy with complete histologic studies should be undertaken, unless the patient's condition precludes surgery or a large retroperitoneal lymphoma occurs in an elderly frail patient. In these cases, every attempt should be made to support the cytologic diagnosis by immunologic studies of the aspirated material. Many patients with non-Hodgkin's lymphomas have generalized disease at the time of diagnosis.[31] Not infrequently, the cytologic diagnosis can be substantiated by a minor procedure such as a bone marrow biopsy. When an abdominal or retroperitoneal NHL is diagnosed by FNAB, careful clinical examination should be made to demonstrate the presence or absence of peripheral adenopathy. If present, a laparotomy can be avoided by surgical biopsy of one of the peripheral nodes.

In the small lymphocytic-type NHL, the cells are morphologically indistinguishable from normal small lymphocytes. The diagnosis is suggested primarily by the observation of a monomorphic population of small lymphocytes. The FNAB diagnosis must be supported by a surgical biopsy or correlated with immunocytochemical studies and examinations of the peripheral blood, serum proteins, and bone marrow. A bone marrow biopsy will be positive in a very high percentage (90–100%) of the cases.[32]

In the small lymphocytic-plasmacytoid NHL and the mixed small and large cell NHL, the cytologic features may simulate reactive hyperplasia because a mixed cell population with a spectrum of cell size is present. These lymphoma types require confirmatory surgical biopsy. On the other hand, a surgical biopsy would not be necessary for large cell malignant lymphoma, malignant lymphoma of small noncleaved cells, and lymphoblastic malignant lymphoma, especially when ancillary marker studies are available to confirm the cytologic diagnosis. However, if there is any uncertainty about the aspiration cytology, one should not hesitate to recommend a confirmatory surgical biopsy.

In some NHLs, particularly the large cell variants, the tumor cells may simulate those of metastatic undifferentiated carcinoma. Cytologic features that favor lymphoma include the dispersed cell pattern, monomorphism of the cell population, and absence of cytoplasmic vacuolation (which aids in its differentiation from adenocarcinoma). An occasional case of lymphoma with the cytologic pattern of carcinoma has been reported.[33] We recently have encountered a case of retroperitoneal lymphoma showing pseudoepithelial clusters (**Fig. 4.16A**). The clue to correct diagnosis is to identify the classic lymphoma pattern (**Fig. 4.16B**) elsewhere in the smear.

Immunoperoxidase and electron microscopic techniques have proved useful in the differential diagnosis.[34,35] Because the majority of NHLs are of monoclonal B-cell origin, immunocytologic demonstration of a monoclonal B-cell population expressing either κ or λ light chain, but not both, confirms the diagnosis of lymphoma. In contrast, lymphocytes derived from a reactive lymphoid hyperplasia consist of polyclonal B cells and T cells. In the diagnosis of lymphoma versus carcinoma, use of antibodies against leukocyte common antigen and cytokeratin will separate lymphoma from carcinoma (see Chapter 16). Ultrastructural identification of cell junctions also confirms the diagnosis of carcinoma.

Hodgkin's Disease

Hodgkin's disease (HD) is a relatively uncommon neoplasm responsible for less than 1% of all newly diagnosed cancers seen in the United States each year. Four histologic subclasses of HD are recognized: lymphocyte predominance, nodular sclerosis, mixed cellularity, and lymphocyte depletion. While the diagnosis of HD can often be made or suggested by FNAB, subclassification is generally

not feasible. In patients with the initial diagnosis already established on surgical biopsy, FNAB can be used in staging, defining the extent of radiation fields, and in recognizing residual disease and relapses after therapy.[36,37]

Aspiration Cytology

In contrast to the NHLs characterized usually by homogeneous populations of tumor cells, Hodgkin's lymphomas have mixed cellular composition in which a substantial part of the component cells are not neoplastic. The neoplastic cells are the Reed-Sternberg (RS) cells and their variants; the nonneoplastic cells are the immunoreactive cells.

The aspirate smears are usually hypercellular and consist of predominantly small benign lymphocytes with variable numbers of plasma cells, eosinophils, and atypical mononucleate and multinucleate histiocyte-like cells with prominent nucleoli. The diagnostic cell is the classic Reed-Sternberg cell (**Fig. 4.17**), which is a large cell, 25–40 μm in diameter, containing two mirror-image nuclei, each having a prominent inclusion-like nucleolus that is markedly eosinophilic when stained with hematoxylin and eosin. Not infrequently, there is peripheral condensation of chromatin, so that the nuclear membrane appears markedly thickened and each nucleolus is surrounded by a halo. Atypical mono- and multinucleate cells with prominent nucleoli, which do not show all the characteristic features of diagnostic RS cells, are often seen. The presence of these RS cell variants should arouse strong concern for Hodgkin's disease, but they should not be regarded as diagnostic RS cell.

Diagnostic Pitfalls. The classic Reed-Sternberg cell is a morphologic marker for Hodgkin's disease. Unfortunately, in the lymphocyte-predominant variant of HD, typical RS cells are infrequent. The diagnosis of HD may be missed unless the cytopathologist has a high index of suspicion and diligently searches for RS cells. Friedman et al.[36] reported that 5.5% of their HD cases were misdiagnosed as benign reactive hyperplasia. In the nodular sclerosis type of HD with marked fibrosis, the lymph node may be difficult to aspirate and the specimen may contain only blood and a few lymphocytes.[38] Such smears are nondiagnostic.

Reed-Sternberg-like cells have been described in infectious mononucleosis and other viral lymphadenopathies, postvaccination reaction, and phenytoin (Dilantin) therapy. Some nonlymphomatous malignancies, such as giant cell carcinoma, choriocarcinoma, melanoma, and sarcomas may produce cells that mimic RS cells.[38–40] To avoid false-positive reports, the diagnosis of HD is made only when typical RS cells are identified in an appropriate cellular milieu and in an appropriate clinical setting. RS-like cells in nonneoplastic lymphadenopathies will disappear after discontinuation of the drug or resolution of the disease.

Finally, the cytologic picture of recurrent HD after intensive multimodality treatment may not resemble the original disease but may mimic large cell NHL because transformation of cell type has occurred. In Friedman's series, 4.4% of HD was erroneously diagnosed as non-Hodgkin's lymphoma as a result of disease progression.[36]

The salient cytologic features that differentiate benign lymphoid hyperplasia, non-Hodgkin's lymphoma, and Hodgkin's disease are summarized in **Table 4.2**.

METASTATIC NEOPLASMS
General Remarks

The most frequent clinical application of FNAB of a lymph node is for the diagnosis of metastatic tumor.[1,2–4,18,41–45] The tech-

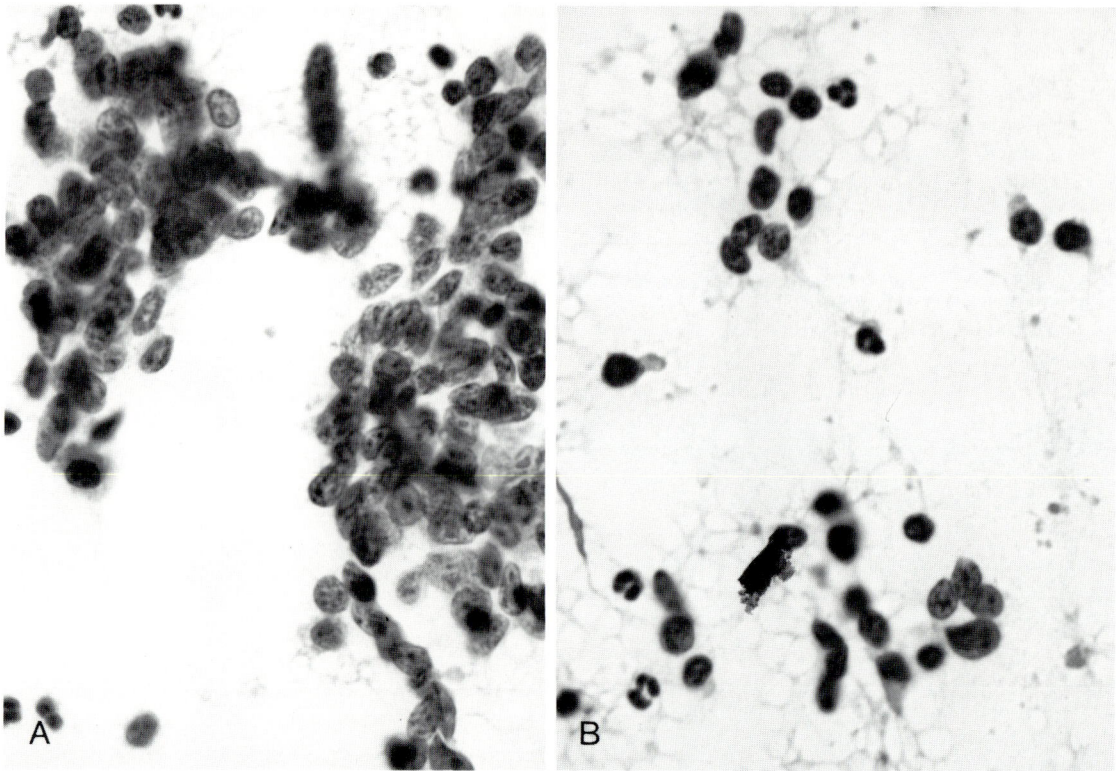

Figure 4.16. Lymphoma with a carcinoma-like pattern, ABC. **A,** Note lymphoma cells in pseudoepithelial clusters. ×500. **B,** Another area from the same smear showing a typical lymphoma pattern of dispersed cells. ×500.

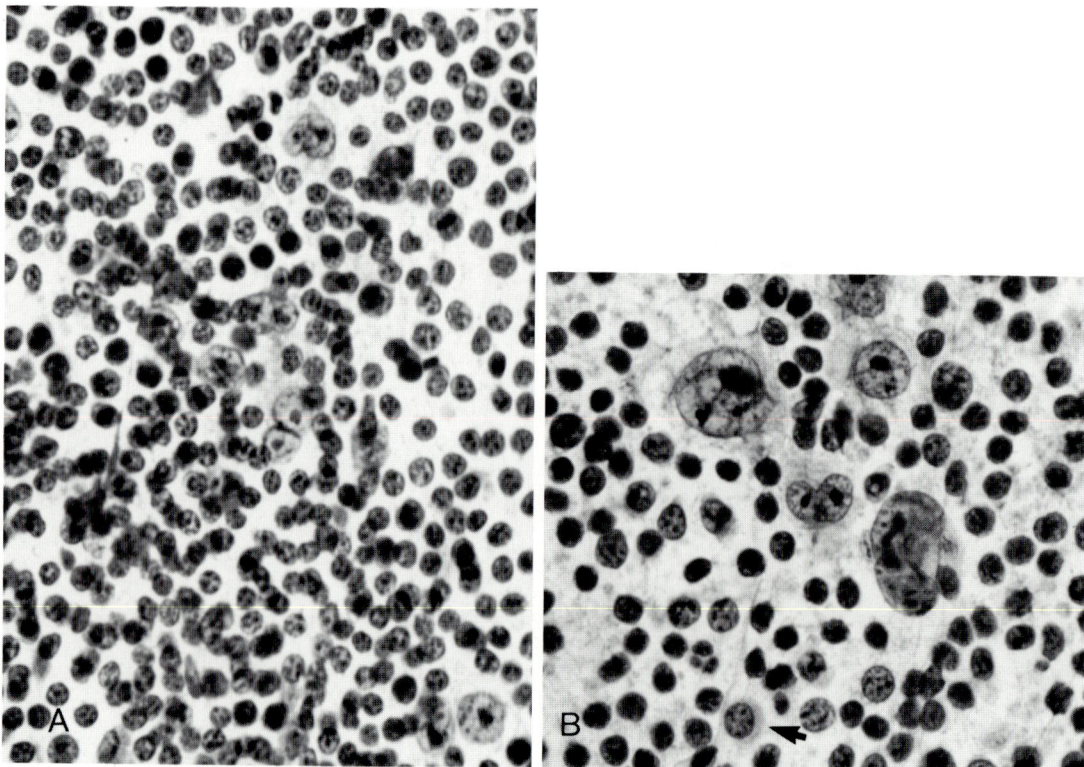

Figure 4.17. Hodgkin's disease, ABC. **A** and **B,** Note atypical large mononucleate cells and classic binucleate Reed-Sternberg cells. The background cells are predominantly small lymphocytes, few eosinophils and plasma cells. *Arrow* indicates a plasma cell. **A,** ×500; **B,** ×1250.

Table 4.2.   Diagnostic Features of Reactive Hyperplasia, Non-Hodgkin's Lymphoma, and Hodgkin's Disease

	Reactive Hyperplasia	Non-Hodgkin's Lymphoma	Hodgkin's Disease
Cell Morphology	Cytologic maturity	Cytologic atypia (except: small lymphocytic NHL)	Reed-Sternberg cells and variants
Cell Composition	Polymorphous (lymphocytes at various stages of maturation, plasma cells and histiocytes)	Monomorphous (except: mixed small and large cell NHL)	Polymorphous (small lymphocytes predominating, some plasma cells and eosinophils)

nique is particularly valuable in evaluating cervical lymph nodes suspected to harbor metastatic carcinoma, because, unlike open biopsy, it does not complicate prospective radical neck surgery. In evaluating metastatic disease involving periaortic or pelvic lymph nodes, FNAB may be used as a substitute to laparotomy.[44,45]

Epithelial cells are not a normal constituent of lymph nodes; therefore, presence of these "alien" cells in an aspirate is indicative of metastatic disease with the following exceptions: salivary gland inclusions in nodes around the angle of the jaw, thyroid inclusions in nodes close to the thyroid gland, melanocyte inclusions in axillary nodes, and glandular inclusions in pelvic nodes in females. Although the cytopathologist should be familiar with these unusual possibilities, in practice these benign inclusions are unlikely to cause problems because first, they are rare, and second, they are generally microscopic in size and do not cause nodal enlargement.

Most of the erroneous diagnoses are caused by inexperience in cytologic interpretation or faulty clinical judgment. The author has reviewed an aspirate in which benign sweat glands in the axilla were interpreted as metastatic carcinoma in a patient who had a previous breast carcinoma. The pathologist was misled by the history and neglected to pay careful attention to the cell morphology.

Identification of the primary site from which the metastasis has arisen can pose a problem with a clinically occult primary tumor. Clinical data, particularly the age and sex of the patient and location of the affected node, provide valuable diagnostic information.[46,47] In cervical lymph nodes, squamous carcinomas are the most common and such metastases nearly always originate from the head and neck region, esophagus, and respiratory tract. In cases of papillary carcinoma, the primary site is almost always the thyroid gland. In low cervical and supraclavicular lymph nodes, most metastases come from the lung and stomach. The latter notably involves the left side more than the right. In axillary nodes, adenocarcinoma of the breast is the most common tumor found in the females and melanoma and lymphoma in the males. Other probable primary sites include lung, stomach, skin, and pharynx.[46] In the inguinal nodes, the metastases for the most part are derived from such obvious sites as the skin of the lower limb and trunk, testicle, penis, ovary, cervix, vulva, anus, and rectum.[47]

Diagnostic Accuracy

Kline and associates[2] showed an accuracy rate of 95% in 376 cases of superficial lymph node aspirations. Lee et al.[43] reported a sensitivity of 89.4%, specificity 90.9%, predictive value of positive results 96.8%, and predictive value of negative results 74.1%. For deep-seated lymph nodes, such as those in the retroperitoneum, the accuracy rate is understandably lower, but FNAB is still the best tool available to make a diagnosis short of a laparotomy. Bonfiglio et al.[3] reported on the FNAB of retroperitoneal lymph nodes in 45 patients; aspirates from 11 patients were positive for malignancy. Only two of the 34 patients with negative aspirations proved to have metastatic nodal disease on follow-up. There were no false-positives. Ewing et al.[44] aspirated 61 cases of abnormal periaortic and pelvic lymph nodes and 48 (79%) were adequate for interpretation. In 28 cases, malignancy was found. Dolan and MacIntosh[45] utilized lymph node aspirations in 50 patients with gynecologic cancer. They reported an overall diagnostic accuracy of 86% in the aspiration of retroperitoneal nodes with the aid of lymphangiography and fluoroscopy, as compared with 38% accuracy for lymphangiography and 66% for surgery.

Squamous Cell Carcinoma

The ABC of squamous cell carcinoma is described in detail elsewhere (see Chapter 7). Briefly, the well-differentiated squamous carcinoma (**Fig. 4.18**) consists of isolated, pleomorphic cells with distinct cell borders. The nuclei are extremely hyperchromatic and contain coarse chromatin. The abundant keratinized cytoplasm is characteristically stained brightly eosinophilic with H & E and orangeophilic or deep green with Pap stain. Some squamous cancer cells do not reveal unequivocal features of malignancy; instead the ABC reveals mature, keratinizing cells with regular, hyperchromatic nuclei, reminiscent of the dysplastic squamous cells from the uterine cervix (**Fig. 4.19**). In a series studied by Engzell and Zajicek, 6% of their cases contained only benign-appearing squamous cells.[48]

When squamous carcinoma metastasizes to lymph nodes, it has a tendency to undergo cystic degeneration (**Fig. 4.20**). In such situations, not only is the cell concentration diluted but also the neoplastic cells may be obscured by inflammatory cells, foamy histiocytes, and necrotic debris, rendering interpretation more difficult.

Moderately and poorly differentiated squamous carcinomas (**Fig. 4.21**) show unequivocal malignant cells distributed singly or in syncytial sheets. The nuclei contain prominent nucleoli, coarsely granular hyperchromatic chromatin, and irregularly thickened nuclear membranes. The cytoplasm is modest and ill defined. In poorly differentiated tumors, keratinization is often minimal or not evident. With a careful search, a few squamous forms may be identified; otherwise, definitive classification may not be possible on the basis of FNAB. The spindle cell variant[49] is a rare form of squamous carcinoma and may simulate sarcoma (see Chapter 11, **Fig. 11.1**). To facilitate diagnosis, the metastatic cells must be compared with those from the primary tumor. Immunocytochemistry and electron microscopy are useful aids in differential diagnosis (see Chapter 16).

Adenocarcinoma

Cells of adenocarcinoma generally exhibit eccentric nuclei, prominent nucleoli, and cytoplasmic vacuolation (**Fig. 4.22**). Determination of the primary site on purely morphologic grounds is not always possible, but certain cytologic features, when present, may be sufficiently characteristic to suggest the origin of the tumor. Colonic adenocarcinomas most often consist of columnar cells arranged in palisades and forming three-dimensional clusters, papillae, and gland-like structures (**Fig. 4.23A**). The mucin-containing signet-ring type is poorly differentiated and most often originates from the stomach, although other sites are possible (**Fig. 4.23B**). Papillary adenocarcinoma with psammoma bodies in neck nodes suggests a thyroid primary, while the same ABC pattern in abdominal or pelvic nodes would indicate ovarian origin. Adenocarcinomas of the lung

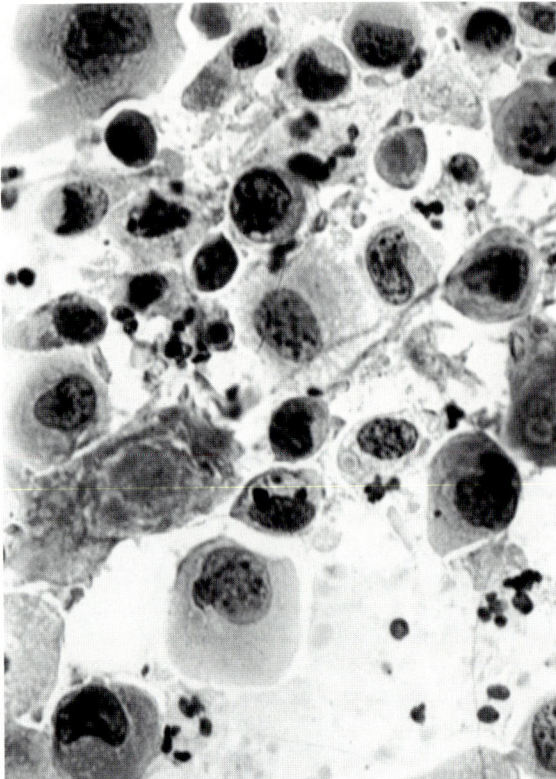

Figure 4.18. Well-differentiated squamous carcinoma metastatic to lymph node, ABC. The squamous cells are large and demonstrate no cell cohesion. The ample cytoplasm is eosinophilic and dense, with sharp cell borders. ×500.

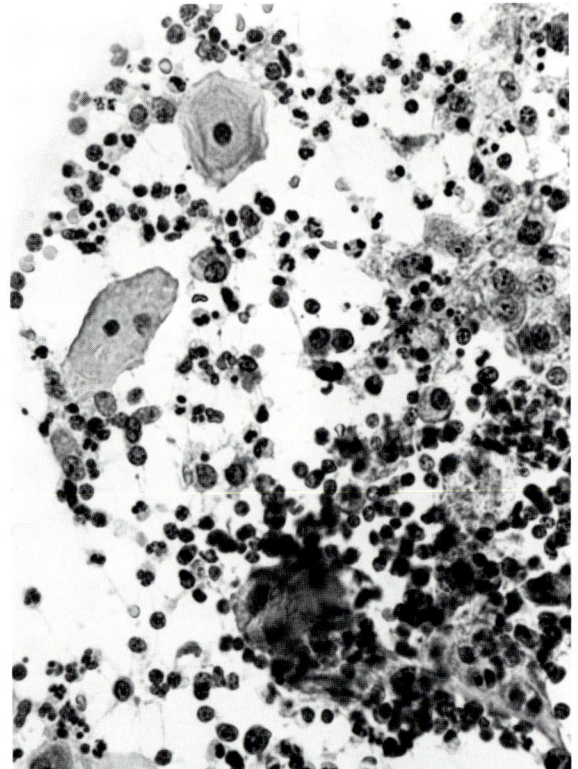

Figure 4.19. Well-differentiated squamous carcinoma metastatic to lymph node, ABC. The tumor cells shown here are mature cells that resemble dysplastic squamous cells of the uterine cervix. ×310.

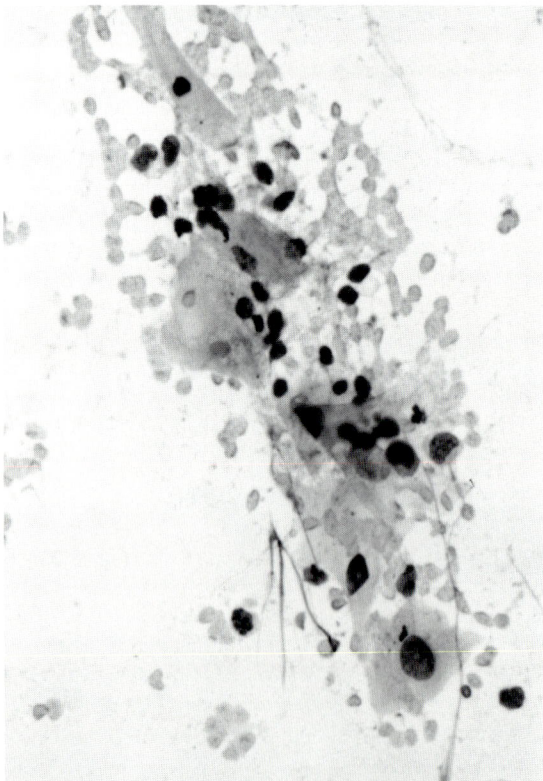

Figure 4.20. Cystic degeneration in a cervical lymph node containing squamous cell carcinoma, ABC. Note few keratinizing squamous cells admixed with lymphocytes and neutrophils in a cystic background. ×310.

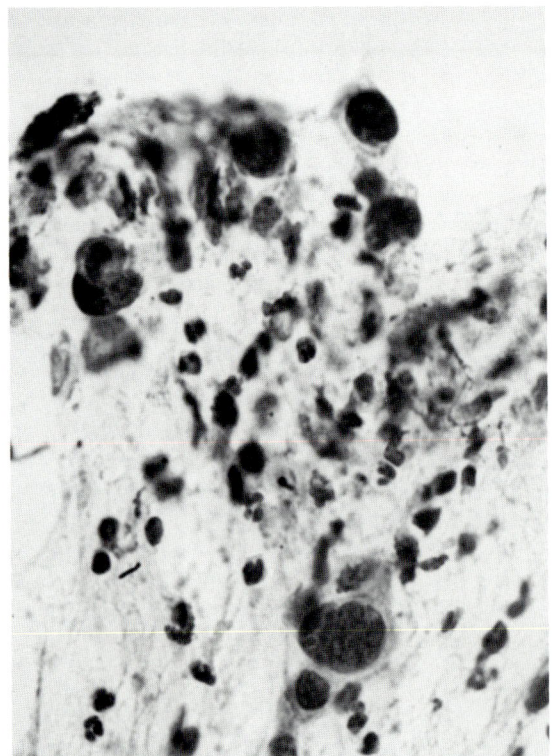

Figure 4.21. Poorly differentiated squamous carcinoma, ABC. Cytoplasmic keratinization is miminal. It is difficult to distinguish this lesion from large cell undifferentiated carcinoma, unless other malignant cells showing better differentiation are identified. ×500.

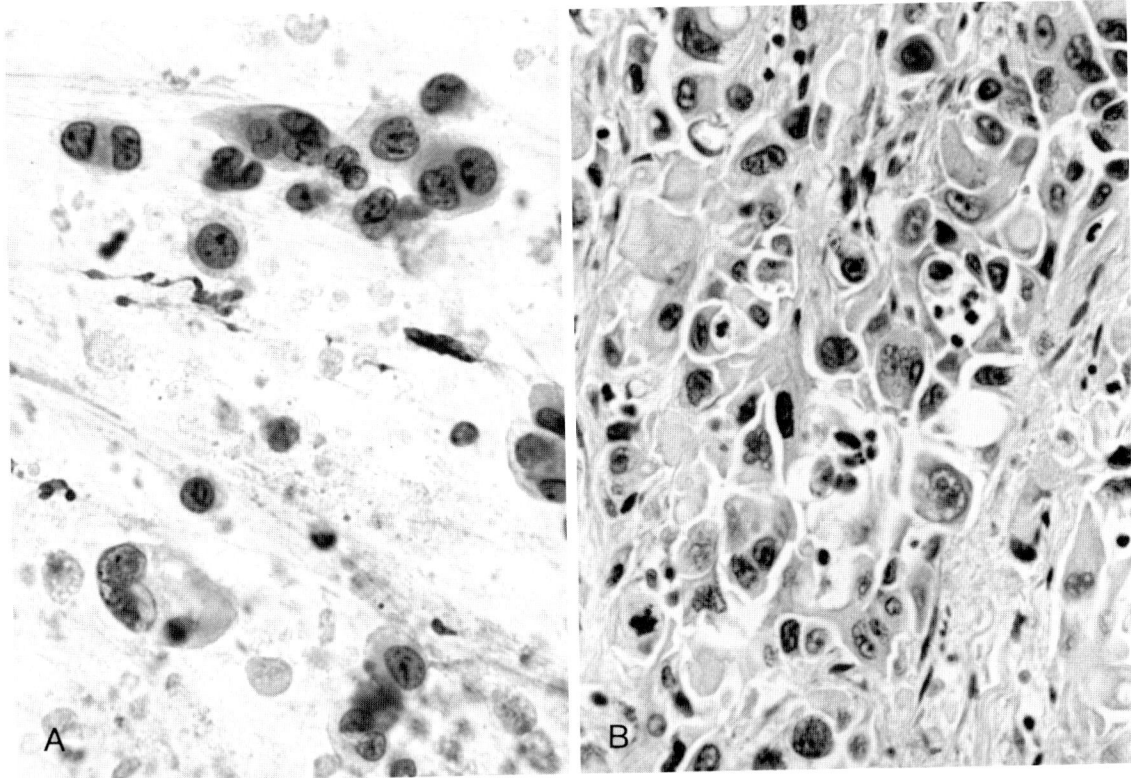

Figure 4.22. Adenocarcinoma metastatic to a celiac lymph node. **A**, ABC. The tumor cells are cuboidal or columnar in shape, have eccentric nuclei, prominant nucleoli, and foamy cyto-plasm. ×310. **B**, Autopsy histology of the primary adenocarci-noma of the stomach. ×310.

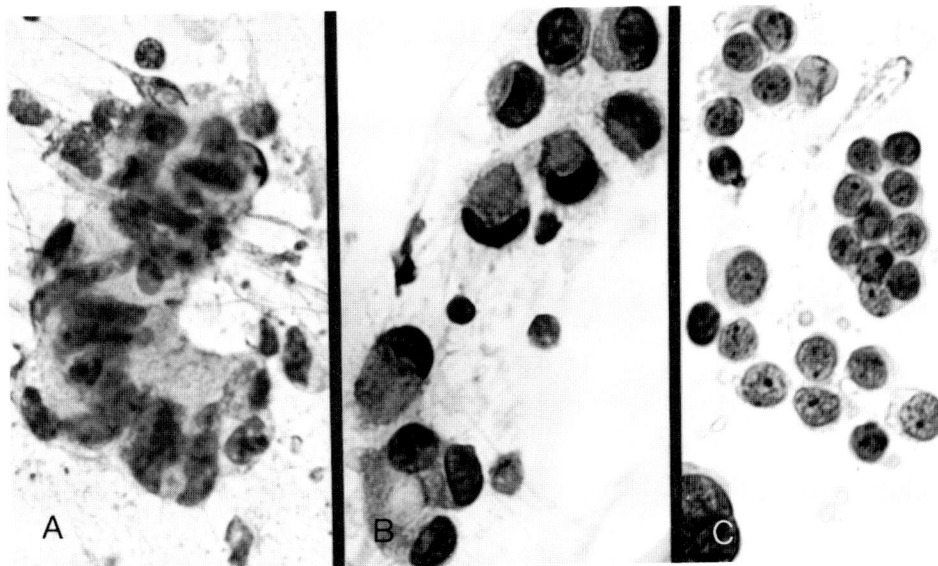

Figure 4.23. Adenocarcinomas, ABC. **A**, Colonic adenocarci-noma. Note tissue fragment composed of columnar cells with basal nuclei, in picket-fence arrangement. ×500. **B**, Signet-ring cell carcinoma from the stomach. Note dispersed tumor cells with eccentric hyperchromatic nuclei, indented by mucin vacu-oles. ×500. **C**, Breast carcinoma. Note uniform, round cells, ar-ranged in small monolayered groups. ×500.

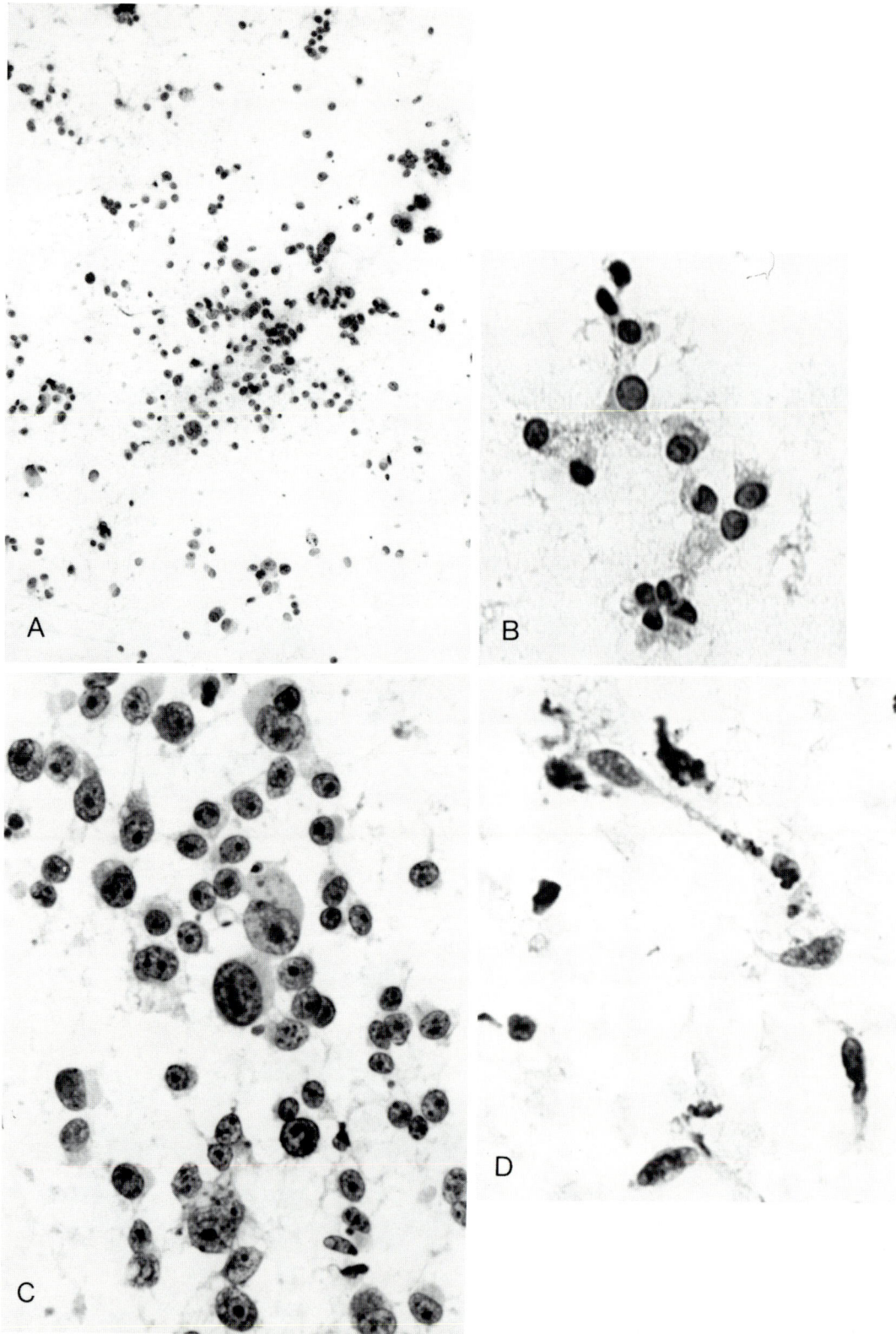

Figure 4.24.   Cytologic spectrum of malignant melanoma, ABC. **A**, Typical low-power view showing tumor cells lying singly and in small loose groups. A trimorphic population of melanoma cells (small, medium, and large cells) is discernable. ×125. **B**, Small-sized melanoma cells, with granulated cytoplasm. ×500. **C**, Ad- mixture of small, medium, and large melanoma cells, together forming a characteristic pattern. Note prominent nucleoli and cytoplasmic pigment granules. Some tumor cells have plasma-cytoid features. ×500. **D**, Spindle-shaped melanoma cells. ×500.

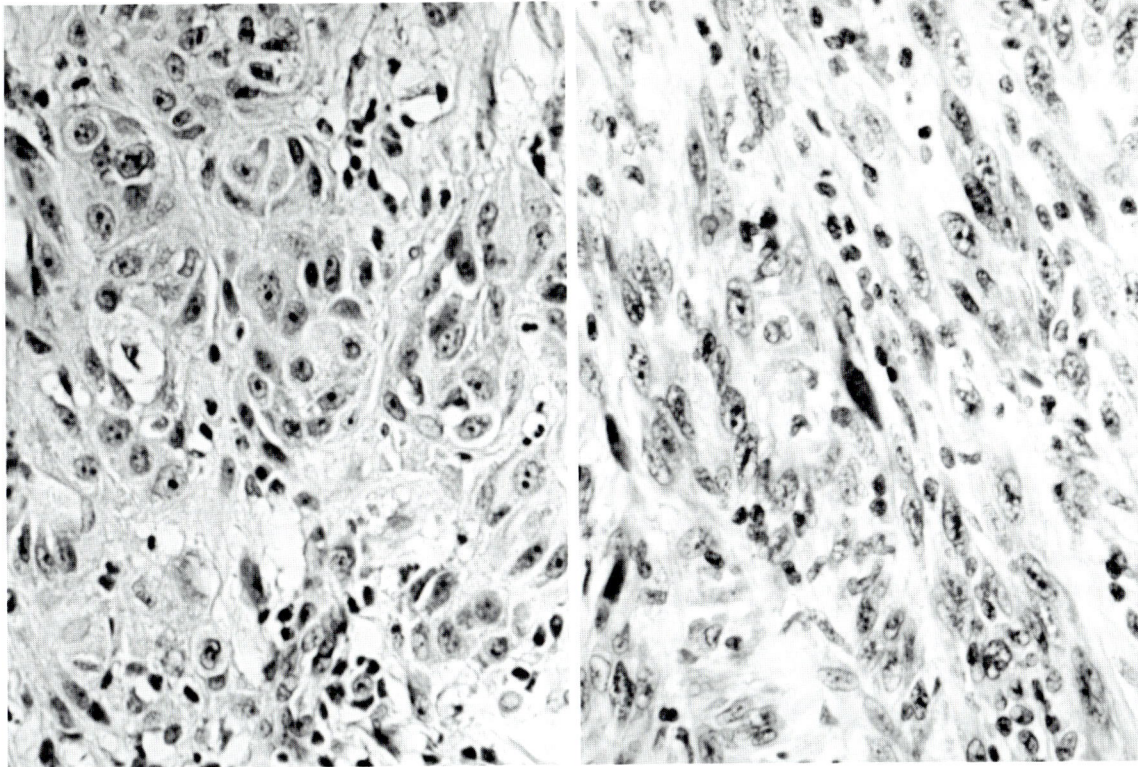

Figure 4.25. Histologic spectrum of malignant melanoma. **A**, Nests of dyshesive, tumor cells with prominent nucleoli and basophilic granulated cytoplasm. ×310. **B**, Spindle cell melanoma. The tumor cells assume a spindle form, otherwise the nuclear and cytoplasmic characteristics are similar to those shown in **A**. ×500.

and the breast generally do not exhibit cytologic features that betray their cellular origin. Nevertheless, ABC of small- to medium-sized malignant cells with intact cytoplasm, having only mild nuclear pleomorphism, in small clusters and single files or in a mononlayer of dyshesive cells suggests metastatic breast carcinoma (**Fig. 4.23C**). A common pattern for prostatic adenocarcinoma consists of relatively small, uniform, glandular cells forming a cribriform or microacinous pattern (see Chapter 14). A specific diagnosis can be made if immunocytochemical studies demonstrate prostatic acid phosphatase or prostatic specific antigen in the tumor cells.[50]

Malignant Melanoma

Malignant melanoma is a very aggressive neoplasm that can metastasize to regional lymph nodes and beyond to become widely disseminated to distant sites. The cytomorphology of this neoplasm (**Figs. 4.24 and 4.25**) has been reported in detail in the literature and is often diagnostic.[51-55] Most cells tend to be isolated but some loose aggregates are also present (**Fig. 4.24A**). The tumor cells are oval to round, and in some cases they are spindle-shaped. Binucleated and multinucleated cells are not infrequent. The nuclei are large. Nucleoli are prominent in many cells, and with the Papanicolaou

stain or hematoxylin and eosin stain perinucleolar halos are often seen. The cytoplasm is moderate to abundant. Melanin granules may be seen intracellularly both in the tumor cells and macrophages and extracellularly. Kline and Kannan[52] have stressed anisocytosis as a characteristic feature. They have recognized three distinct cell populations—small cells about 10 μm in diameter, medium size cells 10–20 μm in diameter, and giant cells. Together they form a characteristic pattern (**Fig. 4.24C**).

Other Metastatic Carcinomas

Metastatic small cell carcinoma is almost always from the lung, but can originate infrequently from diverse locations, such as the esophagus, salivary gland, pancreas, and cervix. The cytologic features are described in Chapter 7. For large cell or giant cell undifferentiated carcinoma, identification of the primary site may not be possible unless the patient is known to have a previously diagnosed cancer. Undifferentiated carcinomas, whether small or large cell, can be confused with malignant lymphoma. Ancillary studies and special stains should be done when indicated. The cytomorphology of hepatocarcinoma and renal cell carcinoma are distinctive and described elsewhere (see Chapters 9 and 12, respectively).

References

1. Bedrossian CWM, Martinez F, Silverberg AB. Fine needle aspiration. In Gnepp DR. Pathology of the head and neck. New York: Churchill Livingstone, 1988:25–99.

1a. Betsill WL, Hajdu SI. Percutaneous aspiration biopsy of lymph nodes. Am J Clin Pathol 1980;73:471–479.
2. Kline TS, Kannan V, Kline IK. Lymphadenopathy and aspiration bi-

opsy cytology. Review of 376 superficial nodes. Cancer 1984;54:1076–1081.

3. Bonfiglio TA, MacIntosh PK, Patten SF Jr, Cafer DJ, Woodworth FE, Kim CW. Fine needle aspiration cytopathology of retroperitoneal lymph nodes in the evaluation of metastatic disease. Acta Cytol 1979;23:126–130.

4. Suen KC. Guides to clinical aspiration biopsy: Retroperitoneum and intestine. New York: Igaku Shoin, 1987.

5. Kardos TF, Kornstein MJ, Frable WJ. Cytology and immunocytology of infectious mononucleosis in fine needle aspirates of lymph nodes. Acta Cytol 1988;32:722–726.

6. Metre MS, Jararam G. Acid-fast bacilli in aspiration smears from tuberculous lymph nodes. Acta Cytol 1987;31:17–19.

7. Bailey TM, Akhtar M, Ali MA. Fine needle aspiration biopsy in the diagnosis of tuberculosis. Acta Cytol 1985;29:732–736.

8. Silverman JF, Marrow HG. Fine needle aspiration cytology of granulomatous diseases of the lung, including nontuberculous mycobacterium infection. Acta Cytol 1985;29:535–541.

9. Silverman JF. Fine needle aspiration cytology of cat scratch disease. Acta Cytol 1985;29:542–547.

10. Christ ML, Feltes-Kennedy M. Fine needle aspiration cytology of toxoplasmic lymphadenitis. Acta Cytol 1982;26:425–428.

11. Stani J. Cytologic diagnosis of reactive lymphadenopathy in fine needle aspiration biopsy specimens. Acta Cytol 1987;31:8–13.

12. Silverberg E, Lubera J. Cancer statistics, 1987. CA 1987;37:2–19.

13. MacMahon B. Epidemiology of Hodgkin's disease. Cancer Res 1966;26:1189–1200.

14. Kern WH. Exfoliative and aspiration cytology of malignant lymphomas. Semin Diagn Pathol 1986;3:211–218.

15. Sneige N, Dekmezian RH, Fanning CV, Manning JT, Ordonez NG, Katz RL. Fine needle aspiration of malignant lymphomas: A cytologic and immunocytochemical study [Abstract]. Acta Cytol 1987;31:651.

16. Orell SR, Skinner JM. The typing of non-Hodgkin's lymphomas using fine needle aspiration cytology. Pathology 1982;14:389–394.

17. Qizilbash AH, Elavathil LJ, Chen V, Young JENM, Archibald SD. Aspiration biopsy cytology of lymph nodes in malignant lymphoma. Diagn Cytolopathol 1985;1:18–22.

18. Ramzy I, Rone R, Schultenover SJ, Buhaug J. Lymph node aspiration biopsy. Diagnostic reliability and limitations—An analysis of 350 cases. Diagn Cytopathol 1985;1:39–45.

18a. Carter TR, Feldman PS, Innes DJ, Frierson HF, Frigy AF. The role of fine needle aspiration cytology in the diagnosis of lymphoma. Acta Cytol 1988;32:848–853.

19. Pontifex AH, Klimo P. Application of aspiration biopsy cytology to lymphomas. Cancer 1984;53:553–556.

20. Jones SE, Butler JJ, Byrne GE, Coltman CA, Moon TE. Histologic review of lymphoma cases from the Southwest Oncology Group. Cancer 1977;39:1071–1076.

21. Rappaport H. Tumors of the hematopoietic system. Atlas of tumor pathology, Section 3, Fascicle 8. Washington D.C.: Armed Forces Institute of Pathology, 1966.

22. Lukes RJ, Collins RD. Immunologic characterization of human malignant lymphomas. Cancer 1974;34:1488–1503.

23. Lennert K. Histopathology of non-Hodgkin's lymphomas. Berlin: Springer-Verlag, 1981.

24. Rosenberg SA. Current concepts in cancer: non-Hodgkin's lymphoma—Selection of treatment on the basis of histologic type. N Engl J Med 1979;301:934–928.

25. Jaffe ES. Relationship of classification to biologic behavior of non-Hodgkin's lymphomas. Semin Oncol 1986;13:3–9.

26. The non-Hodgkin's lymphoma pathologic classification project: National Cancer Institute sponsored study of classification of non-Hodgkin's lymphomas: Summary and description of a working formulation for clinical usage. Cancer 1982;49:2112–2135.

27. Katz RL, Raval P, Manning JT, McLaughlin P, Barlogie B. A morphologic, immunologic, and cytometric approach to the classification of non-Hodgkin's lymphoma in effusions. Diagn Cytopathol 1987;3:91–101.

28. Das DK, Gupta SK, Datta U, Sharma SC, Datta BN. Malignant lymphoma of convoluted lymphocytes: Diagnosis by fine-needle aspiration cytology and cytochemistry. Diagn Cytopathol 1986;2:307–311.

29. George KT, Moriarty AT. Subclassification of non-Hodgkin's lymphoma by fine needle aspiration [Abstract]. Acta Cytol 1987;31:650.

30. Kline TS. Handbook of aspiration biopsy cytology, 2nd ed. New York: Churchill Livingstone, 1988:110.

31. DeVita VT Jr, Hellman S, Rosenberg SA. Cancer: Principles and practice of oncology. Philadelphia: Lippincott, 1982:1348.

32. Evans HL, Butler JJ, Youness EL. Malignant lymphoma, small lymphocytic type. Cancer 1978;41:1440–1455.

33. Selvaggi SM, Greco A, Fazzini E. Percutaneous fine-needle aspiration biopsy in malignant lymphoma: A case report of an unusual cytologic presentation. Diagn Cytolpathol 1986;2:295–300.

34. Robey SS, Cafferty LL, Beschorner WE, Gupta PK. Value of lymphocyte marker studies in diagnostic cytopathology. Acta Cytol 1987;31:453–459.

35. Martin SE, Zhang HZ, Magyarosy E, Jaffe ES, Hsu SM, Chu EW. Immunologic methods in cytology: Definitive diagnosis of non-Hodgkin's lymphomas using immunologic markers for T- and B-cells. Am J Clin Pathol 1984;82:666–673.

36. Friedman M, Kin U, Shimaoka K, Panahon A, Han T, Stutzman L. Appraisal of aspiration cytology in management of Hodgkin's disease. Cancer 1980;45:1653–1663.

37. Dmitrovsky E, Martin SE, Krudy AG, Chu EW, Jaffe ES, Longo DL, Young RC. Lymph node aspiration in the management of Hodgkin's disease. J Clin Oncol 1986;4:306–310.

38. Kardos TF, Vinson JH, Behm FQ, Frable WJ, O'Dowd GJ. Hodgkin's disease: Diagnosis by fine needle aspiration biopsy. Analysis of cytologic criteria from a selected series. Am J Clin Pathol 1986;86:286–291.

39. Strum SB, Park JK, Rappaport H. Observation of cells resembling Sternberg-Reed cells in conditions other than Hodgkin's disease. Cancer 1970;26:176–190.

40. Dorfman RF, Warnke R. Lymphadenopathy simulating the malignant lymphomas. Hum Pathol 1974;5:519–550.

41. Feldman PS, Kaplan MJ, Johns ME, Cantrell RW. Fine-needle aspiration in squamous cell carcinoma of the head and neck. Arch Otolaryngol 1983;109:735–742.

42. Russ JE, Scanlon EF, Christ MA. Aspiration cytology of head and neck masses. Am J Surg 1987;136:342–346.

43. Lee RE, Valaitis J, Kalis O, Sophian A, Schultz E. Lymph node examination by fine needle aspiration in patients with known or suspected malignancy. Acta Cytol 1987;31:563–572.

44. Ewing TL, Buchler DA, Hoogerland DL, Sonek MG, Wirtanen GW. Percutaneous lymph node aspiration in patients with gynecologic tumors. Am J Obstet Gynecol 1982;143:824–828.

45. Dolan TE, MacIntosh PK. Percutaneous retroperitoneal lymph node biopsy: An appraisal for a substitute to laparotomy in far advanced metastatic carcinoma. Gynecol Oncol 1981;11:364–370.

46. Copeland EM, McBride CM. Axillary metastases from an unknown primary site. Ann Surg 1973;178:25–27.

47. Zaren HA, Copeland EM. Inguinal node metastases. Cancer 1978;41:919–923.

48. Engzell U, Zajicek J. Aspiration biopsy of tumors of the neck. I. Aspiration biopsy and cytologic findings in 100 cases of congenital cysts. Acta Cytol 1970;14:51–57.

49. Schantz HD, Ramzy I, Tio FO, Buhaug J. Metastatic spindle-cell carcinoma. Cytologic features and differential diagnosis. Acta Cytol 1985;29:435–441.

50. Kline TS. Guides to clinical aspiration biopsy: Prostate. New York: Igaku Shoin, 1985.

51. Hajdu SI, Savino A. Cytologic diagnosis of malignant melanoma. Acta Cytol 1973;17:320–327.

52. Kline TS, Kannan V. Aspiration biopsy cytology and melanoma. Am J Clin Pathol 1982;77:597–601.

53. Woyke S, Domagala W, Czerniak B, Strokowska M. Fine needle aspiration cytology of malignant melanoma of the skin. Acta Cytol 1980;24:529–538.

54. Friedman M, Forgione H, Shanbhag V. Needle aspiration of metastatic melanoma. Acta Cytol 1980;24:7–15.

55. Perry MD, Gore M, Seigler HF, Johnston WW. Fine needle aspiration biopsy of metastatic melanoma. A morphologic analysis of 174 cases. Acta Cytol 1986;30:385–396.

5

Soft Tissues

Soft tissue is defined as nonepithelial extraskeletal tissue, exclusive of the reticuloendothelial system, glia, and supporting tissue of various parenchymal organs.[1] Virtually all primary soft tissue tumors arise from mesenchymal tissues and, by convention, neoplasms of the peripheral nerves are also considered as soft tissue tumors.

The technique of needle aspiration for soft tissue lesions is essentially the same as for other sites. In superficial lesions, the fascia should not be penetrated by the needle; in tumors located under the fascia, the deeper border of the lesion should not be passed.[2] Various authors[2–8] advocate using FNAB to investigate soft tissue lesions because: (a) the procedure is simple and requires no hospitalization; (b) it may yield sufficient information to distinguish malignant from benign soft tissue lesions; (c) depending on the circumstance, it may help streamline further investigation, facilitate multidisciplinary consultation, or provide a therapeutic approach; and (d) it can be used effectively, as a follow-up procedure, to confirm recurrence and diagnose metastases.

Controversy exists as to whether a formal open biopsy should be performed after a cytologic diagnosis has been obtained. Scandinavian workers[7] have effectively used needle aspiration to avoid many open biopsies; North American pathologists are more cautious. Mirra[8] estimated that, at UCLA, an open biopsy had been performed in approximately 70% of the patients after a needle biopsy or aspirate. At the same time, he found that needle biopsy was very useful in diagnosing lipomas, which are the most common soft tissue tumors. At the Cancer Control Agency of British Columbia, where large numbers of patients with histologically documented sarcomas are being treated and followed, FNAB is indispensable for detecting recurrence and metastases, obviating the need for an open biopsy.

The histologic type of a soft tissue sarcoma generally reflects its behavior. However, some sarcomas are so poorly differentiated that histologic typing is not feasible, and some tumors of the same histologic type, e.g., liposarcomas, may have a diverse biologic behavior. Problems in histologic typing have led some investigators to propose that the ''grade of malignancy'' is as important a prognostic factor as the histologic type of the tumor.[9–10] The American Joint Committee Task Force on Soft Tissue Sarcomas has emphasized the morphologic grade (well, moderately, or poorly differentiated), the size, and the clinical evidence of invasiveness of the primary tumor as important factors in predicting the biologic behavior of soft tissue sarcomas.[10] In general, sarcomas that have an abundant stroma and minimal cytologic atypia tend to be low to intermediate grade; whereas more cellular sarcomas with nuclear pleomorphism and frequent mitoses tend to be high grade.

Approach to Cytologic Interpretation

Due to limited material available in the needle aspirates, it is not always possible to classify soft tissue sarcomas on a histogenetic basis, unless a tumor is a recurrence or metastasis in which previous diagnosis is known. On the other hand, it is frequently possible to categorize soft tissue tumors into three main groups, based on the morphology of the tumor cells: namely, spindle cell tumors, pleomorphic cell tumors, and round cell tumors (**Table 5.1**).[2,3] After a

Table 5.1. Common Categories of Soft Tissue Tumors and Pseudotumors Classified on Fine Needle Aspirates

Benign Lesions
Soft tissue abscess
Lipoma
Spindle cell lesions
Nodular (pseudosarcomatous) fasciitis
Fibromatosis
Dermatofibrosarcoma protuberans[a] (skin and subcutis)
Schwannoma
Leiomyoma
Pleomorphic lesions
Pleomorphic lipoma (skin and subcutis)
Atypical fibroxanthoma (skin and subcutis)

Malignant Lesions
Spindle cell sarcomas
Fibrosarcoma
Leiomyosarcoma
Myxoid liposarcoma
Well-differentiated liposarcoma
Malignant schwannoma
Synovial sarcoma, monophasic
Angiosarcoma
Pleomorphic sarcomas
Malignant fibrous histiocytoma
Pleomorphic liposarcoma
Pleomorphic rhabdomyosarcoma
Round cell sarcomas
Small round cells
Embryonal and alveolar rhabdomyosarcomas
Ewing's sarcoma
Large round cells
Round cell liposarcoma
Epithelioid (tendosynovial) sarcoma
Alveolar soft part sarcoma[b]
Spindle and epithelial cell sarcoma
Synovial sarcoma, biphasic

[a] Not completely benign.
[b] Polyhedral rather than round cells.

soft tissue tumor is classified into one of these three groups, cytochemical, immunocytochemical, and electron microscopic studies may be helpful in further confirming the suspected cytodiagnosis. Irrespective of the histogenesis, tumor grade is an important prognostic feature, and this too can be evaluated on FNAB material. Moreover, this simple cytologic classification has therapeutic implication. According to Rosen,[11] round cell sarcomas, such as those seen in the pediatric age group, and round cell liposarcoma are responsive to alkylating agents and radiation therapy, whereas most spindle cell sarcomas are radiation- and chemotherapy-resistant. Pleomorphic sarcomas are mixed tumors that exhibit the worst characteristics of the spindle cell sarcoma (e.g., resistance to permanent local control with radiation therapy alone) and elements of the round cell sarcoma (e.g., tendency to metastasize and possibly require adjuvant systemic chemotherapy).

Importance of Clinical Correlation

Clinical information is indispensable to accurate FNAB interpretation.[8,12] Most of the sarcomas have their peak incidences beyond 40 years of age. Yet synovial sarcoma and those associated with tendon sheaths (epithelioid sarcoma and clear cell sarcoma) commonly occur in young adults, between 20 and 40 years of age. Embryonal rhabdomyosarcoma, alveolar rhabdomyosarcoma, and Ewing's sarcoma occur in the pediatric and adolescent age groups.

Pseudosarcomas such as nodular fasciitis or proliferative myositis tend to be less than 3 cm in size, while sarcomas tend to be large (>5 cm). The former lesions tend to grow rapidly at the onset and reach maximum size within 6–7 weeks. Any tumor with a history of continuous growth for more than 3 months is rarely, if ever, a reparative pseudosarcoma; on the other hand, swelling with stable growth that has been present for years usually represents a benign soft tissue tumor, such as lipoma.

Deep-seated tumors are usually malignant; whereas, superficial tumors (in dermis or subcutis) are usually benign neoplasms or reparative pseudosarcomas. However, epithelioid sarcoma and angiosarcoma are also superficially situated.[8]

Accuracy of Aspiration Cytology

Layfield and associates[4] reported a sensitivity of 95% and a specificity of 95% for the determination of malignancy in 136 FNAB cases of primary soft tissue tumors. False-positive and false-negative rates were both approximately 2%.

Of the 60 cases of sarcomas studied by Miralles et al.,[2] FNAB was used to correctly make the initial diagnosis of malignancy in 22 patients and confirmed either a local recurrence or the presence of metastases in 38 patients. Among the 57 benign or nonneoplastic lesions, there were two false-positive diagnoses of nonmalignant lesions as low-grade sarcomas.

In our series of 22 cases of retroperitoneal sarcomas,[3] 19 cases were correctly diagnosed or suggested by FNAB, two cases were incorrectly typed as poorly differentiated adenocarcinoma (these occurred in the early part of the study when immunoperoxidase staining technique was not in use), and one case had a false-negative diagnosis. There was one false-positive diagnosis in which a cellular schwannoma was misinterpreted as sarcoma.

BENIGN SOFT TISSUE TUMORS AND PSEUDOTUMORS
Soft Tissue Abscess

A soft tissue abscess as a space-occupying lesion can mimic a soft tissue neoplasm. Experience in the literature[13] indicates that di-

agnosis of soft tissue infections has been delayed or made incorrectly because of reliance on indirect means to determine the etiologic agents. A simple direct method is the needle aspiration of these lesions, combined with Gram stain and culture studies. Proper early diagnosis hastens resolution of the inflammatory process and can be life-saving in some cases. Aspiration yields purulent exudate with numerous polymorphonuclear leukocytes, lymphocytes, and macrophages in a necrotic background (Fig. 5.1).

Lipoma

Lipoma is the most frequently encountered soft tissue tumor and always enters in the differential diagnosis of soft tissue sarcoma. While liposarcomas are deep-seated, lipomas are nearly always superficial. The fat content of a lipoma can be identified by determining its density on computerized tomography. In a patient with a long history of a superficial lesion and a CT scan and a FNAB diagnosis compatible with lipoma, continued observation may be all that is required. On the other hand, if the tumor is not superficial and there is evidence of unabated growth, consideration should be given to the diagnosis of liposarcoma or other sarcomas.

Aspiration Cytology

The needle aspirate of a typical lipoma may contain visible gelatinous fat globules. On microscopic examination, there are fragments of adipose tissue composed of large, mature fat cells (Fig. 5.2). The cytoplasm is voluminous. The nuclei are small and round, displaced toward the periphery of the cytoplasm by a single large lipid vacuole. Neither nuclear pleomorphism nor prominent nucleoli are present.

Several variants of lipoma with overlapping morphologic features are recognized. The spindle cell lipoma is characterized by mature fat cells with variable numbers of spindle cells. The pleomorphic lipoma, which is thought to represent degenerative changes in a preexisting spindle cell lipoma, is characterized by many bizarre atypical giant cells in addition to the mature fat cells and spindle cells. Some of the multinucleated giant cells display circular, peripheral arrangement of the nuclei, an arrangement not unlike the petals of a small flower (Fig. 5.3). These cells are referred to as floret cells and are characteristic, but not specific, for pleomorphic lipoma.[3,14,14a]

Diagnostic Pitfalls and Discussion. Since lipoma cannot be distinguished cytologically from normal adipose tissue, one must make certain that the aspirated material is representative of the lesion and not derived from the normal subcutaneous adipose tissue.

In the rare instances when the lipoma is intramuscular, the inclusion of atrophic muscle fibers in the aspirated samples has caused confusion. The degenerated myocytes have been mistaken for malignant giant cells.[7]

Although the diagnosis of an ordinary lipoma is straightforward, a pleomorphic lipoma may be mistaken for a giant cell malignancy of epithelial or nonepithelial origin. Moreover, on the basis of morphology alone, it is sometimes not possible to separate spindle cell lipoma or pleomorphic lipoma from well-differentiated liposarcoma, since all these lesions contain atypical spindle cells. The observation of the floret cells is a helpful diagnostic clue; they are present characteristically in large numbers in pleomorphic lipomas and are infrequent in well-differentiated liposarcomas. The site of the tumor is another important differentiating feature. Pleomorphic lipomas tend to occur in the head and neck, shoulder and upper back of elderly patients.[14] Azumi et al.[14a] found that the biologic behavior of differentiated lipomatous neoplasms (which include lesions pre-

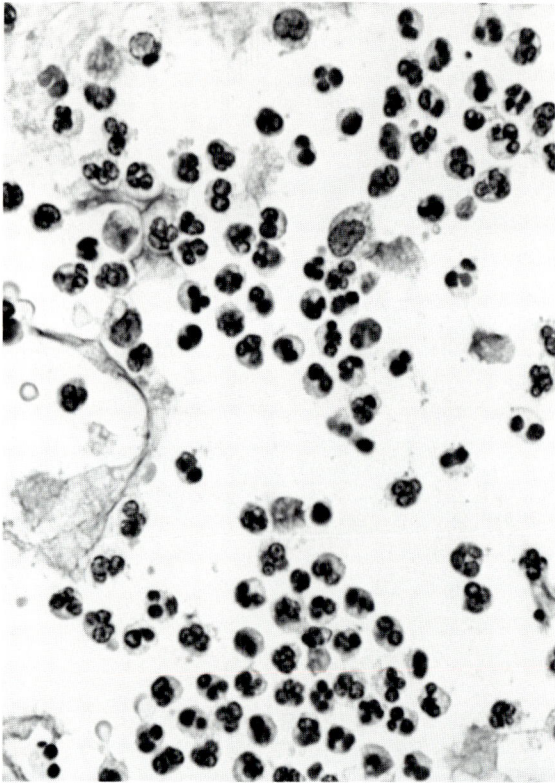

Figure 5.1.   Soft tissue abscess, ABC. Note numerous polymorphonuclear leukocytes and some histiocytes. ×500.

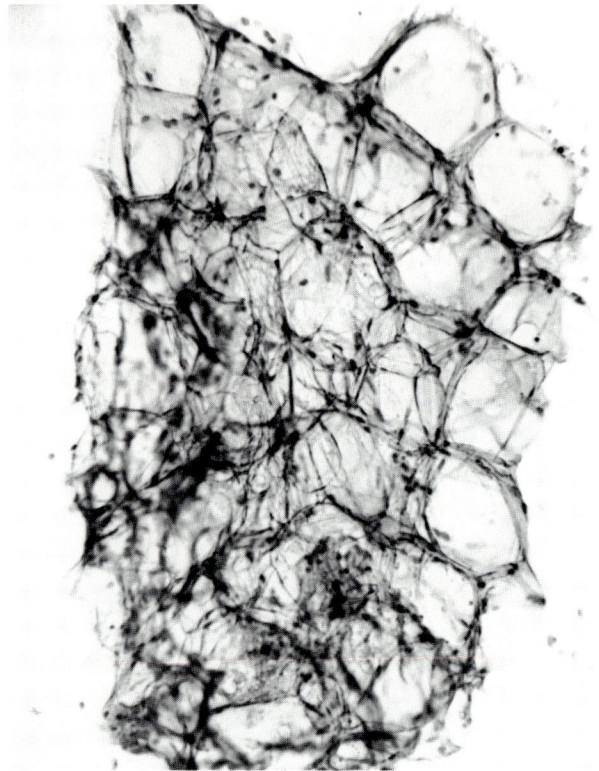

Figure 5.2.   Lipoma, ABC. Note tissue fragment composed of large univacuolar lipocytes with small peripheral nuclei. ×310.

viously called "spindle cell lipoma," "pleomorphic lipoma," and "well-differentiated liposarcoma") correlated better with the location than with the histology of the tumor. Those in the subcutis behaved in a benign manner with no recurrences; those arising in the deep somatic soft tissue and within muscles were more aggressive and tended to recur locally, whereas the retroperitoneal ones behaved like a low-grade liposarcoma, which might kill the host through uncontrolled growth.

Nodular Fasciitis

Nodular fasciitis is a nonneoplastic, exuberant proliferation of fibroblasts and myofibroblasts, accompanied by chronic inflammatory cells. The lesion has a typical clinical presentation: rapid growth, tenderness, and <3 cm size. Enzinger and Weiss[1] have identified three types of nodular fasciitis: the subcutaneous, the intramuscular, and the fascial type. The subcutaneous (superficial) type is four times more common than either the intramuscular or fascial type.

Aspiration Cytology

The aspirates are typically cellular. The basic cells are the fibroblasts, which are generally larger than normal and may vary in size and shape. Some have slender tapered nuclei and variable amount of pink-staining cytoplasm; others have plump, oval nuclei with prominent nucleoli (**Fig. 5.4**). While the majority of the cells are fibroblastic, others may be derived from macrophages. Many cases show a high mitotic activity, which reflects the rapid growth rate of nodular fasciitis and is not an indicator of malignancy. Inflammatory cells including lymphocytes, plasma cells, and macrophages can be seen frequently.

Diagnostic Pitfalls.   The most important thing in the diagnosis of nodular fasciitis is for the cytologist to be cognizant of the

lesion when the clinical history is suggestive. Histologically, the lesion may be mistaken for sarcoma because of its alarmingly high cellularity and increased mitotic activity. Yet Dahl and Akerman[15] stress that on FNAB all the cells lack the cytologic features of malignancy. The fibroblasts resemble those seen in inflammatory and repair processes, rather than those seen in fibrosarcomas.

Fibromatosis

The term *fibromatosis* covers a broad group of fibrous tissue proliferations that have a tendency toward recurrence but do not metastasize like fibrosarcomas. Other synonyms used are desmoid tumor and nonmetastasizing fibrosarcoma or grade I fibrosarcoma. Fibromatosis does not include nonspecific reactive fibrous proliferations that are part of an inflammatory or reparative process. Fibromatoses can be broadly divided into two groups: superficial and deep or musculoaponeurotic.[1] The superficial group includes palmar, plantar, and penile fibromatosis. These lesions are characterized by subcutaneous nodular or plaque-like fibrosis with contracture deformity in the palm, sole, and penile shaft, respectively. The clinical features are rather specific; therefore, aspiration biopsy is seldom performed. The deep, or musculoaponeurotic, group of fibromatosis often attains a large size and involves deeper structures, particularly the musculature of the trunk and the extremities.

Aspiration Cytology

The aspirates vary considerably in cellularity, depending on the amount of extracellular collagenous stroma present in the tumor (**Fig. 5.5**). The more abundant is the collagenous matrix, the less is the cellularity. The four cases reported by McLeod et al.[16] yielded sparsely cellular aspirates.

The cells are fibroblastic in nature, characterized by spindle

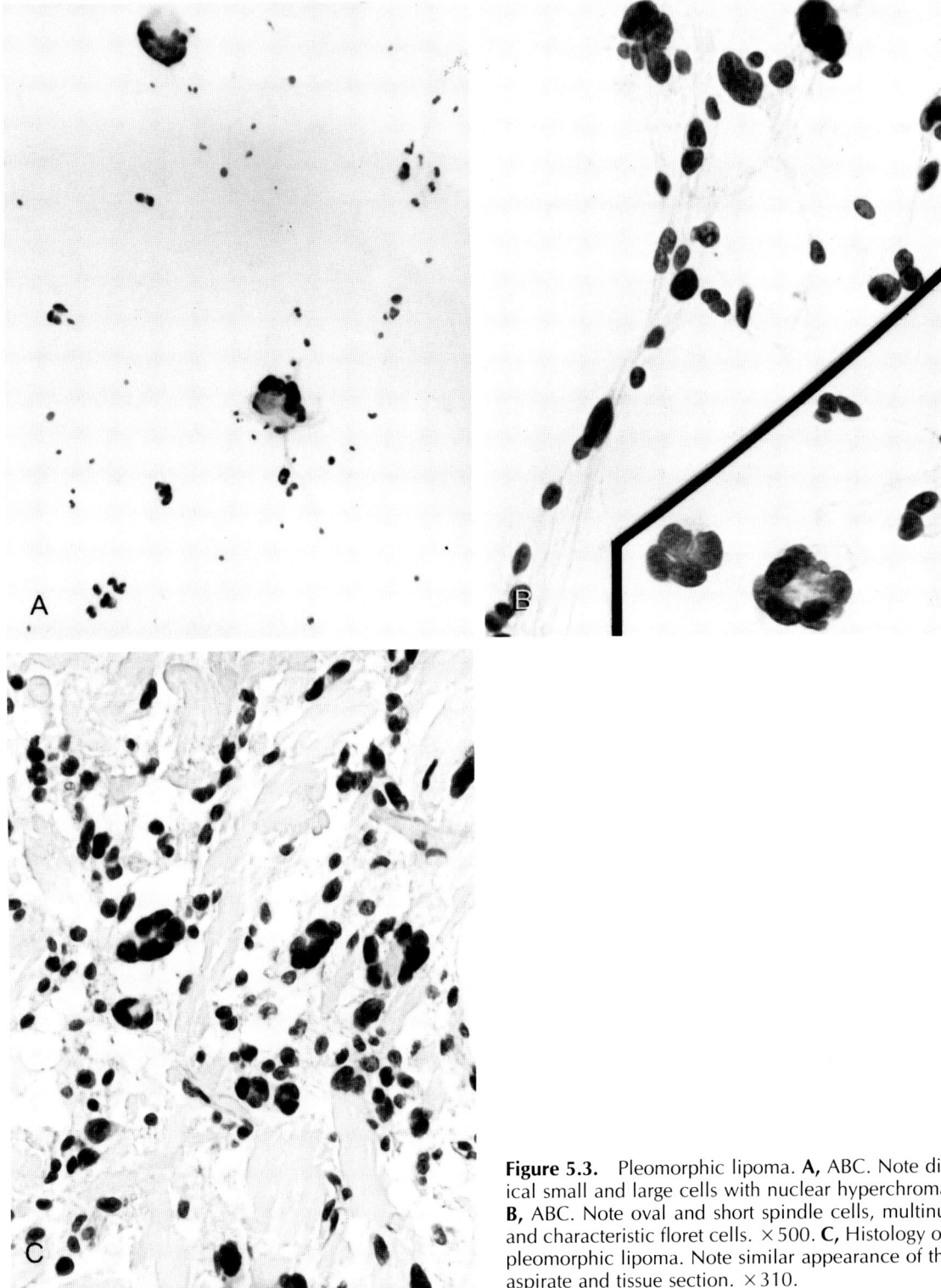

Figure 5.3. Pleomorphic lipoma. **A,** ABC. Note dispersed atypical small and large cells with nuclear hyperchromatism. ×125. **B,** ABC. Note oval and short spindle cells, multinucleated cells and characteristic floret cells. ×500. **C,** Histology of the resected pleomorphic lipoma. Note similar appearance of the cells in the aspirate and tissue section. ×310.

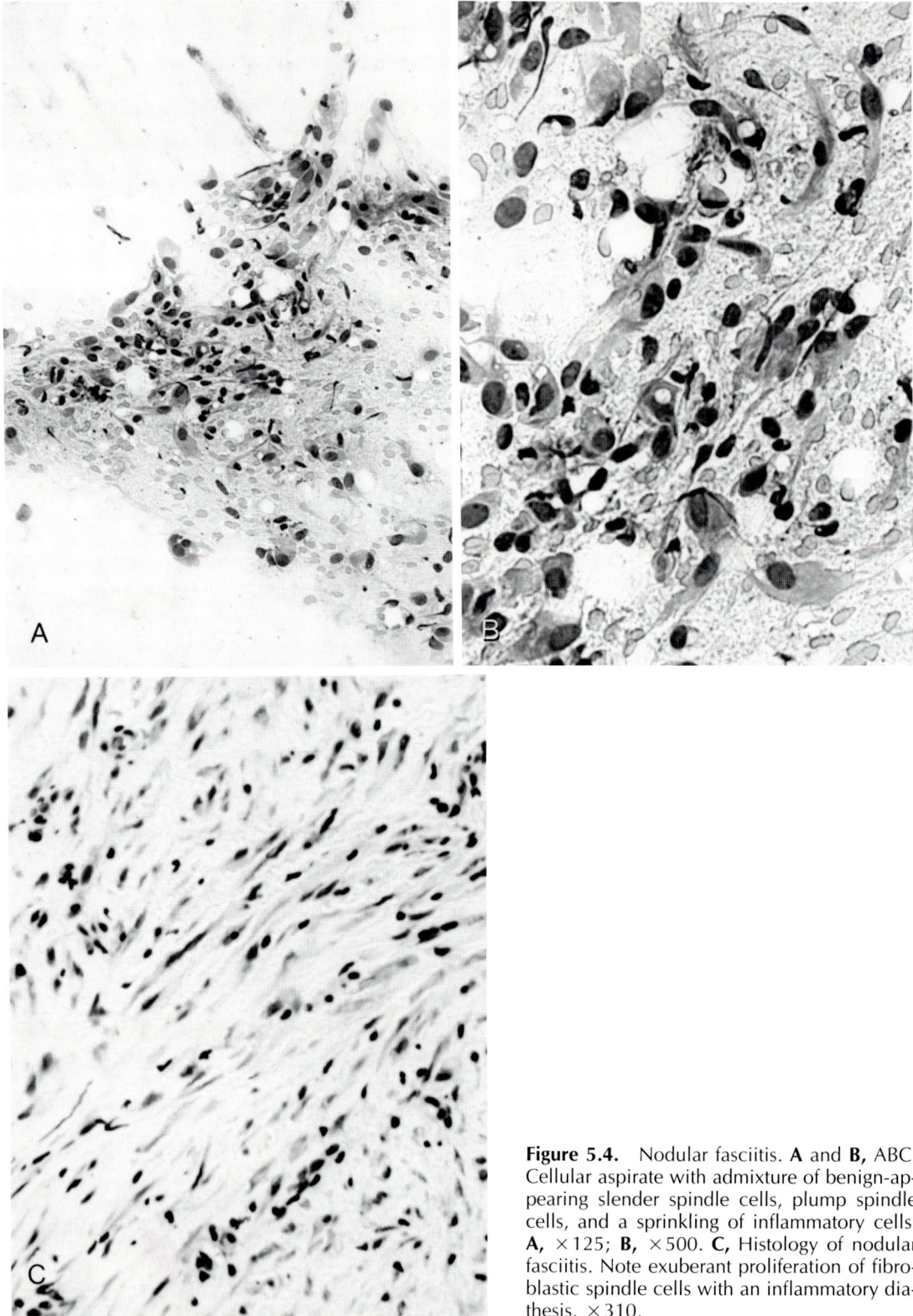

Figure 5.4. Nodular fasciitis. **A** and **B,** ABC. Cellular aspirate with admixture of benign-appearing slender spindle cells, plump spindle cells, and a sprinkling of inflammatory cells. **A,** ×125; **B,** ×500. **C,** Histology of nodular fasciitis. Note exuberant proliferation of fibroblastic spindle cells with an inflammatory diathesis. ×310.

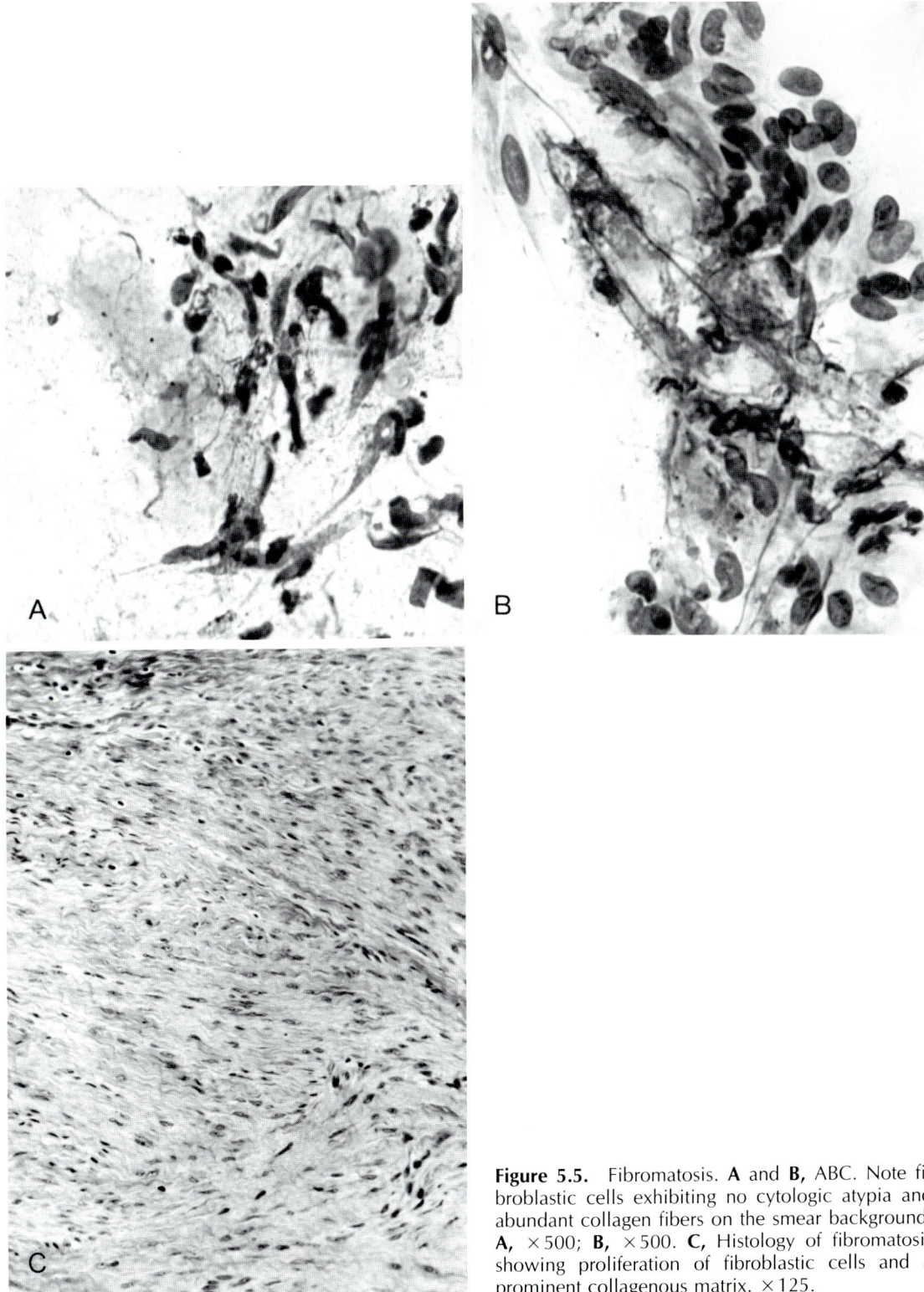

Figure 5.5. Fibromatosis. **A** and **B**, ABC. Note fibroblastic cells exhibiting no cytologic atypia and abundant collagen fibers on the smear background. **A**, ×500; **B**, ×500. **C**, Histology of fibromatosis showing proliferation of fibroblastic cells and a prominent collagenous matrix. ×125.

shape with tapered ends. The nuclei are fusiform, and there are occasional lobated and twisted forms. The chromatin is uniformly distributed; some cells contain small nucleoli. Atypical hyperchromatic or bizarre nuclei are not observed. Unlike nodular faciitis, mitotic activity is either rare or absent, and inflammatory cells are not present. On the other hand, an appreciable collagen diathesis is usually present on the background.

Diagnostic Pitfalls. In some instances, the distinction between a fibromatosis and a well-differentiated fibrosarcoma is very difficult or even impossible. In general, the lack of abnormal mitoses and nuclear atypia is valuable in indicating that the lesion is not a sarcoma.

Dermatofibrosarcoma Protuberans

Dermatofibrosarcoma protuberans is a low-grade malignancy that has a propensity for local recurrence but rarely metastasizes. A fully developed dermatofibrosarcoma protuberans has a typical gross appearance that is characterized by a nodular cutaneous growth that often protrudes above the skin surface, which may be reddish or bluish in color and is liable to ulcerate. Histologically, the tumor is composed of compact bundles of spindle fibroblast-like cells, arranged radially in a cartwheel or storiform pattern. There is usually little nuclear pleomorphism and only low to moderate mitotic activity.

Aspiration Cytology

The aspirates consist of fascicles of benign-appearing, slender spindle cells cytologically indistinguishable from those seen in fibromatosis, but extracellular collagenous material is not as prominent **(Fig. 5.6)**. The spindle cells have a tendency to swirl, mirroring the storiform pattern seen in histologic sections.[17] A correct diagnosis can be made if the cytological picture is correlated with the typical gross appearance of the lesion.

Schwannoma (Neurilemoma)

Schwannoma is a benign, slow-growing, encapsulated neoplasm of the Schwann cells. These tumors are seldom larger than 3–4 cm in diameter. Although many exceptions occur, small tumors are often homogeneously fibrous and solid, whereas large variants tend to be cystic with myxoid degeneration.

Aspiration Cytology

ABC shows variable numbers of isolated spindle cells and tissue fragments composed of spindle cells. Although the classic slender nuclei of the Schwann cells are described as being bent or wavy and having pointed ends, in fact many of the nuclei are indistinguishable from those of the fibroblastic cells. The cytoplasm is moderately abundant and may show tangled hairline cytoplasmic pro-

cesses. Both Antoni type A and Antoni type B tissues can be seen in the aspirates **(Figs. 5.7 and 5.8)**. The Antoni type A tissue **(Fig. 5.8A)** is represented by compact tissue fragments composed of fascicles of spindle cells in palisade orientation, with little intervening stromal tissue. Within the Antoni type A tissues, one may see Verocay bodies **(Fig. 5.8B)**, which consist of a central core of fibrillar material lying between two bundles of spindle cells.[18] The Antoni type B tissue, on the other hand, is repesented by loosely textured, myxofibrillar stroma with few spindle cells **(Fig. 5.8C)**.

Diagnostic Pitfalls. Schwannomas are distinguished from fibroblastic lesions by cells having palisading nuclei, fibrillary cytoplasm, and a myxofibrillary smear background. S100 protein reactivity is demonstrable in Schwann cells but absent in fibroblasts. Schwannomas are frequently associated with a nerve, and thus sharp radiating pain experienced by the patient during the aspiration would suggest a schwannoma rather than a fibroblastic tumor.

We misinterpreted a case of retroperitoneal schwannoma as spindle cell sarcoma **(Fig. 5.9)**. One must bear in mind that an occasional schwannoma can be very cellular and contains bizarre cells.[3,19] These bizarre cells probably represent a degenerative phenomenon. Caution is needed in the interpretation of these tumors. Cellular atypia in a schwannoma does not necessarily denote malignancy unless it is associated with tumor necrosis and increased mitotic activity.

Myxoma

This is an uncommon benign tumor whose histologic features resemble those of the core of the umbilical cord of the mature fetus.[20] Some of these tumors are located intramuscularly, mostly in the thigh, buttock, shoulder, and upper arm, and generally measure 5–10 cm in diameter. Despite its rarity, intramuscular myxoma is important because clinically and pathologically it may be confused with a soft tissue sarcoma, particularly myxoid liposarcoma.[20]

Aspiration Cytology

The ABC reveals a large amount of myxomatous material in which a small number of cells are embedded. The latter are spindle or stellate in shape with drawn out cytoplasmic processes and have regular fusiform nuclei **(Fig. 5.10)**. The paucity of cells and their innocuous appearance serve to distinguish myxomas from well-differentiated myxoid liposarcomas.

Leiomyoma

Cutaneous leiomyomas are small tumors that generally fall into the domain of the dermatologists. These tumors can be readily excised in toto and aspiration biopsy is superfluous. Larger leiomyomas occur in the uterus and stomach. For cytologic description, see under ''Smooth Muscle Tumors'' in Chapter 11.

Figure 5.6. Dermatofibrosarcoma protuberans. **A,** ABC. Note tangled mass of swirling spindle cells. × 500. **B,** Histology of the resected dermatofibrosarcoma protuberans showing a cellular tumor composed of spindle cells in storiform arrangement. Note similarity between cytologic and histologic features. × 125.

Figure 5.7. A large schwannoma arising in the groin of a 54-year-old man. **A,** ABC. Note many small cellular tissue fragments

(Antoni type A tissue) as well as isolated spindle cells in a myxoid background (Antoni type B tissue). × 125. **B,** Histologic features of the resected schwannoma. Note morphologic resemblance to the cytologic features seen in the aspirate. The cellular Antoni A area is seen in the *upper half* of the figure and the Antoni B area, composed of myxoid stroma with sparse spindle cells, is seen in the *lower half.* × 100.

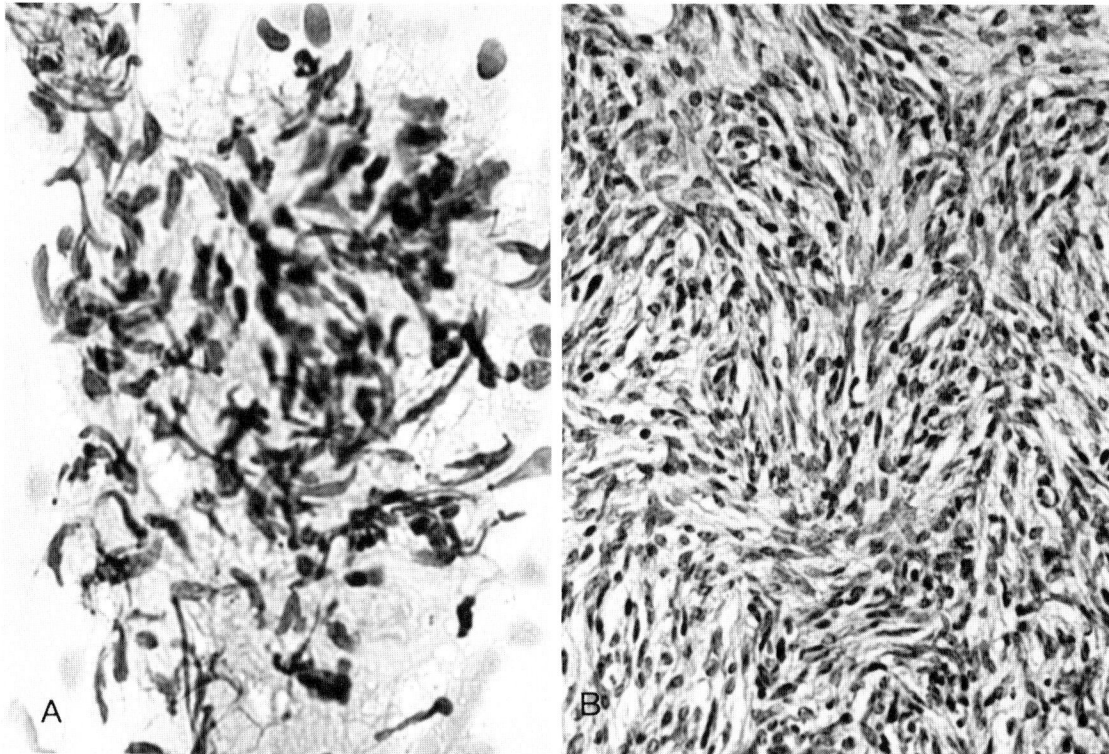

Figure 5.6.

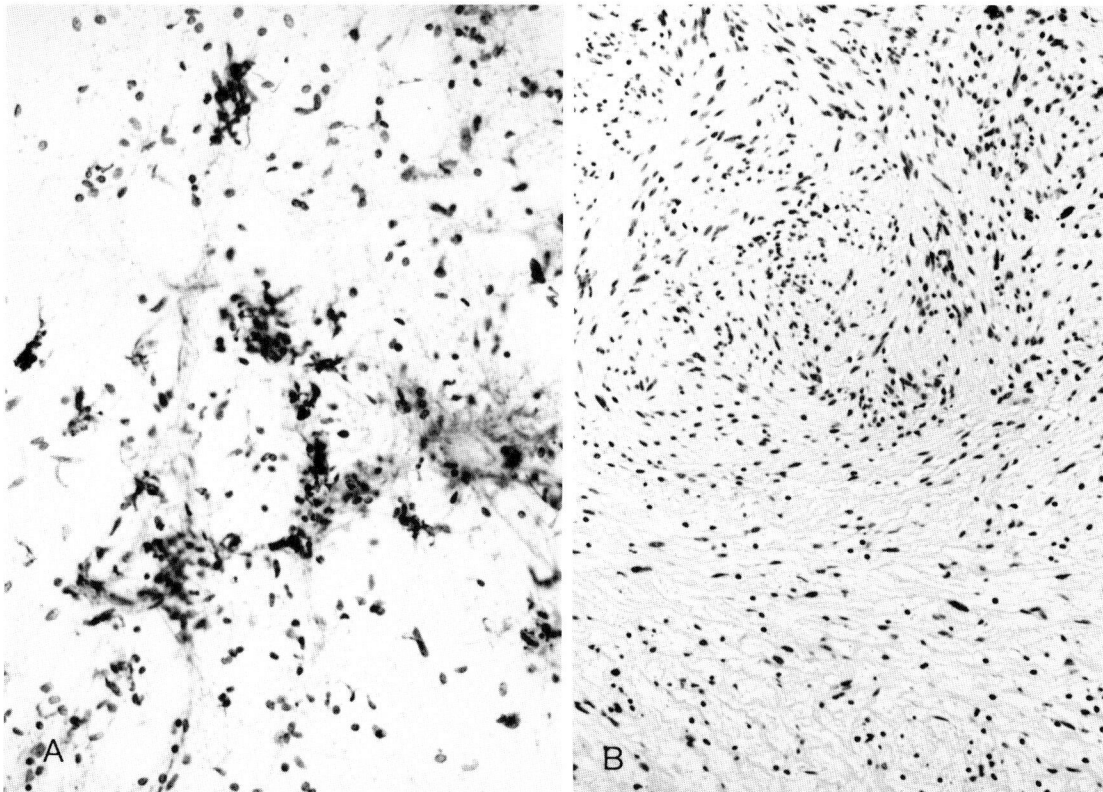

Figure 5.7.

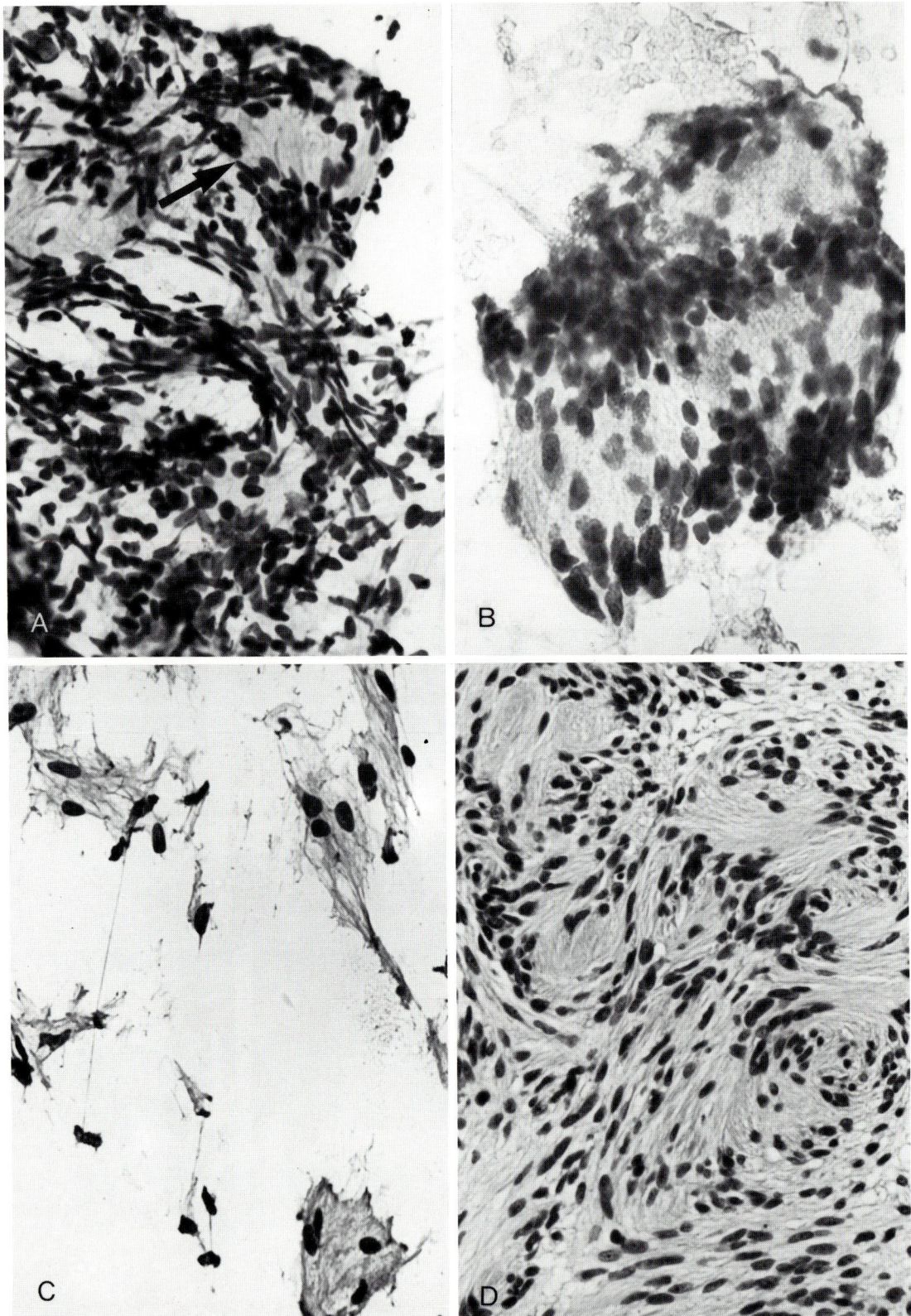

Figure 5.8.   Schwannoma. **A,** ABC. Antoni type A tissue show-ing hypercellularity and palisading nuclei. *Arrow* shows fibrillary background. ×500. **B,** ABC. Verocay bodies. ×600. **C,** ABC. Antoni type B tissue showing paucity of spindle cells. Also note characteristic fibrillary cytoplasmic processes. ×500. **D,** Histol-ogy of schwannoma showing Antoni A area with Verocay bod-ies. Note characteristic fibrillary cytoplasm and matrix. ×310.

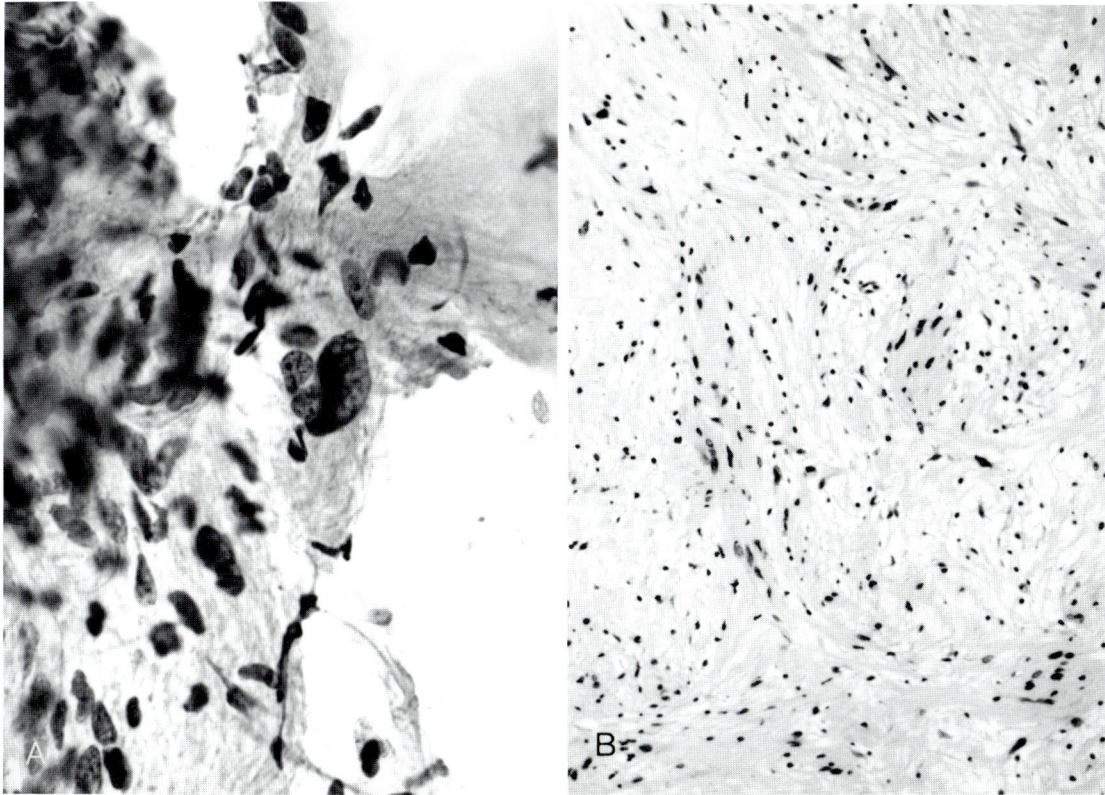

Figure 5.9. Schwannoma with cellular atypia (false-positive diagnosis). **A,** ABC. Note large cells with atypical hyperchromatic nuclei. The fibrillary appearance of the cytoplasm is typical of neurogenic cells. ×500. **B,** Tissue section of the resected schwannoma showing atypical cells. ×125.

SPINDLE CELL SARCOMAS
Fibrosarcoma

Fibrosarcoma may arise at any site, but most occur in the extremities. The vast majority are deep, large tissue masses. Up to 15 years ago, almost all spindle cell collagen-producing sarcomas were classified as fibrosarcomas. Today, the apparent incidence of fibrosarcomas has greatly decreased because the diagnosis is made less often due to the emergence of malignant fibrous histiocytoma as a defined entity.

Aspiration Cytology

Cells of well-differentiated fibrosarcomas are elongated and readily recognized as fibroblastic. The individual cells are distinguished from those derived from fibromatosis by their atypical hyperchromatic nuclei and mitotic activity **(Fig. 5.11)**. Poorly differentiated fibrosarcomas are easily recognized as spindle cell sarcoma because the tumor cell nuclei show obvious malignant characteristics.

Diagnostic Pitfalls. The cytopathologist must keep in mind that even though FNAB of the tumor may show the appearance of a fibrosarcoma, this does not necessarily mean that the primary line of differentiation is indeed fibroblastic, as fibrosarcomatous foci are a common feature of malignant fibrous histiocytomas, synovial sarcomas, and liposarcomas. Multiple aspirations from different parts of the lesion can minimize sampling errors. For example, bizarre multinucleated giant cells are not a feature of fibrosarcomas, and their presence in a sarcoma usually means that the lesion is more likely malignant fibrous histiocytoma or liposarcoma.

Myxoid Liposarcoma

The major sites of occurrence of liposarcomas are the extremities, particularly the thigh, and the retroperitoneum. These tumors are generally between 7 and 10 cm in size, although some may be larger. The myxoid and the well-differentiated liposarcoma are the commonest types of liposarcomas, each constituting about 30–40% of all the liposarcomas. The less common types are the pleomorphic and the round cell variant. In terms of clinical behavior, the well-differentiated and myxoid types are much less aggressive than the other two types.[1,21] Myxoid liposarcoma is discussed here; other types will be described separately in later sections.

Aspiration Cytology

Cellular Pattern. Myxoid liposarcomas have three basic components: cellular, vascular, and myxoid **(Figs. 5.12 and 5.13)**.[7,22,23] The ABC characteristically shows abundant filmy, basophilic, myxoid material derived from the tumor matrix, which is rich in acid mucopolysaccharides. Embedded within the myxoid matrix are the tumor cells and small tubular blood vessels with sharply angulated branches. The proportions of tumor cells and stroma vary considerably from case to case. Even within the same tumor, certain areas may contain numerous tumor cells and others may exhibit a myxoid stroma with few cells.

Cell Morphology. Most of the tumor cells are rather bland, short, and spindly or stellate, and the cytoplasm is not vacuolated. These nonvacuolated cells are referred to as prelipoblasts.[21] In some aspirates, classic lipoblasts are scarce, but, if diligently searched for, they will be seen. A lipoblast is a lipogenic cell whose cytoplasm is

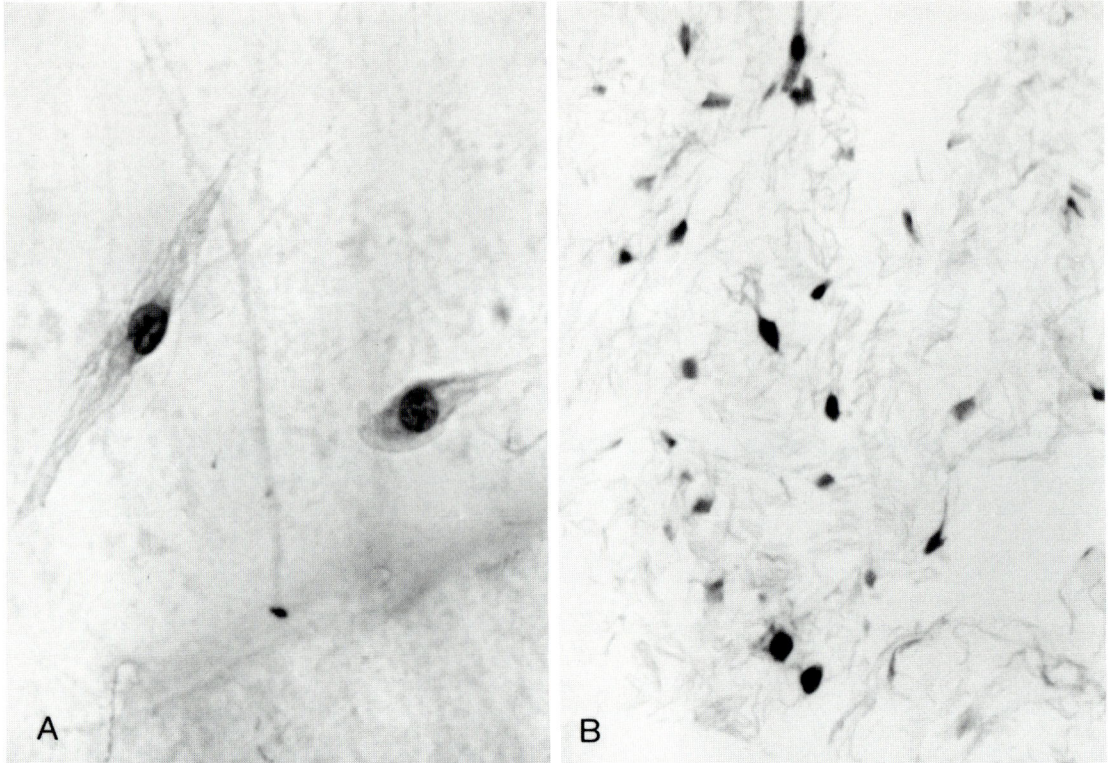

Figure 5.10.

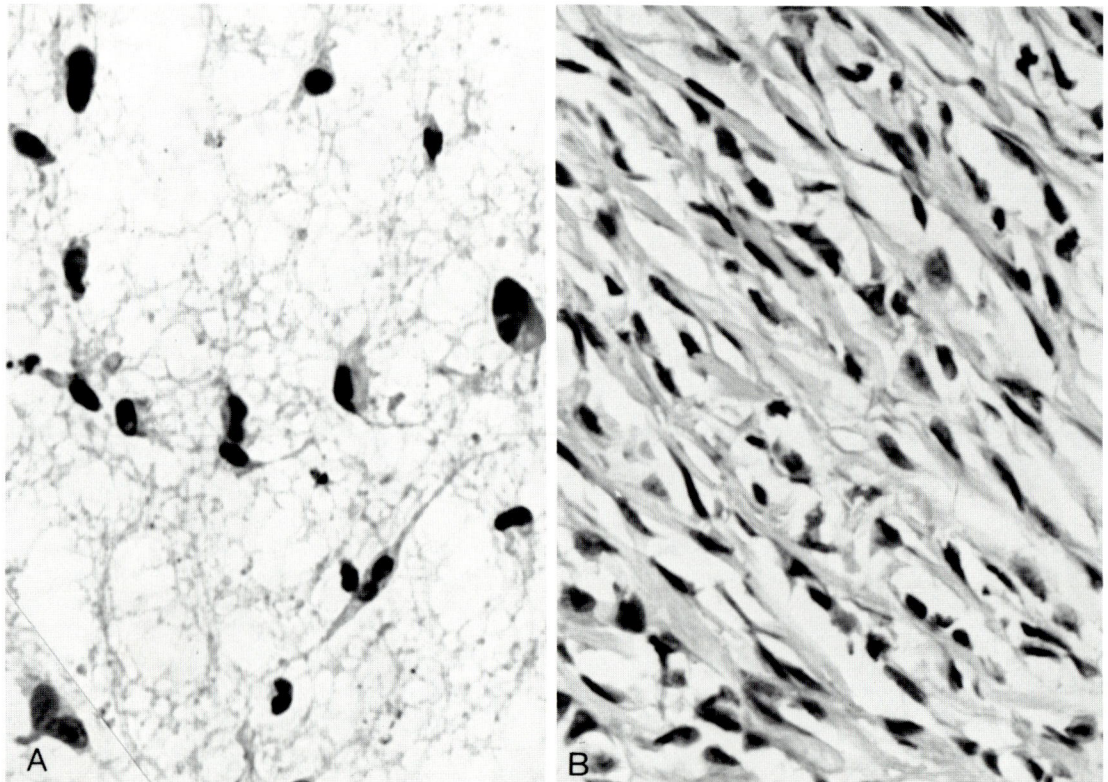

Figure 5.11.

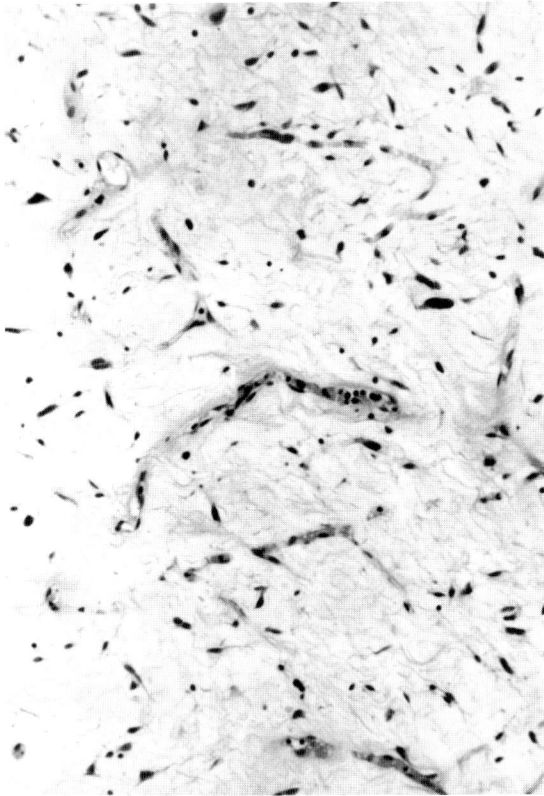

Figure 5.12. Tissue section of myxoid liposarcoma. Note spindle- and stellate-shaped cells, plexiform (chicken wire) vascular pattern, and extracellular myxoid material. ×125.

Table 5.2. Comparative Cytology of Selected Myxoid Soft Tissue Tumors[a]

Intramuscular Myxoma	Myxoid Schwannoma	Myxoid Liposarcoma	Myxoid MFH
Very uncommon	Quite uncommon	Common	Quite common
Low cellularity	Variable cellularity	Variable cellularity	High cellularity
Component cells similar to benign fibroblasts in appearance	Schwannian pattern with nuclear palisading	Variegated appearance from atypical spindle cells to prelipoblasts to vacuolated lipoblasts	Admixture of atypical spindle cells and multinucleate giant cells
		Prominent capillary network	

[a]Other myxoid soft tissue tumors, including the myxoid variant of dermatofibrosarcoma protuberans and extraskeletal myxoid chondrosarcoma, are uncommon and have not been encountered in our FNAB material.

characterized by rounded, "punched out," single or multiple lipid vacuoles that typically indent or compress the nucleus (**Figs. 5.13**).

Diagnostic Pitfalls. The cellularity of myxoid liposarcomas is quite variable. If the aspirate is obtained from a hypocellular myxoid area, a false-negative diagnosis may result. The observation of myxoid stromal substance in an aspirate is an important clue to an alert pathologist that the tumor may be a myxoid liposarcoma. In a proper clinical context, the combined cytologic features of spindle cells, branching vascular network, and myxoid stroma is so typical that a diagnosis of myxoid liposarcoma must be seriously considered even without finding acceptable lipoblasts. On the other hand, it should be noted that a myxoid stroma can also be seen in various benign as well as malignant soft tissue tumors (**Table 5.2**).

Lipoblasts must be differentiated from the following benign or malignant cells. *(a)* Lipid-laden histiocytes show foamy cytoplasm. The cytoplasmic lipid in histiocytes is more finely dispersed and

Figure 5.10. Intramuscular myxoma. **A,** ABC. The aspirate is hypocellular with a few benign spindle cells in a filmy myxoid background. ×500. **B,** Histologic section of the myxoma with sparse spindle cells in a myxomatous matrix. ×310.

Figure 5.11. Well-differentiated fibrosarcoma in the distal forearm of a 74-year-old man. The lesion had been excised 7 years previously and now recurred. The aspiration biopsy was obtained from the recurrence. **A,** ABC. Atypical spindle cells with coarse hyperchromatic chromatin and irregular nuclear membranes. ×500. **B,** Histology of the previously excised fibrosarcoma. Note fibroblastic cells showing nuclear hyperchromasia and atypia. ×500.

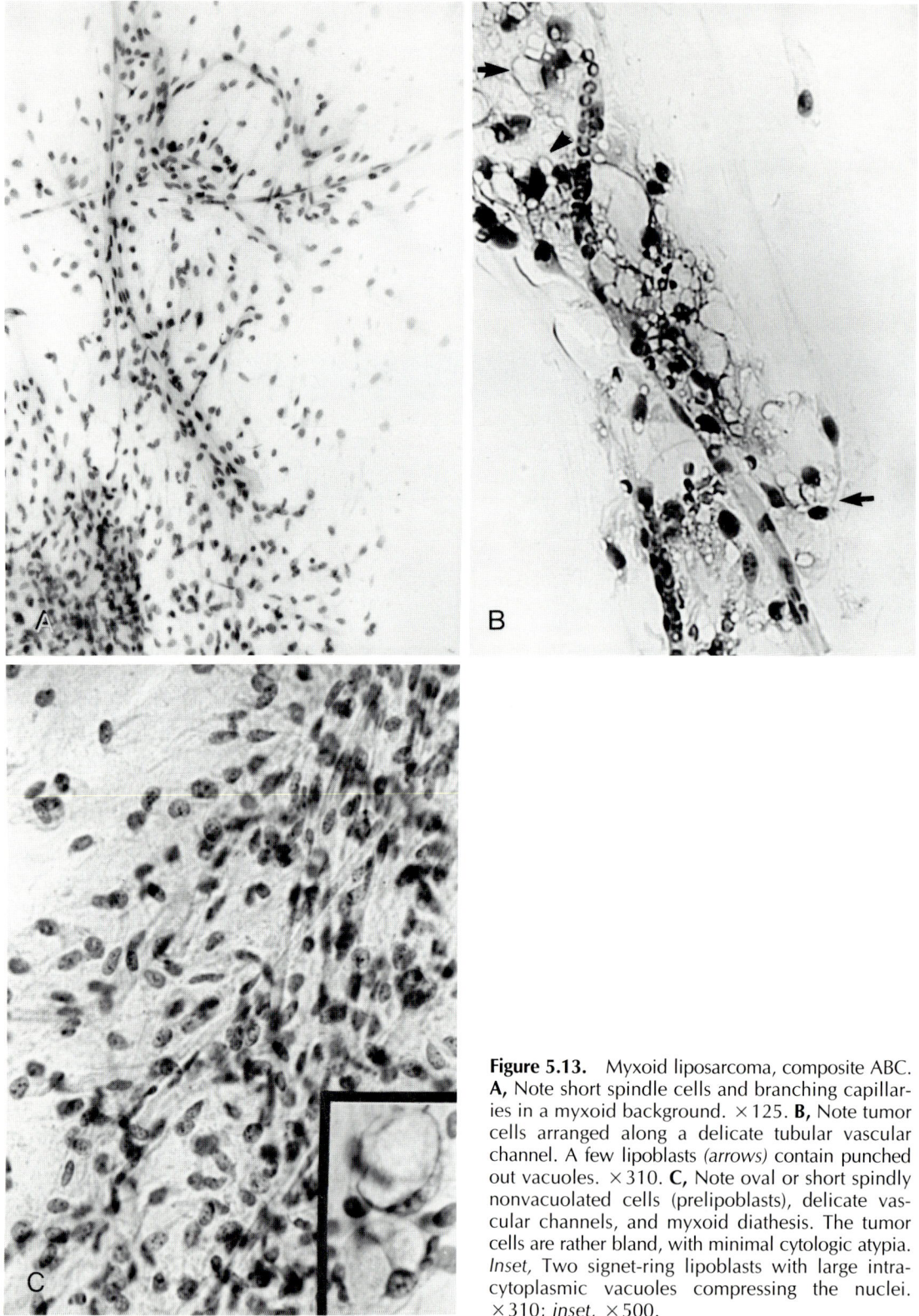

Figure 5.13.   Myxoid liposarcoma, composite ABC. **A,** Note short spindle cells and branching capillaries in a myxoid background. ×125. **B,** Note tumor cells arranged along a delicate tubular vascular channel. A few lipoblasts *(arrows)* contain punched out vacuoles. ×310. **C,** Note oval or short spindly nonvacuolated cells (prelipoblasts), delicate vascular channels, and myxoid diathesis. The tumor cells are rather bland, with minimal cytologic atypia. *Inset,* Two signet-ring lipoblasts with large intracytoplasmic vacuoles compressing the nuclei. ×310; *inset,* ×500.

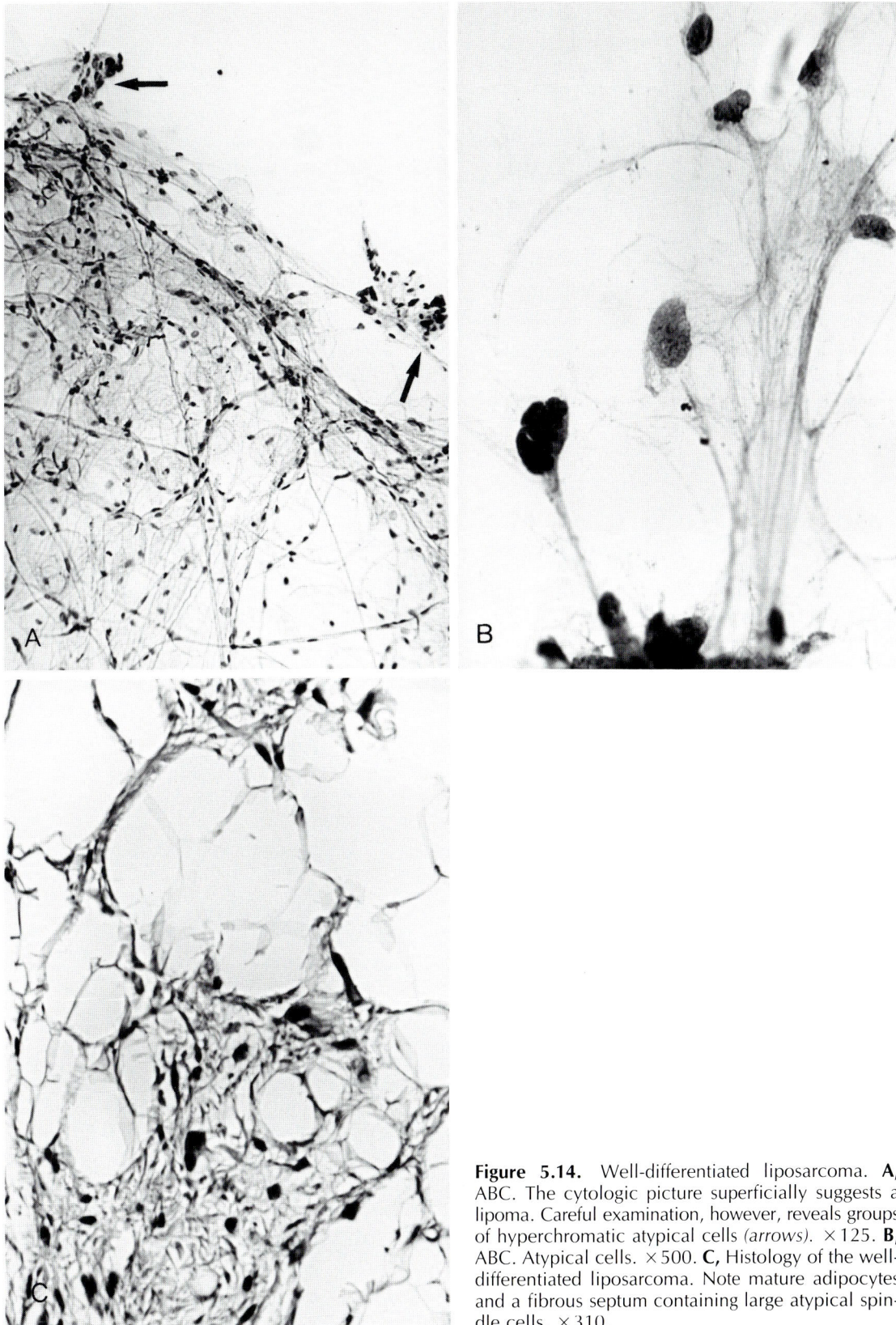

Figure 5.14. Well-differentiated liposarcoma. **A,** ABC. The cytologic picture superficially suggests a lipoma. Careful examination, however, reveals groups of hyperchromatic atypical cells *(arrows).* ×125. **B,** ABC. Atypical cells. ×500. **C,** Histology of the well-differentiated liposarcoma. Note mature adipocytes and a fibrous septum containing large atypical spindle cells. ×310.

does not distort the nuclei. *(b)* Poorly preserved or degenerated benign or malignant cells of any origin may show cytoplasmic vacuolation and may simulate lipoblasts. Usually other features of degeneration are also present, such as nuclear and cytoplasmic swelling with hyperchromasia, loss of chromatin crispness, and wrinkling of the nuclear membrane. *(c)* Benign atypical lipoblasts may be seen in fat necrosis and atypical and pleomorphic lipomas.[23,24] *(d)* Lipoblast-like cells can be found in chordoma, signet-ring cell carcinoma, and malignant fibrous histiocytoma.

Well-differentiated Liposarcoma

The ABC of well-differentiated liposarcoma closely resembles that of a lipoma (although the clinical presentation is different). The correct cytologic diagnosis is contingent on finding adult fat intersected by irregular bands of fibrous tissue in which there are variable amounts of mucoid changes and lipoblasts having atypical, hyperchromatic nuclei **(Fig. 5.14)**. The diagnosis of well-differentiated liposarcoma is not possible if only mature adipose tissue is aspirated.

Leiomyosarcoma

Compared with leiomyosarcomas of the visceral organs such as the uterus and gastrointestinal tract, leiomyosarcomas of soft tissues are uncommon. The more frequent sites of occurrence in the soft tissues are the retroperitoneum and extremities. Smooth muscle tumors of the skin are small and almost always benign.[25]

Aspiration Cytology

Well-differentiated leiomyosarcomas **(Fig. 5.15)** are characterized by small and large tissue fragments composed of spindle cells arranged in parallel rows. Nuclear pleomorphism is not pronounced. The elongated or ovoid nuclei are similar to those in fibrosarcoma except for a greater tendency of nuclear palisading.

Poorly differentiated leiomyosarcomas **(Fig. 5.16)** show more dissociated cells than coherent cell clumps. There are bizarre giant cell forms in addition to spindle cells. Mitotic activity is high. Intense phagocytic activity may result in bubbly or vacuolated cells, simulating liposarcoma or malignant fibrous histiocytoma.

Diagnostic Pitfalls. The well-differentiated leiomyosarcoma resembles leiomyoma and is separated from the latter by atypical nuclear features, such as irregular nuclear membrane, abnormal chromatin pattern, prominent nucleoli, and increased mitotic figures. Nonetheless, some examples of leiomyosarcoma are so well differentiated that clear-cut features of malignancy are not apparent.[26] **Table 5.3** shows the principal features that help in separating leiomyoma from leiomyosarcoma.

Cellular nodular fasciitis was mistaken in the past for leiomyosarcoma even on histologic examination.[27] Although cells in nodular fasciitis may exhibit increased mitotic activity, they lack cytologic features of malignancy. Nowadays, nodular fasciitis is a well-defined entity, with a rather characteristic clinical presentation.

Other Spindle Cell Sarcomas

Neurogenic sarcoma (malignant schwannoma) is uncommon, and it is difficult to distinguish it from fibrosarcomas, unless microscopic Schwannian features are present or clinically the patient has Von Recklinghausen's disease or the tumor can be shown to have arisen from a nerve.[28,29] The two cases I have studied, like the case reported by Hood et al.,[29] showed obviously malignant spindle cells not capable of further characterization on ABC **(Fig. 5.17)**. Immunoperoxidase staining for S100 protein, a marker for Schwann cells, is helpful in the identification of neurogenic tumors when interpreted judiciously within the clinical context.

Synovial sarcoma usually occurs in the paraarticular regions, in close association with the joint capsules and tendon sheaths, but it is uncommon in joint cavities. There are two histologic forms: monomorphic and biphasic. The monomorphic variant consists of a monotonous population of spindle cells resembling fibrosarcoma. Nuclear pleomorphism is not pronounced, and mono- or multinucleated giant cells are not a feature of synovial sarcoma. An occasional case may have predominant rounded or ovoid, rather than spindled, cells.[30] The biphasic synovial sarcoma has an epithelial gland-like component in addition to the spindle cell component.[31] The ABC of the biphasic form resembles a carcinosarcoma **(Figs. 1.6 and 5.18)**.

PLEOMORPHIC SARCOMAS
Malignant Fibrous Histiocytoma

Malignant fibrous histiocytomas (MFHs) are the most common soft tissue sarcomas of late adult life.[32] These tumors occur principally in the extremities or in the abdominal cavity or retroperitoneum. There has been much controversy over the histogenesis of MFH. Recent studies[33] have provided support for the view that MFH is part of the spectrum of neoplasms of fibroblasts. Another problem is the use of the diagnosis of MFH as a wastebasket for any morphologically unclassifiable pleomorphic sarcoma.

Aspiration Cytology

The aspirates are generally hypercellular and reveal a mixture of spindle cells and mononucleated and multinucleated grotesque giant cells **(Fig. 5.19)**.[34–37] For the most part, the tumor cells occur singly, but they sometimes form small, rather flat, loosely cohesive clusters. Three-dimensional cell balls or clusters like those seen in epithelial neoplasms are not seen. The nuclei of the tumor cells are hyperchromatic, with irregular coarse chromatin and prominent nucleoli. The cytoplasm shows varying degrees of foaminess. Some of the spindle cells and a few multinucleated giant cells show a "comet" configuration, which is characterized by an eccentrically positioned nucleus at one end of the cell and a long tapering cytoplasmic tail at the other end **(Fig. 5.19B)**. These comet cells are a characteristic, but not a specific, feature of MFH.[34]

Myxoid MFH is a common variant, constituting about 25% or more of MFHs. In the past, this tumor was probably diagnosed as myxofibrosarcoma or myxoid liposarcoma. The tumor cells generally exhibit minimal to moderate nuclear pleomorphism in a myxoid background **(Fig. 5.20)**.[37] Lipoblasts should not be present.

Diagnostic Pitfalls. Not all morphologically pleomorphic soft tissue neoplasms are malignant. The pleomorphic morphology of atypical fibroxanthoma of the skin may be indistinguishable from

Table 5.3. Well-differentiated Leiomyosarcomas versus Leiomyomas of Soft Tissues[a]

	Leiomyoma	Leiomyosarcoma
Size	<2.5 cm	>2.5 cm
Located in skin	Some	0
Aspiration cytology		
Cellularity	Variable	Generally cellular
Nuclear atypia	Absent	Subtle to obvious
Mitotic activity	0 to low	Increased

[a]Data partly based on Stout AP, Hill WT. Leiomyosarcoma of the superficial soft tissues. Cancer 1958;11:844–854.

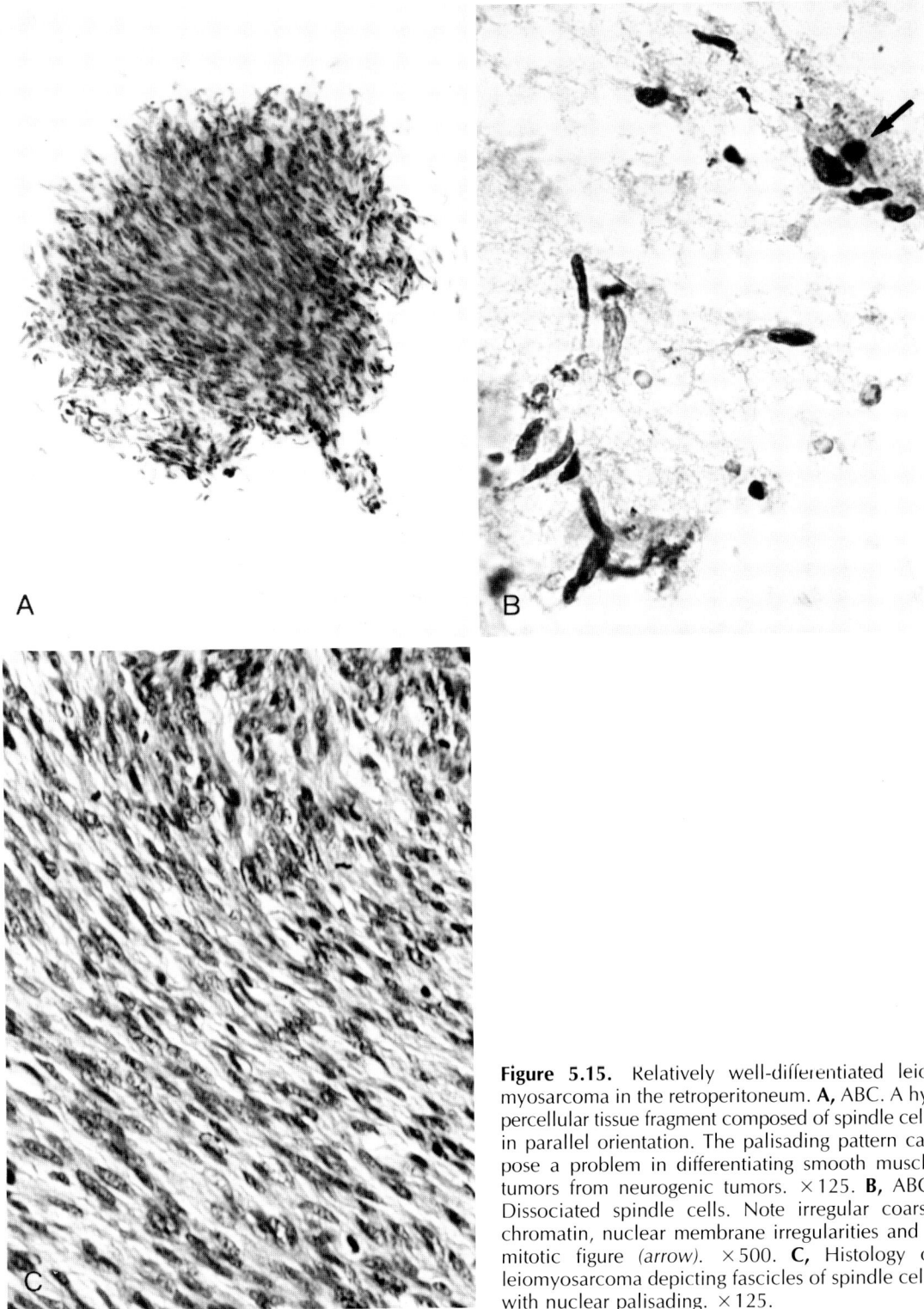

Figure 5.15. Relatively well-differentiated leiomyosarcoma in the retroperitoneum. **A,** ABC. A hypercellular tissue fragment composed of spindle cells in parallel orientation. The palisading pattern can pose a problem in differentiating smooth muscle tumors from neurogenic tumors. ×125. **B,** ABC. Dissociated spindle cells. Note irregular coarse chromatin, nuclear membrane irregularities and a mitotic figure *(arrow)*. ×500. **C,** Histology of leiomyosarcoma depicting fascicles of spindle cells with nuclear palisading. ×125.

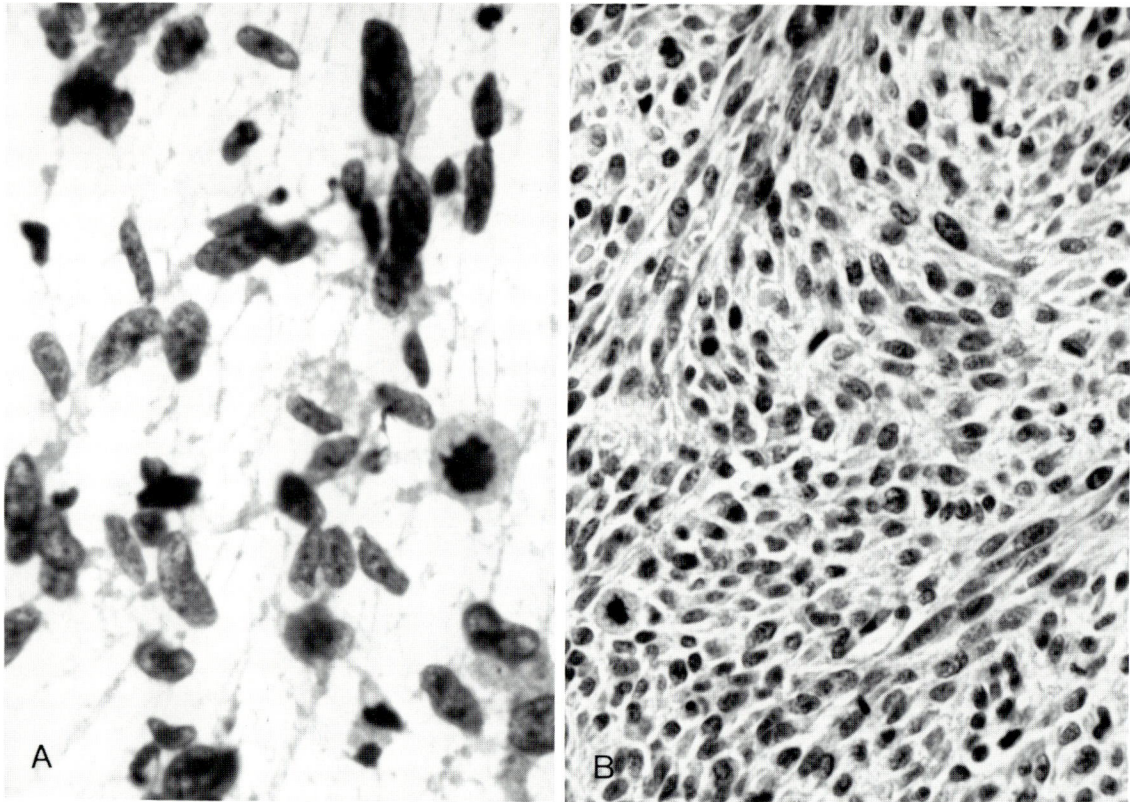

Figure 5.16. Poorly differentiated leiomyosarcoma. **A,** ABC. Mitotically active, malignant spindle cells lying singly. ×500. **B,** Histology of the resected leiomyosarcoma showing fascicles of pleomorphic spindle cells intersecting one another at right angle. ×310.

MFH and yet it almost invariably pursues a benign course.[38] It is distinguished from MFH by its superficial location and its preference for the sun-damaged skin of the head and neck in elderly persons.

MFH can be mistaken for anaplastic giant cell carcinoma. In general, the giant cells in carcinoma are less pleomorphic than those in MFH; the enormous size and grotesque appearance of some of the cells in MFH are rarely attained in carcinoma. The comet cells with foamy cytoplasmic tails are not a feature seen in carcinomas, whose cells tend to be more polygonal and have granular cytoplasm. In difficult cases, additional aspirated material should be procured for immunocytochemical and electron microscopic studies.

Pleomorphic Liposarcoma

Pleomorphic liposarcoma is a high-grade sarcoma, accounting for about 12% of all liposarcomas.[21] The commonest location is deep within the soft tissues of the thigh. The hypercellular aspirates contain many large atypical cells assuming a variety of shapes and sizes, with marked hyperchromasia and nuclear pleomorphism. Multinucleated giant cells with vacuolated or deeply eosinophilic cytoplasm are not uncommon. The diagnosis of pleomorphic liposarcoma is contingent upon the identification of characteristic lipoblasts **(Fig. 5.21),** which are univacuolated or multivacuolated cells whose nuclei are typically compressed or indented by well-defined cytoplasmic fat vacuoles.

Pleomorphic Rhabdomyosarcoma

Pleomorphic rhabdomyosarcoma is an extremely rare tumor. It is now realized that most cases originally reported as such in adults are not muscle tumors at all, but pleomorphic forms of malignant fibrous histiocytoma or liposarcoma.[32] In Enzinger and Weiss's series,[1] there were only a few examples of pleomorphic rhabdomyosarcomas in adults, and in nearly all of them, the authors expressed doubt as to the correctness of diagnosis. According to these authors,[1] cells with cross-striations are virtually nonexistent in adult pleomorphic rhabdomyosarcomas.

The one case we studied **(Fig. 5.22)** showed scattered pleomorphic oval, strap-shaped, and racquet-shaped cells with a sprinkling of multinucleated giant cells. The cytoplasm was densely eosinophilic and contained granules or fibrils, but cross-striations were equivocal. The cytoplasmic borders were well-defined. Subsequent histologic examination of the resected tumor showed areas of malignant osteoid in addition to the rhabdomyoblastic elements; it was, by strict criteria, a malignant mesenchymoma rather than a rhabdomyosarcoma.

ROUND CELL SARCOMA
Embryonal Rhabdomyosarcoma

Embryonal rhabdomyosarcoma is the most common soft tissue sarcoma in children. The preferred sites are the head, neck, and genitourinary region. Those tumors developing from the mesenchyme of the mucous membranes lining hollow viscera, such as the urinary bladder and vagina, assume a polypoid, grape-like configuration, and are referred to as sarcoma botryoides.

Aspiration Cytology

The ABC shows moderate to marked cellularity, with tumor cells scattered singly or in small loose clusters. The predominant

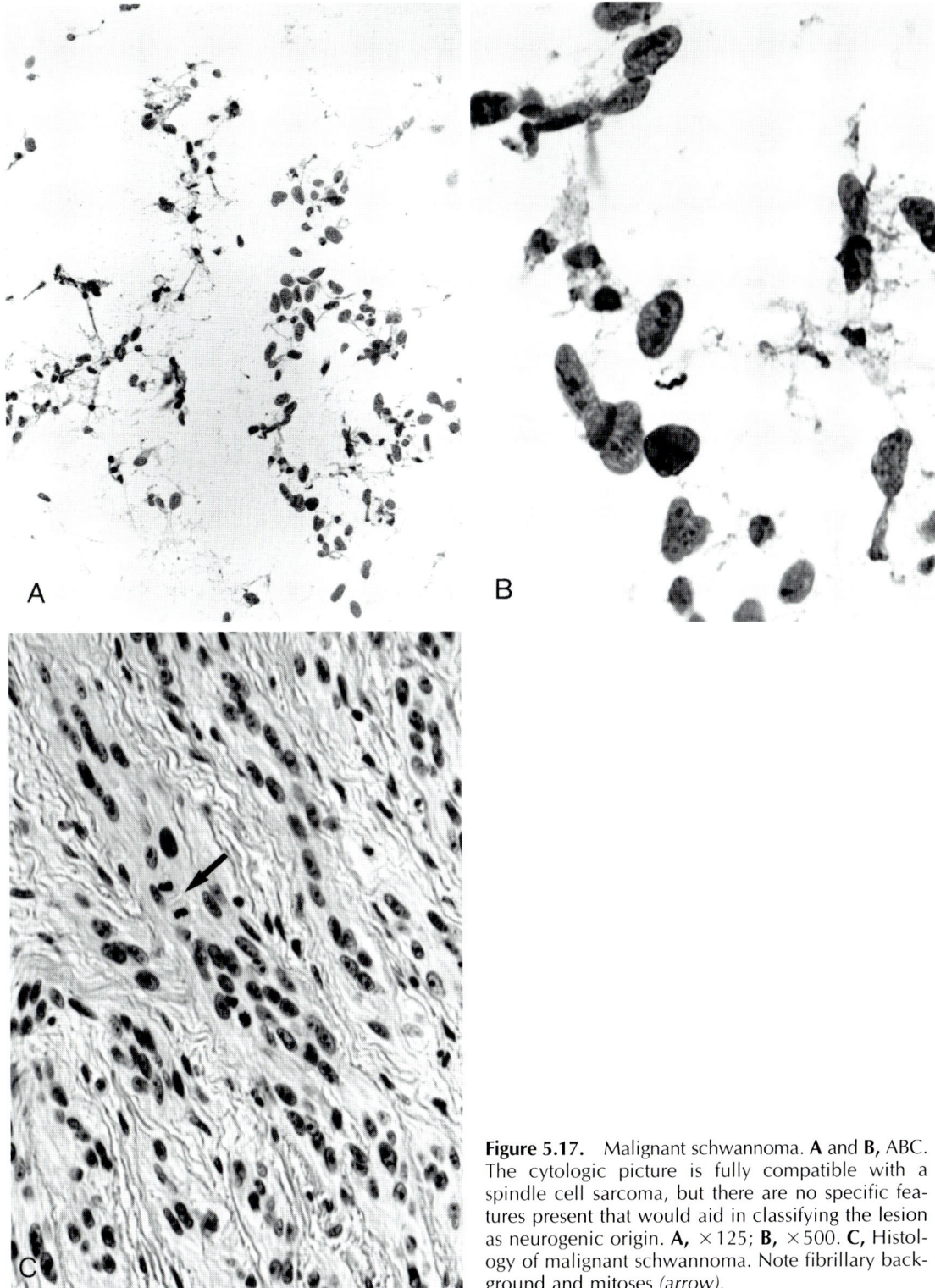

Figure 5.17. Malignant schwannoma. **A** and **B,** ABC. The cytologic picture is fully compatible with a spindle cell sarcoma, but there are no specific features present that would aid in classifying the lesion as neurogenic origin. **A,** ×125; **B,** ×500. **C,** Histology of malignant schwannoma. Note fibrillary background and mitoses *(arrow)*.

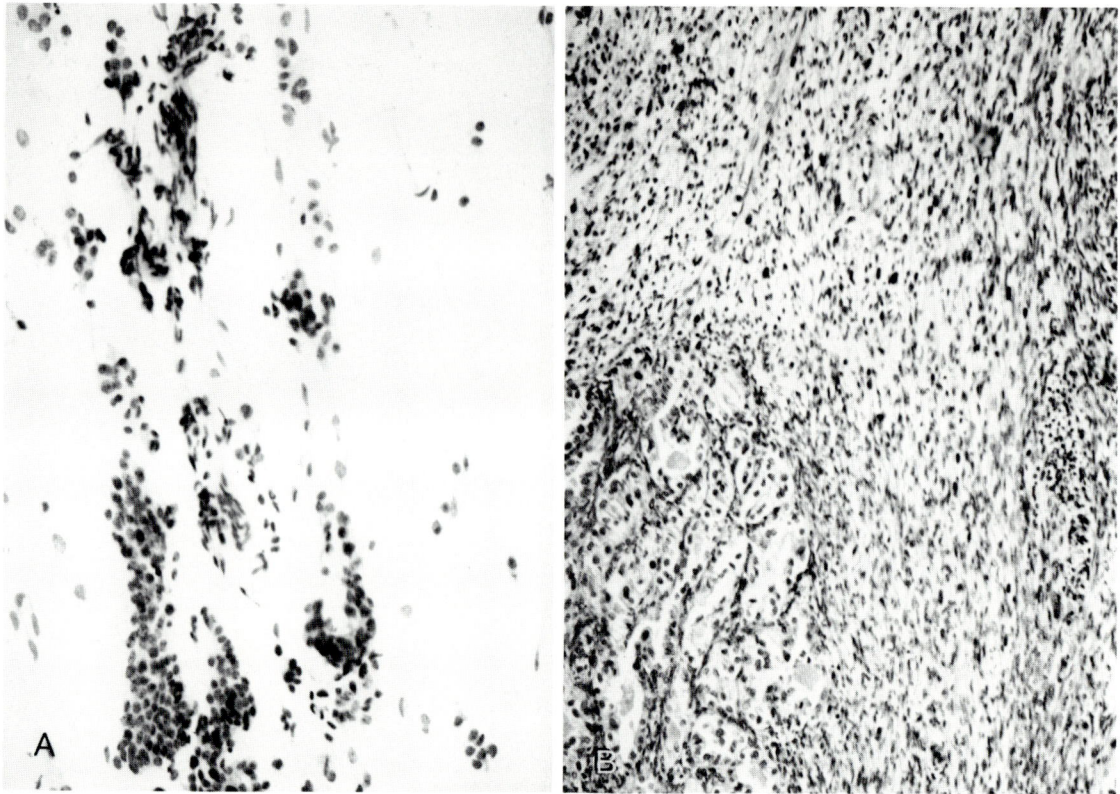

Figure 5.18.   Synovial sarcoma, biphasic form. **A,** ABC. Note admixture of spindle cells and epithelial cells. ×125. **B,** Histology of synovial sarcoma depicting a fibrosarcoma pattern admixed with glandular formations *(left lower corner)*. ×125.

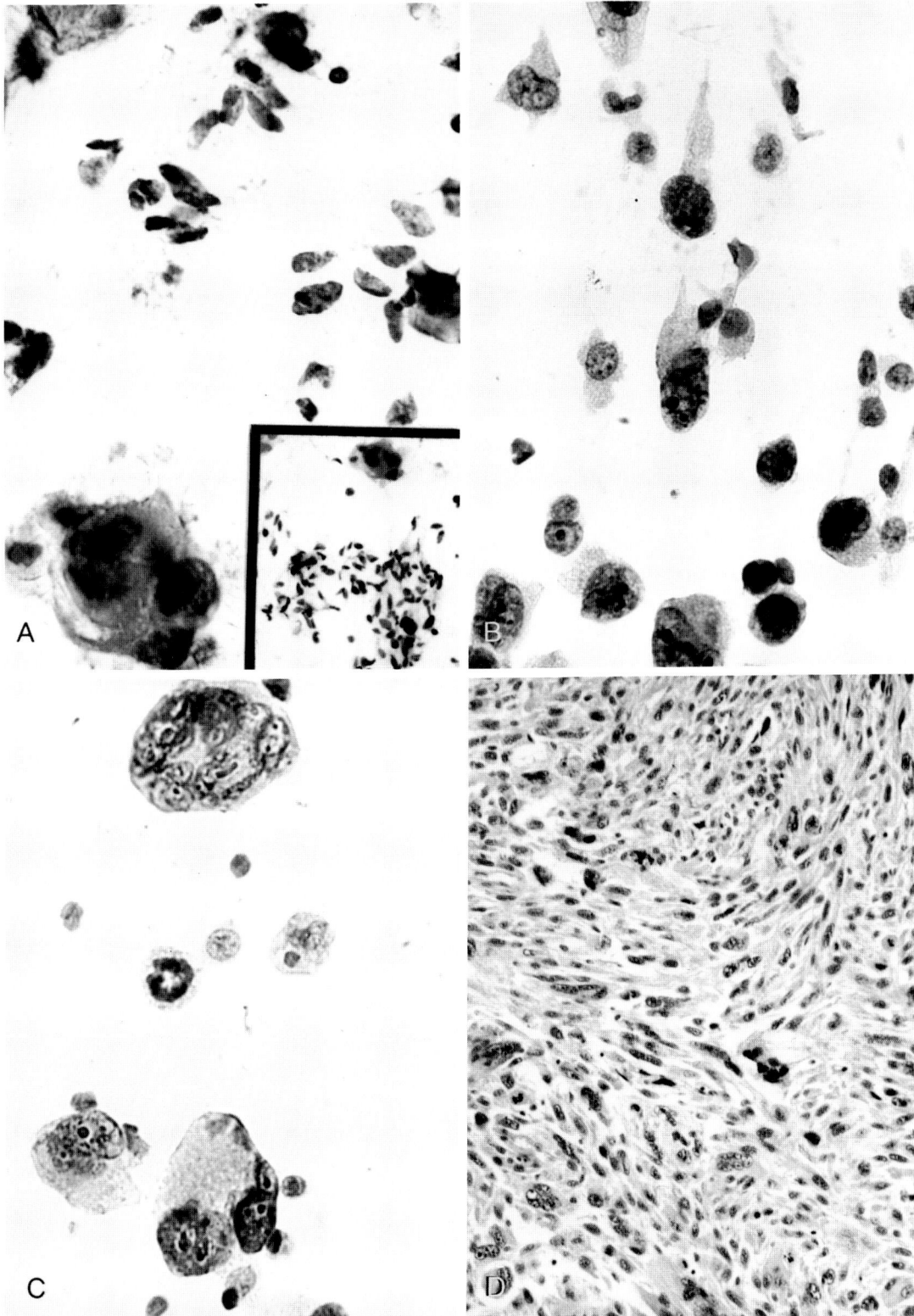

Figure 5.19. Malignant fibrous histiocytoma. **A,** ABC. Note admixture of malignant spindle cells and pleomorphic giant cells. ×500; *inset,* ×125. **B,** ABC. Note rounded cells and comet cells with cytoplasmic tails. ×500. **C,** ABC. Bizarre multinucleated giant cells with finely foamy cytoplasm. ×500. **D,** Histology of malignant fibrous histiocytoma depicting giant cells and spindle cells. ×310.

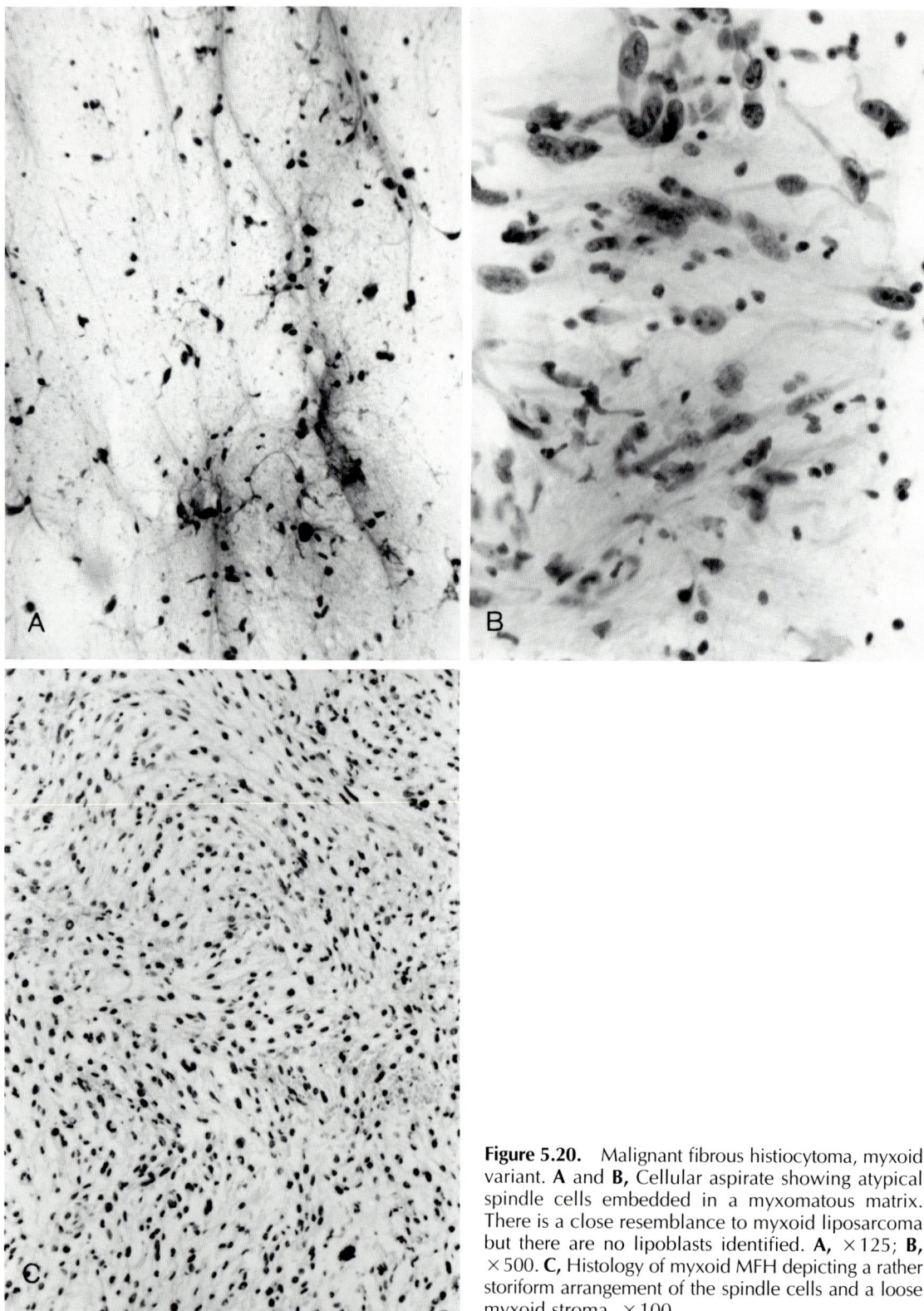

Figure 5.20.   Malignant fibrous histiocytoma, myxoid variant. **A** and **B,** Cellular aspirate showing atypical spindle cells embedded in a myxomatous matrix. There is a close resemblance to myxoid liposarcoma but there are no lipoblasts identified. **A,** ×125; **B,** ×500. **C,** Histology of myxoid MFH depicting a rather storiform arrangement of the spindle cells and a loose myxoid stroma. ×100.

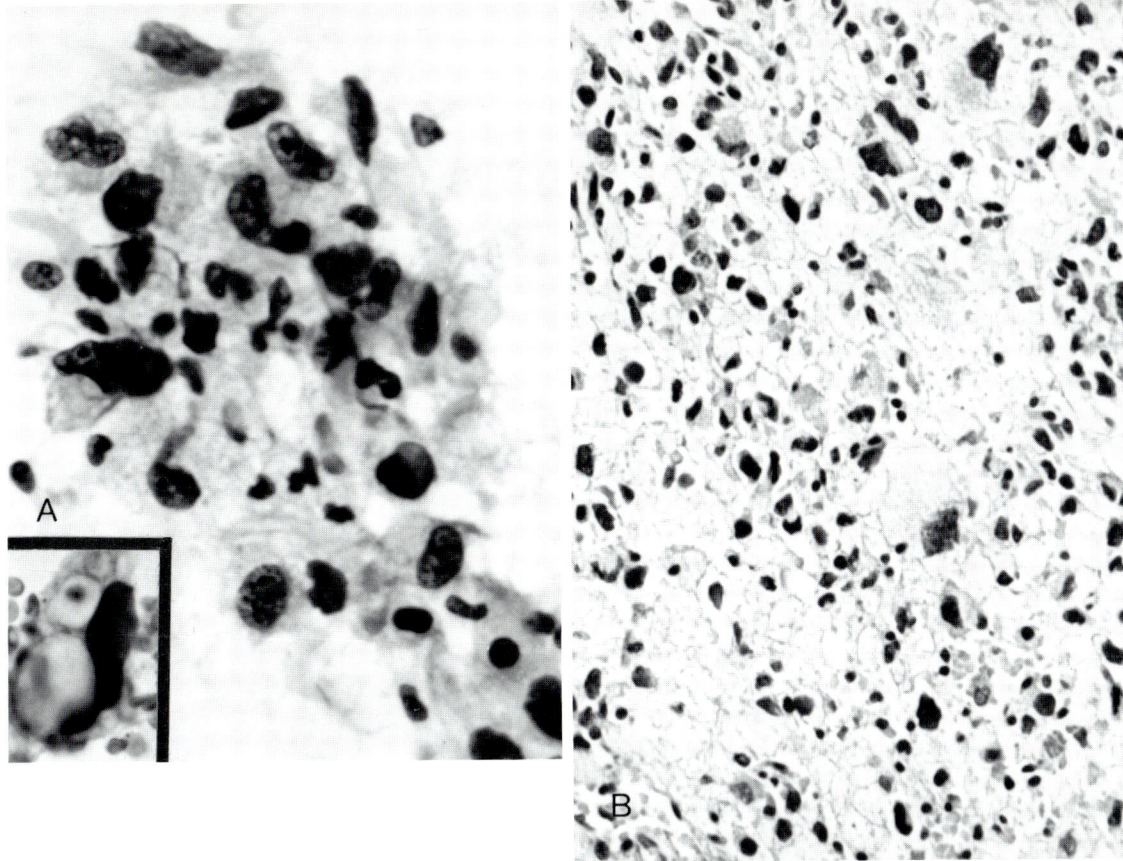

Figure 5.21. Pleomorphic liposarcoma. **A,** ABC. Note pleomorphic cells with abnormal chromatin pattern and prominent nucleoli. *Inset* shows a multivacuolated lipoblast with a scalloped nucleus. ×500. **B,** Histology of pleomorphic liposarcoma showing malignant lipoblasts with marked cytologic pleomorphism. ×310.

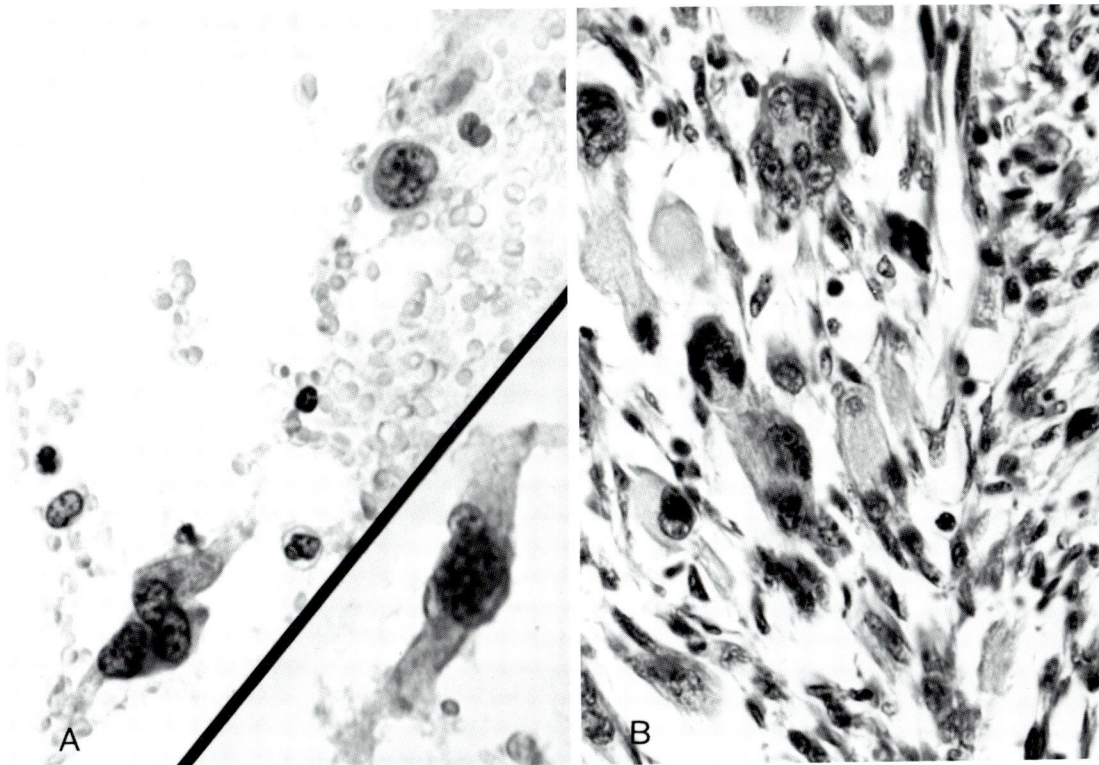

Figure 5.22. Pleomorphic rhabdomyosarcoma. **A,** ABC. Note variably sized malignant cells with eosinophilic granular or fibrillar cytoplasm and well-defined cytoplasmic borders. *Inset* shows a strap-shaped cell. ×500. **B,** Histology of the resected tumor showing a rhabdomyoblastic area. However, areas of malignant osteoid are present elsewhere in the tumor and, strictly speaking, the tumor is a malignant mesenchymoma. ×310.

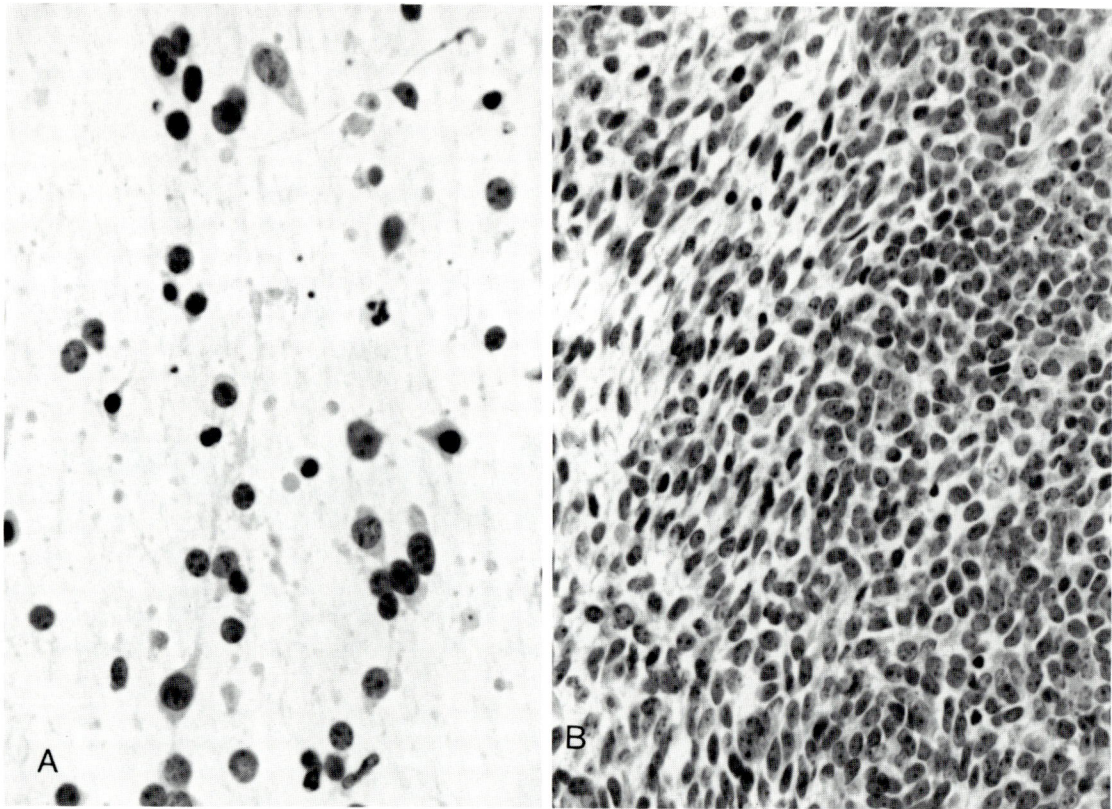

Figure 5.23.

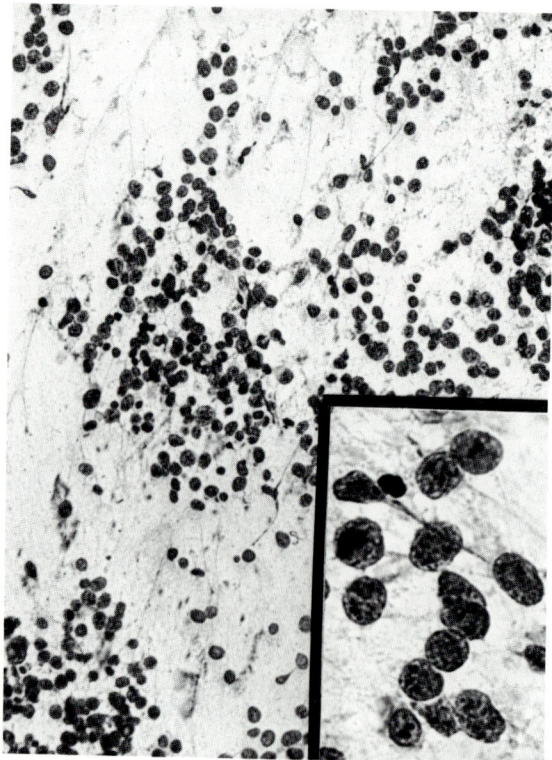

Figure 5.24.

Figure 5.23. Embryonal rhabdomyosarcoma. **A,** ABC. Note small round cells resembling lymphocytes and other cells with moderate amount of pink cytoplasm, consistent with rhabdomyoblastic differentiation. Note also nuclear pleomorphism and nucleoli. ×500. **B,** Histology of the resected embryonal rhabdomyosarcoma. Note pleomorphic small cells. ×310.

Figure 5.24. Soft tissue Ewing's sarcoma, ABC. Small round cells displaying a vague pseudorosette pattern. *Inset,* High-power detail of tumor cells. Compared to cells of embryonal rhabdomyosarcoma, these cells are more uniform. ×125; *inset,* ×500.

cells are the undifferentiated small round cells with scanty cytoplasm, resembling lymphocytes but slightly larger. The nuclei are hyperchromatic or vesicular, with irregular nuclear membranes and prominent nucleoli (**Fig. 5.23**).

Other cells include oval cells, short spindle cells, and elongated, strap-shaped cells. These cells have more cytoplasm, which is eosinophilic granular or fibrillar. Cross-striations, however, are difficult to recognize on routine stains at the light microscopic level.[39]

Differential Diagnosis and Diagnostic Pitfalls. From the morphologic point of view, embryonal rhabdomyosarcoma belongs in the group of tumors designated as "small round cell malignancy."[40] Other neoplasms included in this group are neuroblastoma, Ewing's sarcoma, malignant lymphoma, and oat cell carcinoma. Diagnosis of embryonal rhabdomyosarcoma is based on the identification of cells with rhabdomyoblastic differentiation. The finding of cells having deeply eosinophilic and fibrillar cytoplasm should alert the cytopathologist to the possibility that the tumor may be of myogenic origin, which can be confirmed by immunostaining the tumor cells for desmin, actin, or myosin.[39] Neuroblastoma is recognized by its rosette pattern and a neurofibrillary background (see Chapter 13). Periodic acid-Schiff (PAS)-positive cytoplasmic granules are found typically in Ewing's sarcoma and sometimes in rhabdomyosarcoma in small amount. The tumor cells of Ewing's sarcoma (see below) are more uniform than those of rhabdomyosarcoma. Racquet and strap cells with eosinophilic cytoplasm are not present in Ewing's sarcoma. Malignant lymphoma enters into the differential diagnosis because of the undifferentiated appearance of the round cells. Immunoperoxidase staining of tumor cells for leukocyte common antigen is useful in confirming their lymphocytic origin. False-positive results are extremely uncommon.

Many of these small round cell malignancies affect a specific age range and show a specific site of predilection; thus, a full knowledge of the clinical data including the age and site of the tumor is crucial for correct identification of these tumors (**Table 5.4**).

Extraskeletal Ewing's Sarcoma

Extraskeletal Ewing's sarcoma occurs as a primary tumor in the soft tissue without bone involvement.[41] The sites of predilection are the soft tissues of the paravertebral region, chest wall, retroperitoneum, and lower extremities. The tumor affects predominantly adolescents and young adults. The histogenesis of these neoplasms is uncertain. Interestingly, recent ultrastructural studies have demonstrated neurosecretory granules in a few cases, and some cases have shown neuron-specific enolase immunoreactivity, suggesting neuroblastic differentiation.[42,43]

Aspiration Cytology

The ABC (**Fig. 5.24**) is usually cellular and shows uniform round cells arranged singly or in a loose, imperfect rosette-like pattern. The vesicular nuclei have finely divided chromatin, and frequently a single minute nucleolus. The cytoplasm is ill-defined, scanty, and pale staining and may be irregularly vacuolated due to the presence of intracytoplasmic glycogen. There are no spindled cells or giant cells.[44,45]

Diagnostic Pitfalls. Ewing's sarcoma must be distinguished from other small round cell tumors. Cytologic features characteristic of Ewing's sarcoma cells are nuclear uniformity, cytoplasmic glycogen (**Fig. 5.25**) and positive immunoreaction to vimentin antibody. Cells of rhabdomyosarcomas show more anisocytosis and have a greater amount of chromatin, more irregular nuclear membranes, and prominent nucleoli (see under "Embryonal Rhabdomyosarcoma" and **Table 5.4**.).

Other Round Cell Sarcomas

Round cell liposarcoma is a rare variant of liposarcoma and is a highly aggressive tumor. The ABC shows rather cohesive sheets of round cells with moderate degree of nuclear atypia. These cells

Table 5.4. Differential Diagnosis of Small Round Cell Tumors

Neoplasm	Age Group	Primary Sites	Cytologic Features	Cytochemical and Immunoperoxidase Stains	Electron Microscopy
Embryonal rhabdomyosarcoma	Infants and children	Head and neck, urogenital tract	Small cells with fibrillar eosinophilic cytoplasm	Vimentin (+) Desmin (+)	Myofilaments
Ewing's sarcoma	Children and adolescents	Bone and soft tissue	Small uniform round cells	Vimentin (+) PAS[a] (+) NSE (±)	Glycogen (+) cell junctions (+)
Neuroblastoma	Infants and children	Adrenal and sympathetic chain	Small round cells; rosette formation; neurofibrillary matrix	NSE (+)	Microtubules; cell processes; neurosecretory granules
Small cell anaplastic carcinoma	Adult	Lung and occasionally other sites	Cell groups with nuclear molding; cell necrosis	NSE (+)	Scant numbers of neurosecretory granules; desmosomes (+)
Carcinoid tumor	Adult	Lung and gastrointestinal tract	Uniform cells in mosaic and organoid patterns	NSE (+) Grimelius (+)	Abundant neurosecretory granules; desmosomes (+)
Malignant lymphoma	Any age	Lymphoid tissue	Atypical lymphocytes	LCA (+)	Lymphoid cells; desmosomes (−)

[a]PAS, periodic acid-Schiff stain; NSE, neuron-specific enolase; LCA, leukocyte common antigen.

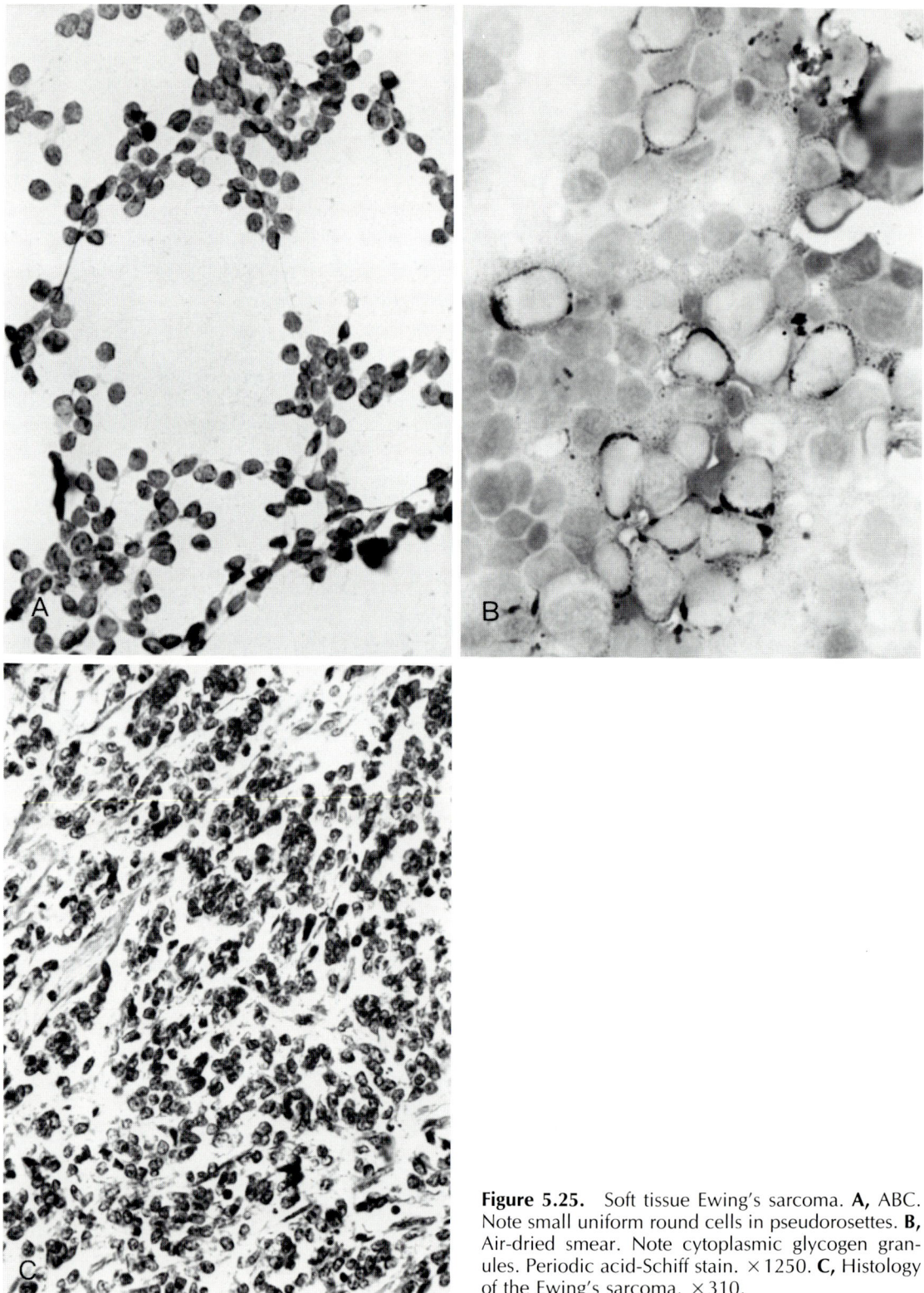

Figure 5.25. Soft tissue Ewing's sarcoma. **A,** ABC. Note small uniform round cells in pseudorosettes. **B,** Air-dried smear. Note cytoplasmic glycogen granules. Periodic acid-Schiff stain. ×1250. **C,** Histology of the Ewing's sarcoma. ×310.

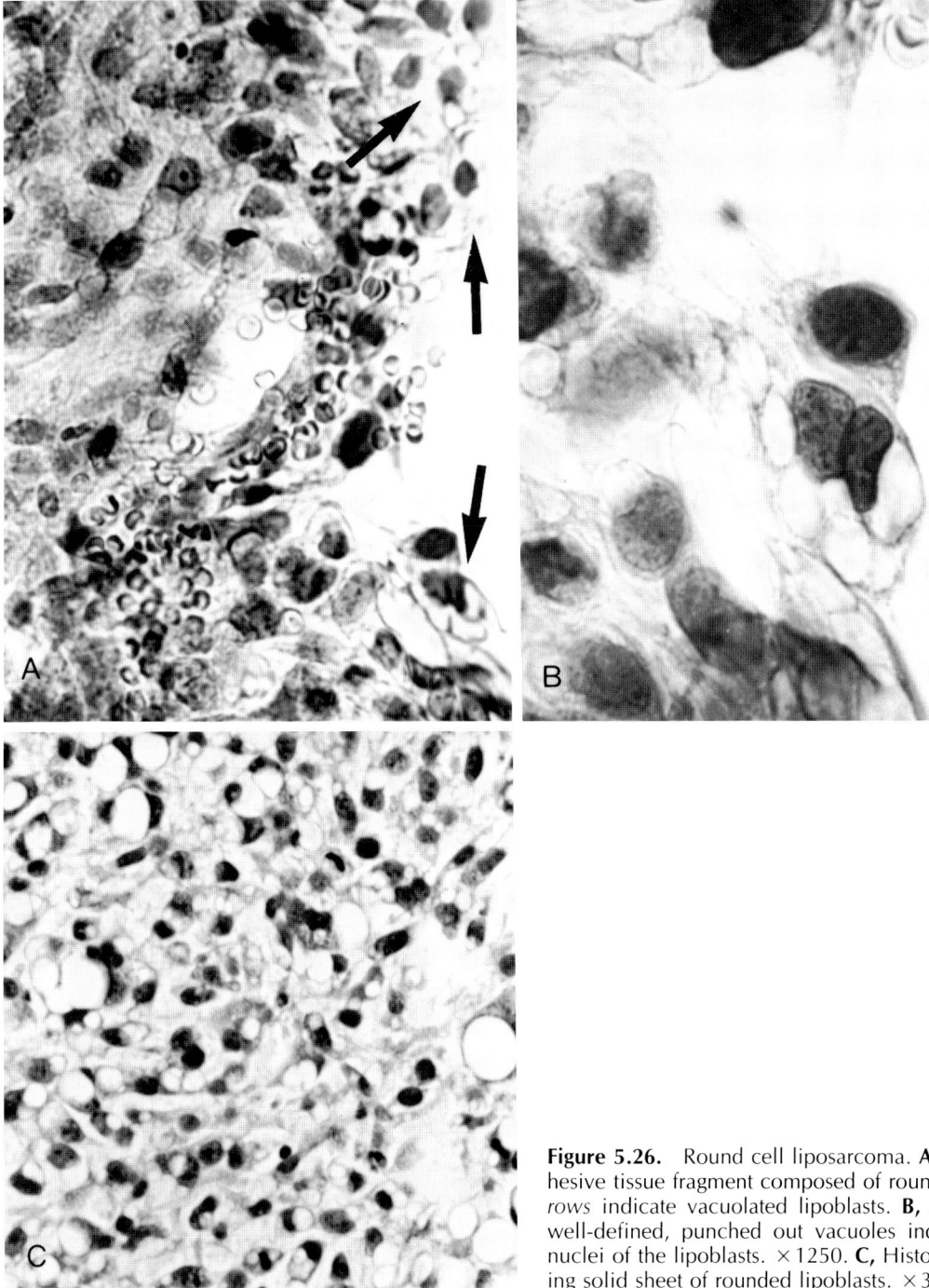

Figure 5.26. Round cell liposarcoma. **A,** ABC. Cohesive tissue fragment composed of round cells. *Arrows* indicate vacuolated lipoblasts. **B,** ABC. Note well-defined, punched out vacuoles indenting the nuclei of the lipoblasts. ×1250. **C,** Histology showing solid sheet of rounded lipoblasts. ×310.

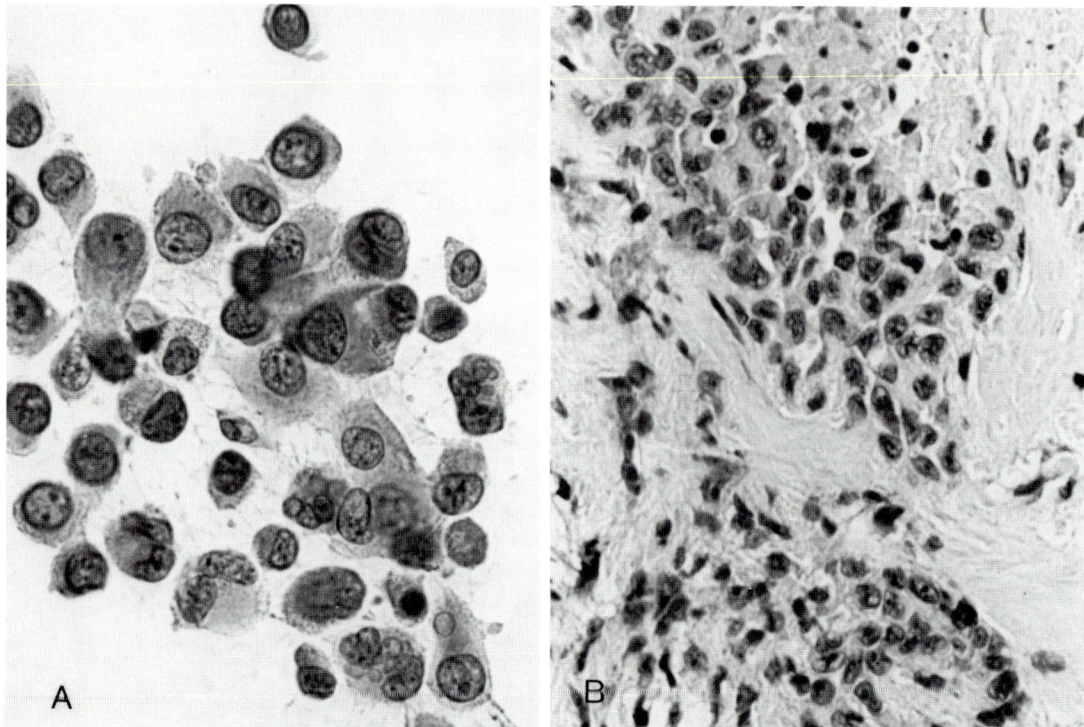

Figure 5.27. Epithelioid sarcoma. **A,** ABC. Numerous dyshesive, round cells with strikingly eosinophilic cytoplasm. The cells are much larger in size than cells of embryonal rhabdomyosarcoma or Ewing's sarcoma. There is only a moderate degree of nuclear pleomorphism. ×500. **B,** Histology of epithelioid sarcoma showing islands of tumor cells with fibrosis and an area of necrosis. ×310.

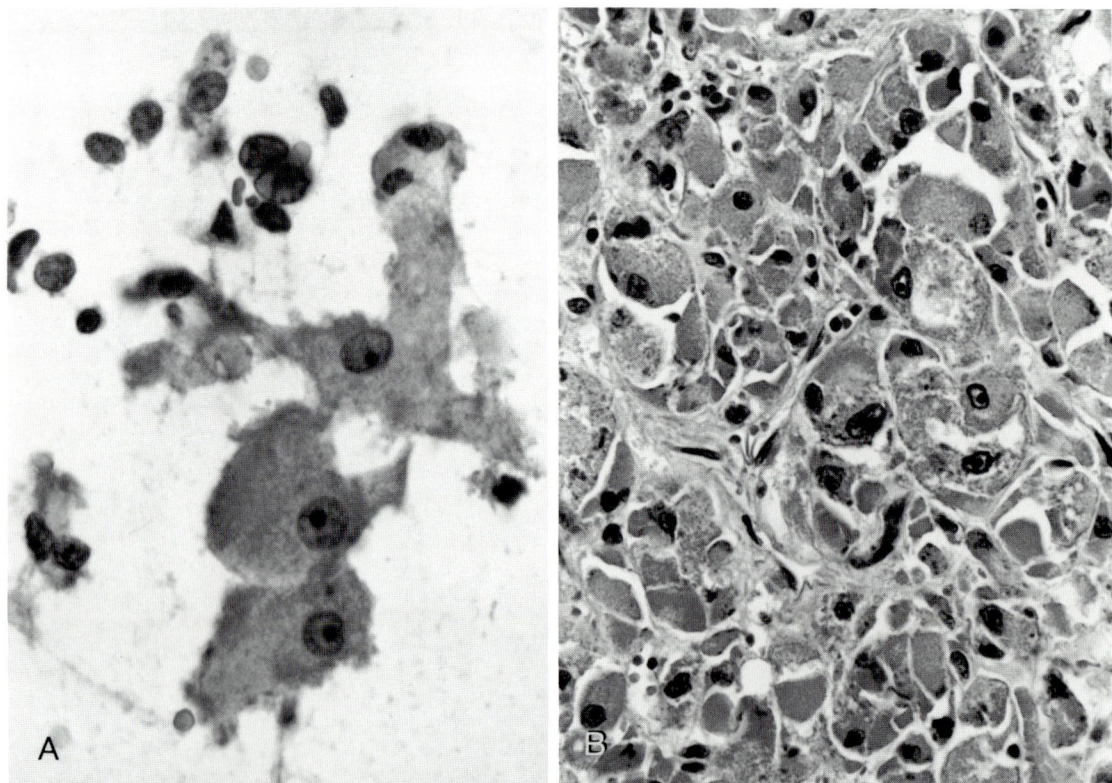

Figure 5.28. Alveolar soft part sarcoma. **A,** Note large polyhedral cells with prominent nucleoli and abundant granular cytoplasm. ×500. **B,** Histologic section of the alveolar soft part sarcoma. Note tumor cells arranged in alveolar nests. ×310.

are much larger than those of embryonal rhabdomyosarcoma and Ewing's sarcoma. Many show lipoblastic differentiation (**Fig. 5.26**). Myxoid stroma and capillary network may be present but are not as striking as in myxoid liposarcoma.

Synovial sarcoma may show medium-sized round cells to the exclusion of spindle cells.[30] Other forms of tendosynovial neoplasms (epithelioid sarcoma and clear cell sarcoma)[46] also exhibit predominantly round cells on fine needle aspirates. The ABC of epithelioid sarcoma (**Fig. 5.27**) shows moderately large, dispersed, rounded, or polygonal tumor cells with eosinophilic cytoplasm, similar to epithelial cells such as those from breast carcinoma or epithelioid cells

from a granulomatous process. Plump spindle cells may also be seen but bizarre giant cells are absent. Extreme cellular pleomorphism is uncommon.

Finally, aspirates of alveolar soft part sarcoma show large, polyhedral or round tumor cells with vesicular nuclei, prominent central nucleoli, and abundant coarsely granulated cytoplasm (**Fig. 5.28**).[47] PAS-positive, diastase-resistant intracytoplasmic needle-shaped inclusions have been reported in an aspirate of alveolar soft part sarcoma.[48] The tumor is extremely uncommon, highly malignant, and most often occurs in the deep soft tissues of the thigh and leg of young adults.

References

1. Enzinger FM, Weiss SW. Soft tissue tumors. St. Louis: CV Mosby, 1983.
2. Miralles TG, Gosalbez F, Menendez P, Astudillo A, Torre C, Buesa J. Fine needle aspiration cytology of soft-tissue lesions. Acta Cytol 1986;30:671–678.
3. Suen KC. Guides to clinical aspiration biopsy. Retroperitoneum and intestine. New York: Igaku Shoin, 1987:28–51.
4. Layfield LJ, Anders KH, Glasgow BJ, Mirra JM. Fine needle aspiration of primary soft-tissue lesions. Arch Pathol Lab Med 1986;110:420–424.
5. Crosby JH, Hoeg K, Hager B. Transthoracic fine needle aspiration of primary and metastatic sarcomas. Diagn Cytopathol 1985;1:221–227.
6. Kim K, Naylor B, Han IH. Fine needle aspiration cytology of sarcomas metastatic to the lung. Acta Cytol 1986;30:688–694.
7. Walaas L, Kindblom LG. Lipomatous tumors. A correlative cytologic and histologic study of 27 tumors examined by fine needle aspiration cytology. Hum Pathol 1985;16:6–18.
8. Mirra JM. Pathology of soft tissue sarcomas. In Eilber FR, Morton DL, Sondak VK, Economou JS. The soft tissue sarcomas. Orlando: Grune & Stratton, 1987:11–50.
9. Costa J, Wesley RA, Glatstein NE, Rosenberg SA. The grading of soft tissue sarcomas: Results of a clinico-histopathologic correlation in a series of 163 cases. Cancer 1984;53:530–541.
10. Russell WO, Cohen J, Enzinger FM, et al. A clinical and pathological staging system for soft tissue sarcomas. Cancer 1977;40:1562–1570.
11. Rosen G. Chemotherapy of sarcomas. In Eilber FR, Morton DL, Sondak VK, Economou JS. The soft tissue sarcomas. Orlando: Grune & Stratton, 1987:83–98.
12. Eilber FR. Sarcomas of bone and soft tissue. In Pilch YH. Surgical oncology. New York: McGraw-Hill, 1984:897.
13. Uman SJ, Kunin CM. Needle aspiration in the diagnosis of soft tissue infections. Arch Intern Med 1975;135:959–961.
14. Shmookler BM, Enzinger FM. Pleomorphic lipoma: A benign tumor simulating liposarcoma. Cancer 1981;47:126–133.
14a. Azumi N, Cutis J, Kempson RL, Hendrickson MR. Atypical and malignant neoplasms showing lipomatous differentiation. Am J Surg Pathol 1987;11:161–183.
15. Dahl I, Akerman M. Nodular fasciitis. A correlative cytologic and histologic study of 13 cases. Acta Cytol 1981;25:215–223.
16. McLeod DL, Geisinger KR, Hopkins MB III, Silverman JF. Fine needle aspiration cytology of the fibromatosis: A clinical and cytopathologic assessment [Abstract]. Acta Cytol 1987;31:683.
17. Perry MD, Furlong JW, Johnston WW. Fine needle aspiration cytology of metastatic dermatofibrosarcoma protuberans. A case report. Acta Cytol 1986;30:507–512.
18. Ramzy I. Benign schwannoma: Demonstration of Verocay bodies using fine-needle aspiration. Acta Cytol 1977;21:316–319.
19. Ryd W, Mugal S, Ayyash K. Ancient neurilemoma: A pitfall in the cytologic diagnosis of soft-tissue tumors. Diagn Cytopathol 1986;2:244–247.
20. Ireland DCR, Soule EH, Ivins JC. Myxoma of somatic soft tissues. Mayo Clin Proc 1973;48:401–410.
21. Allen PW. Tumors and proliferations of adipose tissue. New York: Masson Publishing, 1981:131–171.
22. Akerman M, Rydholm A. Aspiration cytology of lipomatous tumors. A 10–year experience at an orthopedic oncology center. Diagn Cytopathol 1987;3:295–302.
23. James LP. Myxoid liposarcoma: Diagnosis by fine needle aspiration cytology. Am Soc Clin Pathol Check Sample 1983;C–9.
24. James LP. Cytopathology of mesenchymal repair. Diagn Cytopathol 1985;1:91–104.
25. Stout AP, Hill WT. Leiomyosarcoma of the superficial soft tissues. Cancer 1958;11:844–854.
26. Dahl I, Hagmar B, Angervall L. Leiomyosarcoma of the soft tissue. A correlative cytologic and histologic study of 11 cases. Acta Pathol Microbiol Scand Sect A Pathol 1981;89:285–291.
27. Allen PV, Nodular fasciitis. Pathology 1972;4:9–26.
28. Harkin JC, Reed RJ. Tumors of the peripheral nervous system. Atlas of tumor pathology, 2nd Series, Fascicle 3. Washington D.C.: Armed Forces Institute of Pathology, 1969.
29. Hood IC, Qizilbash AH, Young JEM, Archibald SD. Needle aspiration cytology of a benign and a malignant schwannoma. Acta Cytol 1984;28:157–164.
30. Hajdu SI, Hajdu EO. Exfoliative cytology of malignant lymphoreticular, soft tissue and bone neoplasms. Pathol Annu 1977;11:317–334.
31. Koivuniemi A, Nickels J. Synovial sarcoma diagnosed by fine needle aspiration biopsy. A case report. Acta Cytol 1978;22:515–518.
32. Weiss SW, Enzinger FM. Malignant fibrous histiocytoma. Cancer 1978;41:2250–2266.
33. Wood GS, Beckstead JH, Turner RR, Hendrickson MR, Kempson RL, Warnke RA. Malignant fibrous histiocytoma tumor cells resemble fibroblasts. Am J Surg Pathol 1986;10:323–335.
34. Hsiu JG, Kreuger JK, D'Amato NA, Morris JR. Primary malignant fibrous histiocytoma of the lung. Fine needle aspiration cytologic features. Acta Cytol 1987;31:345–350.
35. Walaas L, Angervall L, Hagmar B, Save-Soderbergh J. A correlative cytology and histologic study of malignant fibrous histiocytoma: An analysis of 40 cases examined by fine-needle aspiration cytology. Diagn Cytopathol 1986;2:46–54.
36. Kim K, Goldblatt PJ. Malignant fibrous histiocytoma. Cytologic, light microscopic and ultrastructural studies. Acta Cytol 1982;26:507–511.
37. Nguyen GK, Jeannot A. Cytopathologic aspects of pulmonary metastasis of malignant fibrous histiocytoma, myxoid variant. Fine needle aspiration biopsy of a case. Acta Cytol 1982;26:349–353.

38. Fretzin DF, Helwig EB. Atypical fibroxanthoma of the skin. Cancer 1973;31:1541–1552.
39. de Jong ASH, van Kessel-van Vark M, van Heerde P. Fine needle aspiration biopsy diagnosis of rhabdomyosarcoma. An immunocytochemical study. Acta Cytol 1987;31:573–577.
40. Akhtar M, Ali MA, Sabbah R, Bakry M, Nash JE. Fine needle aspiration biopsy diagnosis of round cell malignant tumors of childhood. Cancer 1985;55:1805–1817.
41. Gillespie JJ, Roth LM, Wills ER, Einhorn LH, Willman J. Extraskeletal Ewing's sarcoma. Am J Surg Pathol 1979;3:99–108.
42. Mierau GW. Extraskeletal Ewing's sarcoma (peripheral neuroepithelioma). Ultrastruct Pathol 1985;9:91–98.
43. Cavazzana AO, Miser JS, Jefferson J, et al. Experimental evidence for a neural origin of Ewing's sarcoma of bone. Am J Pathol 1987:127:507–518.
44. Brehaut LE, Anderson LH, Taylor DA. Extraskeletal Ewing's sarcoma. Diagnosis of a case by fine needle aspiration cytology. Acta Cytol 1986;30:683–687.
45. Kontozoglou T, Krakauer K, Qizilbash AH. Ewing's sarcoma. Cytologic features in fine needle aspirates in two cases. Acta Cytol 1986;30:513–518.
46. Hajdu SI, Shiu MH, Fortner JG. Tendosynovial sarcomas. Cancer 1977;39:1201–1217.
47. Nieberg RK. Fine needle aspiration cytology of alveolar soft-part sarcoma. A case report. Acta Cytol 1984;28:198–202.
48. Zaleski S, Setum C, Benda J. Cytologic presentation of alveolar soft-part sarcoma of the vagina. A case report. Acta Cytol 1986;30:665–670.

6

Breast

The breast is one of the most common sites for aspiration biopsy.[1-6] Breast lumps are not only frequent but are also readily palpable. The technique of breast aspiration is so simple, rapid, and free of major complications that many physicians perform the procedure in their offices.[7,8] Like most other centers in North America, at our institution we aspirate mainly palpable breast masses, but other workers have shown that nonpalpable, mammographically demonstrable lesions also can be successfully needled with a stereotaxic device.[9,10]

Initially, most workers limited the use of aspiration to breast cysts[11] and breast masses that were clinically suspected to be malignant,[12,13] but a recent study shows convincingly that the routine use of FNAB in the evaluation of both benign and malignant breast nodules can lower medical costs by allowing the surgeon to triage which patients should have an outpatient excisional biopsy under local anesthesia and which patients should have a one-stage inpatient surgery.[14] In addition to these advantages, a positive preoperative diagnosis of carcinoma reduces patient uncertainty and anxiety, allows full discussion of treatment options, and permits preoperative metastatic workup on an outpatient basis. Moreover, when tissue sample is not available, estrogen receptor determination can be carried out on aspirated material.[15]

Diagnostic Accuracy

The accuracy rate of breast aspiration biopsy depends very much on the experience and previous training of the aspirator and the interpreter. The reported sensitivity of FNAB in the diagnosis of breast cancer varies considerably from just over 50% to approximately 95%.[1-8,12,13,16] Lee and associates[17] reported that the technical failure rate to obtain a positive diagnosis in cases of carcinoma was 9.8% for the single experienced aspirator and 45.9% for the group with many aspirators. Cohen and associates[18] showed that experienced interpreters had achieved statistically a significantly higher level of sensitivity and specificity than nonexpert interpreters. In general, reports from centers where FNAB is widely used have shown that the mean value for sensitivity is about 90%, specificity 95%, and predictive value for positive results 95%.[19,20] The statistics also vary as to whether or not the frozen section procedure is used after a positive cytologic diagnosis has been made. Understandably, the pathologist will be much more conservative in rendering a malignant cytologic diagnosis (hence, the sensitivity rate is lower) if mastectomy is to be performed without frozen section or surgical biopsy. At our institution, the frozen section procedure is considered unnecessary if the cytologic diagnosis is reported as definitely malignant by the author (six surgical pathologists are on rotation to sign-out FNAB). Among the 5713 breast aspirations, including both solid and cystic lesions, performed from January 1981 to December 1985,

there were 529 cases of carcinoma, of which a cytologic diagnosis of malignancy was made in 79%, a "suspicious" diagnosis in 11%, and a benign diagnosis in 10%. Among the 5184 benign cases, there was one false-positive diagnosis (the surgeon in this case elected to do an open biopsy, which showed florid ductal hyperplasia) and 28 "suspicious" cytologic diagnoses.

Pragmatic Approach

From a practical viewpoint, aspirates obtained from palpable breast carcinomas can be divided into three cytologic categories. The first category consists of aspirates that can be diagnosed unequivocally as positive for carcinoma, and an intraoperative frozen section becomes superfluous. In other words, the false-positive rate is zero in this group. In our experience, about 70–80% of breast carcinomas fall into this category; but for novices the percentage is understandably lower, making up about 50% or less of breast carcinomas.

The second category consists of aspirates with cytologic features suspected of carcinoma. About 15–20% of the carcinomas (mostly invasive lobular carcinomas) belong in this category and occasional cases of ductal hyperplasia and cellular fibroadenoma are also included. Prior to mastectomy, a frozen section examination is always required for confirmation of carcinoma in this group.

The third category consists of false-negative cases, which constitute about 10% of the carcinomas. This group comprises mostly desmoplastic carcinomas, small-sized carcinomas, and well-differentiated and tubular carcinomas. Hence, failure to identify carcinoma on aspiration biopsy cannot be considered definitive.

It is important to remember that there are many types of breast carcinoma and there is a wide range of morphologic expressions, ranging from the innocuous to the obviously malignant. **Figure 6.1** shows diagrammatically the cytology spectrum of the various types of malignant and benign lesions of the breast and that there is a significant overlap in cytologic appearance between the benign and malignant conditions. The cytopathologist should aim at diagnosing conclusively 75–85%, but not 100%, of breast carcinomas so that he or she can maintain at all times a wide margin of safety and a zero false-positive rate (see later discussion).[3,12] It is not crucial whether the smears are alcohol-fixed or air-dried, because "fine-tuning" of diagnosis is not necessary and may even lead to overdiagnosis. The air-dried method of fixation is indeed more convenient and preferred when aspirations are performed by surgeons in their offices. Subtle nuclear changes that are important in separating malignant from benign lesions in other sites are not as important in the diagnosis of palpable breast carcinoma, because if the slightest doubt exists, the pathologist must refrain from diagnosing the lesion as carcinoma and defer the diagnosis to open biopsy or frozen section.

The fact that aspiration cytology is unable to differentiate be-

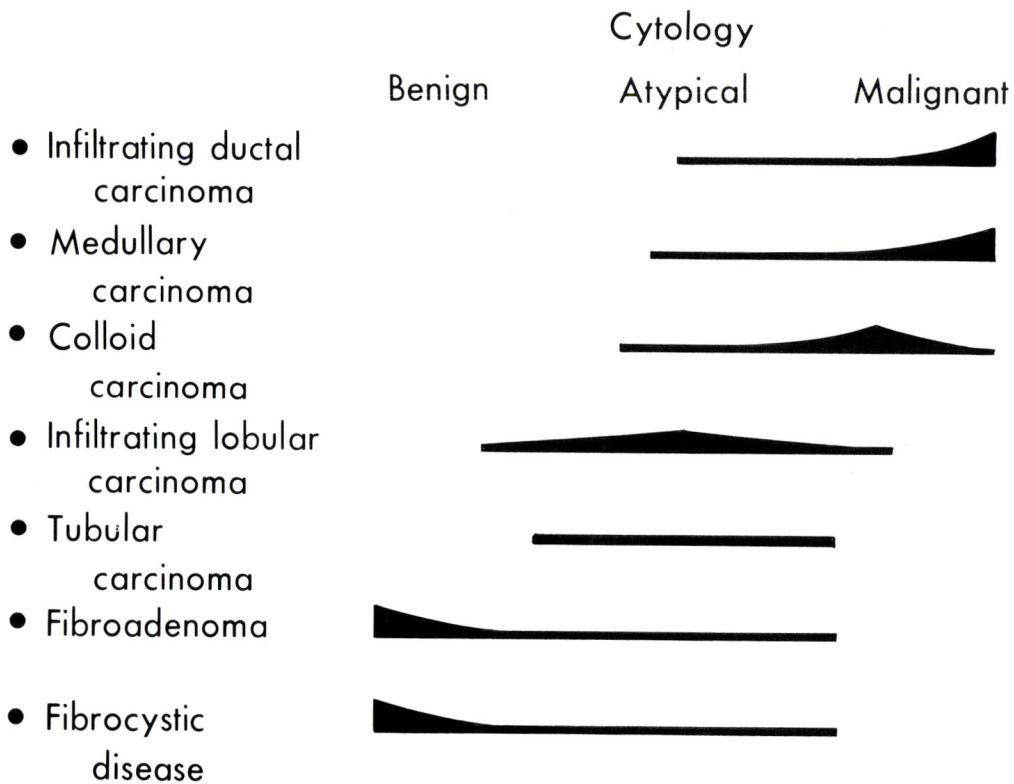

Figure 6.1. Cytology spectrum of various malignant and benign lesions of the breast.

tween intraductal and invasive ductal carcinoma is a moot point since the type of surgical treatment to be carried out is primarily contingent on the size of the palpable tumor and stage of the disease.[21,22]

MALIGNANT NEOPLASMS

Cancer of the breast is the most common malignancy encountered in women,[23] and the great majority of these cancers are infiltrating ductal carcinomas of the nonspecific type.[24] Breast carcinomas that have specific microscopic features or have a specific clinical behavior are classified separately. **Table 6.1** shows with some slight modifications the classification of breast carcinomas published in the Armed Forces Institutes of Pathology fascicle: *Tumors of the Breast*.[24]

Table 6.1.   Histologic Classification of Breast Carcinomas

Carcinomas of mammary ducts
  Intraductal
    Papillary carcinoma
    Comedocarcinoma
  Infiltrating
    Ductal carcinoma, nonspecific type
    Medullary carcinoma
    Colloid carcinoma
    Papillary carcinoma
    Tubular carcinoma
Carcinomas of mammary lobules
  In situ lobular carcinoma
  Infiltrating lobular carcinoma
Unusual types
  Intracystic carcinoma
  Squamous carcinoma
  Adenoid cystic carcinoma
  Sarcomatoid metaplastic carcinoma

Infiltrating Ductal Carcinoma, Nonspecific Type

Ductal carcinomas of the nonspecific type account for about 70–80% of all breast carcinomas. To make an unequivocal diagnosis of carcinoma so that definitive operation can be performed without frozen section examination, or radiation or chemotherapy can be given in inoperable cases, a set of strict cytologic criteria must be observed. Any false-positive report not only invalidates this valuable function of FNAB but may also prove harmful to the patient.

Aspiration Cytology

Cellular Pattern.   An increased cellularity is the first prerequisite for the diagnosis of breast carcinoma. The classic malignant pattern should show numerous tumor cells present as isolated cells in addition to clusters of various sizes **(Fig. 6.2)**.

Attempts at making the diagnosis on sparsely cellular material should be discouraged. Moreover, one should insist on seeing dyshesive or isolated malignant cells before a categoric diagnosis of carcinoma is made.[25] Cohesive cell clusters by themselves, no matter how atypical cytologically, are not an absolute criterion for carcinoma, because similar elements may be derived from atypical ductal hyperplasia, cellular papillomas, and fibroadenomas.

Cell Morphology.   In general, the malignant cells show nuclear enlargement, and considerable anisonucleosis may be present **(Fig. 6.2B)**. The nuclei are hyperchromatic and have irregularly distributed coarse chromatin. Nucleolar prominence is observed in poorly differentiated carcinomas, but may not be seen in other cases and is not required for diagnosis. Cytoplasm is visible, as opposed to the naked oval nuclei seen in benign lesions (discussed later). In some cases, the nuclei of the neoplastic cells may show little cytologic atypia in the usual sense **(Fig. 6.3)**. Nonetheless, a confident diag-

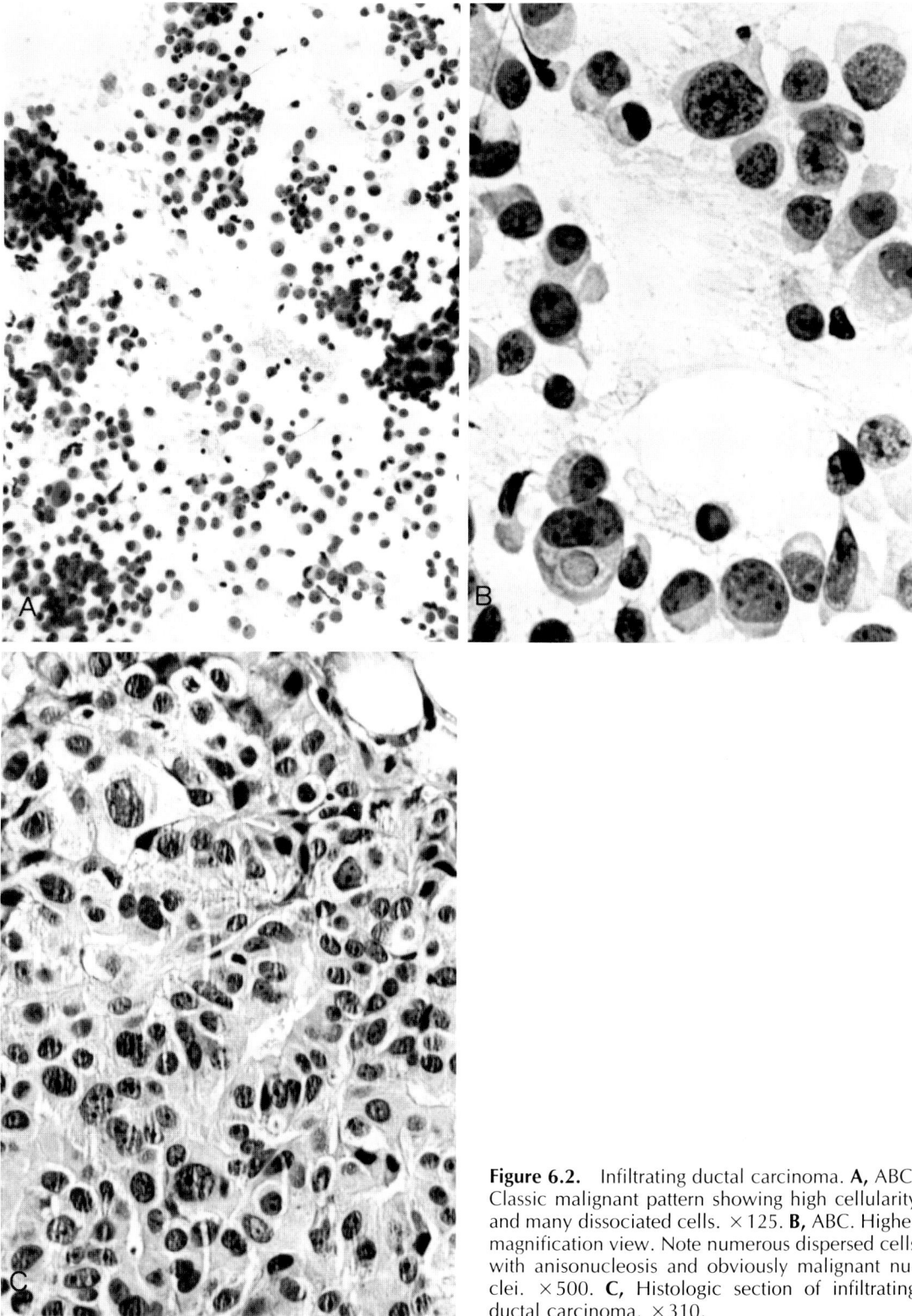

Figure 6.2. Infiltrating ductal carcinoma. **A,** ABC. Classic malignant pattern showing high cellularity and many dissociated cells. ×125. **B,** ABC. Higher magnification view. Note numerous dispersed cells with anisonucleosis and obviously malignant nuclei. ×500. **C,** Histologic section of infiltrating ductal carcinoma. ×310.

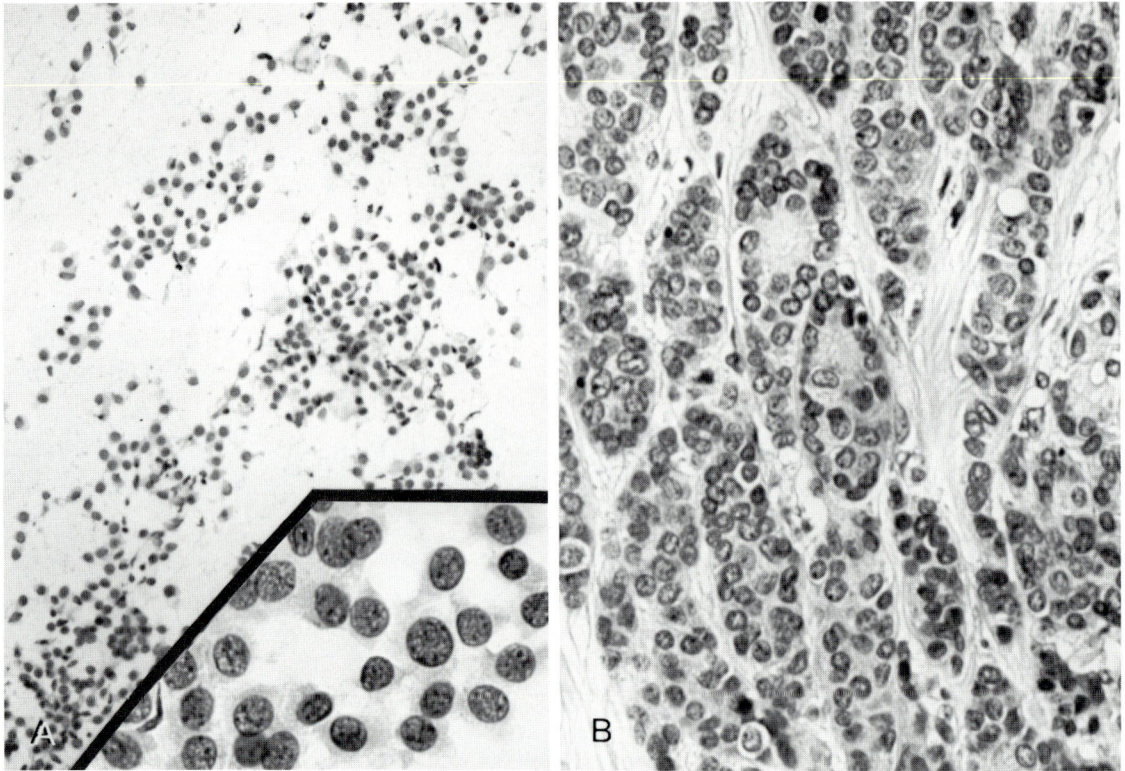

Figure 6.3.

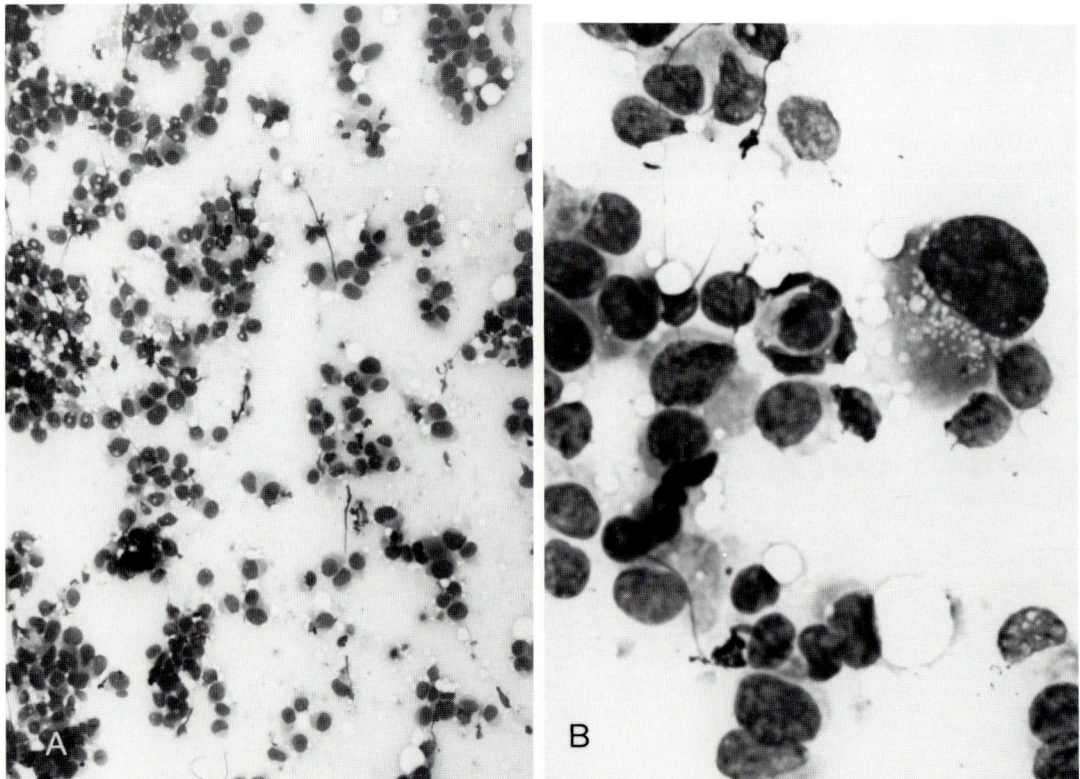

Figure 6.4.

nosis of carcinoma can still be made in the presence of hypercellularity and a dispersed cell pattern. Air-dried smears (**Fig. 6.4**) are also suitable for interpretation.

Diagnostic Pitfalls. If one adheres to the strict cytologic criteria outlined above (high cellularity and pronounced cell dyshesion), about 10–15% of breast carcinomas will have a false-negative diagnosis. This conservatism is mandatory if the cytologic diagnosis is the basis for a radical mastectomy.[3,12] A negative cytologic report, therefore, should not preclude an open surgical biopsy if clinical or mammographic evidence suggests malignancy.

The common causes for false-negative cytologic reports are: (a) sampling problems in small lesions and markedly fibrotic lesions, and (b) interpretive problems, especially in well-differentiated carcinomas (e.g., tubular carcinoma and intraductal papillary carcinoma) and in carcinomas with small uniform cells (e.g., lobular carcinoma).

False-positive cytologic reports are largely interpretive errors. These may result from inexperience, an over-zealous pathologist, or making a diagnosis on insufficient material.

More recently, as more mammary carcinomas are treated with local irradiation following a partial mastectomy, benign irradiated cells constitute a diagnostic problem in evaluating tumor recurrence. Two important cytologic features aid in separating irradiated cells from malignant cells, in addition to the clinical history. First, the smears are characterized by poor cellularity and second, some benign bipolar naked nuclei (myoepithelial cell nuclei) can be seen in close proximity to the atypical cell clusters.[26,27]

Medullary Carcinoma

Medullary carcinoma of the breast, accounting for less than 5% of breast carcinomas, has a distinctive microscopic picture and a prognosis better than infiltrating ductal carcinoma of the nonspecific type. The tumor cells are large, rather uniform, and exhibit a syncytial growth pattern. An important part of the histologic picture is a prominent lymphoid component within the tumor.

Aspiration Cytology

Aspirates from medullary carcinomas are cell-rich. The ABC shows neoplastic cells admixed with lymphocytes (**Fig. 6.5**). The neoplastic cells are large and polygonal in shape, with round or cleaved, vesicular nuclei and distinct nucleoli. Cytoplasm is abundant. The cytoplasmic borders are often poorly demarcated and some cells appear as naked nuclei. In addition to the single cells, syncytial groups of tumor cells are present. The number of lymphocytes is variable, but at times they may present in such large numbers that they can obscure the neoplastic cells and render interpretation difficult.

Colloid Carcinoma

Massive mucin production characterizes colloid carcinoma, which represents about 2–3% of all breast cancers. Like medullary carcinoma, it has a better prognosis than the ordinary invasive ductal carcinoma.

Aspiration Cytology

The number of tumor cells present is quite variable. A copious amount of mucous material with few tumor cells may be aspirated. The tumor cells are generally small and fairly uniform with minimal atypia (although in an occasional case the tumor cells can be quite pleomorphic). The cytoplasm is frequently vacuolated. The cells occur singly and in small loose clusters and are seen floating in a sea of mucin (**Fig. 6.6**). The finding of a large amount of mucin in a breast aspirate should alert the pathologist to the possibility of colloid carcinoma even though the neoplastic cells present may have a relatively innocuous appearance.[28]

Tubular Carcinoma

Tubular carcinoma is a very well-differentiated form of carcinoma, characterized by orderly ducts and tubules. The tumors tend to be small in size when first diagnosed and have a favorable prognosis.

The smears are moderately cellular and show variably sized tubules and cords, formed by small uniform cuboidal or columnar cells. The nuclear appearance may be quite bland (**Fig. 6.7**). Dissociated cells are not prominent. A definitive cytologic diagnosis of carcinoma should not be made and an excisional biopsy or frozen section is called for.

Papillary Carcinoma

Papillary carcinoma of the breast is a circumscribed, slow-growing tumor with malignant cells forming papillary projections. The tumor can be intraductal or infiltrating, and the papillary configuration is often maintained even in the infiltrating stage.

The aspirates show a variable cellularity, consisting of isolated cells and small papillae or large clusters with three-dimensional papillary projections. The background frequently shows hemosiderin-laden macrophages and blood. The papillary clusters may predominate the smear, and the component cells are cohesive (**Fig. 6.8**). Because of the cohesive cell pattern and the frequently innocuous appearance of the malignant cells, this tumor may be difficult to differentiate from benign papilloma or fibroadenoma.[29] A cytologic diagnosis of papillary carcinoma must be confirmed by frozen section or excisional biopsy. Even in tissue sections, its separation from papilloma may be difficult.

Figure 6.3. Infiltrating ductal carcinoma. **A,** ABC. Note cellular dyshesion and hypercellularity. Compared with the case shown in **Figure 6.2,** the tumor cells here are smaller and more uniform, with much less cytologic atypia. **A,** ×100; *Inset,* ×500. **B,** Histologic section of the ductal carcinoma. Note small, uniform cells ×310.

Figure 6.4. Infiltrating ductal carcinoma, air-dried smear. **A** and **B,** The diagnosis of carcinoma can be made because the basic malignant pattern is present, even though the chromatin pattern is not as well preserved as in alcohol-fixed smears. May-Grünwald Giemsa stain, **A,** ×125; **B,** ×500.

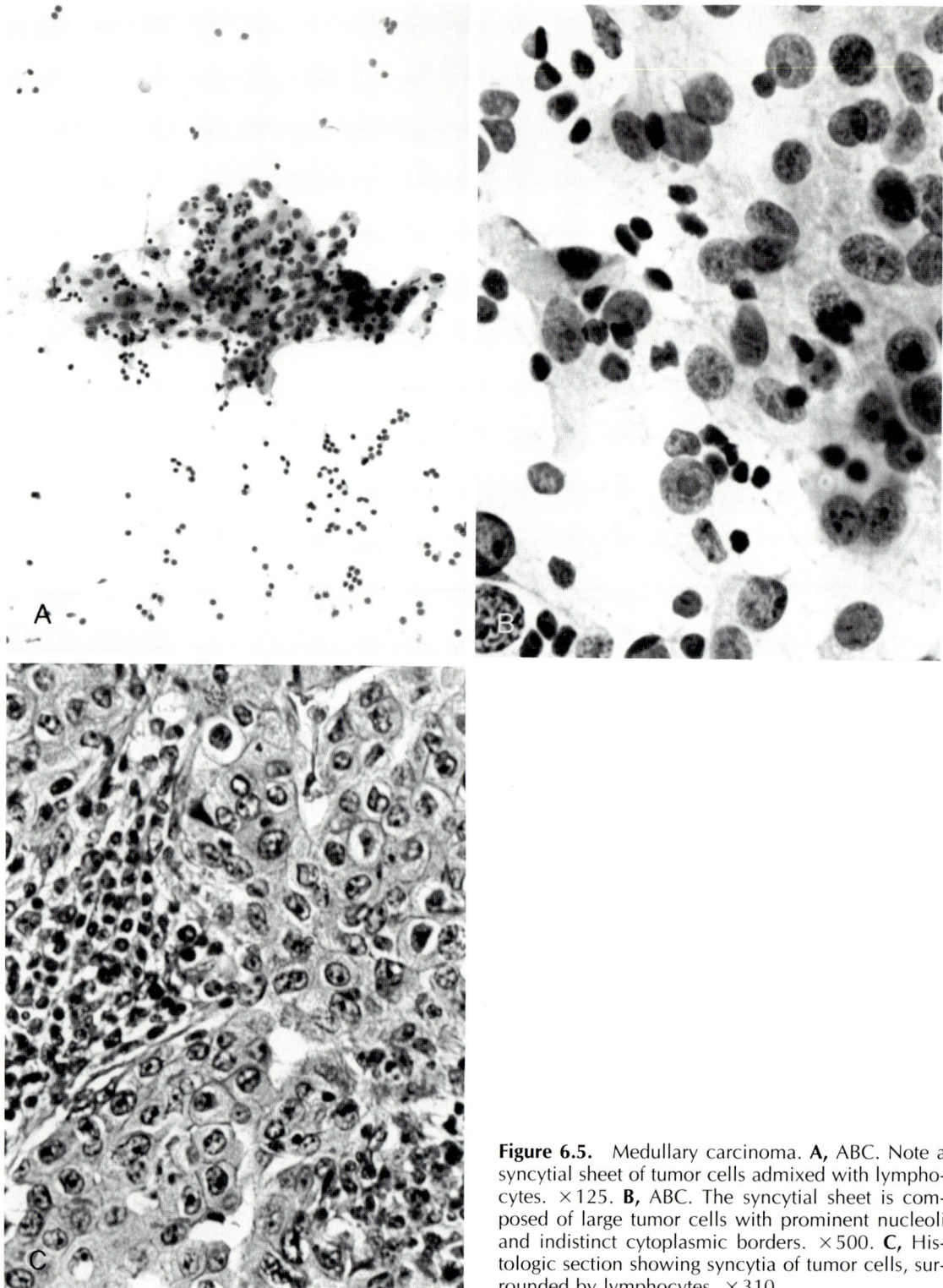

Figure 6.5. Medullary carcinoma. **A,** ABC. Note a syncytial sheet of tumor cells admixed with lymphocytes. ×125. **B,** ABC. The syncytial sheet is composed of large tumor cells with prominent nucleoli and indistinct cytoplasmic borders. ×500. **C,** Histologic section showing syncytia of tumor cells, surrounded by lymphocytes. ×310.

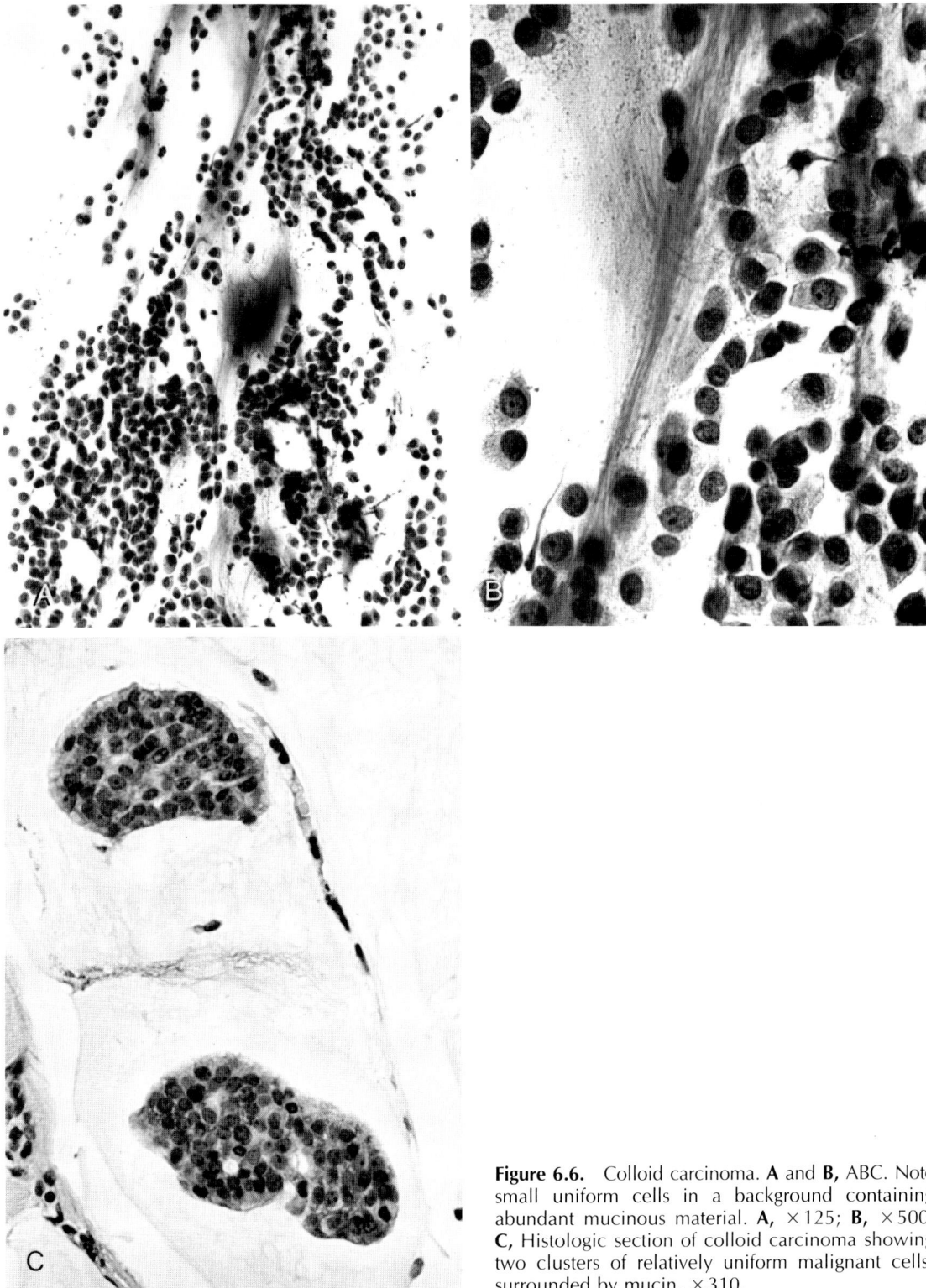

Figure 6.6. Colloid carcinoma. **A** and **B,** ABC. Note small uniform cells in a background containing abundant mucinous material. **A,** ×125; **B,** ×500. **C,** Histologic section of colloid carcinoma showing two clusters of relatively uniform malignant cells, surrounded by mucin. ×310.

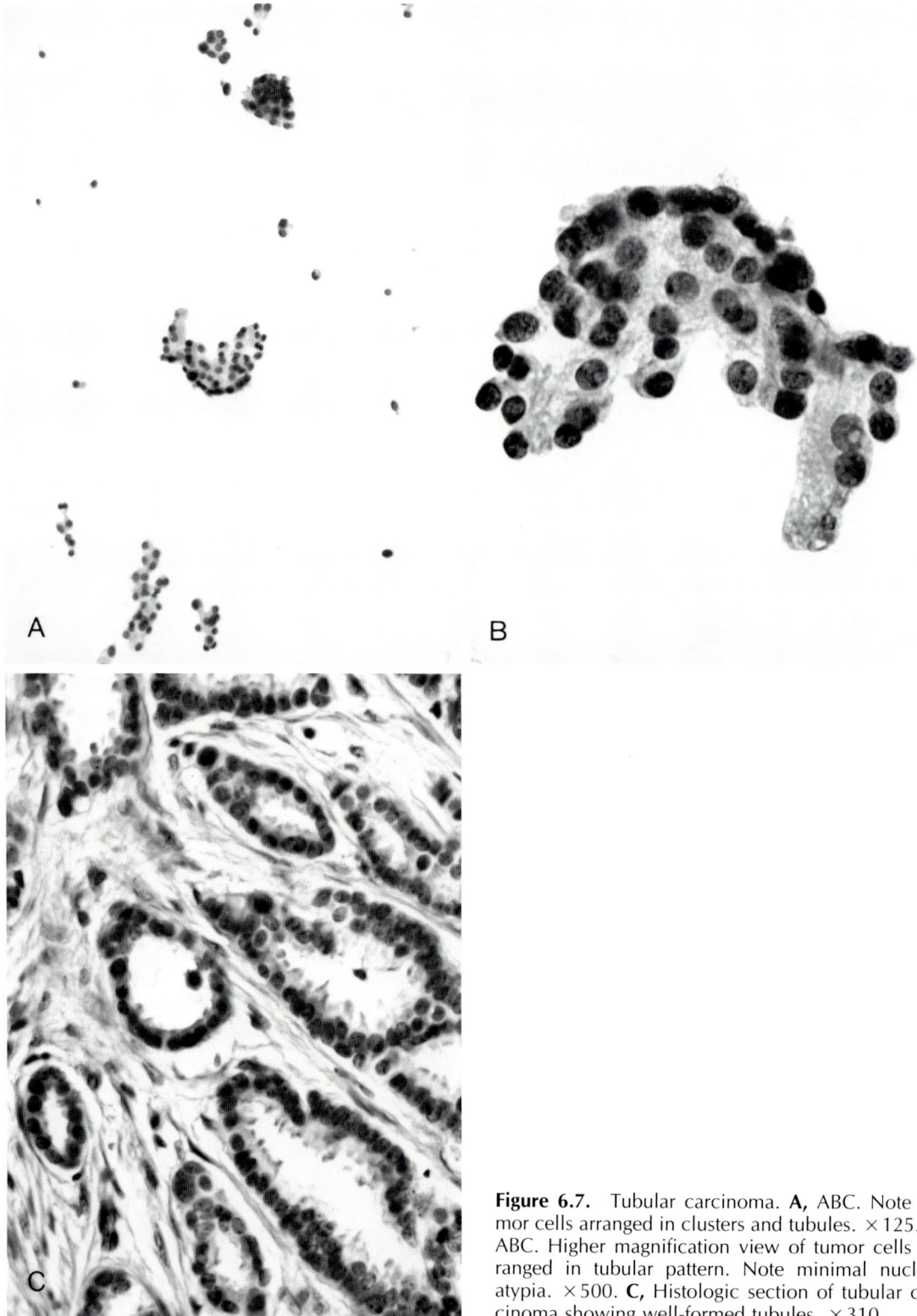

Figure 6.7. Tubular carcinoma. **A,** ABC. Note tumor cells arranged in clusters and tubules. ×125. **B,** ABC. Higher magnification view of tumor cells arranged in tubular pattern. Note minimal nuclear atypia. ×500. **C,** Histologic section of tubular carcinoma showing well-formed tubules. ×310.

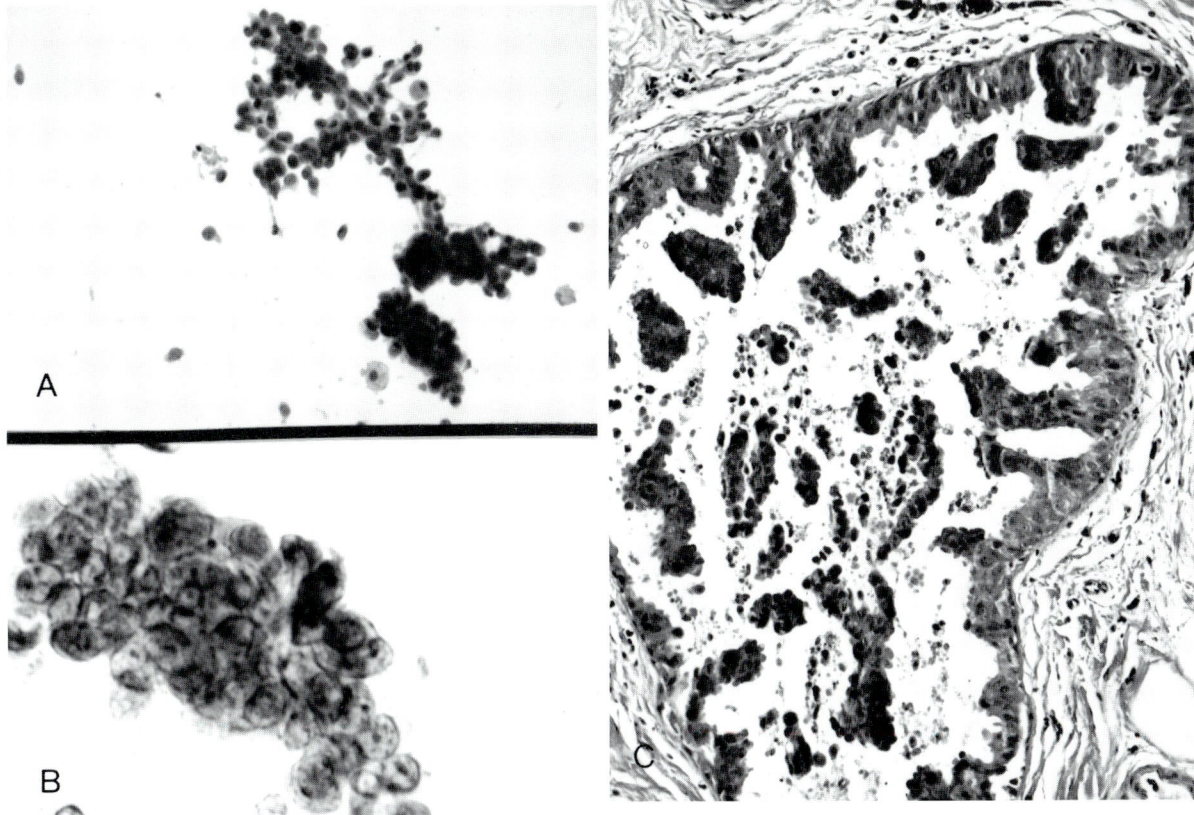

Figure 6.8. Intraductal papillary carcinoma. **A,** ABC. Papillary clusters. ×125. **B,** ABC. A three-dimensional papillary cluster of cohesive cells showing moderate degree of nuclear atypia. ×500.

C, Histologic section showing neoplastic papillae growing within a duct. Note hemosiderin-laden macrophages and blood in the duct lumen. ×125.

In the literature, Naran et al.[30] described nuclear membrane irregularity in one-third of cases; in contrast, Kline and Kannan[29] reported minimal nuclear abnormalities and cellular monomorphism in their cases. Moderate anisonucleosis, however, is a common feature seen in all of the reported cases.[29,30]

Infiltrating Lobular Carcinoma

Infiltrating lobular carcinoma, constituting about 5–10% of all breast tumors, is much less common than infiltrating ductal carcinoma. It is frequently multifocal and is as lethal as the ordinary infiltrating ductal carcinoma. Histologically, it is characterized by small neoplastic cells that diffusely infiltrate a dense fibrous stroma. The single-file (also called ''Indian file'') arrangement of the neoplastic cells is a well-known characteristic of this tumor.

Aspiration Cytology

The aspiration cytology of invasive lobular carcinoma has been discussed in detail by various authors[31,32] and is summarized below.

Cell Morphology. The cells are relatively small, rounded, and may superficially resemble lymphocytes **(Fig. 6.9)**. Anisonucleosis is minimal but the nuclear membrane is irregular. Prominent nucleoli may be seen in some of the cells. The N/C ratio is high. In some cases, the tumor cells contain cytoplamic mucin vacuoles **(Fig. 6.10)**.

Cellular Pattern. The ABC presents a cell-sparse pattern due to marked stromal desmoplasia, which is a feature present in most of invasive lobular carcinomas. The dense fibrous stroma binds down the tumor cells and prevents them from being aspirated. In the smears the tumor cells occur in small loose clusters, in short Indian files, or lying singly **(Fig. 6.9)**. At times, larger sheets of dyshesive tumor cells can also be seen **(Fig. 6.10)**.

Diagnostic Pitfalls. In a study from Memorial Sloan-Kettering Cancer Center, only 25% of the 87 lobular carcinomas could be interpreted as positive.[7] In view of the cell-sparse pattern and the uniformity and the small size of the tumor cells, we do not advocate making a definite diagnosis of lobular carcinoma on aspirates. With increased experience, one may be able to suspect the diagnosis with a high degree of confidence. For the novice, this tumor type is a frequent source of false-negative reports.

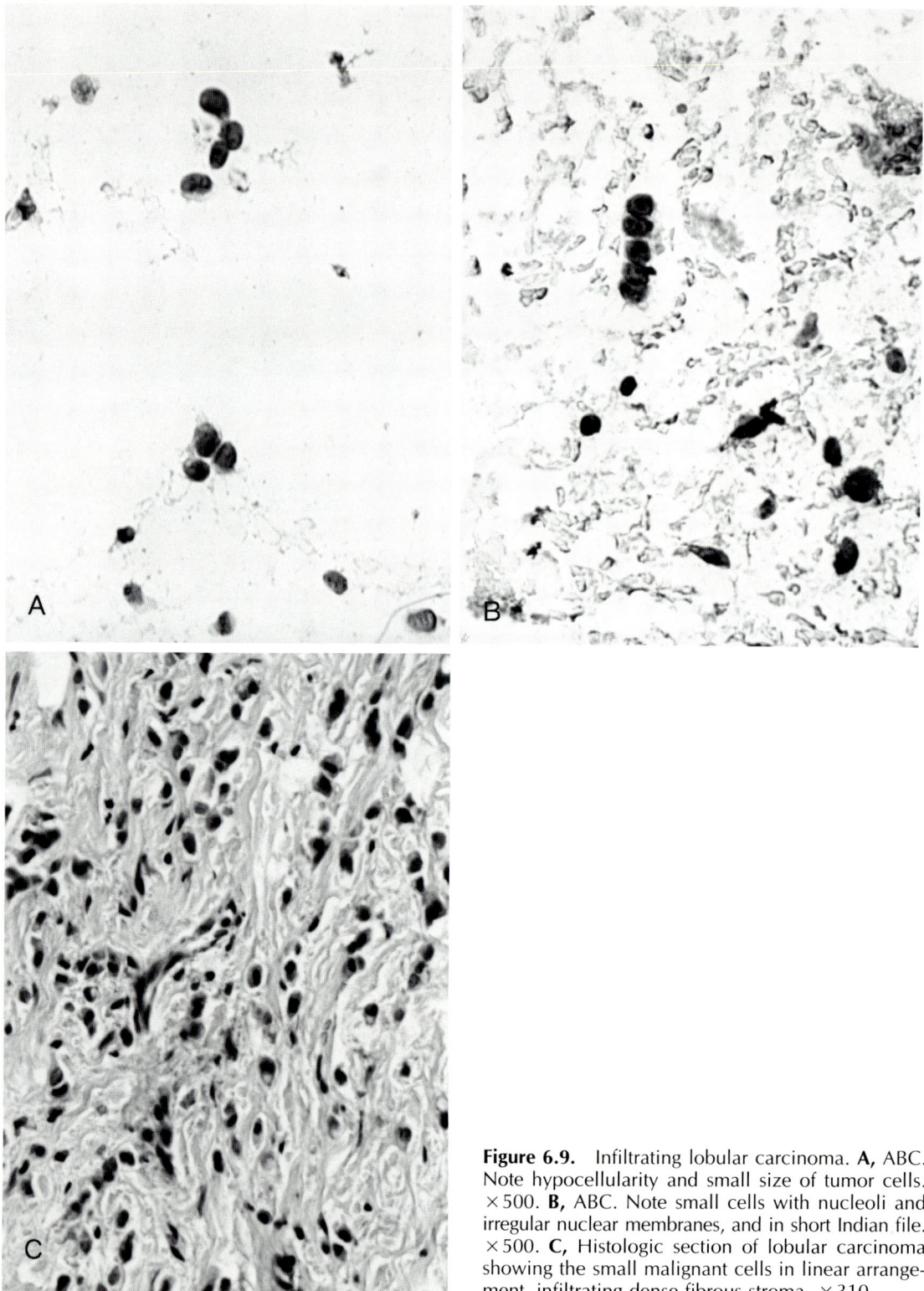

Figure 6.9. Infiltrating lobular carcinoma. **A,** ABC. Note hypocellularity and small size of tumor cells. ×500. **B,** ABC. Note small cells with nucleoli and irregular nuclear membranes, and in short Indian file. ×500. **C,** Histologic section of lobular carcinoma showing the small malignant cells in linear arrangement, infiltrating dense fibrous stroma. ×310.

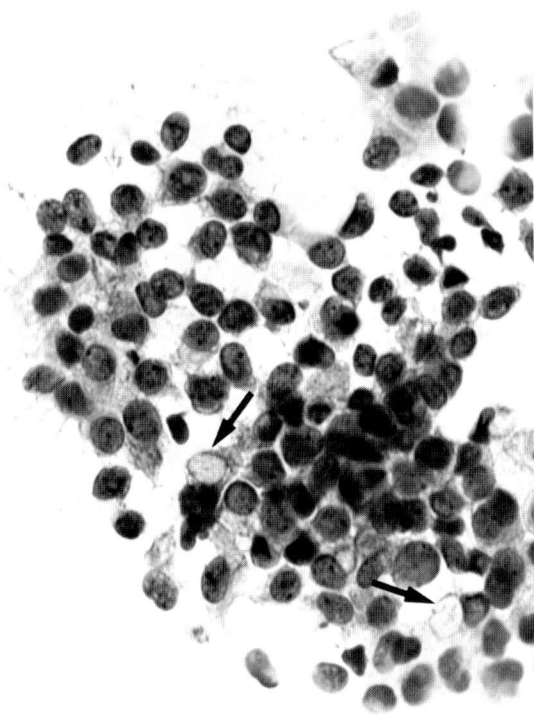

Figure 6.10. Infiltrating lobular carcinoma, ABC. Large cell sheet composed of dyshesive tumor cells with small, round, rather uniform nuclei. A few cells show cytoplasmic mucin vacuoles *(arrows).* ×500.

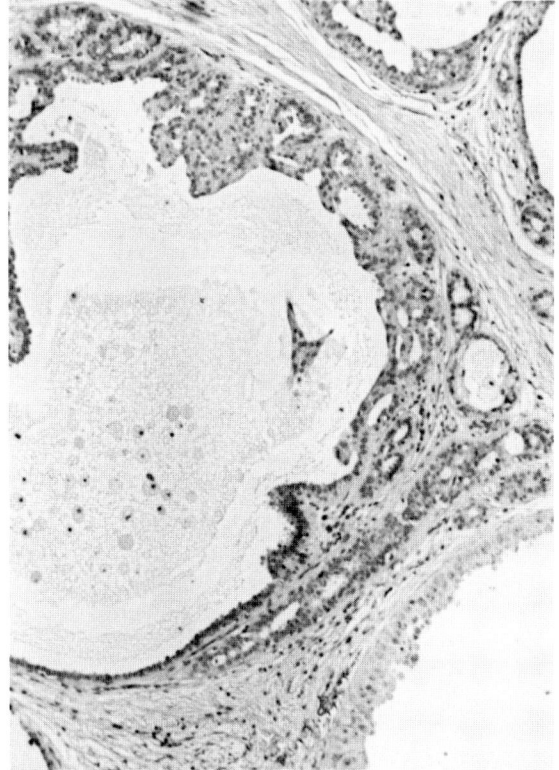

Figure 6.11. Histology of fibrocystic disease. Note cystic dilatation of mammary ducts, containing foamy macrophages and focal apocrine metaplasia of ductal epithelium. ×125.

BENIGN TUMORS AND TUMOR-LIKE LESIONS

Fibrocystic Disease

Mammary fibrocystic disease is the most common abnormality of the breast in women of reproductive age. The disease is usually bilateral and the breasts are characteristically lumpy, with soft to rubbery firm, ill-defined nodules. The histologic changes are protean **(Fig. 6.11).** Ducts and ductules may be dilated to variable degree. Large cysts may develop and are lined with atrophic or flattened epithelium. Apocrine metaplastic change in ductal epithelium is common. Foci of epithelial hyperplasia and papillomatosis are observed, but epithelial involution is also usual. The stroma is usually dense.

Aspiration Cytology

The aspirates are hypocellular to moderately cellular **(Fig. 6.12A).** The most common cellular element is the benign epithelial duct cell. These cells are small, uniform, and low columnar to cuboidal. The nuclei are bland and the nucleoli are tiny or absent. They are characteristically arranged in well-organized clusters with a honeycomb pattern **(Fig. 6.12B),** although some degree of nuclear crowding can be seen especially in cases of ductal hyperplasia.

Another characteristic feature is the small oval naked nuclei, lying singly in the background. These naked nuclei have smooth nuclear membranes, a uniformly stained chromatin pattern, and in-

visible nucleoli **(Fig. 6.12C).** The exact origin of these naked nuclei are uncertain; it is believed that they are derived from myoepithelial cells or stromal connective tissue cells.[33] The fibrous matrix, although abundant in mammary fibrocystic disease, is not easily aspirated and is thus poorly represented in aspirated material. Another cell type, which is frequently but not always present, is the apocrine metaplastic cell **(Fig. 6.12D).** These are large, cohesive cells with abundant eosinophilic granular cytoplasm. The nuclei are round and moderate to large in size. The nucleoli may at times be quite prominent.

Diagnostic Pitfalls. In one series of breast FNABs, 82% of 210 cases of fibrocystic disease showed few or no epithelial cells.[34] The question then comes up as to what represents an adequate sample. According to Kline[20] an aspirate specimen is considered adequate if it is vigorously and competently taken and includes punctures from different representative areas. There must be at least two or three epithelial groups per slide.

On the other hand, in cases of fibrocystic disease in which ductal hyperplasia dominates, the smears are rich in cells. In atypical hyperplasia **(Fig. 6.13),** the aspirate may consist of many sheets of epithelial cells that are cytologically atypical.[35] In such situations, it is important to study carefully the appearance of the scattered isolated cells. The presence of isolated benign naked oval nuclei should suggest a benign diagnosis; isolated carcinoma cells, on the other hand, show nuclear abnormalites and visible cytoplasm.

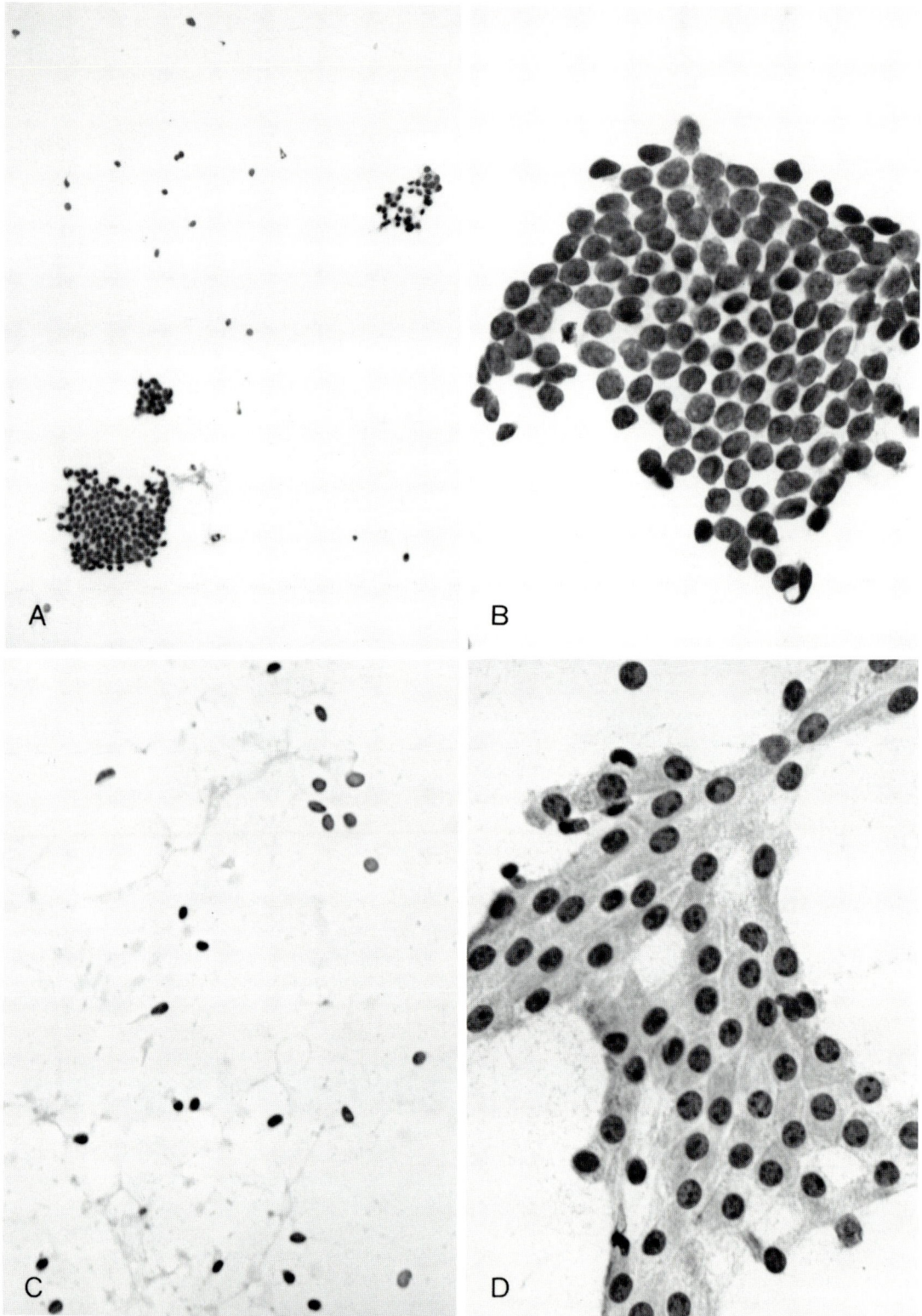

Figure 6.12. Fibrocystic disease, ABC. **A,** Note clusters of uniform cells and a few naked oval nuclei scattered in the background. ×125. **B,** Well-organized cell cluster containing small, uniform cells in honeycomb arrangement. ×500. **C,** Many naked oval nuclei lying singly. ×310. **D,** Sheet of apocrine metaplastic cells. These cells are cohesive, with nucleoli and abundant eosinophilic granular cytoplasm. ×500.

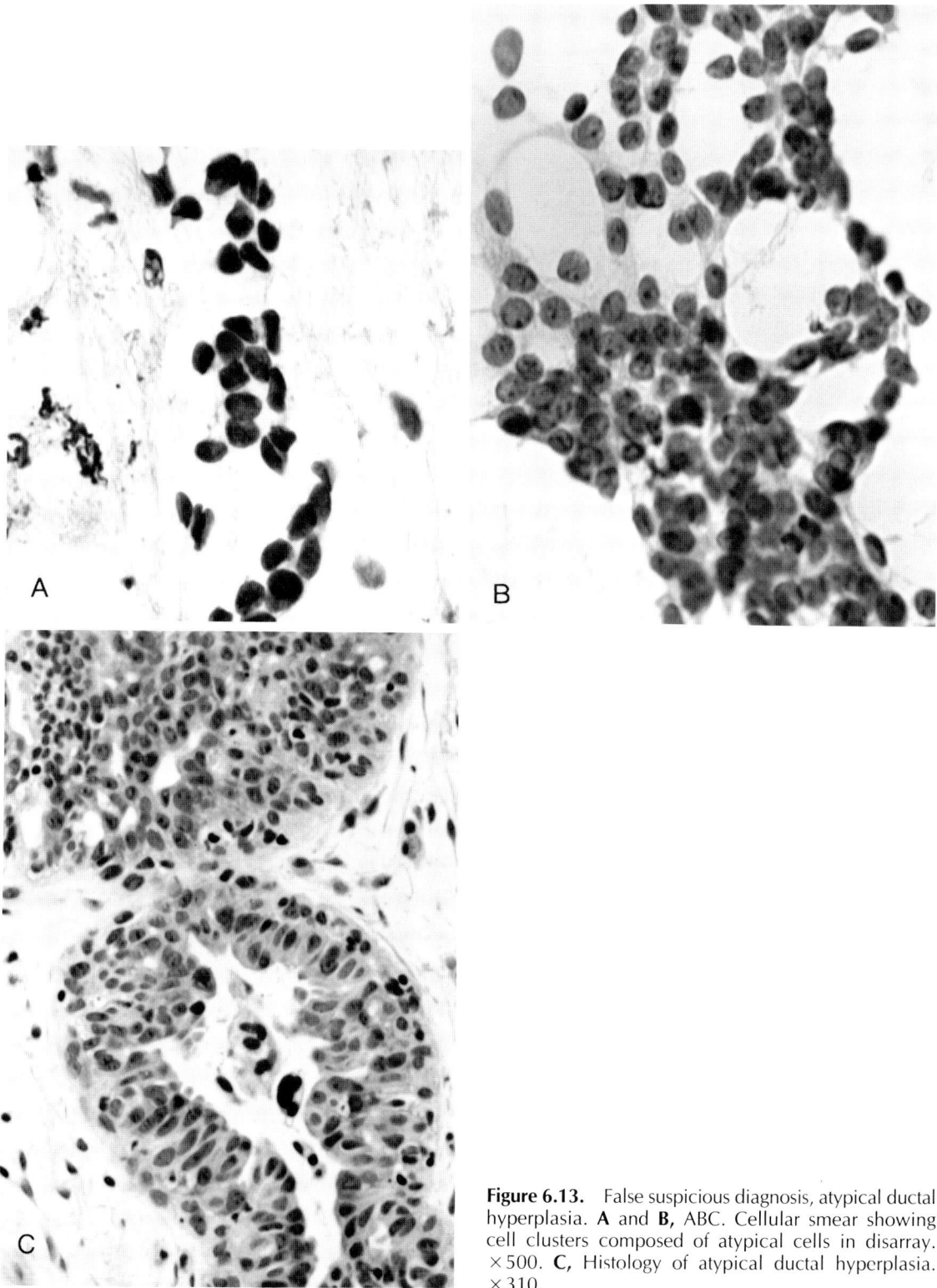

Figure 6.13. False suspicious diagnosis, atypical ductal hyperplasia. **A** and **B,** ABC. Cellular smear showing cell clusters composed of atypical cells in disarray. ×500. **C,** Histology of atypical ductal hyperplasia. ×310.

Cysts

Breast cysts are common and are part of the fibrocystic disease spectrum. Needle aspiration biopsy is not only used for diagnosis but also is used as a therapeutic tool for evacuation of cyst content.[36,37] This is the most common condition in which malignancy can be excluded by FNAB and a surgical excision can be avoided because a malignant breast cyst is a rare occurrence (see "Diagnostic Pitfalls").

Aspiration Cytology

The aspirated fluid may be clear or turbid, straw-colored, green, or brown. The fluid may contain a few small clumps of benign duct cells and apocrine metaplastic cells as in fibrocystic disease, and sometimes leukocytes. The major cell type is the foamy histiocyte (**Fig. 6.14**) and in many instances these are the only cells present in the fluid.

Diagnostic Pitfalls. If the cyst fluid is grossly bloody, one must keep in mind the possibility of malignancy, although it may simply be due to bleeding into the benign cyst. Cystic material containing papillary cell clusters, fronds, or large sheets of more than 100 ductal cells may be an indication of an intraductal papilloma or carcinoma.[36,38] On the other hand, benign apocrine cells are not seen in cancer cases, but are frequently encountered in benign cysts.[36]

Intracystic carcinomas are rare. Rosemond et al.[11] reported a 0.1% incidence in 3000 breast cysts. In two of the three cases reported by the same authors[37] the cyst reappeared within 2 weeks of the time of the original aspiration, and in the third case it was not completely eliminated by the original aspiration attempt.

A separate carcinoma may be present adjacent to a cyst. If any solid lump can still be palpable after the cyst has been evacuated, this must be reaspirated.

Fibroadenoma

Fibroadenomas are common benign neoplasms of the breast and generally occur in women between 20 and 35 years of age. Clinically they are single, demarcated lumps, with a rubbery firm consistency and are usually no more than 3 cm in diameter.

Aspiration Cytology

The cytologic features of fibroadenomas resemble those of fibrocystic disease.[39] The differences are mainly quantitative; aspirates of fibroadenomas contain aggregates of benign ductal epithelial cells and isolated naked oval nuclei in greater numbers (**Fig. 6.15**). The epithelial cells occur in small and large cell sheets, composed of tightly packed, uniform, round cells, with scant cytoplasm, often arranged as branching ducts, resulting in a characteristic antler horn pattern.[40] The isolated naked oval nuclei are bipolar, cigar-shaped, and benign-appearing; they are seen scattered on the background. Apocrine metaplastic cells, so often seen in fibrocystic disease, are much less frequent. When a fibroadenoma is rich in stroma, fragments of pink collagenous tissue also may be present in the smear.

Diagnostic Pitfalls. Cytologically, it is not always possible to separate fibroadenoma from florid fibrocystic disease, unless fluid is also aspirated. Clinically, the former is a discrete solid lump, while the latter is usually associated with diffuse lumpy breasts.

Aspirates from fibroadenomas may be misinterpreted as carcinoma because of hypercellularity of the smears or presence of atypical ductal cells or both (**Fig. 6.16**).[35] The cytopathologist should pay attention to the benign naked oval nuclei and the uniform cohesive cell sheets. Their presence should preclude the diagnosis of malignancy.

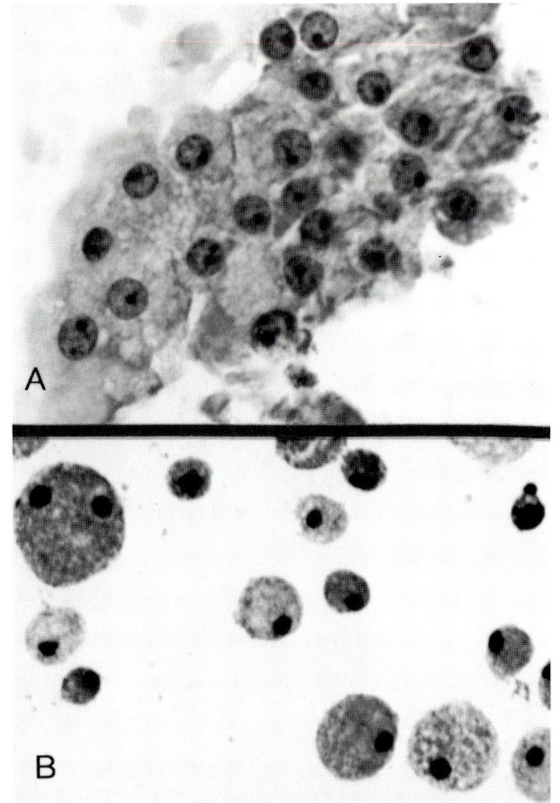

Figure 6.14. Benign breast cyst, ABC. **A,** Sheet of degenerated apocrine cells with distinct nucleoli and granular cytoplasm. ×500. **B,** Foamy histiocytes. May-Grünwald Giemsa stain, ×500.

Conversely, some well-differentiated mammary carcinomas, such as tubular carcinoma and papillary carcinoma, may be mistaken for fibroadenoma on cytology, because aspirations of all these lesions yield tight, orderly cell clusters.

Cystosarcoma Phyllodes

Cystosarcoma phyllodes, also known as giant fibroadenoma, is a rare type of mammary neoplasm. The tumor generally occurs in women older than those with fibroadenoma and attains a much greater size (as large as 15 cm or more).[41] Histologically, it differs from fibroadenoma in that the stromal or mesenchymal cells show marked proliferation and sometimes may be pleomorphic. The epithelial component of the tumor, on the other hand, is similar to that of fibroadenoma. The continued use of the term giant fibroadenoma is undesirable, because some of these tumors (about 20%) behave in a malignant fashion. In the malignant tumors, the stromal cells are morphologically malignant, reminiscent of fibrosarcoma; whereas in the benign tumors, the stroma is like that of a fibroma. In practice, however, the distinction between the two groups is not always that clear-cut. Borderline cases are therefore encountered and local recurrence is not uncommon.[42]

Aspiration Cytology

The ABC (**Figs. 6.17** and **6.18**) of benign and borderline cystosarcomas show many sheets of epithelial duct cells, stromal tissue fragments, and isolated mesenchymal cells (including bipolar naked nuclei).[43] The epithelial cells are arranged in cohesive sheets, resembling those seen in fibroadenomas. Both bipolar naked nuclei and spindle-shaped fibrocytes with visible cytoplasm can be seen in the background. The presence of the latter cells favors the diagnosis of

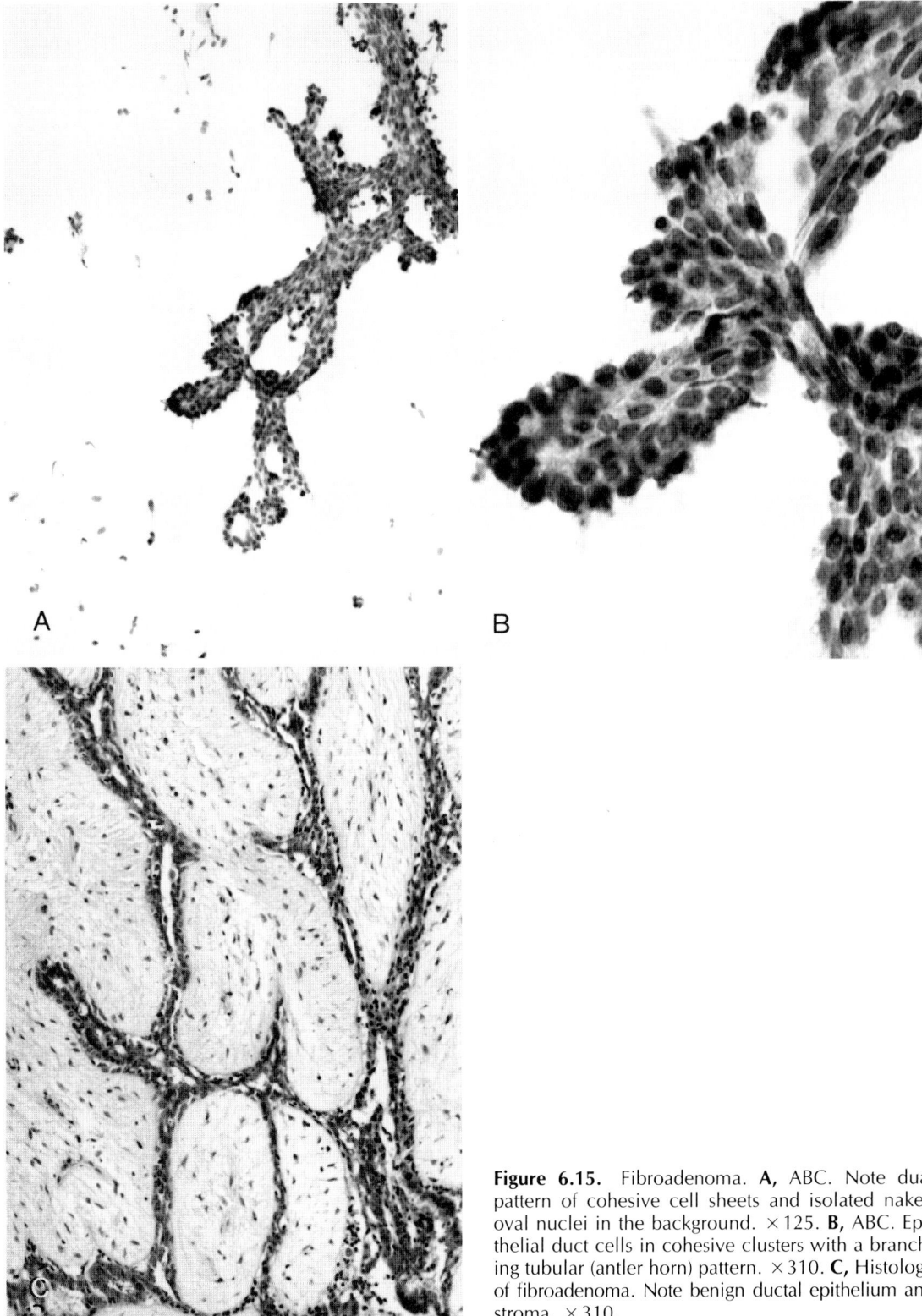

Figure 6.15. Fibroadenoma. **A,** ABC. Note dual pattern of cohesive cell sheets and isolated naked oval nuclei in the background. ×125. **B,** ABC. Epithelial duct cells in cohesive clusters with a branching tubular (antler horn) pattern. ×310. **C,** Histology of fibroadenoma. Note benign ductal epithelium and stroma. ×310.

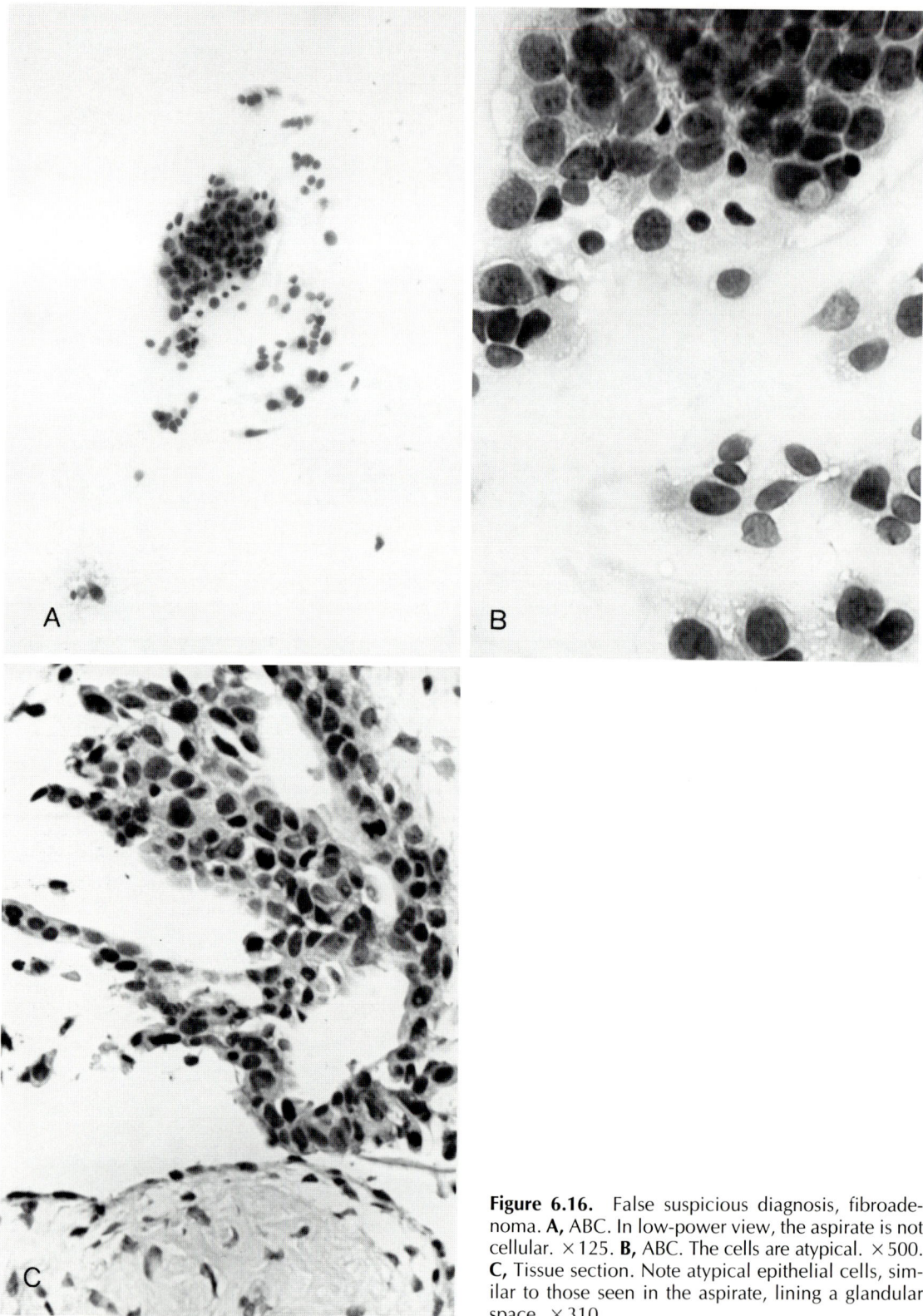

Figure 6.16. False suspicious diagnosis, fibroadenoma. **A,** ABC. In low-power view, the aspirate is not cellular. ×125. **B,** ABC. The cells are atypical. ×500. **C,** Tissue section. Note atypical epithelial cells, similar to those seen in the aspirate, lining a glandular space. ×310.

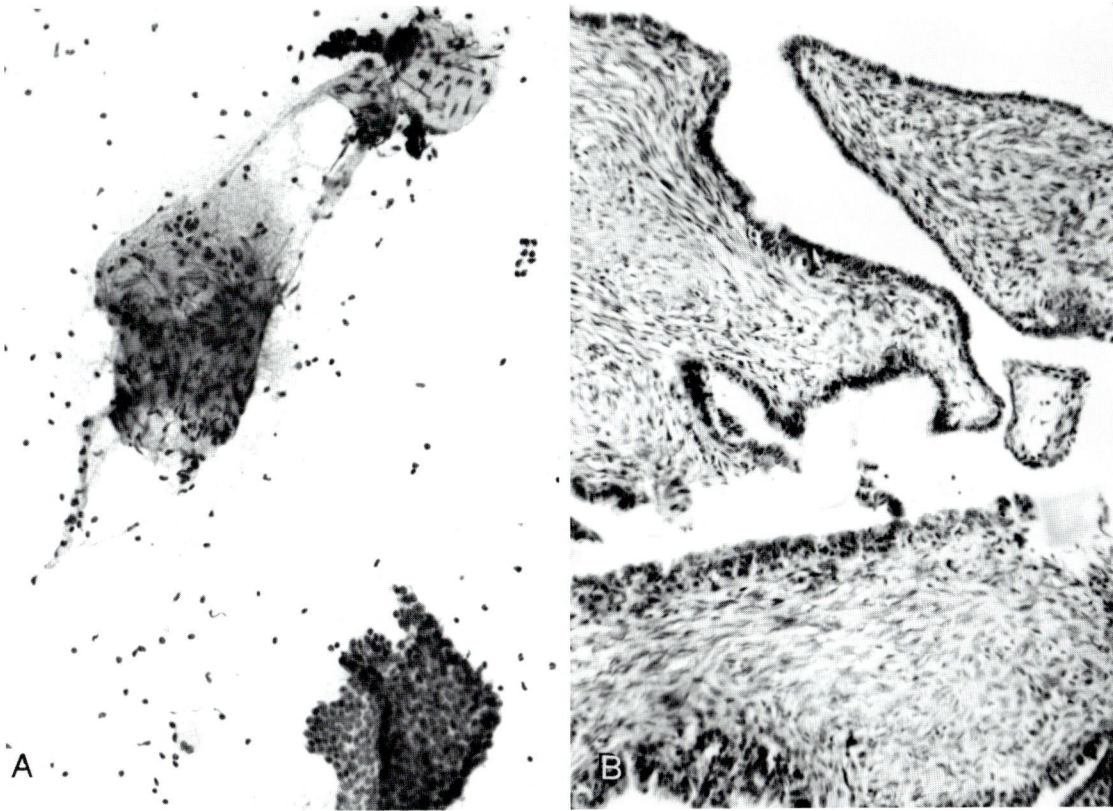

Figure 6.17.

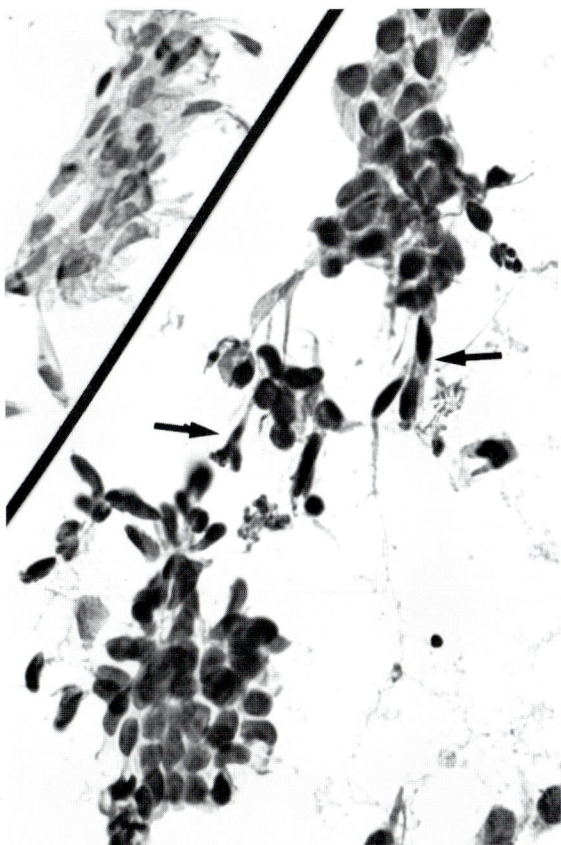

Figure 6.18.

Figure 6.17. Benign cystosarcoma phyllodes. **A,** ABC. Note a benign epithelial tissue fragment, two large stromal tissue fragments, and many naked oval nuclei in the background. ×125. **B,** Histology of benign cystosarcoma phyllodes. Note polypoid, hypercellular, stromal overgrowths protruding into large spaces. ×125.

Figure 6.18. Benign cystosarcoma phyllodes, ABC. Note admixture of epithelial cells and spindle stromal cells with visible cytoplasm (arrows and inset). ×500.

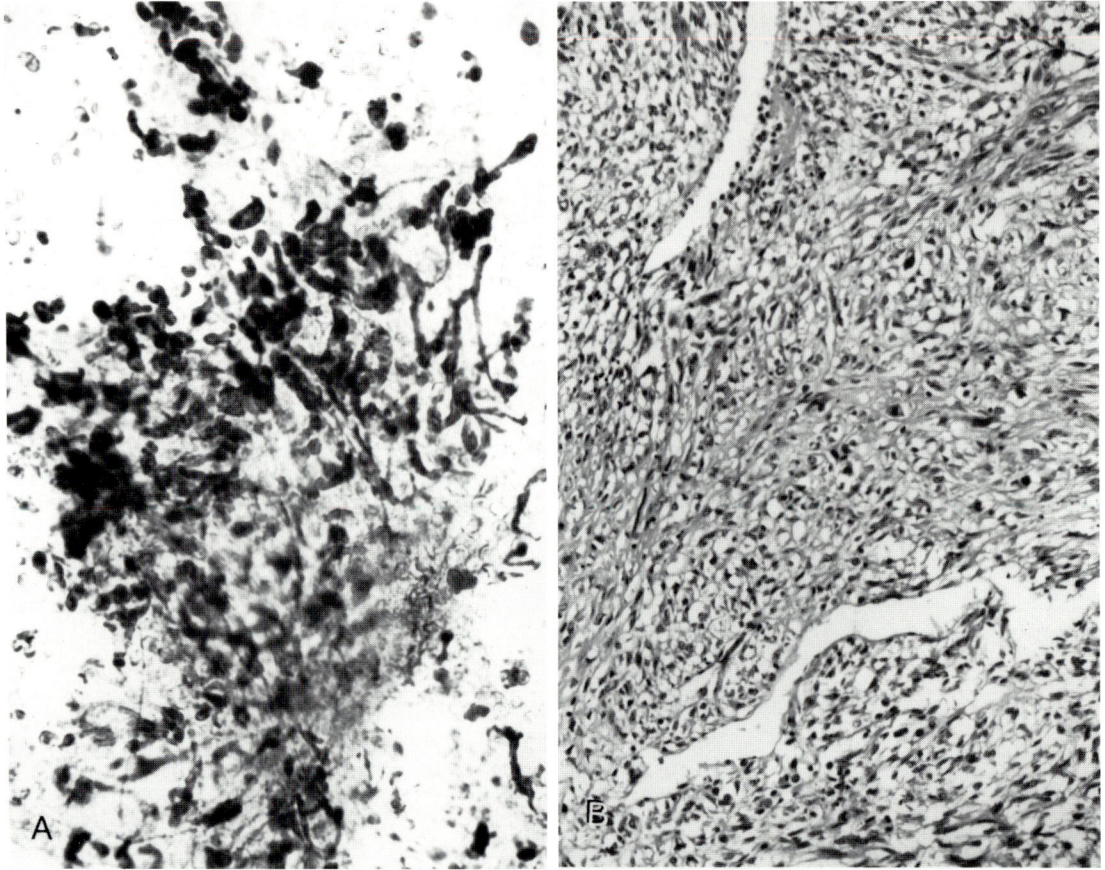

Figure 6.19.

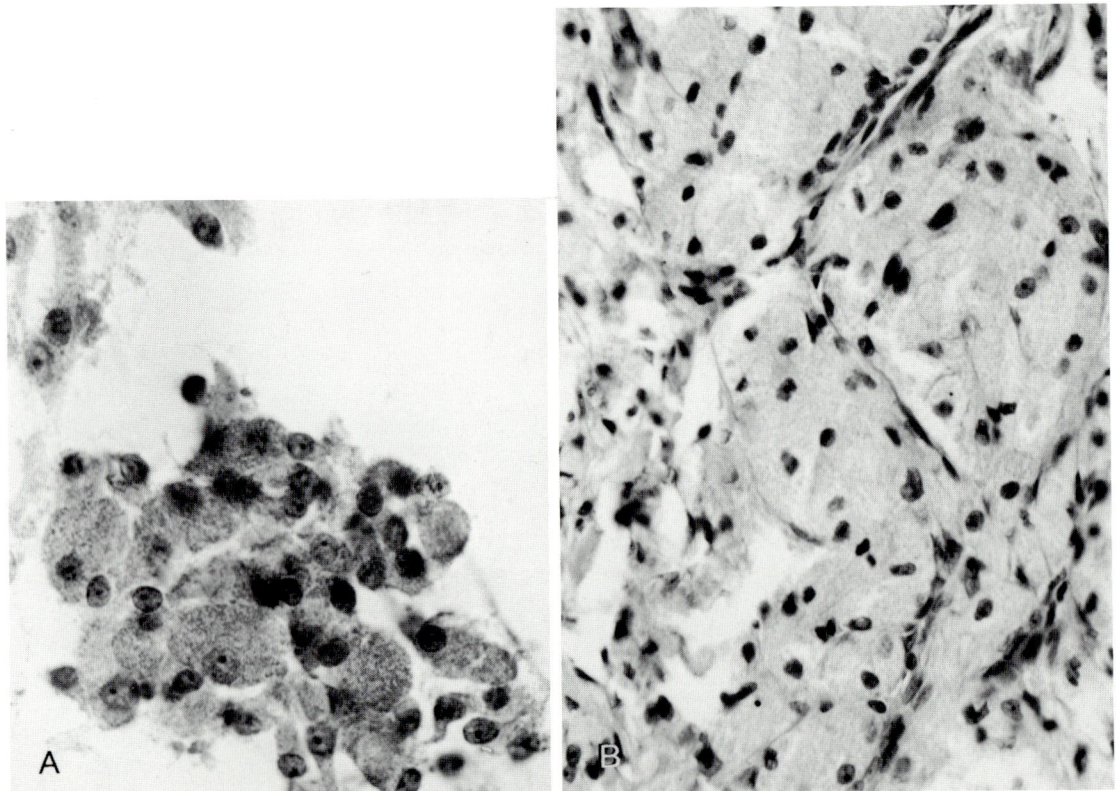

Figure 6.20.

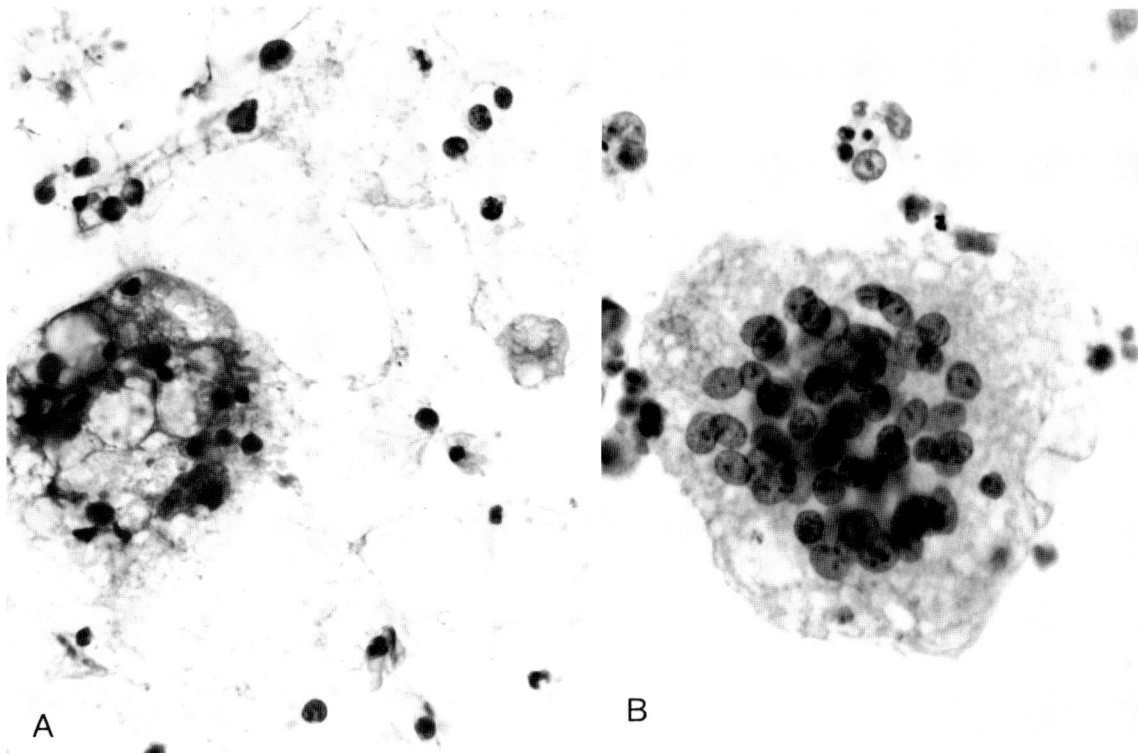

Figure 6.21. Fat necrosis, ABC. **A,** Note a large group of lipid-laden histiocytes, lymphocytes, and plasma cells. ×310. **B,** A large multinucleate histiocyte containing numerous cytoplasmic lipid vacuoles. ×500.

phyllodes tumor over fibroadenoma.[44] In addition, stromal tissue fragments, which are rare in aspirates of fibroadenomas, are readily discernible and show varying degrees of cytologic atypia in borderline cases.

Malignant cystosarcoma phyllodes is characterized by a sarcomatous appearance of the stromal cells and the ductal formations are distorted or obliterated by the stromal overgrowth. The stromal cells, haphazardly arranged, are oval or spindle-shaped with marked nuclear atypia **(Fig. 6.19)**.[5,43]

Diagnostic Pitfalls. Hajdu and Hajdu[42] have pointed out that in aspiration cytology it may be difficult to differentiate the benign phyllodes tumors from fibroadenomas, and the malignant phyllodes tumors from other sarcomas and pseudosarcomatous metaplastic carcinoma of the breast. Kline[20] has stressed the importance of clinical correlation and team approach in the diagnosis of phyllodes tumors.

Granular Cell Tumor

Granular cell tumors are uncommon, yellow-tan, firm lesions rarely more than 1–2 cm. They can be found in the skin, breast, tongue, and many other sites. When occurring in the breast, granular cell tumor may clinically simulate a carcinoma. The histogenesis of this tumor is still unclear. In the past, the granular cells were thought to be derived from muscle cells, but subsequent ultrastructural and histochemical studies have favored the argument that the lesion is of Schwann cell origin.[45,46]

ABC shows many round to polygonal tumor cells having small round nuclei, a uniformly granular eosinophilic cytoplasm, and indistinct cytoplasmic borders **(Fig. 6.20)**. The cells appear in small loose clusters and as single cells. The granular cells must be distinguished from reactive histiocytes and apocrine cells.

Gynecomastia

Gynecomastia is an endocrine-related disorder characterized by benign enlargement of breast(s) in a male. The typical histologic picture consists of hyperplasia of the ductal epithelium, with or without accompanying stromal proliferation. The aspiration cytology resembles that of fibroadenoma and, like fibroadenoma, a large number of epithelial cell sheets may be aspirated. Attention to the clinical presentation prevents interpreting these cohesive cell sheets as malignant.

Inflammatory Lesions

The most frequent inflammatory lesion of the breast that may be clinically confused with carcinoma is fat necrosis. Characteristically, the lesion presents as a hard lump, often with a history of trauma. However, when the trauma history is absent or indefinite, clinical confusion with carcinoma arises. The ABC shows a mixture of lymphocytes, fibrocytes, lipid-laden macrophages with marked cytoplasmic vacuolation (lipophages), and sometimes multinucleated giant histiocytes **(Fig. 6.21)**.

Figure 6.19. Malignant cystosarcoma phyllodes. **A,** ABC. Stromal tissue fragment composed of pleomorphic spindle cells. ×500. **B,** Histologic section of malignant cystosarcoma phyllodes showing proliferation of pleomorphic stromal cells. ×310.

Figure 6.20. Granular cell tumor. **A,** ABC. Note tumor cells with small, round nuclei and abundant granular cytoplasm. ×500. **B,** Tissue section of granular cell tumor. ×310.

Figure 6.22. Breast abscess, ABC. Note large atypical cells with prominent nucleoli, admixed with polymorphonuclear leukocytes. The source of origin of these atypical cells is not apparent and may be epithelial or fibroblastic. ×500.

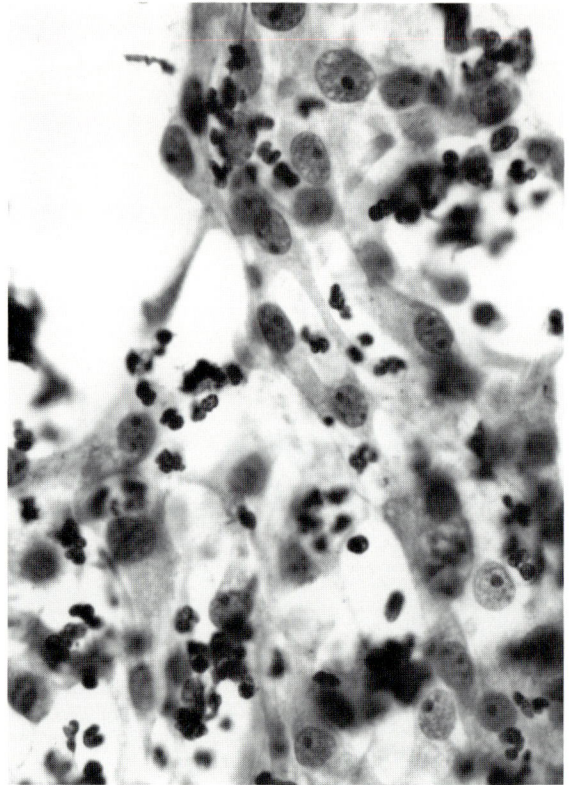

Breast abscesses are caused by pyogenic organisms. Clinical presentation is either as a fluctuant, tender mass or a poorly defined lump in the breast. Aspiration yields numerous polymorphonuclear leukocytes and necrotic debris. Semifluid or purulent material (pus) may be aspirated. During the resolution phase, ABC may reveal highly reactive epithelial cells or reactive fibroblasts. Both types of cells have large nuclei and prominent nucleoli (**Fig. 6.22**), simulat-

ing cancer cells. However, these reactive cells are arranged in sheets rather than as single cells and are frequently admixed with acute inflammatory cells.

Tuberculosis of the breast diagnosed by aspiration cytology has been reported.[47] The cytologic picture, characterized by clusters of plump epithelioid histiocytes, lymphocytes, and necrotic debris, is the same as tuberculosis elsewhere (see Chapters 4 and 7).

References

1. Bottles K, Miller TR, Cohen MB, et al. Fine needle aspiration biopsy: Has its time come? Am J Med 1986;81:525–531.
2. Frable WJ. Needle aspiration of the breast. Cancer 1984;53:671–676.
3. Kern WH. The diagnosis of breast cancer by fine needle aspiration smears. JAMA 1979;241:1125–1127.
4. Kline TS. Breast lesions. Diagnosis by fine needle aspiration biopsy. Am J Diagn Gynecol Obstet 1979;1:11–16.
5. Oertel YC, Galblum LI. Fine needle aspiration of the breast: Diagnostic criteria. Pathol Annu 1983;18 (Part I):375–407.
6. Wilson SL, Ehrmann RL. The cytologic diagnosis of breast aspirations. Acta Cytol 1978;22:470–475
7. Bell DA, Hajdu SI, Urban JR, Gaston JP. Role of aspiration cytology in the diagnosis and management of mammary lesions in office practice. Cancer 1983;51:1182–1189.
8. Kline TS, Joshi LP, Neal HS. Fine needle aspiration of the breast: Diagnosis and pitfalls. A review of 3545 cases. Cancer 1979;44:1458–1464.
9. Nordenstrom B, Zajicek J. Stereotaxic needle biopsy and preoperative indication of non-palpable mammary lesions. Acta Cytol 1977;21:350–351.
10. Bibbo M, Scheiber M, Cajulis R, Keebler CM, Wied GL, Dowlatshahi K. Stereotaxic fine needle aspiration cytology of clinically occult malignant and premalignant breast lesions. Acta Cytol 1988;32:193–201.
11. Rosemond GP, Maier WP, Brobyn TJ. Needle aspiration of breast cysts. Surg Gynecol Obstet 1969;128:351–354.
12. Rosen PP, Hajdu SI, Robbins G, Foote FW. Diagnosis of carcinoma of the breast by aspiration biopsy. Surg Gynecol Obstet 1972;134:837–838.
13. Hajdu SI, Melamed MR. The diagnostic value of aspiration smears. Am J Clin Pathol 1973;59:350–356.
14. Silverman JF, Lannin DR, O'Brien K, Norris HT. The triage role of fine needle aspiration biopsy of palpable breast masses. Acta Cytol 1987;31:731–736.
15. Silfversward B, Gustafsson JA, Gustafsson SA, Nordenskjold B, Wallgren A, Wrange O. Estrogen receptor analysis on fine needle aspirates and on histologic biopsies from human breast cancer. Eur J Cancer 1980;16:1351–1357.
16. Elston CW, Cotton RE, Davies CJ, Blamey RW. A comparison of the use of the "Tru-Cut" needle and fine needle aspiration cytology in the preoperative diagnosis of carcinoma of the breast. Histopathology 1978;2:239–254.
17. Lee KR, Foster RS, Papillo JL. Fine needle aspiration of the breast. Importance of the aspirator. Acta Cytol 1987:31:281–284.
18. Cohen MB, Rodgers C, Hales MS, et al. Influence of training and

experience in fine needle aspiration biopsy of breast. Arch Pathol Lab Med 1987;111:518–520.

19. Pilotti S, Rilke F, Delpiano C, Di Pietro S, Guzzon A. Problems in fine needle aspiration biopsy cytology of clinically or mammographically uncertain breast tumors. Tumori 1982;68:407–412.

20. Kline TS. Handbook of fine needle aspiration biopsy cytology, 2nd ed., New York: Churchill Livingstone, 1988:199–252.

21. Atkins H, Hayward JL, Klugman DJ, Wayte AB. Treatment of early breast cancer: A report after ten years of a clinical trial. Br Med J 1972;2:423–429.

22. Veronesi U. Current status of primary surgery in the management of breast cancer. In Bonadonna G. Breast cancer: Diagnosis and management. Chichester, NY: John Wiley & Sons, 1984:169–203.

23. Silverberg E, Lubera JA. Cancer Statistics, 1988. CA 1988;38:5–22.

24. McDivitt RW, Stewart FW, Berg JW. Tumors of the breast. Atlas of tumor pathology, 2nd Series, Fascicle 2. Washington, D.C.: Armed Forces Institute of Pathology, 1968.

25. Koss LG, Woyke S, Olszewski W. Aspiration biopsy. Cytologic interpretation and histologic bases. New York: Igaku Shoin, 1984:76.

26. Pedio G, Landolt U, Zobeli L. Irradiated benign cells of the breast: A diagnostic pitfall in fine needle aspiration cytology. Acta Cytol 1988;32:127–128.

27. Bendeson L. Aspiration cytology of radiation-induced changes of normal breast epithelium. Acta Cytol 1987;31:309–310.

28. Duane GB, Kanter MH, Branigan T, Chang C. A morphologic and morphometric study of cells from colloid carcinoma of the breast by fine needle aspiration. Distinction from other breast lesions. Acta Cytol 1987;31:742–750.

29. Kline TS, Kannan V. Papillary carcinoma of the breast: A cytomorphologic analysis. Arch Pathol Lab Med 1986;110:189–191.

30. Naran S, Simpson J, Gupta RJ. Cytologic diagnosis of papillary carcinoma of the breast in needle aspirates. Diagn Cytopathol 1988;4:33–37.

31. Kline TS, Kannan V, Kline IK. Appraisal and cytomorphologic analysis of common carcinomas of the breast. Diagn Cytopathol 1985;1:188–193.

32. Antoniades K, Spector HB. Similarities and variations among lobular carcinoma cells. Diagn Cytopathol 1987;3:55–59.

33. Tsuchiya S, Maruyama Y, Koike Y, Yamada K, Kobayashi Y, Kagaya A. Cytologic characteristics and origin of naked nuclei in breast aspirate smears. Acta Cytol 1987;31:285–290.

34. Linsk JA, Kreuzer G, Zajicek J. Cytologic diagnosis of mammary tumors from aspiration biopsy smears. II. Studies on 210 fibroadenomas and 210 cases of benign dysplasia. Acta Cytol 1972;16:130–138.

35. Kline TS. Masquerades of malignancy. A review of 4241 aspirates from the breast. Acta Cytol 1981;25:263–266.

36. Takeda T, Suzuki M, Sato Y, Hase T, Yamada S. Aspiration cytology of breast cysts. Acta Cytol 1982;26:37–38.

37. Rosemond GP. Differentiation between cystic and solid mass by needle aspiration. Surg Clin N Am 1963;43:1433–1437.

38. Abramson DJ. A Clinical evaluation of aspiration of cysts of the breast. Surg Gynecol Obstet 1974;139:531–537.

39. Zajicek J, Capersson T, Jakobsson P, Kudinowski J, Linsk J, Us-Krasovec M. Cytologic diagnosis of mammary tumor from aspiration biopsy smears. Comparison of cytologic and histologic findings in 2111 lesions and diagnostic use of cytophotometry. Acta Cytol 1970;14:370–376.

40. Bottles K, Chan JS, Holly EA, Chiu SH, Miller TR. Cytologic criteria for fibroadenoma. A step-wise logistic regression analysis. Am J Clin Pathol 1988;89:707–713.

41. Azzopardi JG. Problems in breast pathology. Philadelphia: WB Saunders, 1979:346–364.

42. Hajdu SI, Hajdu EO. Cytopathology of sarcomas. Philadelphia: WB Saunders, 1976:246–253.

43. Simi U, Moretti D, Iacconi P, Arganini M, Roncella M, Miccoli P, Giacomini G. Fine needle aspiration cytomorphology of phyllodes tumor. Differential diagnosis with fibroadenoma. Acta Cytol 1988;32:63–66.

44. Mottot C, Pouliquen ×, Bastien H, Cava E, Cayot F, Marsan C. Fibroadenomes de tumeurs phyllodes: Approche cytopathologique. Ann Anat Pathol 1978;23:233–240.

45. Fisher ER, Wechsler H. Granular cell myoblastoma—a misnomer: Electron microscopic and histochemical evidence concerning its Schwann cell derivation and nature (granular cell schwannoma). Cancer 1962;15:936–954.

46. Bangle R Jr. A morphological and histochemical study of the granular cell myoblastoma. Cancer 1952;5:950–965.

47. Vassilakos P. Tuberculosis of the breast: Cytologic findings with fine needle aspiration. Acta Cytol 1973;17:160–165.

7

Lung

Fine needle aspiration biopsy (FNAB) of the lung is a useful diagnostic procedure that can be carried out on an outpatient basis, provided the expertise of a thoracic surgical service is readily available to handle the more serious but rare complications. The technique is particularly rewarding in situations where a thoracotomy is diagnostic rather than therapeutic, i.e., in unresectable lung cancers, metastatic cancers to the lung, small cell anaplastic carcinomas that are not treated surgically, and confirmation of suspected benign or inflammatory lesions. Prompt use of FNAB also expedites surgical decisions in some atypical cases, which may otherwise be followed conservatively. If an infection is suspected, the aspirated material can be used for culture of organisms. The sensitivity for this technique, in our hands, has been 94%, the specificity 100%, and predictive value of a positive report 100%.[1] Other experienced workers also have reported high diagnostic accuracy: sensitivity being 82–91%, and specificity 95–100%.[2–5]

At our institution, transthoracic FNABs are performed by radiologists under fluoroscopic guidance. A Chiba 22–gauge needle was used for aspiration before 1980, but since then we have used the Greene needle single-pleural-puncture technique. The Greene needle combination consists of a 22–gauge inner and a 19–gauge outer needle. The outer needle is advanced through the chest wall and pleura but not into the lesion. The inner aspiration needle is advanced into the lesion through the lumen of the outer needle, which acts as a conduit and as a guide. The guide needle remains in position while the pathologist examines the aspirate so that, if the aspirate is inadequate, multiple aspirations can be performed with no further plural or pulmonary punctures, thereby reducing the risk of pneumothorax. In contrast, the Chiba needle only permits a single aspiration per puncture. The Greene needle is manufactured by the same company (Cook Inc., Box 489, Bloomington, IN 47401) as the Chiba needle.

Contraindications to pulmonary FNAB include bleeding diathesis, severe emphysema, and pulmonary hypertension. Complications of pulmonary FNAB include pneumothorax, hemoptysis, air embolism, and implantation of malignant cells.[6] All of these complications are extremely uncommon, with the exception of pneumothorax. At our hospital, pneumothorax has occurred in 33% of our cases, but only 6% have required intercostal tube drainage.[1] In a large series of 5300 cases reported by Sinner,[6] there were no fatalities; however, he recorded one death as the result of untreated tension pneumothorax occurring at another hospital. This was most unfortunate since the death was preventable.

NORMAL CYTOLOGY

In a lung aspirate specimen, there is a variety of normal cell types that must be distinguished from neoplastic cells. When the needle traverses a large- or medium-sized bronchus, the aspirate may contain variable numbers of ciliated bronchial epithelial cells. These cells are columnar in shape and have round basal nuclei and cyanophilic cytoplasm. They occur often in small palisaded clusters having a ciliated border (**Fig. 7.1**). A second, less commonly encountered bronchial epithelial cell is the mucin-producing, or goblet, cell whose cytoplasm is distended by a large apical mucin vacuole. Bronchiolar and alveolar epithelial cells (**Fig. 7.2**) are nonciliated low-cuboidal cells, with round uniform nuclei and a relatively high nuclear/cytoplasmic (N/C) ratio. In the nonreactive state, their identification may not be always possible because they may resemble mesothelial cells or small histiocytes. In many reactive or inflammatory conditions, hyperplasia and atypia of bronchiolar and alveolar epithelial cells may occur and these cells should be distinguished from cells derived from bronchioloalveolar carcinoma (see discussion below).

Alveolar macrophages (**Fig. 7.2**) occur as dispersed, single cells with abundant, pale, and finely vacuolated cytoplasm, often containing carbon pigment. The nuclei are small, round or reniform, and frequently eccentric. Nuclear chromatin is finely granular and evenly distributed.

The polygonal mesothelial cells occur singly or in monolayered sheets (**Fig. 7.3**). The nuclei are oval and regular, with fine stippled chromatin. In the normal nonreactive state, the nucleoli are small and the cytoplasmic borders are well-defined. The cells are characteristically separated from each other by clear gaps due to the presence of numerous long surface microvilli, which can be readily appreciated on electron microscopic examination.

REACTIVE ATYPIA OF EPITHELIAL CELLS

Severe atypia of the bronchial, bronchiolar, and alveolar epithelium can occur in a variety of benign conditions, including tuberculosis, organizing pneumonia, pulmonary infarction, fungal and viral infections, and effects of irradiation and chemotherapy.[7–9] These atypical cytologic changes may at times cause confusion with malignancy. **Figure 7.4A** shows a crowded cluster of atypical bronchiolar cells in a pulmonary aspirate obtained from a case of tuberculosis. The source of origin of these atypical benign bronchiolar cells is clearly depicted in the histologic section in **Figure 7.4B**.

Figure 7.5, A and **B**, shows a group of atypical cells from a case of organizing pneumonia. These cells were interpreted by a pathologist as being suspicious for malignancy. Although there was nuclear and nucleolar enlargement, there were no significant chromatin abnormalities and no nuclear membrane irregularities. The histologic examination of the lobectomy specimen (**Fig. 7.5C**) revealed an organizing pneumonia, in which atypical bronchial epithelial cells were noted. To avoid a false-positive FNAB diagnosis, it

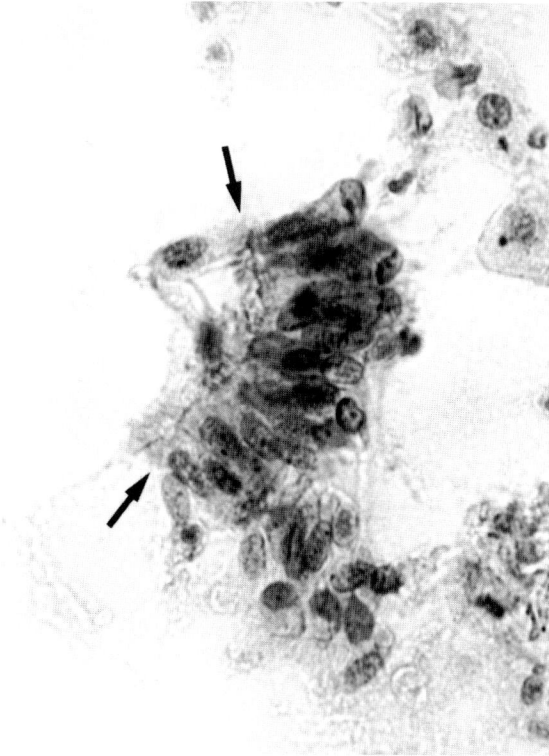

Figure 7.1.

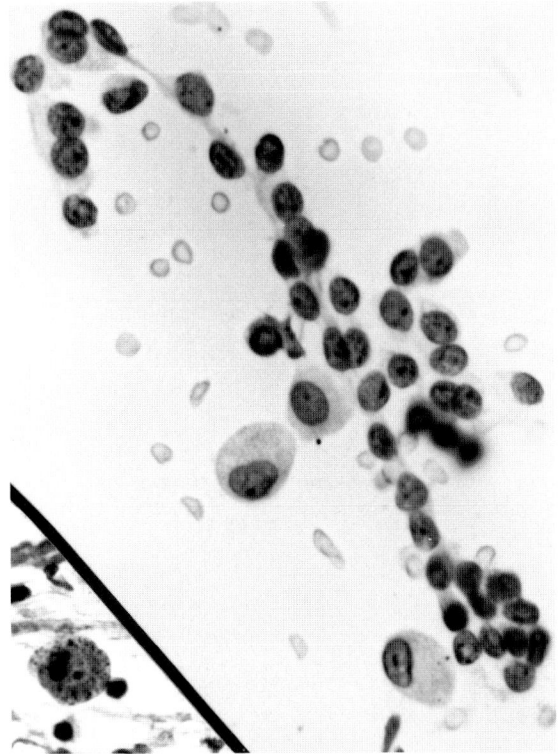

Figure 7.2.

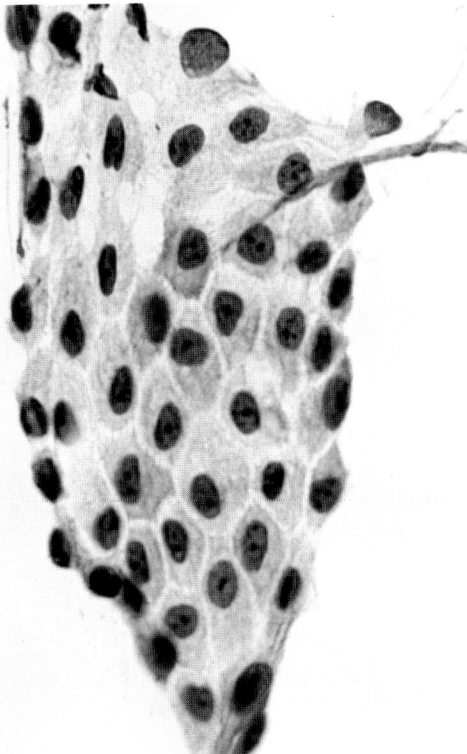

Figure 7.3.

Figure 7.1. Normal columnar bronchial cells arranged in a palisade fashion, ABC. Note numerous cilia *(arrows)* perpendicular to the terminal plates. Cuboidal reserve cells are seen at the basal portion of the cell sheet. ×500.

Figure 7.2. Normal bronchioloalveolar epithelial cells and macrophages, ABC. The bronchiolar and alveolar cells are small cuboidal nonciliated cells with a high nuclear cytoplasmic ratio. They tend to occur in small, loosely formed groups. The alveolar macrophages are large cells with abundant foamy cytoplasm. *Inset* shows a macrophage with ingested carbon particles. ×500.

Figure 7.3. Mesothelial cells in a monolayer, ABC. Note polygonal shape, small nucleoli, and distinct intercellular spaces. ×500.

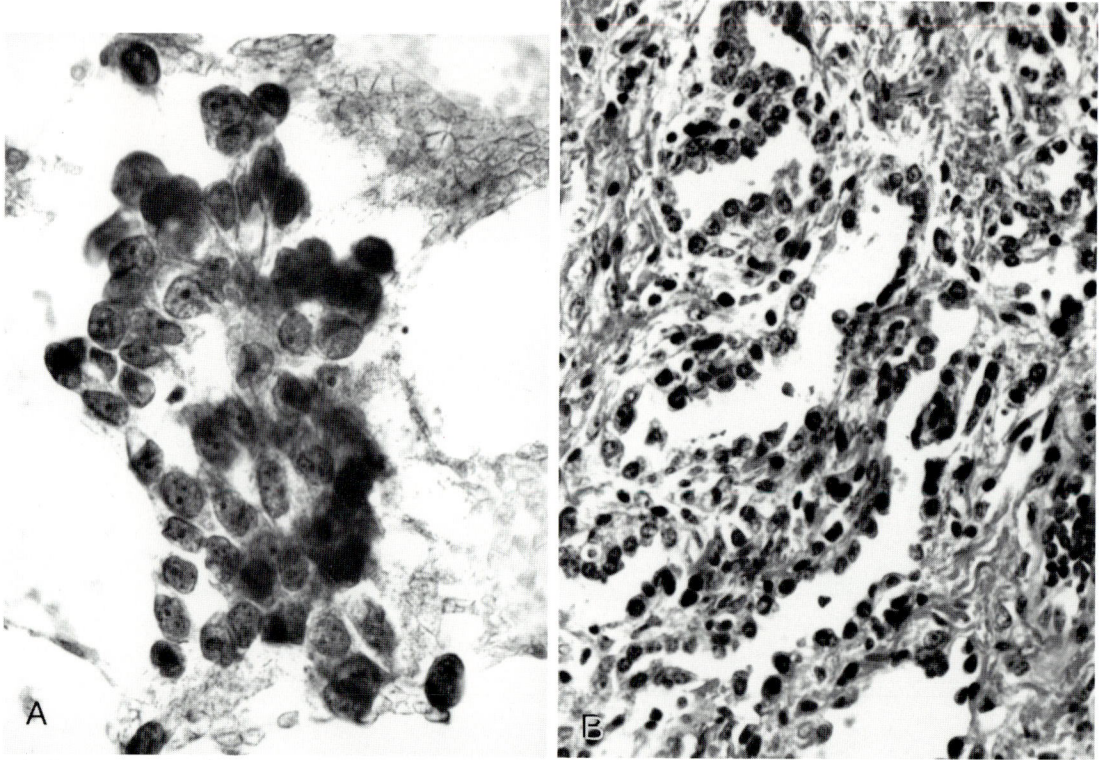

Figure 7.4. **A,** Lung aspirate showing a cluster of atypical bronchiolar cells from a case of pulmonary tuberculosis. ×500. **B,** Histologic section showing the reactive atypical bronchiolar cells and pulmonary fibrosis. ×310.

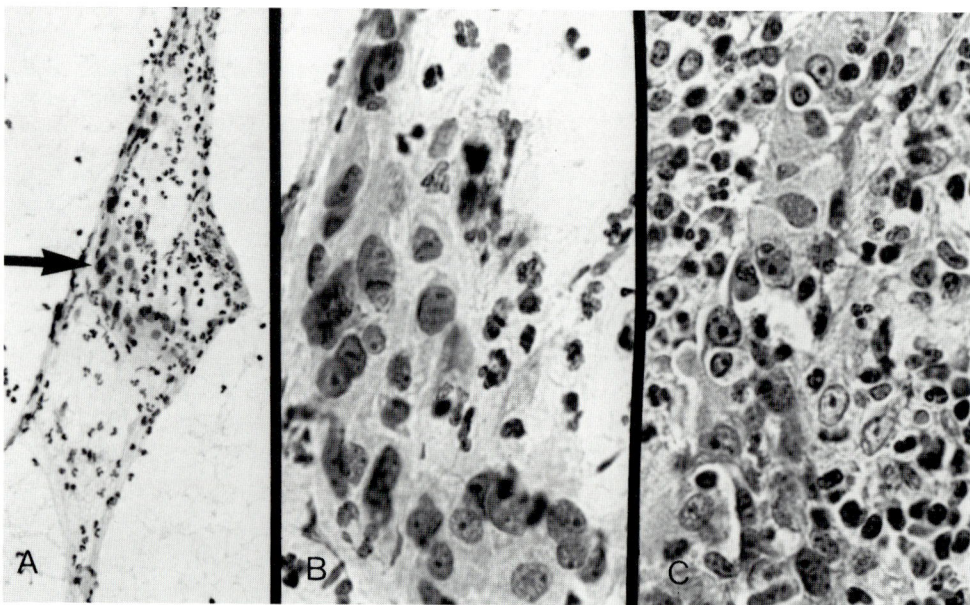

Figure 7.5. Organizing pneumonia, ABC. **A,** A loose group of atypical epithelial cells *(arrow)* in an inflammatory background. ×125. **B,** Higher magnification view of the atypical cells, admixed with inflammatory cells. ×500. **C,** Histology of the organizing pneumonia. It is apparent that the atypical bronchial cells with enlarged nucleoli are the source of the abnormal cells seen in the aspirate. ×500.

is important to evaluate not just the cell morphology but also the overall smear pattern. An aspirate obtained from a malignancy generally contains a large number of abnormal cells of similar cytologic appearance and they are present in large sheets as well as smaller clusters (see **Figs. 7.10A** and **7.13A**); whereas an aspirate from a reactive condition contains only few troublesome cells and they occur in smaller groups, often dominated by an inflammatory background **(Fig. 7.5)**. Additionally, one may observe a spectrum of atypical cellular changes ranging from mild, to moderate, to marked atypia.

Figure 7.6 depicts a pulmonary aspirate from a patient who received busulfan for treatment of leukemia. In addition to a carefully taken history including the use of chemotherapeutic agents and radiation, the cytologic features listed below are also clues to the pathologist that the atypical changes may have been the effects of radiation or chemotherapy:

1. Enlarged hyperchromatic nuclei with prominent nucleoli;
2. Proportional increase in amount of cytoplasm (hence a low N/C ratio is maintained);
3. No nuclear membrane irregularity;
4. "Smudgy" chromatin;
5. Cytoplasmic degeneration (vacuolation).

Furthermore, Johnston et al.[9] have pointed out that a major key to the correct recognition of these cells lies in the tendency for many of them to be roughly rectangular in shape **(Fig. 7.6)**.

PRIMARY MALIGNANT NEOPLASMS
Squamous Cell Carcinoma

Squamous cell carcinoma is the most common type of primary lung cancer, comprising slightly less than half the cases seen in clinical practice. Most of these cancers originate from the segmental bronchi. Hence, they are more centrally located, as opposed to ad-

enocarcinomas, which are usually peripheral lesions. Histologically, squamous carcinomas exhibit a spectrum of appearances from well-differentiated with obvious keratinization to poorly differentiated with polygonal and spindle cells exhibiting little or no keratinization. We usually describe two types as though they were distinct from one another, but in reality any squamous carcinoma may combine the features of both types.

Aspiration Cytology of Well-differentiated (Keratinizing) Squamous Cell Carcinoma

Cell Pattern. The aspirates are cellular. Dispersed, single cells are common **(Fig. 7.7)**; cohesive tissue fragments are rare.

Cell Morphology. The tumor cells are characterized by marked pleomorphism in size and shape. There are bizzare cells, polygonal cells, and tadpole and elongate cells **(Fig. 7.7)**. The nuclei are dark staining or opaque. Nucleoli, while not as common as in poorly differentiated malignancies, may occasionally be large. Nuclear/cytoplasmic ratios vary from very high to very low because of the extreme variablity in the amount of cytoplasm produced by these cells. The cytoplasmic borders are typically sharply defined. Cytoplasmic keratinization is characterized by dense, glassy cytoplasm, which usually stains deep orange (sometimes deep green) with the Papanicolaou (Pap) stain or brightly eosinophilic with hematoxylin and eosin stain.

Diagnostic Pitfalls. Degeneration and necrosis of cells of other types of carcinoma may result in nuclear opacity (pyknosis) and cytoplasmic eosinophilia that may lead to confusion with squamous carcinoma. In this respect, Pap stain is superior to H & E stain because keratin appears orangeophilic in the former.

Aspiration Cytology of Poorly Differentiated (Nonkeratinizing) Squamous Cell Carcinoma

Cell Pattern. The aspirates are rich in cells. The tumor cells are more apt to be present as syncytial tissue fragments in addition to single cells. The nuclei have a tendency to orient in the same

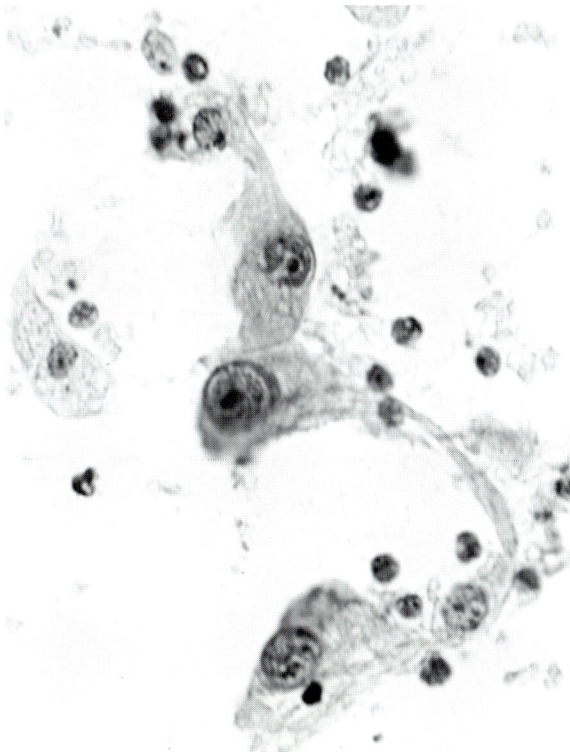

Figure 7.6. Epithelial changes secondary to busulfan therapy, ABC. The cells are large, rectangular in shape, and have a prominent nucleolus. Degenerative changes, such as smudged chromatin pattern and cytoplasmic vacuolation, are evident. × 500.

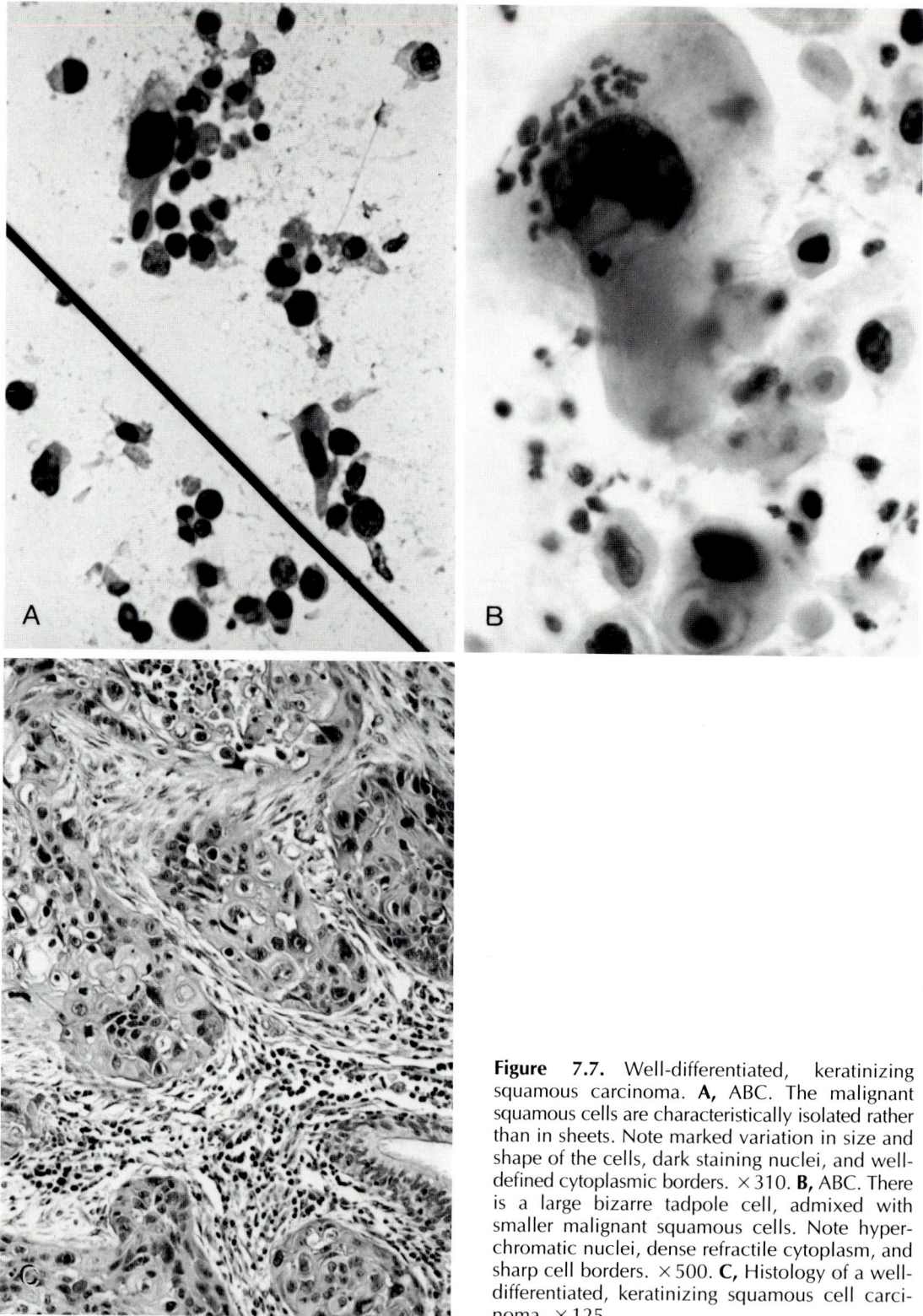

Figure 7.7. Well-differentiated, keratinizing squamous carcinoma. A, ABC. The malignant squamous cells are characteristically isolated rather than in sheets. Note marked variation in size and shape of the cells, dark staining nuclei, and well-defined cytoplasmic borders. ×310. B, ABC. There is a large bizarre tadpole cell, admixed with smaller malignant squamous cells. Note hyperchromatic nuclei, dense refractile cytoplasm, and sharp cell borders. ×500. C, Histology of a well-differentiated, keratinizing squamous cell carcinoma. ×125.

direction along the long axis of the tissue fragments, which often show jagged borders **(Fig. 7.8)**.

Cell Morphology. The cells derived from nonkeratinizing squamous carcinoma show much less nuclear and cytoplasmic pleomorphism than its keratinizing counterpart. The tumor cells are smaller, more uniform, but have a high N/C ratio. The nuclei are less opaque, with coarsely granular chromatin and prominent macronucleoli, although many cells without macronucleoli are also present. The cytoplasmic borders of the cells are poorly defined **(Fig. 7.8)**.

Diagnostic Pitfalls. Nonkeratinizing squamous cell carcinoma must be distinguished from poorly differentiated adenocarcinoma and small cell undifferentiated carcinoma. In general, the spatial arrangement of the tumor cells in each of these tumor types is different, although in some cases distinction may not be possible. The tissue fragments of poorly differentiated nonkeratinizing squamous carcinoma differ from those of adenocarcinomas (discussed below) in that they lack a smooth outer border and the component cells are oriented in one direction rather than arranged radially to enclose glandular lumina. Identification of a few scattered, better differentiated squamous cells, which may accompany the less-differentiated tumor cells, also aids in diagnosing the tumor as squamous carcinoma.

In small cell undifferentiated carcinoma, the small tumor cells lack visible cytoplasm and exhibit considerable crowding and nuclear molding with no nuclear orientation.

Occasionally, poorly differentiated squamous carcinoma may consist focally or entirely of spindle cells, mimicking a spindle cell sarcoma. Immunoperoxidase staining of these spindle cells usually shows positivity for cytokeratin. Likewise, electron microscopy can aid in the positive diagnosis of poorly differentiated squamous carcinoma by identification of tonofilaments and desmosomes **(Fig. 7.8D)**.

Adenocarcinoma

In most reported series of primary lung cancer, adenocarcinomas account for 15–20% of the cases, but their incidence has been increasing in recent years.[10] Unlike squamous cell and small cell carcinomas, most adenocarcinomas are found more pripherally in the lung. In the WHO classification[11] two main forms of adenocarcinoma are included, namely bronchogenic and bronchioloalveolar. Bronchogenic adenocarcinomas have a broad morphologic spectrum and may form acinar, glandular, papillary, and sheet-like structures. In rare instances when the bronchogenic adenocarcinoma is predominately papillary, it may be difficult to separate it from bronchioloalveolar carcinoma (discussed below). In other instances when the tumor is very poorly differentiated, it may not be separable from large cell undifferentiated carcinoma.

Bronchioloalveolar carcinomas (BACs) are well-differentiated adenocarcinomas whose cells characteristically grow on preexisting alveolar surface without destroying the lung parenchyma. The tumor cells are bland and frequently form papillary tufts that project into the alveolar space. Two histologic subtypes of BAC are recognized. One subtype originates from either type II alveolar pneumocytes or Clara cells and is composed of cells that vary from cuboidal to columnar, with little or no mucin. The other subtype is derived from metaplastic bronchiolar mucous cells, and the tumor cells are tall columnar with abundant supranuclear cytoplasmic mucin. The patients with mucinous BACs tend to do poorly, while the nonmucinous BACs tend to be solitary tumors and the patients have a better prognosis.[12]

Traditionally, BAC is defined as a well-differentiated adeno-

carcinoma; therefore, if one encounters considerable nuclear pleomorphism, it is more likely that the tumor is a bronchogenic adenocarcinoma than bronchioloalveolar carcinoma. Interestingly, Tao et al.[13] have reported a poorly differentiated variant of BAC, which cytologically and biologically resembles poorly differentiated bronchogenic adenocarcinoma or large cell undifferentiated carcinoma rather than its better differentiated counterpart.

Aspiration Cytology of Bronchogenic Adenocarcinoma

Cell Pattern. Cells of bronchogenic adenocarcinoma are arranged in multilayered tissue fragments **(Fig. 7.9)**, monolayered sheets **(Fig. 7.10)**, or cell clusters of various sizes **(Fig. 7.11)**. Single cells are also present, being seen more often in poorly differentiated than in well-differentiated adenocarcinomas.

The tissue fragments and clusters often exhibit characteristic spatial arrangements that aid in their identification as adenocarcinoma. Tumor cells within such tissue fragments may palisade around empty spaces, which represent glandular lumina **(Fig. 7.9A)**. Some cells may display a side-by-side arrangement **(Fig. 7.9B)**. The large, monolayered sheets, composed of haphazardly arranged tumor cells, probably represent the walls of larger glands **(Fig. 7.10)**. Smaller clusters of tumor cells are commonly present **(Fig. 7.11)**. Not infrequently, the external aspect of a tissue fragment or cell cluster is sharply defined due to the formation by the tumor cells of a continuous, or "community," border **(Fig. 7.11)**.

Papillary carcinoma is a rarer form of pulmonary adenocarcinoma, with psammoma bodies seen in some cases. The ABC reveals three-dimensional tissue fragments with a frond-like configuration and sharply defined outer borders **(Fig. 7.12)**. Unlike in tissue sections where the papillary fronds frequently show a central connective tissue core **(Fig. 7.12, *inset*)**, in aspirate specimens the fronds often appear as thick, solid structures without visible connective tissue cores because they are not sectioned as in histologic sections.

Cell Morphology. Cells of bronchogenic adenocarcinomas exhibit far less variation and pleomorphism than those of keratinizing squamous cell carcinoma and usually have a columnar or round shape with moderately well-defined cytoplasmic membranes **(Figs. 7.10 and 7.11)**. The nuclei are round and exhibit the general features of malignancy. In well-differentiated lesions, micronucleoli and/or macronucleoli are present, whereas in poorly differentiated lesions, macronuclei predominate. The cytoplasm is foamy or vacuolated. A mucin stain demonstrates intracytoplasmic mucin in some cells.

Diagnostic Pitfalls. Severe atypia of respiratory epithelial cells, which can be caused by infectious, postradiation, and drug-induced processes, may simulate adenocarcinoma and is the main source of false-positive cytologic reports. The cytologic criteria for separating reactive atypia from adenocarcinoma have been referred to above (see "Reactive Atypia of Epithelial Cells").

In some instances, an adenocarcinoma is so poorly differentiated that it may not be possible to differentiate it from large cell undifferentiated carcinoma on FNAB. It may be necessary to take a large number of tissue blocks from the resected specimen before glandular differentiation is apparent.

Whenever a primary adenocarcinoma of the lung is diagnosed, it is important to rule out a metastatic adenocarcinoma. This is usually possible because a history of carcinoma from another site is given. With some exceptions (see "Metastatic Carcinoma"), it is generally not possible to separate primary from metastatic adenocarcinomas on morphologic grounds alone.

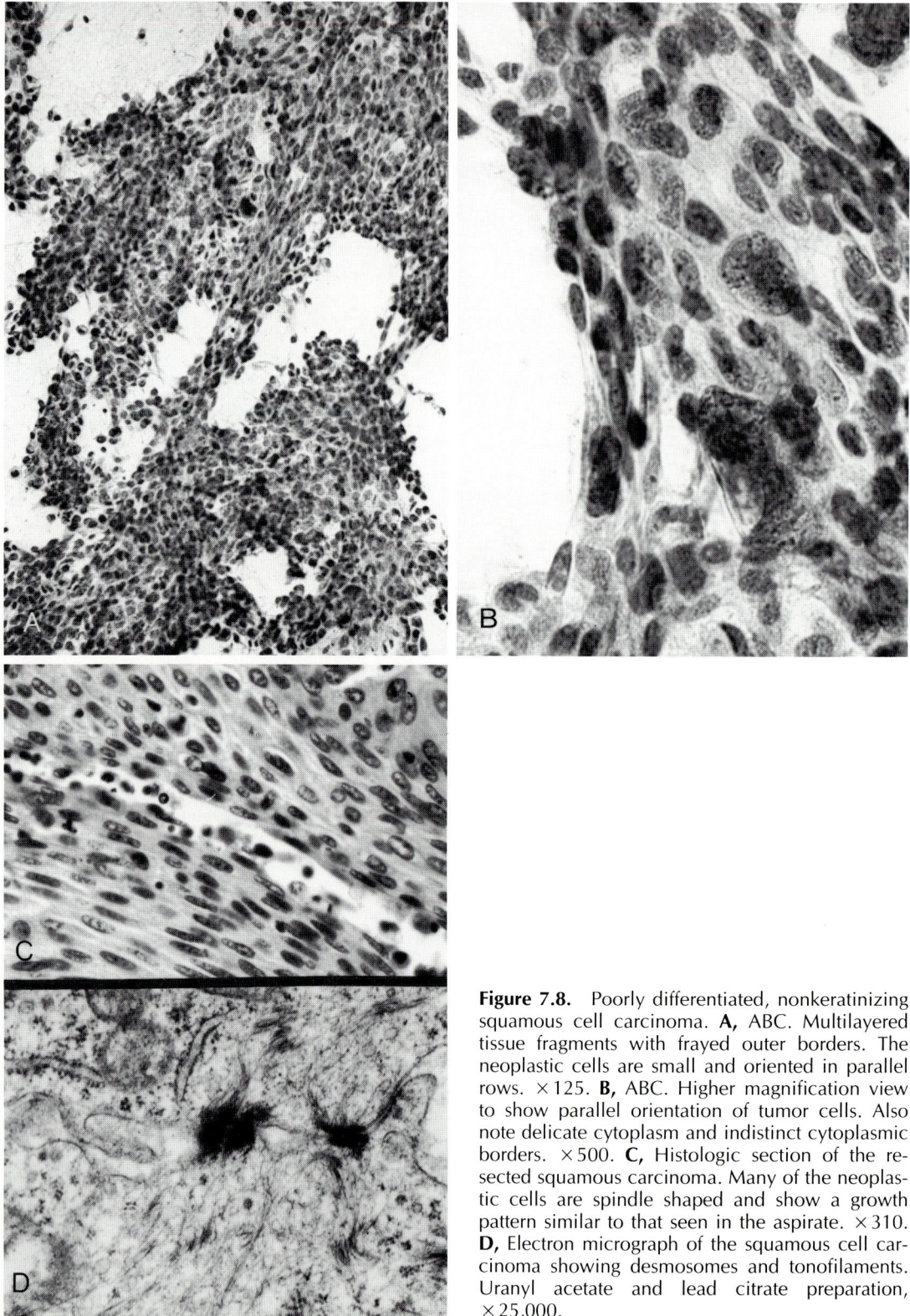

Figure 7.8. Poorly differentiated, nonkeratinizing squamous cell carcinoma. **A,** ABC. Multilayered tissue fragments with frayed outer borders. The neoplastic cells are small and oriented in parallel rows. ×125. **B,** ABC. Higher magnification view to show parallel orientation of tumor cells. Also note delicate cytoplasm and indistinct cytoplasmic borders. ×500. **C,** Histologic section of the resected squamous carcinoma. Many of the neoplastic cells are spindle shaped and show a growth pattern similar to that seen in the aspirate. ×310. **D,** Electron micrograph of the squamous cell carcinoma showing desmosomes and tonofilaments. Uranyl acetate and lead citrate preparation, ×25,000.

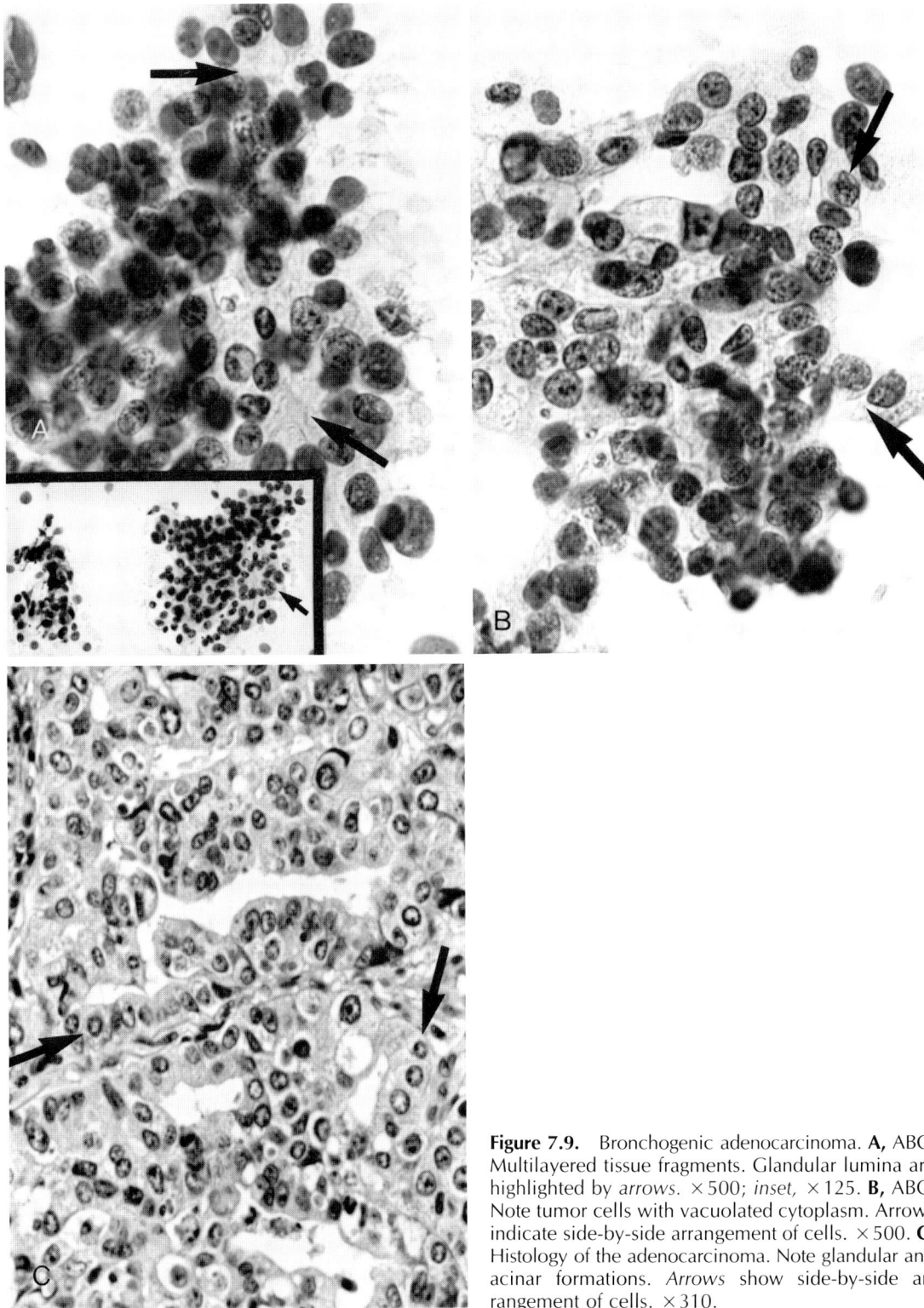

Figure 7.9. Bronchogenic adenocarcinoma. **A,** ABC. Multilayered tissue fragments. Glandular lumina are highlighted by *arrows.* ×500; *inset,* ×125. **B,** ABC. Note tumor cells with vacuolated cytoplasm. Arrows indicate side-by-side arrangement of cells. ×500. **C,** Histology of the adenocarcinoma. Note glandular and acinar formations. *Arrows* show side-by-side arrangement of cells. ×310.

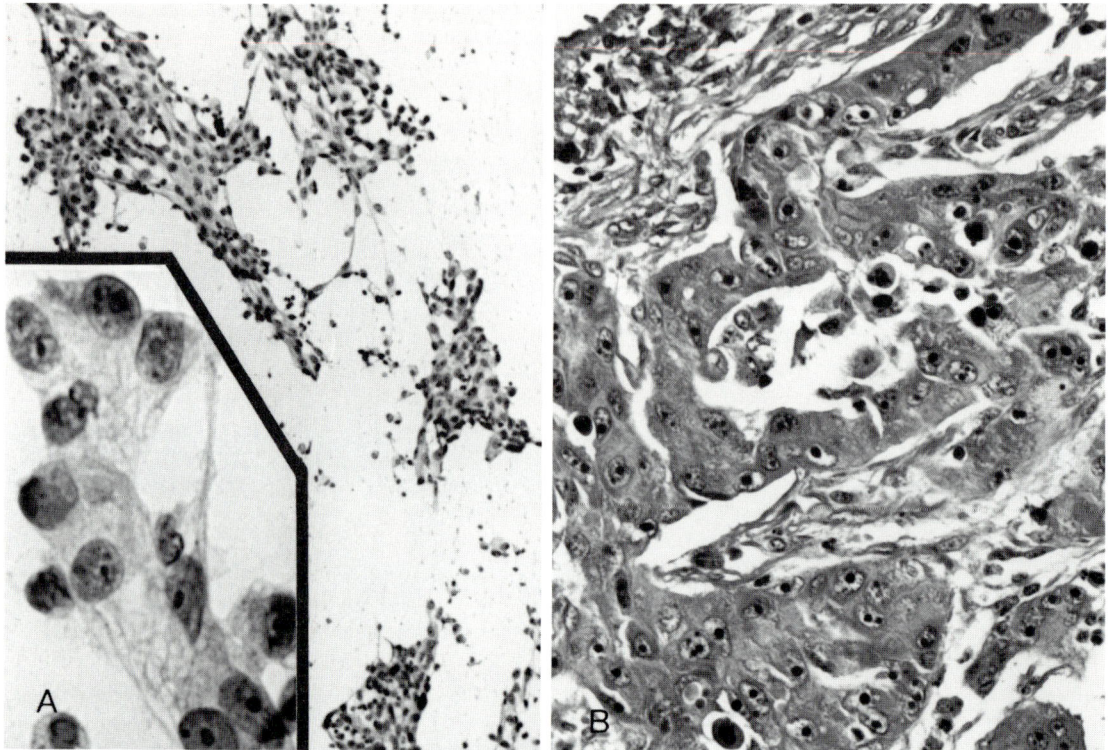

Figure 7.10.

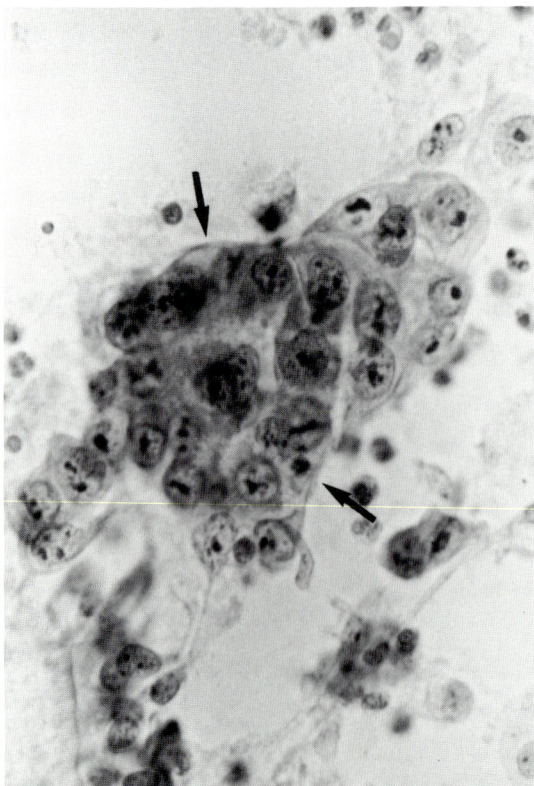

Figure 7.11.

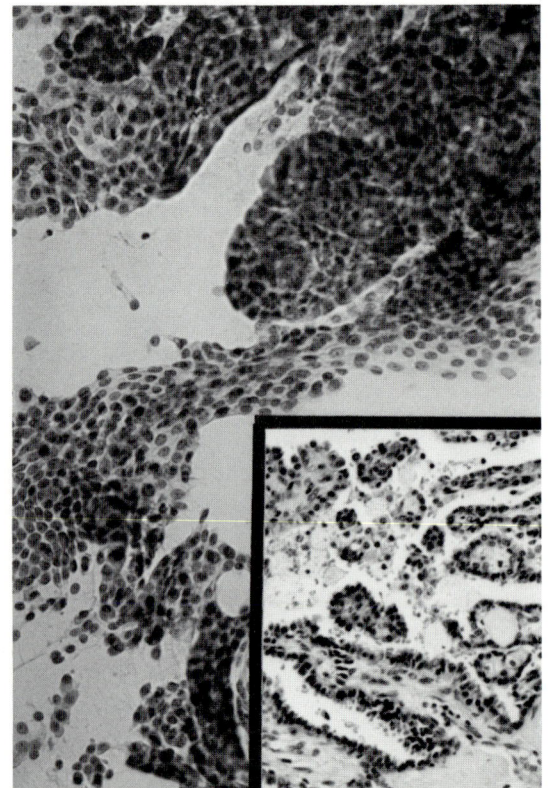

Figure 7.12.

Aspiration Cytology of Bronchioloalveolar Carcinoma

Cell Pattern. Smears are cell-rich. There are many small and large cell sheets as well as cell clusters (**Fig. 7.13A**). The latter occur as cell balls with a considerable depth of focus (**Figs. 7.13–7.15**). Cell-ball formations are characteristic of BAC (but not specific) and correspond in histologic sections to the papillary tufts that are formed on the surface of the alveolar walls (**Figs. 7.13C, 7.14B, and 7.15D**).

In the mucous cell subtype, the smear background contains an abundant mucin and macrophages attracted to the mucin (**Fig. 7.15A**).

Cell Morphology. Tumor cells of the nonmucous cell subtype are small, fairly uniform, and cuboidal to columnar in shape. The nuclei are hyperchromatic, relatively bland, and the N/C ratio is high (**Fig. 7.13**). Intranuclear cytoplasmic inclusions, similar to those seen in papillary thyroid carcinoma (Chapter 2), are also seen. Neoplastic cells derived from the Clara cells tend to have a ''hobnail'' appearance, are generally more pleomorphic, and show prominent nucleoli (**Fig. 7.14**).

Tumor cells of the mucin-secreting subtype (**Fig. 7.15**) are tall columnar and show bland basal nuclei and prominent supranuclear mucin vacuoles. The N/C ratio is generally low.

Diagnostic Pitfalls. Severe atypia of epithelial cells induced by various nonneoplastic conditions can mimic carcinoma; conversely, an extremely well-differentiated BAC can be mistaken for reactive atypia. Generally an aspirate is likely to be derived from BAC, if a large amount of material is present, including many sheets of several hundred cells, as opposed to few worrisome cells in nonneoplastic cases.[14] Other helpful criteria for diagnosing BAC include architectural three-dimensionality, distinct communal borders, intranuclear cytoplasmic inclusions, and relative nucleolar size.[15–17]

Colonic and pancreatic adenocarcinomas metastatic to the lung may cytologically simulate mucin-producing BACs, and metastatic breast adenocarcinomas and mesotheliomas may simulate the nonmucinous BACs. History of previous malignancy or asbestos exposure along with evaluation of the radiologic appearance of the lesion and its relationship to the underlying lung is important (see ''Mesothelioma'' in Chapter 8).

Small Cell Undifferentiated Carcinoma

Small cell undifferentiated carcinomas, which constitute 15–20% of the primary lung carcinomas, are highly aggressive tumors. Mediastinal and extrathoracic metastases are common by the time of clinical presentation. Based on the WHO classification,[11] there are two basic histologic groups: the classic lymphocyte-like (oat cell) subtype and the intermediate cell subtype. In cytologic material, this distinction cannot always be made because their morphologies seem to merge imperceptibly with one another. Even on histologic sections, interobserver variation with regard to subtyping is great, and it is still debatable whether there is any significant difference in survival between the subtypes.[18] Irrespective of subtype, small cell undifferentiated carcinomas are sensitive to chemotherapy and radiation, while non-small cell carcinomas of the lung do not. Hence, correct diagnosis of small cell carcinoma has significant clinical relevance.

Aspiration Cytology

Cell Pattern. Tumor cells are plentiful, distributed singly and in aggregates of various sizes (**Fig. 7.16A**). The tumor cells within the aggregates do not display obvious nuclear orientations as in adenocarcinomas or squamous cell carcinomas. Instead, the cells tend to mold haphazardly one on the other (**Fig. 7.16B**). The background commonly contains necrotic nuclear debris.

Cell Morphology. Classic oat cells (**Fig. 7.16**) are small, round or oval, and about twice the size of lymphocytes. In properly fixed material, nuclear chromatin is finely distributed in a ''salt and pepper'' appearance, and nucleoli are invisible or very small. There are irregularities of nuclear membranes, and nuclear molding is common. Cytoplasm is scanty or invisible. In the intermediate cell variant (**Fig. 7.17**), tumor cells may be polygonal or fusiform in shape and are often intermixed with smaller oat-type cells. Intermediate-type cells have larger nuclei and a larger rim of cytoplasm. Chromatin shows a similar salt and pepper pattern, but some nuclei may show more pleomorphism, coarsely granular hyperchromatic chromatin, and visible nucleoli. Despite more cytoplasm, cytoplasmic fragility often results in many bare nuclei stripped of cytoplasm. Thus, one of the criteria distinguishing the intermediate subtype from the oat cell subtype is lost.

Diagnostic Pitfalls. Small cell undifferentiated carcinoma may superficially resemble lymphoma. In well-fixed material, the salt and pepper appearance of the chromatin, invisible nucleoli, and cell clustering with nuclear molding are features that distinguish this tumor from lymphoma. In doubtful cases, a positive immunoperoxidase reaction for leukocyte common antigen will identify cells of lymphoid origin (see Chapter 16, ''Diagnostic Immunocytochemistry'').

Figure 7.10. Bronchogenic adenocarcinoma. **A,** ABC. Large, monolayered sheets of neoplastic cells. *Inset,* The neoplastic cells show prominent nucleoli and vacuolated cytoplasm. Some cells are somewhat columnar in shape. ×125; *Inset,* ×500. **B,** Histology of the resected adenocarcinoma showing large glands. ×310.

Figure 7.11. Bronchogenic adenocarcinoma, ABC. A small cluster of malignant cells with prominent nucleoli and irregular, coarse chromatin. Note smooth curved border *(arrows)* of the cell cluster. ×500.

Figure 7.12. Bronchogenic adenocarcinoma, papillary variant, ABC. Tissue fragments with three-dimensional, papillary configuration and sharply defined external borders. ×180. *Inset,* Histologic section of bronchogenic papillary adenocarcinoma showing numerous papillary fronds. ×125.

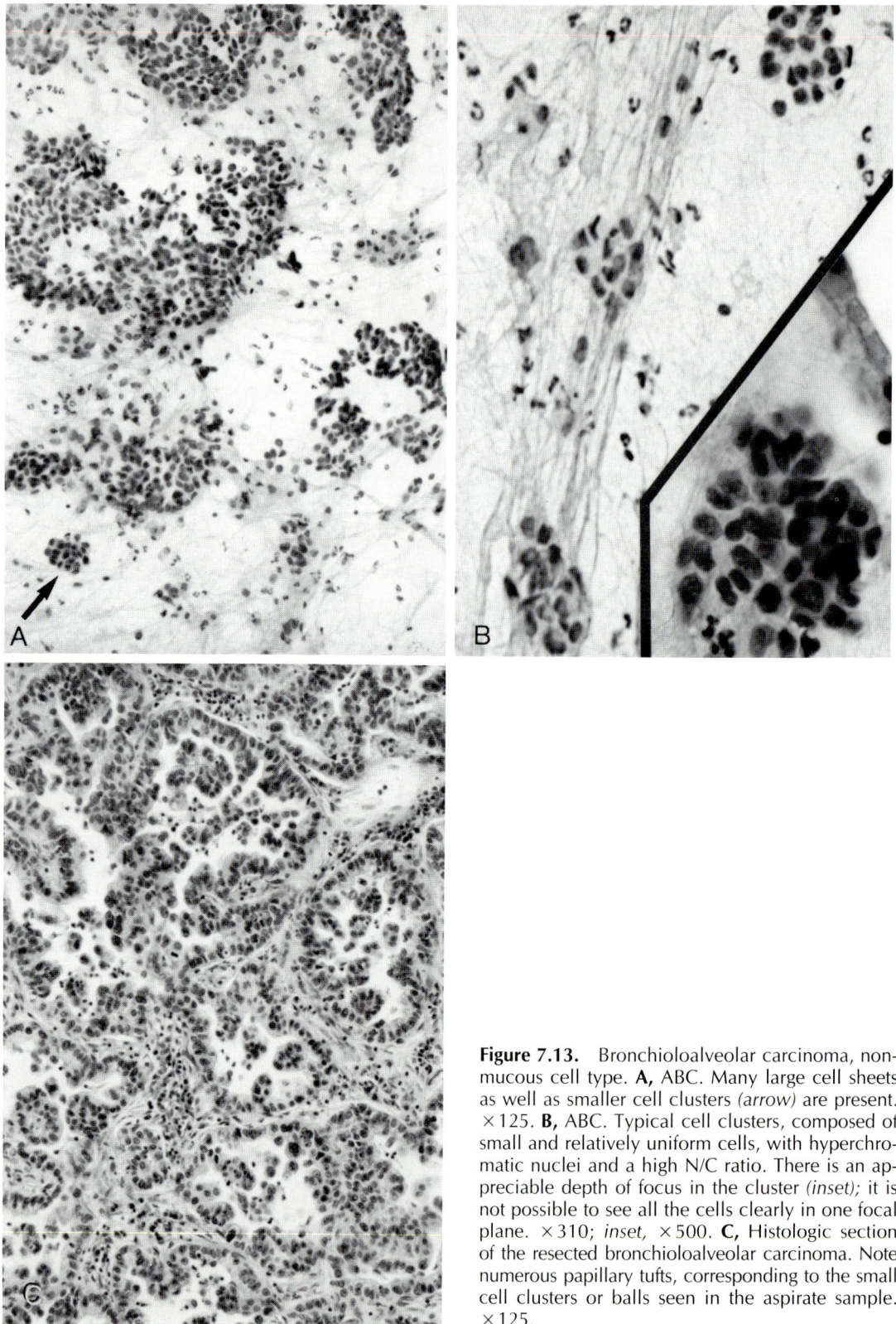

Figure 7.13. Bronchioloalveolar carcinoma, non-mucous cell type. **A,** ABC. Many large cell sheets as well as smaller cell clusters *(arrow)* are present. ×125. **B,** ABC. Typical cell clusters, composed of small and relatively uniform cells, with hyperchromatic nuclei and a high N/C ratio. There is an appreciable depth of focus in the cluster *(inset);* it is not possible to see all the cells clearly in one focal plane. ×310; *inset,* ×500. **C,** Histologic section of the resected bronchioloalveolar carcinoma. Note numerous papillary tufts, corresponding to the small cell clusters or balls seen in the aspirate sample. ×125.

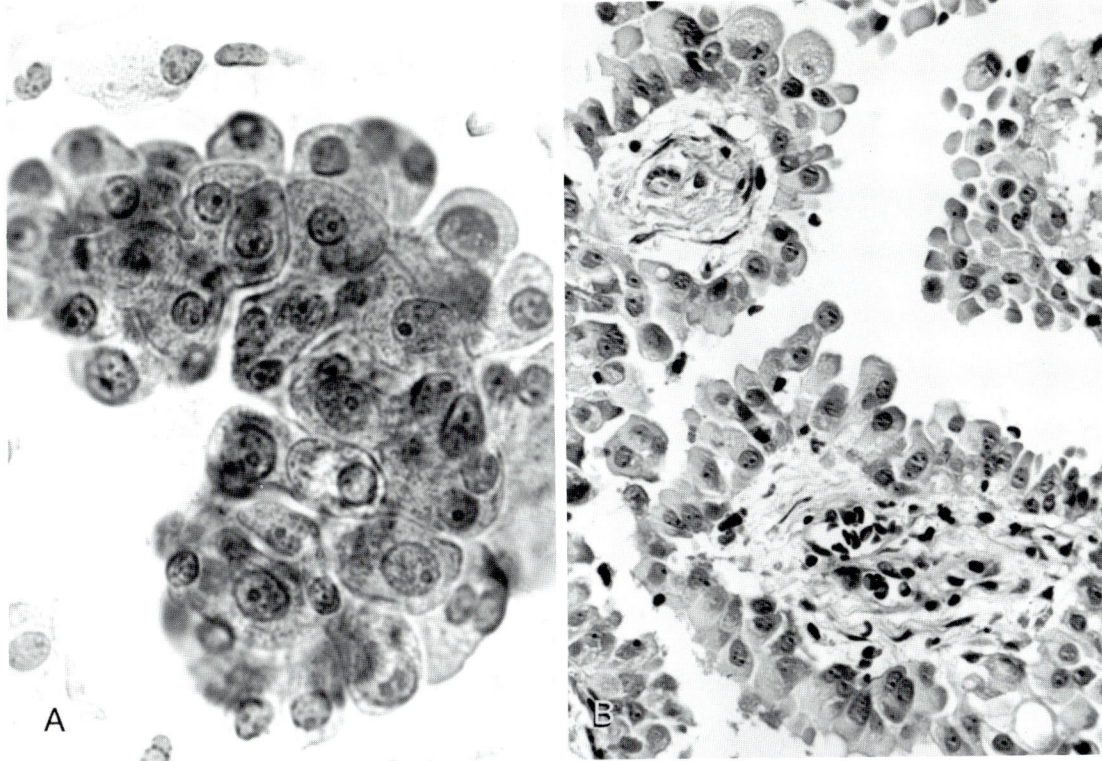

Figure 7.14. Bronchioloalveolar carcinoma, nonmucous cell type. **A,** ABC. Cluster of tightly packed tumor cells. Note hobnail appearance of the cells and prominent nucleoli. ×500. **B,** His-tologic section of the bronchioloalveolar carcinoma showing similar hobnail cells forming papillae. ×310.

When tumor cells of an adenocarcinoma or squamous carcinoma are small, they may mimic small cell undifferentiated carcinoma. Glandular cells and squamous cells, however, have different nuclear characteristics and more cytoplasm. The tumor cells within the tissue fragments often, though not always, show spatial arrangements that are characteristic for that particular tumor type (see "Squamous Cell Carcinoma" and "Adenocarcinoma"). Some tumors classified as the intermediate type of small cell undifferentiated carcinoma by routine light microscopy may, indeed, be small cell adenocarcinomas or squamous carcinomas.[19]

The difficulty of separating carcinoid tumor of the lung from small cell undifferentiated carcinoma has been reported (see "Carcinoid Tumor"). Mistakes have happened more frequently in sputum than in FNAB specimens where cells are well-fixed.

Large Cell Undifferentiated Carcinoma

Large cell undifferentiated carcinoma comprises approximately 10% of cases in most series. This tumor shows solid sheets of large cells with no evidence of squamous, glandular, or small cell differentiation. Hence, it is essentially a diagnosis made by exclusion. It is interesting to note that studies by electron microscopy have demonstrated that many of the large cell undifferentiated carcinomas are in fact glandular or squamous in origin.[20]

Aspiration Cytology

Cellular Pattern. The aspirates are hypercellular. The tumor cells are lying singly or loosely grouped as unstructured tissue fragments **(Fig. 7.18).** Tumor necrosis is a common finding and this is reflected by the presence of necrotic debris in the smear background.

Cell Morphology. The cytologic diagnosis of the tumor cells as malignant is seldom difficult because they show obvious criteria of malignancy. The neoplastic cells **(Fig. 7.18)** are large and the cytoplasm is usually abundant and may be clear, granular, or solidly eosinophilic. The nuclear pattern may take on a variety of forms but does not have the intense hyperchromasia of the squamous cell nucleus. The chromatin is irregular in distribution and a prominent nucleolus is usually present.

The giant cell carcinoma is a variant in which malignant bizarre giant cells are present. Since a few giant cells may be seen as a nonspecific finding in many forms of carcinoma, giant cells must be a conspicuous component of the neoplasm to justify the term giant cell carcinoma **(Fig. 7.19).**

Diagnostic Pitfalls. Undoubtedly there are cases of both squamous carcinoma and adenocarcinoma that have become so undifferentiated that distinguishing morphologic features are no longer apparent to permit classification into one of the differentiated categories. When confronted with such a situation, it has been suggested that it is both reasonable and accurate in respiratory cytologic material to simply regard the lesion as large cell undifferentiated carcinoma.[21]

Sometimes, a large cell carcinoma is so degenerated that tumor cells may appear as naked nuclei and a large cell lymphoma will enter into the differential diagnosis. The naked tumor nuclei may even lead to a confusion with small cell undifferentiated carcinoma, especially the intermediate cell variant. In general, the prominent nucleoli serve to distinguish them from cells of small cell undifferentiated carcinoma.

Carcinoid Tumor

Pulmonary carcinoid tumors are relatively rare neoplasms, accounting for only 2–3% of all lung tumors. These tumors arise from

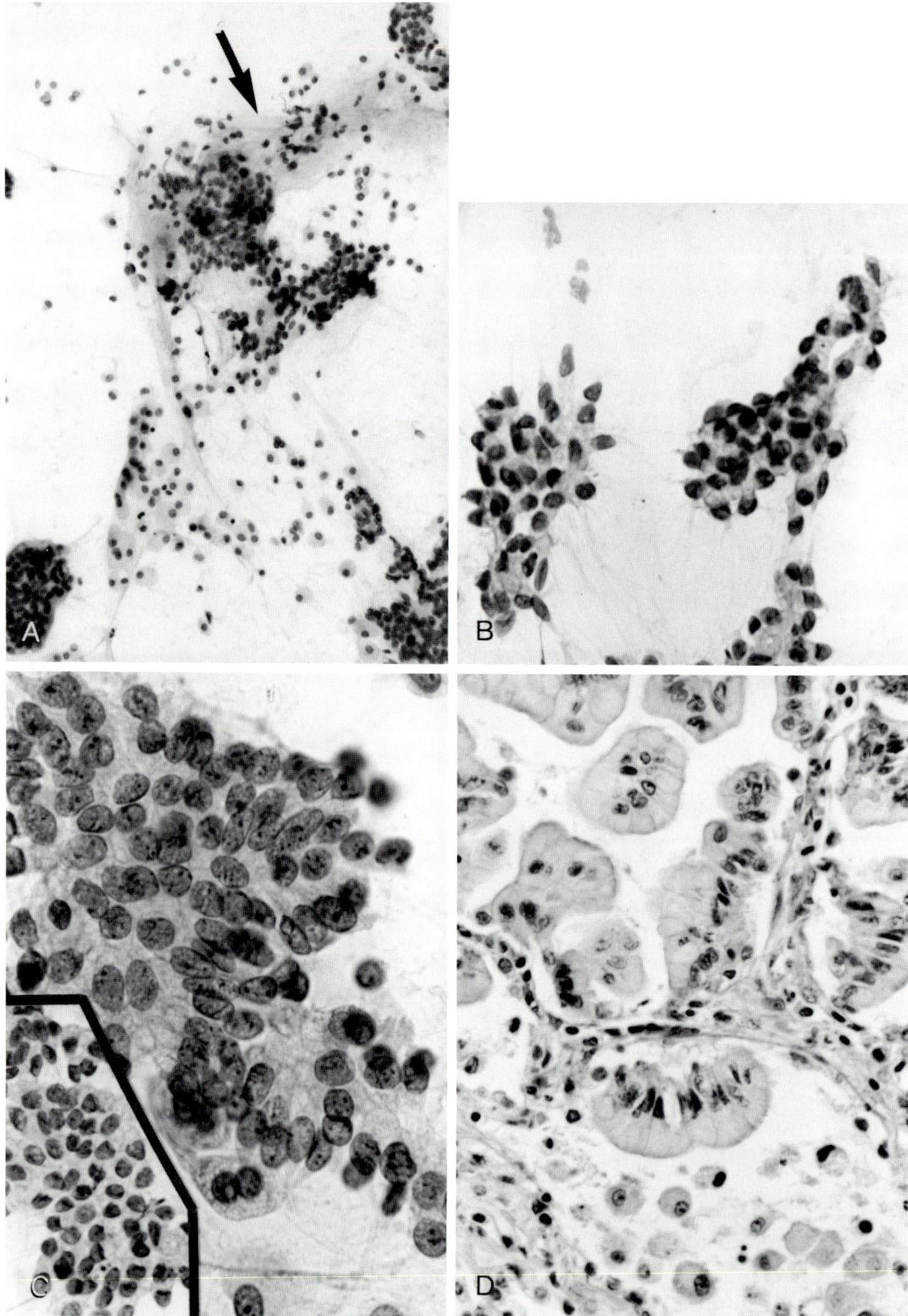

Figure 7.15. Bronchioloalveolar carcinoma, mucin-producing type. **A,** ABC. Note varying sized tissue fragments in a background of abundant mucus *(arrow)*. The scattered single cells in the background are macrophages, responding to the mucin production. ×125. **B** and **C,** ABC. Note clusters of columnar cells with deceptively bland nuclei and cytoplasmic mucin vacuoles. **B,** ×310; **C,** ×500; *inset,* ×310. **D,** Histologic section of bronchioloalveolar carcinoma. Note similar bland appearance of the neoplastic cells. The isolated cells in the alveolar space are macrophages. ×310.

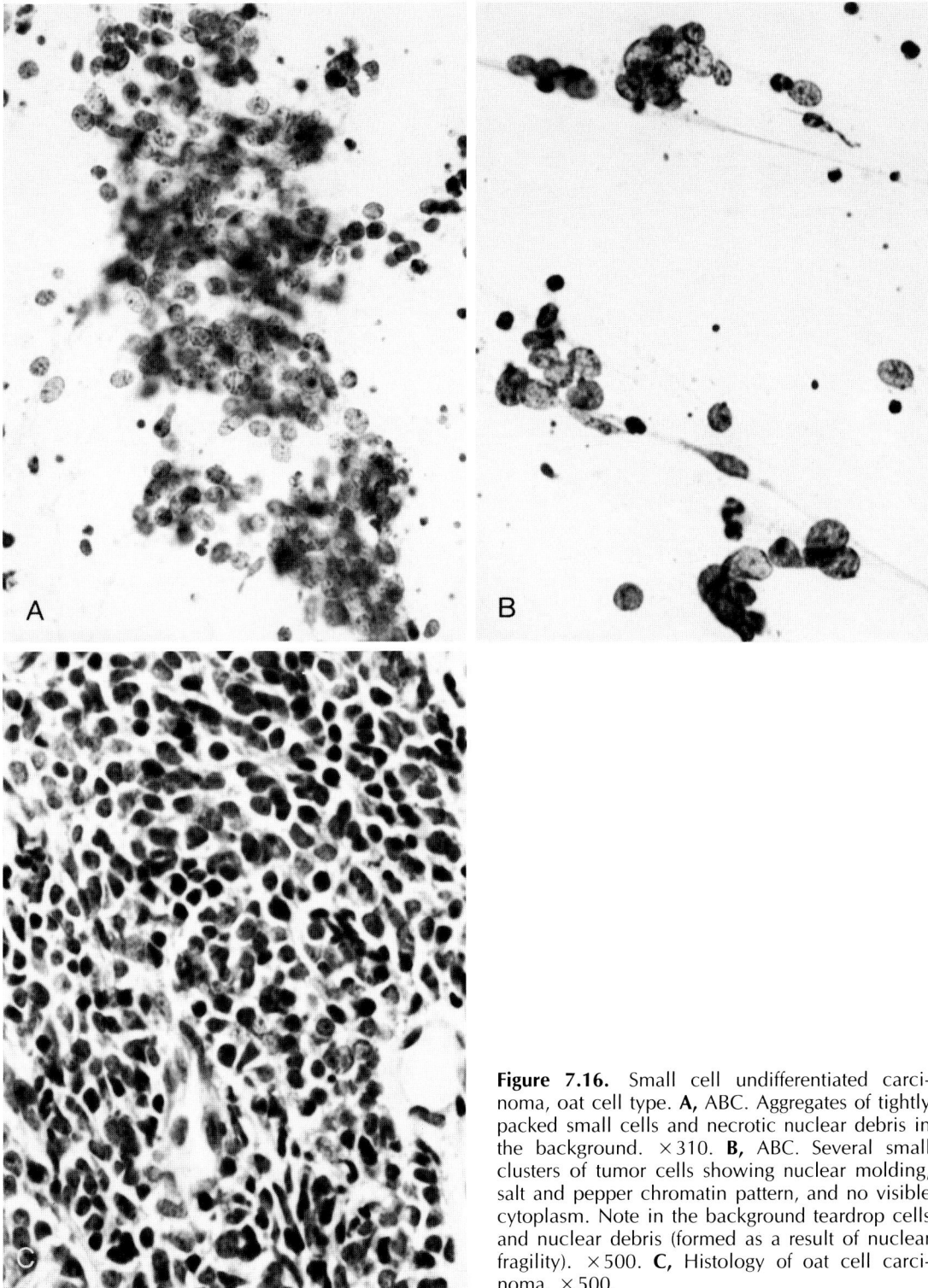

Figure 7.16. Small cell undifferentiated carcinoma, oat cell type. **A,** ABC. Aggregates of tightly packed small cells and necrotic nuclear debris in the background. ×310. **B,** ABC. Several small clusters of tumor cells showing nuclear molding, salt and pepper chromatin pattern, and no visible cytoplasm. Note in the background teardrop cells and nuclear debris (formed as a result of nuclear fragility). ×500. **C,** Histology of oat cell carcinoma. ×500.

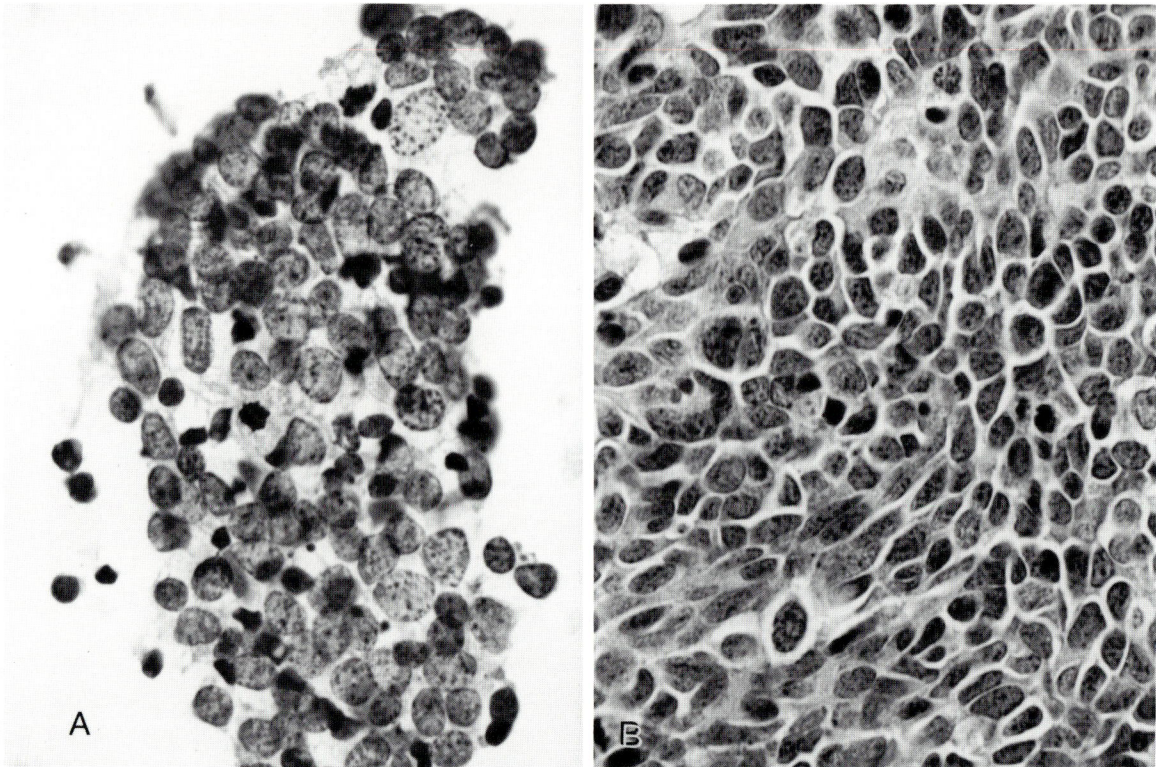

Figure 7.17. Small cell undifferentiated carcinoma, intermediate type. **A,** The neoplastic cells are larger and show more cytoplasm than those depicted in **Figure 7.16.** The salt and pepper chromatin pattern is retained. ×500. **B,** Histology of small cell undifferentiated carcinoma, intermediate type. The majority of the cells are larger than oat cells and are polygonal or fusiform in shape. There are also a few small oat cells. ×500.

the bronchial endocrine cells (the Kulchitsky cells), which belong to the APUD system. APUD cells are endocrine cells having the cytochemical properties of **a**mine **p**recursor **u**ptake and **d**ecarboxylation.[22] Carcinoid tumor is often viewed as the more benign counterpart of the small cell undifferentiated carcinoma because cells from both tumors are shown ultrastructurally to contain neurosecretory granules in the cytoplasm, and both tumors are capable of producing Cushing's syndrome. Unlike small cell undifferentiated carcinomas, carcinoid tumors **(Fig. 7.20)** are histologically bland neoplasms, consisting of uniform cells with moderately abundant, finely granular cytoplasm and a low nucleus-to-cytoplasm ratio. The tumors are only slowly invasive and metastases occur infrequently.

Aspiration Cytology

Cell Pattern. Aspirates are cell-rich, and the smear background is clean. The most striking low-power view is the uniformity of the tumor cells **(Fig. 7.21)**. The cells are commonly displayed in flat, loose sheets forming a mosaic pattern. Acini, or pseudorosettes, are also common **(Fig. 7.22)**. Cells arranged in thin ribbons (trabecular pattern) is the least common pattern **(Fig. 7.23)**, and may not be appreciated by the novice.

Cell Morphology. The classic carcinoid tumor **(Figs. 7.21 and 7.22)** is composed of uniform cuboidal or polygonal cells with pale, delicate, finely granular cytoplasm. The nuclei are regular and round, with evenly distributed chromatin granules. Nucleoli are frequently visible but small. In general, the N/C ratio is low, but we have encountered a few cases in which the cells are small and have scanty cytoplasm **(Fig. 7.24)**. Another cell type is the spindle cell; it is most often seen in carcinoid tumors that are peripherally located in the lung.[23] In some cases, the tumor may be composed exclusively of spindle cells **(Fig. 7.25)**.

Diagnostic Pitfalls. Because the cells of carcinoid tumors are cytologically bland, they must be distinguished from hyperplastic bronchial and bronchiolar cells.[24,25] The benign cells are in general more cohesive, whereas tumor cells are more loosely arranged, with mosaic, acinar, trabecular, or mixed pattern. Observation of spindle cells is helpful in diagnosing carcinoid tumor.

At times, differentiating bronchioloalveolar carcinoma from carcinoid tumor may be difficult since both tumors may exhibit extremely well-differentiated and uniform cells. Carcinoid tumor cells generally have more cytoplasm, which is finely granular; whereas cells in BACs (except the mucinous subtype) have a high N/C ratio. The cell clusters in BACs are more or less papillary in configuration, whereas the acini or pseudorosettes in carcinoid tumors have less depth of focus and have a central lumen.

An occasional carcinoid tumor may consist entirely or focally of small neoplastic cells **(Fig. 7.24)**, mimicking small cell undifferentiated carcinoma.[26,27] Cells in the former are cytologically bland, with delicate granular cytoplasm, while those in the latter have hyperchromatic nuclei, with irregular nuclear membranes and nuclear molding. A necrotic background is characteristic of small cell undifferentiated carcinoma.

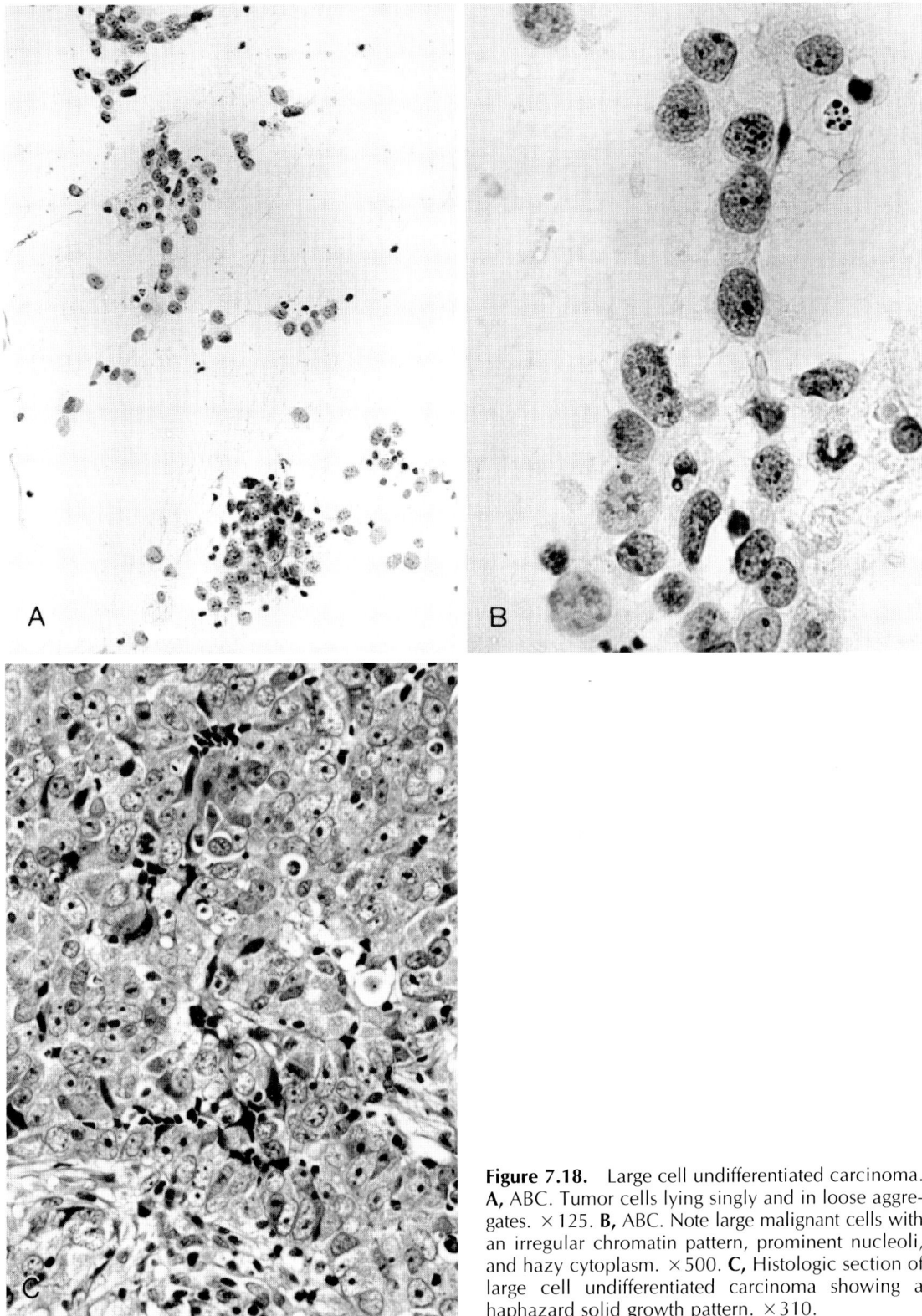

Figure 7.18. Large cell undifferentiated carcinoma. **A,** ABC. Tumor cells lying singly and in loose aggregates. ×125. **B,** ABC. Note large malignant cells with an irregular chromatin pattern, prominent nucleoli, and hazy cytoplasm. ×500. **C,** Histologic section of large cell undifferentiated carcinoma showing a haphazard solid growth pattern. ×310.

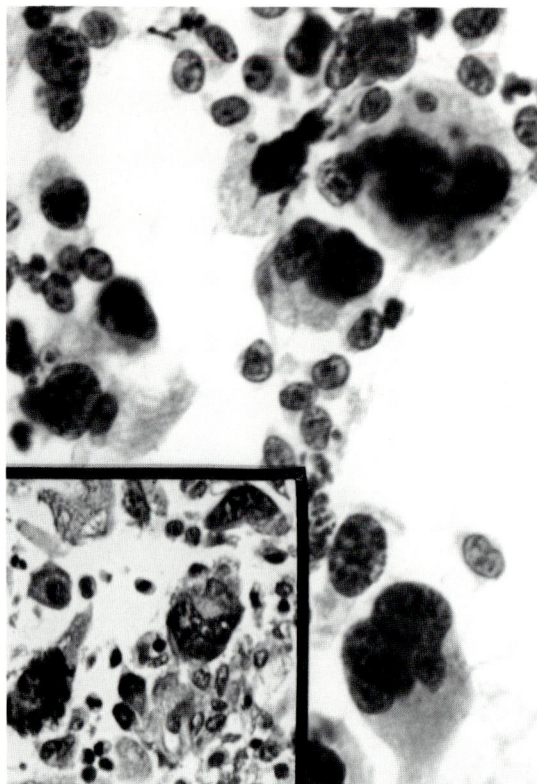

Figure 7.19. Giant cell carcinoma, ABC. Note numerous bizarre multinucleate giant cells. *Inset* shows the corresponding histology. ×500; *inset,* ×310.

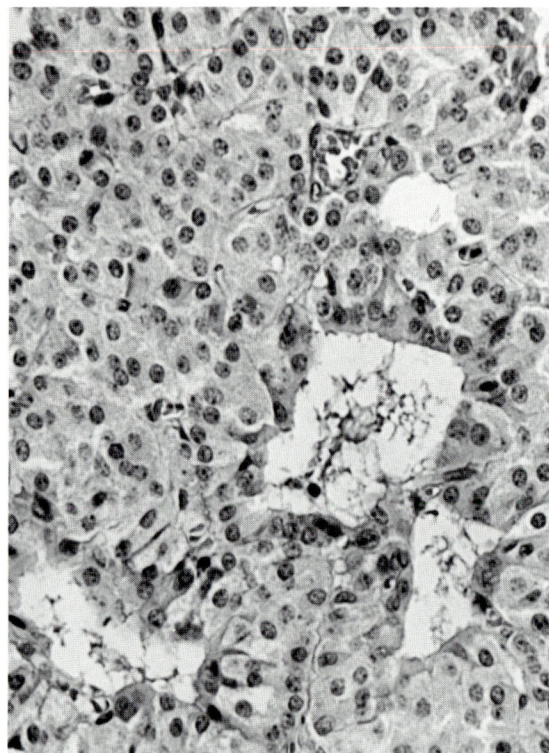

Figure 7.20. Histologic section of a prototypic carcinoid tumor. Note uniform rounded nuclei, finely granular cytoplasm, and low N/C ratio. Also note sheet-like mosaic pattern, trabeculae, and glandular spaces. ×310.

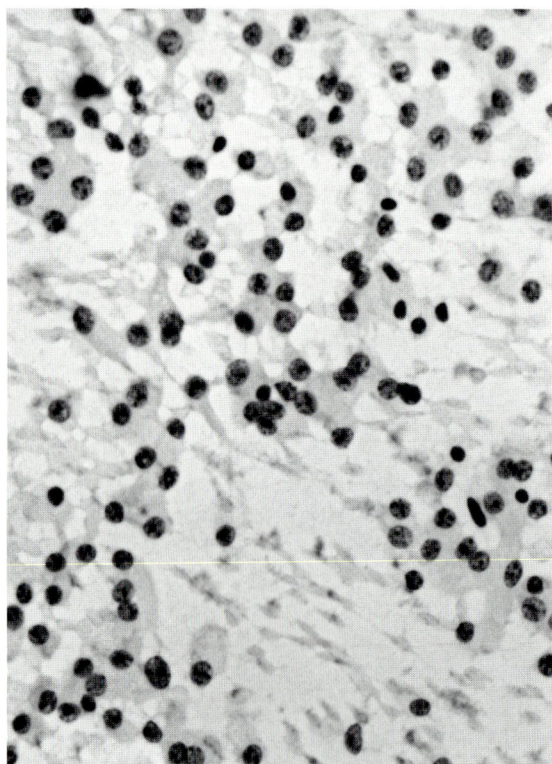

Figure 7.21. Carcinoid tumor, ABC. Note cellular uniformity and mosaic arrangement of cells. Same case as in **Figure 7.20.** ×310.

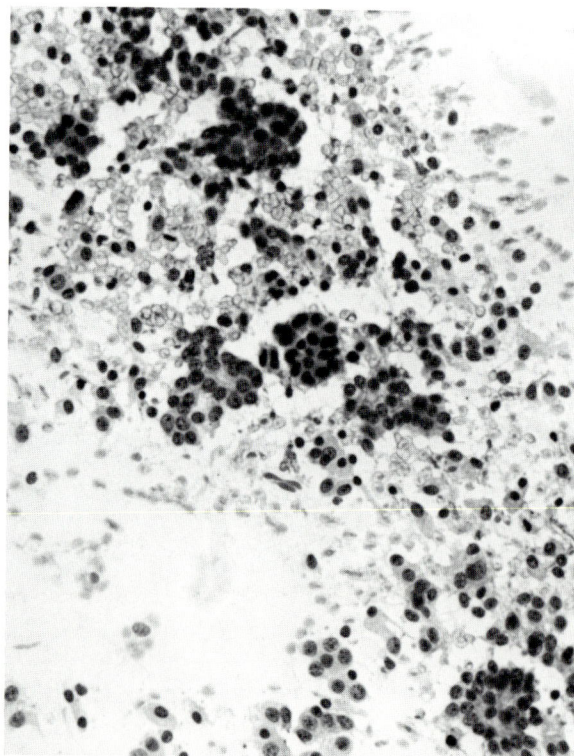

Figure 7.22. Carcinoid tumor with an acinar pattern, ABC. Tumor cells are arranged radially to encircle tiny lumina. ×160.

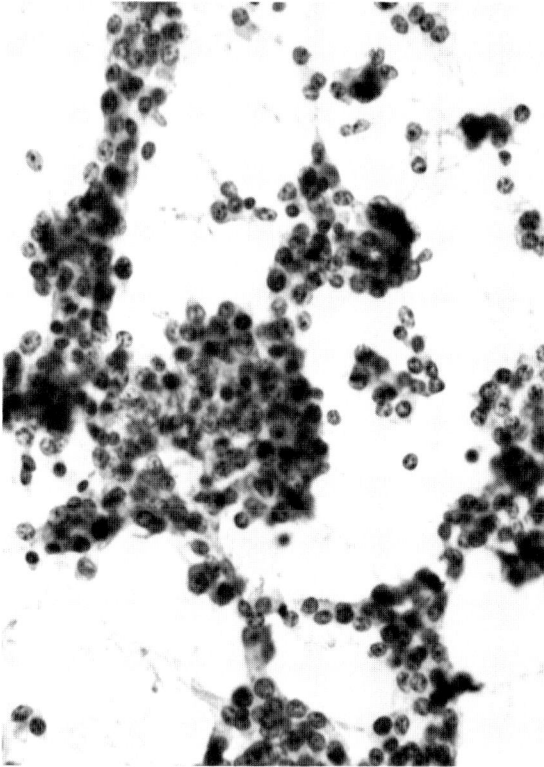

Figure 7.23.

Figure 7.23. Carcinoid tumor, ABC. Tumor cells are arranged in anastomosing ribbons of varying widths and in larger solid sheets. ×310.

Figure 7.24. Carcinoid tumor, small cell variant. **A,** ABC. A pathology resident mistook this lesion for small cell undifferentiated carcinoma. Clearly visible cytoplasm in some tumor cells *(arrows)* and relatively bland nuclei distinguish this tumor from small cell undifferentiated carcinoma. ×500. **B,** Histology of the resected carcinoid tumor. There is a predominance of small cells, but necrosis and mitoses are conspicuously absent. ×310.

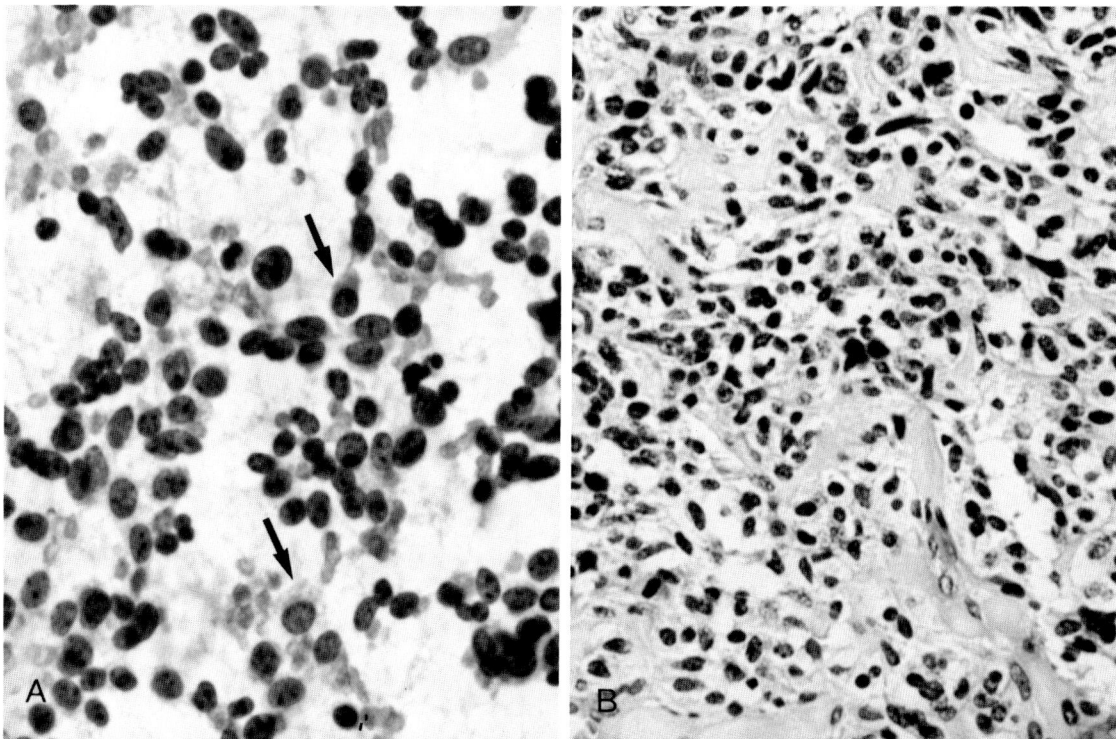

Figure 7.24.

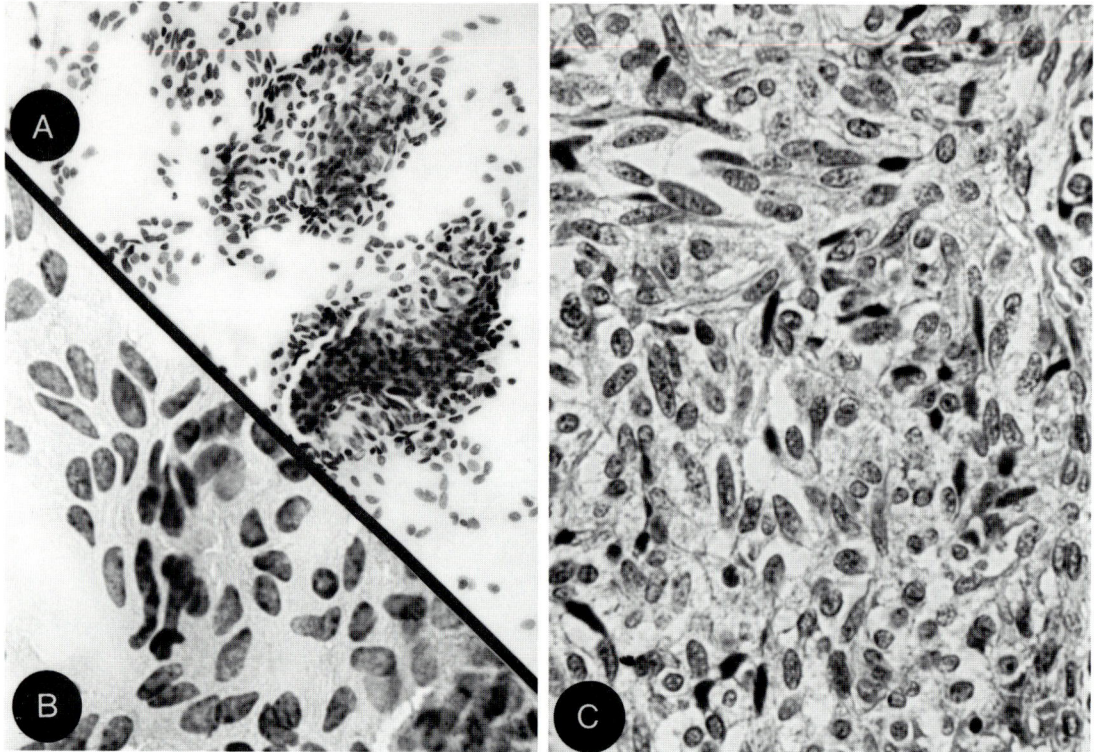

Figure 7.25.

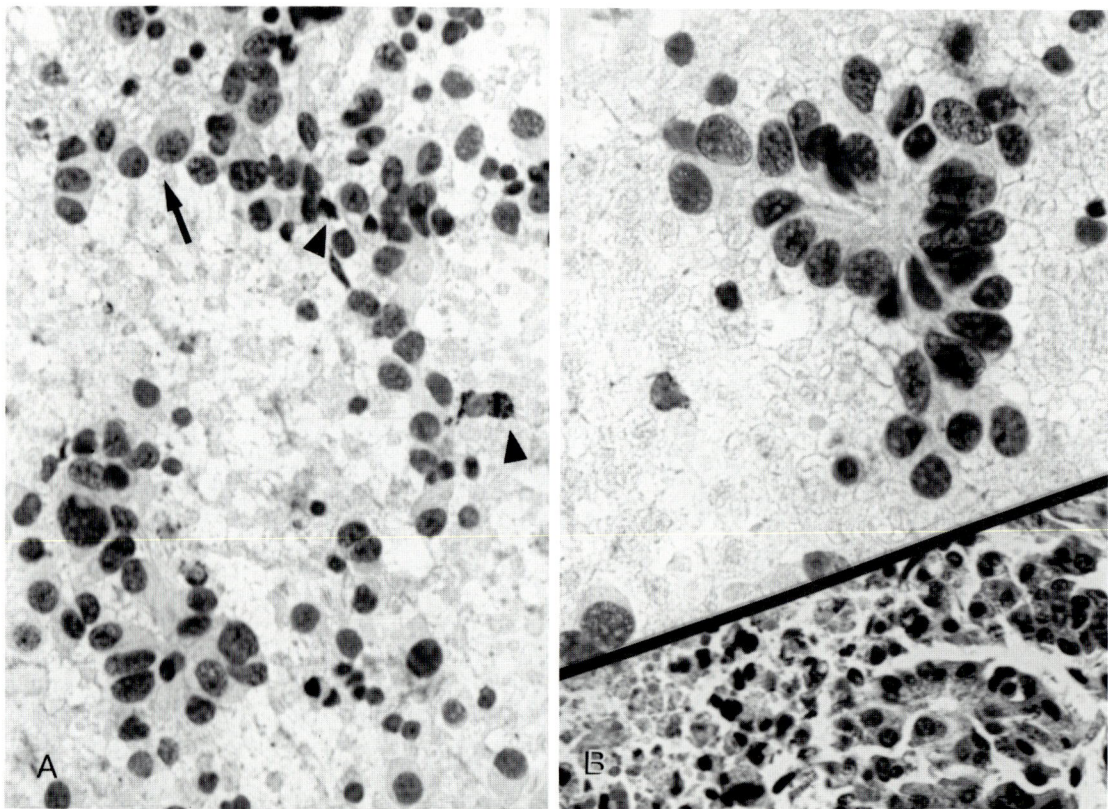

Figure 7.26.

Atypical Carcinoid Tumor

The classic carcinoid tumors as described above have a low malignant potential, but occasionally one may encounter a tumor that is quite aggressive, with a clinical course intermediate between the typical carcinoid and small cell undifferentiated carcinoma. These aggressive carcinoid tumors are referred to by various authors as atypical carcinoid tumor, malignant carcinoid tumor, or well-differentiated neuroendocrine carcinoma.[28–30] These tumors are cytologically more pleomorphic than typical carcinoid tumors and show areas of necrosis and mitoses.

Aspiration Cytology

The following criteria are characteristic of atypical carcinoid tumors (**Fig. 7.26**). *(a)* The tumor cells are more pleomorphic. Bland cellular monomorphism, a hallmark for typical carcinoid tumors, is no longer observed. *(b)* Mitotic figures can be readily identified. *(c)* The smear background shows necrosis.

Cells of atypical carcinoids are distinguished from those of small cell undifferentiated carcinoma by their larger size and more cytoplasm. Nuclear molding is minimal or absent. In our experience and that of others,[29] well-formed acini (**Fig. 7.26B**) are quite common in atypical carcinoids but are rare in small cell undifferentiated carcinomas.

Diagnostic Pitfalls. Cytologic diagnosis of atypical carcinoid is difficult. At various times, the tumors have been confused with typical carcinoid, adenocarcinoma, poorly differentiated squamous carcinoma, and small cell undifferentiated carcinoma.[28,29] Since atypical carcinoid and small cell undifferentiated carcinoma may be difficult to separate in FNA specimens, it is recommended that surgical resection be performed for all stage 1 neoplasms of the lung with cytologic features evocative of either neoplasm.[28]

We have mistaken one case of atypical carcinoid for adenocarcinoma because of the predominance of acini in the FNAB.

Malignant Lymphoma

Malignant lymphoma comprises only 0.5% of malignancies arising in the lung.[31] Involvement of the lung as the primary site is much less common than are pulmonary lesions forming part of more widespread disease. Any of the morphologic types may be seen in the lung, although most cases have been of small lymphocytic type, with relatively low aggressiveness.[32] The same set of cytologic criteria for diagnosing nodal lymphoma can be applied to the diagnosis of extranodal lymphoma (see Chapter 4). Hodgkin's disease arising primarily in the lung is very rare.

METASTATIC TUMORS

The lung is a common site for metastatic tumors. These metastases may be single or be restricted to a single lobe of the lung and thereby be curable by resection. The most common source of metastases in women is breast cancer, and in men colonic cancer.[33] Sarcomas also frequently metastasize to the lung. The interpretation of the pulmonary aspirate from a patient with a past history of malignancy can be greatly facilitated by review of the previous slides. Ancillary procedures, such as immmunocytochemistry and electron microscopy, may provide useful diagnostic information.

Recognition of a specific cytologic feature in the malignant cells is extremely helpful in making the correct diagnosis. For example, the cytopathologist may be able to observe the clear cytoplasm of a renal cell carcinoma (**Fig. 7.27**) or melanin pigment granules in the cells of a malignant melanoma (see Chapter 4).

There are no absolute criteria for separating primary from metastatic adenocarcinomas. Observation of large tissue fragments consisting of strikingly palisaded, columnar cells with elongated nuclei is a feature characteristic, although by no means specific, of well-differentiated colonic adenocarcinomas (**Fig. 7.28**). Metastatic breast adenocarcinomas generally present no specific cytologic pattern that can be distinguished from other adenocarcinomas; often the tumor cells form small cell clusters simulating bronchioloalveolar carcinoma. In some cases the cells are arranged in the characteristic "Indian file" pattern as depicted in **Figure 7.29**.

Metastatic squamous carcinomas to the lung originate most commonly from the head and neck region, larynx, esophagus, and uterine cervix. The cytologic features of these tumors are similar to those of primary squamous carcinoma of the lung. In cases of non-keratinizing squamous carcinoma of the small cell variety, the aspirate may mimic primary small cell undifferentiated carcinoma. **Figure 7.30** illustrates such a case, but a review of the original biopsy of the uterine cervix (**Fig. 7.30**, *inset*) permits a cytologic diagnosis of metastatic carcinoma from the cervix to be made. It is interesting to note that a recent study[34] has shown neurosecretory granules in some poorly differentiated carcinomas of the cervix.

The lung is frequently involved by metastatic sarcomas and there is usually a history of previous surgery for a soft tissue tumor. However, the observation of spindle cells in an aspirate does not necessarily denote a sarcoma. As discussed earlier, some carcinoid tumors are composed of spindle cells, and poorly differentiated squamous carcinomas can have pseudosarcomatous features. The cytopathology of sarcomas is discussed in detail in Chapter 5.

TUMOR-LIKE LESIONS AND INFLAMMATORY LESIONS

Although FNAB is mainly used for the diagnosis of malignant disease, some investigators[35] have estimated that almost 70–75% of the benign lesions of the lung may be diagnosed by this technique. Dahlgren and Ekström[36] successfully diagnosed tuberculosis in up to 80% of the cases. Jackson et al.[37] reported a 75% success rate in identifying microorganisms from lung aspirations in their series of 229 cases.

Figure 7.25. Carcinoid tumor, spindle cell variant. **A** and **B,** ABC. Note elongated, bland nuclei and finely granular cytoplasm. **A,** ×125; **B,** ×500. **C,** Histology of the spindle cell carcinoid. Note spindle cells with granular cytoplasm. ×310.

Figure 7.26. Atypical carcinoid. **A,** Some tumor cells still retain the appearance of classic carcinoid cells *(arrow),* while others show much pleomorphism. *Arrowheads* indicate mitotic figures. ×310. **B,** ABC. Atypical carcinoid cells forming a small acinar structure. Compared with classic carcinoid, there is much more nuclear pleomorphism. *Inset,* Histology of the resected tumor. Note prominent necrosis, a feature not seen in classic carcinoid. ×500; *inset,* ×310.

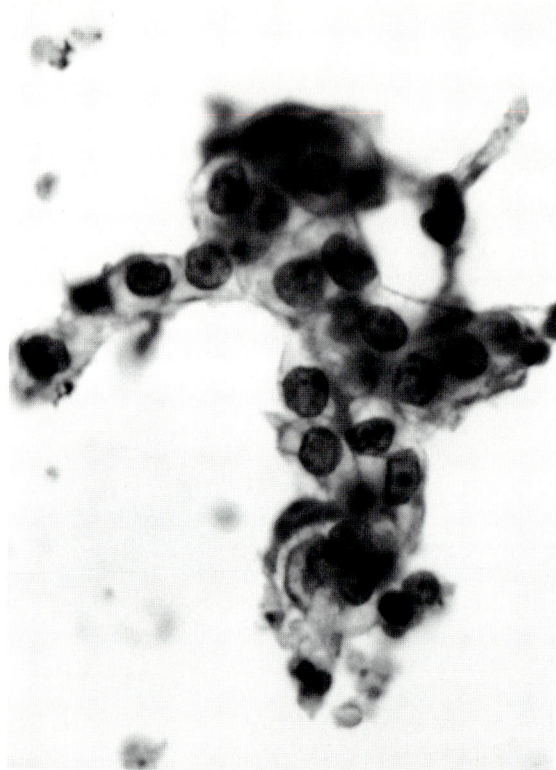

Figure 7.27. Metastatic renal cell carcinoma, ABC. Note tumor cells characterized by clear cytoplasm and prominent nuclei. ×500.

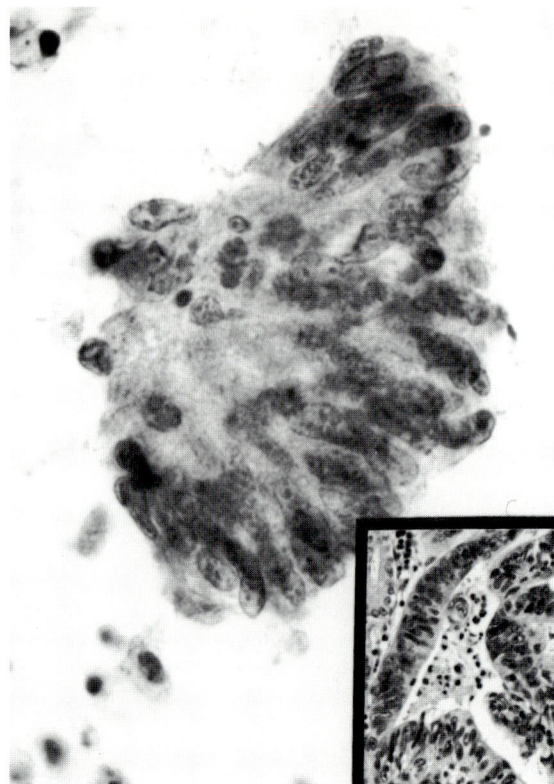

Figure 7.28. Metastatic colonic adenocarcinoma, ABC. Note palisading columnar cells. This feature is commonly seen in well-differentiated colonic adenocarcinomas. *Inset* shows the histology of the primary adenocarcinoma. Note nuclear palisading. ×500; *inset,* ×125.

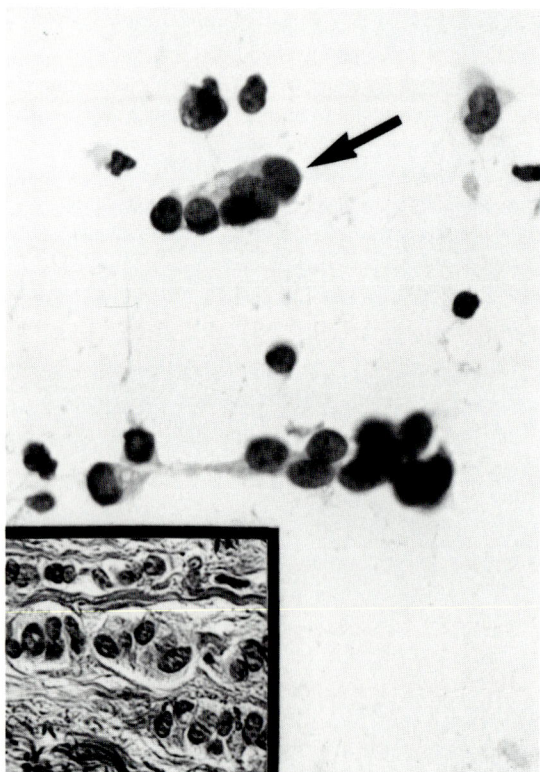

Figure 7.29. Metastatic breast adenocarcinoma, ABC. Note tumor cells in Indian file arrangement *(arrow)* and small cell cluster. *Inset,* Histology of the mammary ductal adenocarcinoma. Note identical cellular arrangement to that seen in the aspirate. ×500; *inset,* ×310.

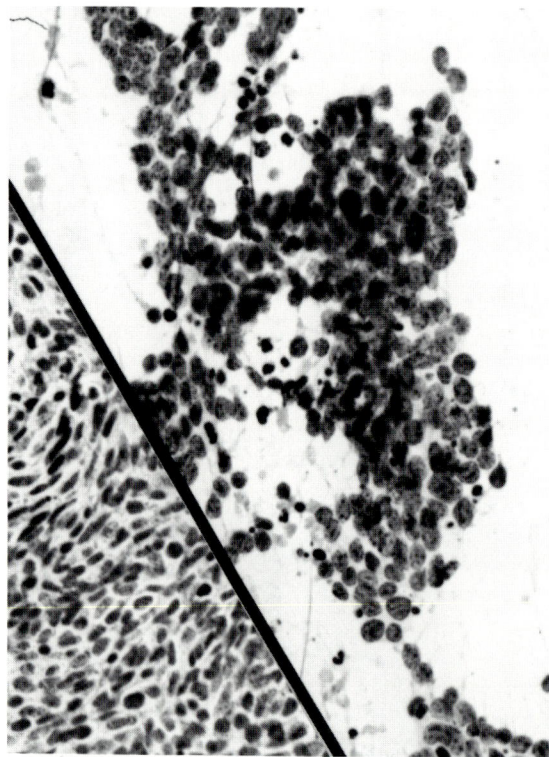

Figure 7.30. Metastatic nonkeratinizing squamous carcinoma from uterine cervix, ABC. The tumor is composed of small cells, which can easily be mistaken for primary small cell undifferentiated carcinoma of the lung. *Inset,* Histology of the original biopsy of the uterine cervix showing a poorly differentiated nonkeratinizing squamous carcinoma. ×310; *inset,* ×310.

146

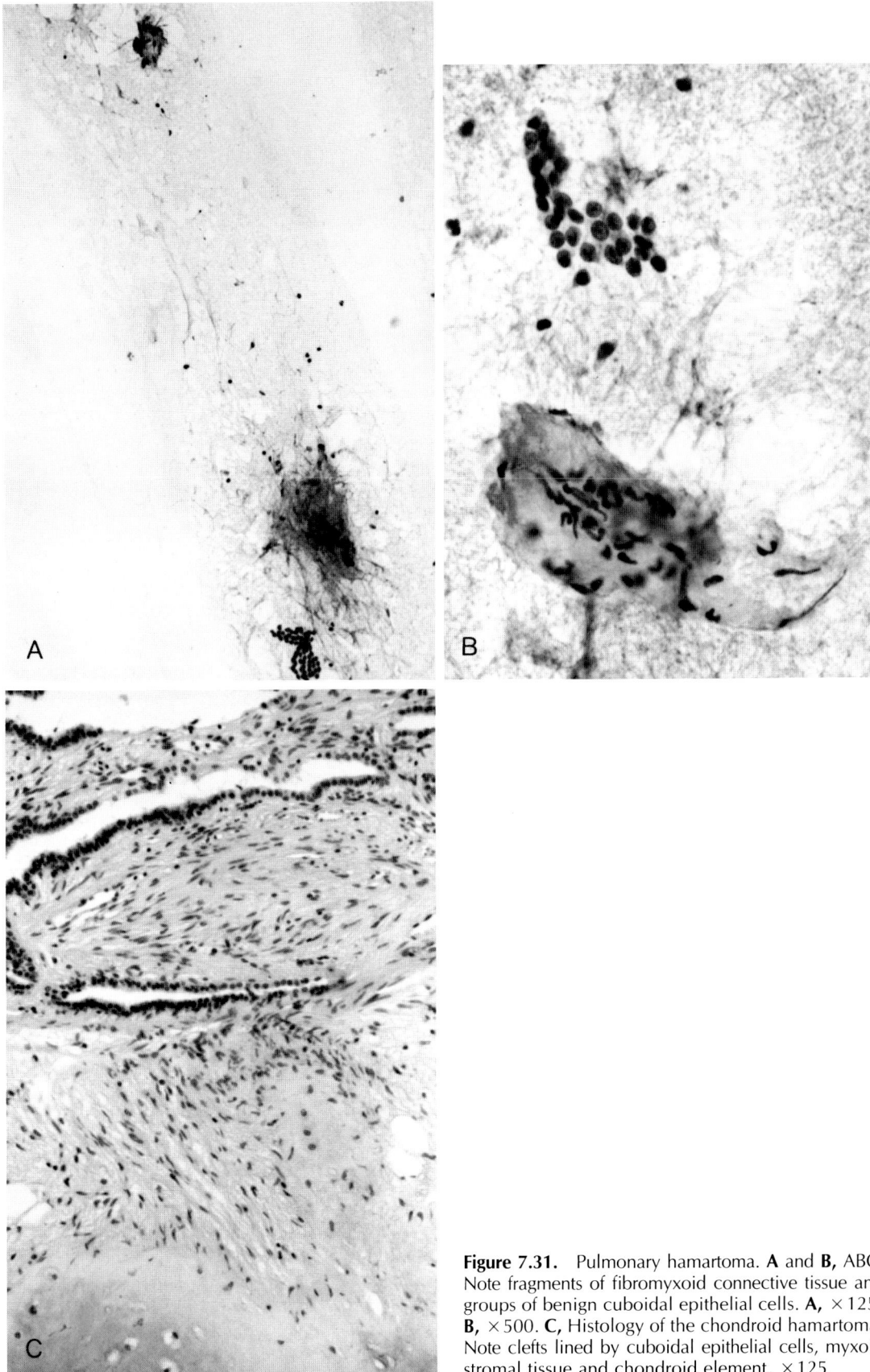

Figure 7.31. Pulmonary hamartoma. **A** and **B,** ABC. Note fragments of fibromyxoid connective tissue and groups of benign cuboidal epithelial cells. **A,** ×125; **B,** ×500. **C,** Histology of the chondroid hamartoma. Note clefts lined by cuboidal epithelial cells, myxoid stromal tissue and chondroid element. ×125.

Hamartoma

Hamartoma is the most frequent benign tumor-like lesion of the lung and can be diagnosed by FNAB.[38,39] They are circumscribed nodules and may mimic malignant neoplasms on chest roentgenography. Histologically, they reveal columnar or cuboidal bronchial epithelium lining cleft-like spaces and an abundant stroma that frequently includes a prominent chondroid or myxoid mesenchymal component.

Aspiration Cytology

Cellularity of the smears is variable. A characteristic feature is the presence of small fragments of myxofibrillar stromal tissue, as well as groups of benign epithelial cells (**Fig. 7.31**). Failure to recognize the myxofibrillar tissue leads the cytologist to render a nondiagnostic diagnosis. On the other hand, if large numbers of the benign epithelial cells lining the clefts are aspirated, the smears will be cellular and may be mistaken for carcinoid tumor.[38–40]

Amyloidosis

Pulmonary amyloidosis is rare but important, as it may clinically and radiologically mimic lung neoplasm. It can occur as a diffuse infiltrate or as single or multiple nodules. The cytopathology of pulmonary amyloidosis has been described.[41] The case we encountered occurred as multiple pulmonary nodules. The aspirate contained irregular masses of acellular, amorphous, waxy material that stained eosinophilic with hematoxylin and eosin and bluish green with the Papanicolaou technique (**Fig. 7.32**). The amyloid material showed characteristic apple-green birefringence with Congo red stain.

Tuberculoma

Of all the inflammatory lesions that may simulate a neoplasm, the most common one is a tuberculoma. The aspirates may be sparsely cellular if a necrotic area is aspirated; otherwise it is cell-rich, with many chronic inflammatory cells and histiocytes. Cohesive, syncytial clumps of epithelioid histiocytes, reminiscent of epithelial cell clusters, are a characteristic feature. Epithelioid histiocytes have plump, elongated nuclei with finely granular chromatin and pale-pink, indistinct cytoplasm (**Fig. 7.33**). Multinucleated Langhans' giant cells (**Fig. 7.33B,** *inset*) may or may not be seen. The smear background contains necrotic debris and various types of chronic inflammatory cells, with small lymphocytes predominating. Caseous material appears granular and eosinophilic and lacks recognizable cell remnants. Sometimes acid-fast bacilli can be demonstrated in the smears or cell blocks with the Ziehl-Neelsen stain or fluorescence technique.[42,43]

Specific Infections Other Than Tuberculosis

Besides tuberculoma, other pulmonary granulomas are usually fungal. Many of these fungi stain well enough to be directly visualized with routine smears if the pathologist is alert. Further morphologic details can be demonstrated with either Grocott-Gomori methenamine-silver stain or periodic acid-Schiff stain. Care should also be taken to insure that appropriate cultures are carried out.

Aspiration Cytology

Pathogenic fungi are present in the smears either in yeast or hyphal form. The smear background usually contains scattered benign respiratory cells, acute inflammatory cells, lymphocytes, and histiocytes. In **Figure 7.34** are shown the yeast cells of *Cryptococcus neoformans*. The organisms are ovoid to spherical, measure 8–12 μm in diameter, and have a thick capsule that does not stain with hematoxylin and eosin or with the Papanicolaou technique, thus leaving a characteristic halo around the centrally stained area. The capsule, however, can be stained with mucicarmine. Single budding is char-

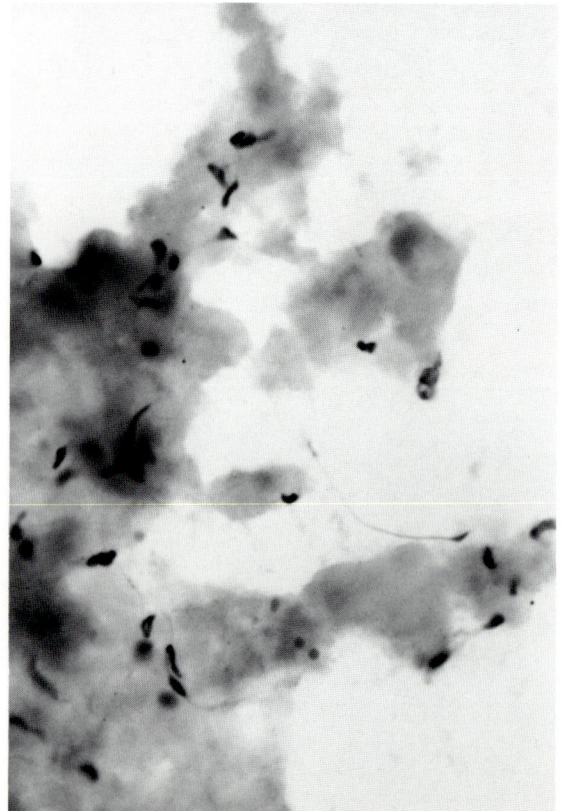

Figure 7.32. Pulmonary amyloidosis, ABC. Fragments of amorphous, acellular material, stained eosinophilic with hematoxylin and eosin or blue-green with the Papanicolaou technique. × 310.

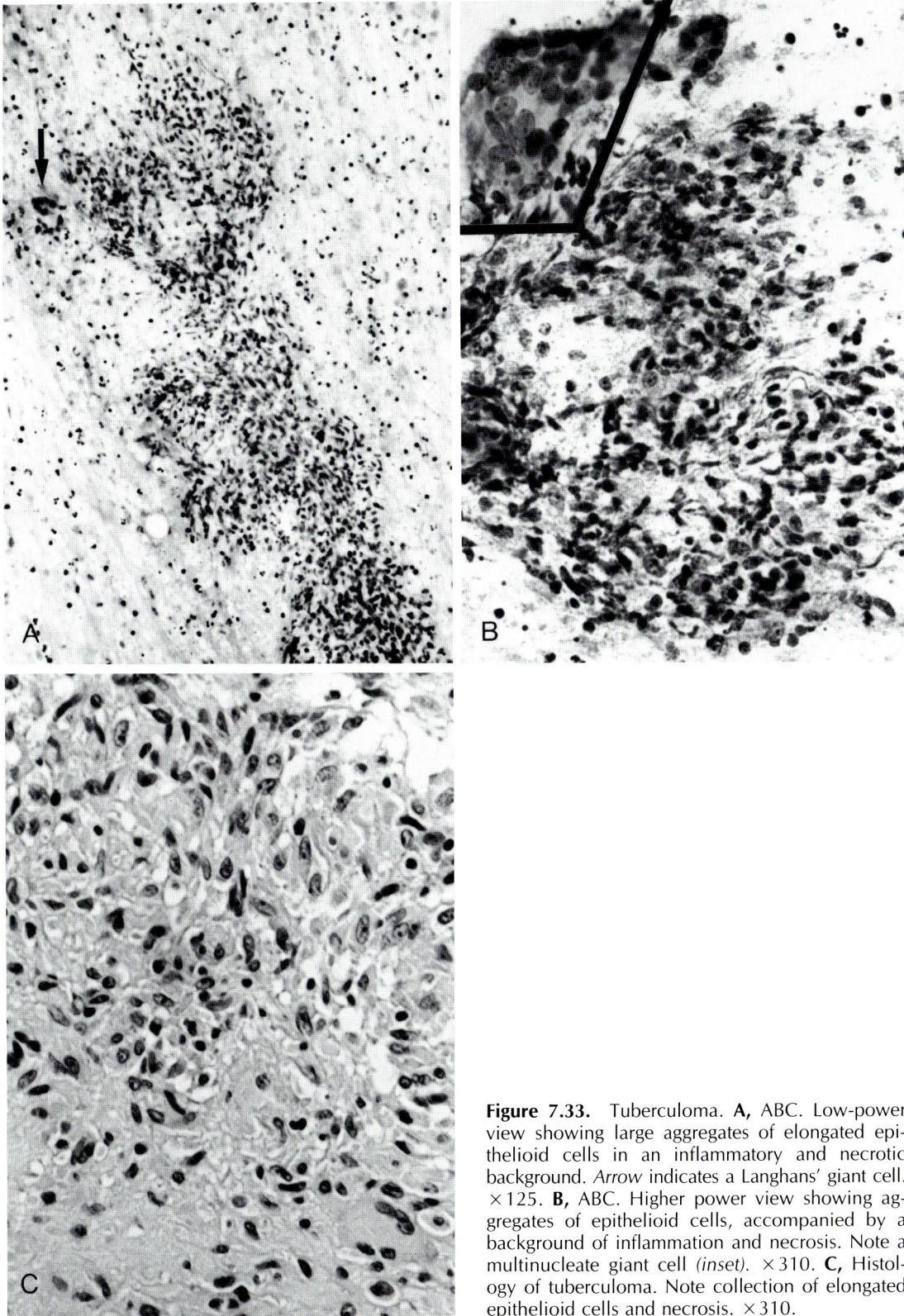

Figure 7.33. Tuberculoma. **A,** ABC. Low-power view showing large aggregates of elongated epithelioid cells in an inflammatory and necrotic background. *Arrow* indicates a Langhans' giant cell. ×125. **B,** ABC. Higher power view showing aggregates of epithelioid cells, accompanied by a background of inflammation and necrosis. Note a multinucleate giant cell *(inset).* ×310. **C,** Histology of tuberculoma. Note collection of elongated epithelioid cells and necrosis. ×310.

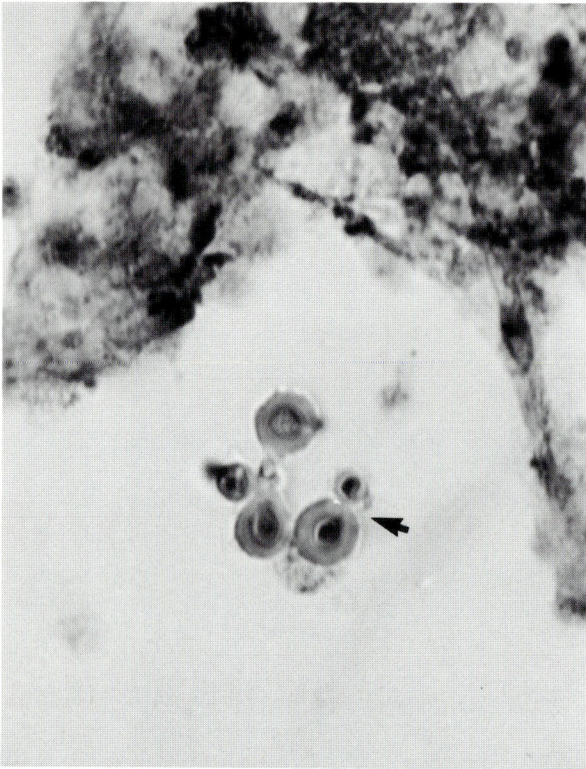

Figure 7.34. *Cryptococcus neoformans,* ABC. The organisms occur in yeast form and have a thick, gelatinous, nonstaining capsule. Single budding *(arrow)* is characteristic. Gomori's methenamine-silver stain. × 1200.

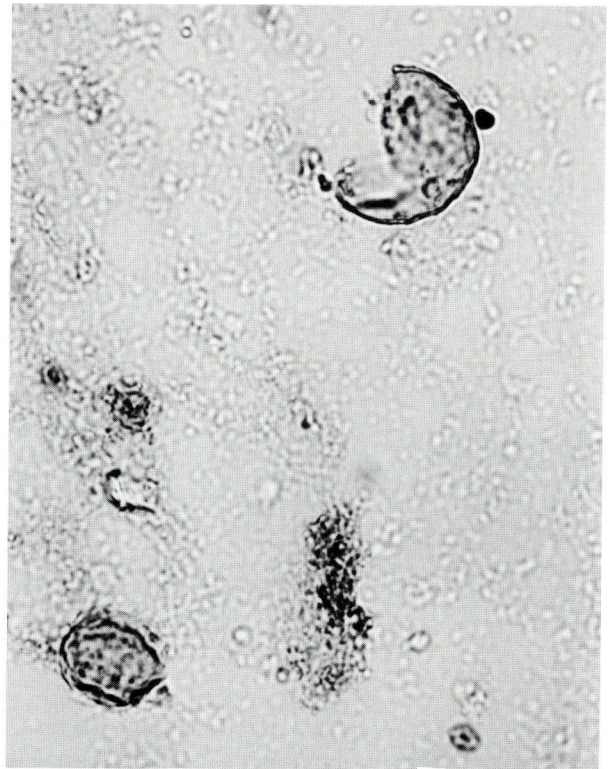

Figure 7.35. *Coccidioides immitis,* ABC. Two large spherules containing endospores. Note characteristic double contour walls. The wall of the larger spherule has ruptured, while the wall of the smaller one has collapsed. × 500.

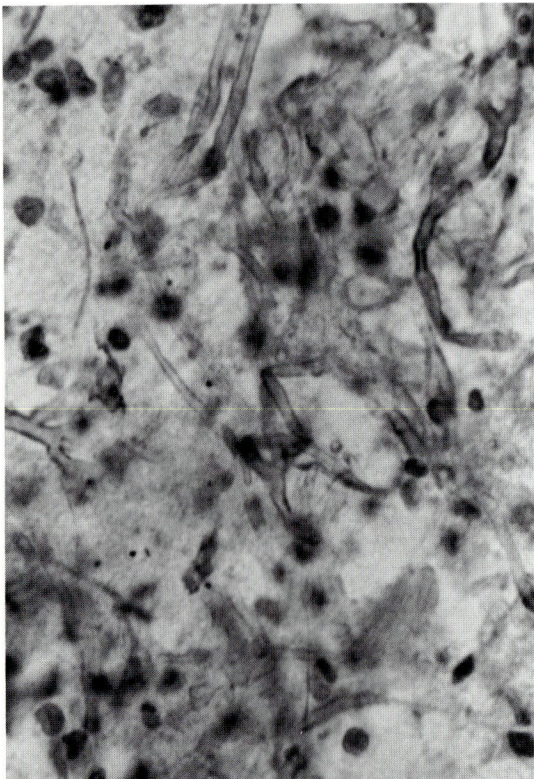

Figure 7.36. *Aspergillus fumigatus,* ABC. Numerous septate hyphae, branching at 45° angle. × 500.

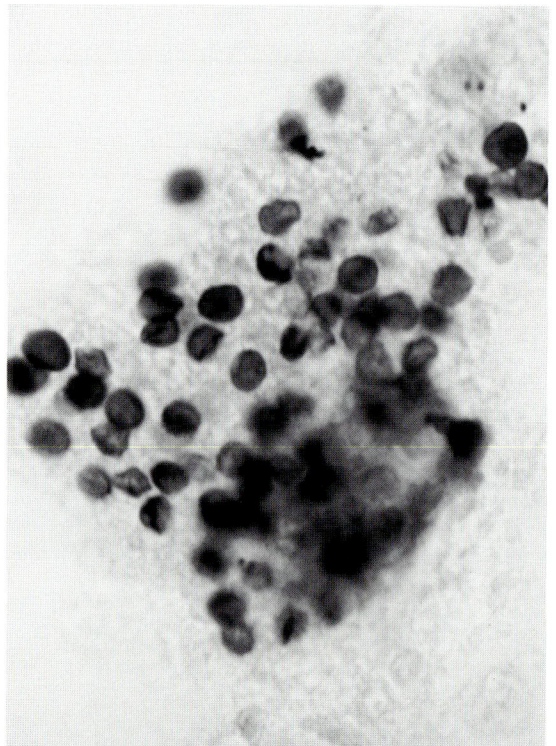

Figure 7.37. *Pneumocystis carinii,* ABC. These organisms appear as 5–8 μm-diameter cysts, some of which contain a dark-staining central globoid structure. The cysts are spherical, but some have collapsed with a cup-shaped contour. Gomori's methenamine-silver stain. × 1200.

acteristic and there is a tendency for the bud to pinch off, leaving a markedly attenuated neck attached to the mother yeast. **Figure 7.35** shows spherules (sporangia) of *Coccidioides immitis*, with a characteristic round, doubly contoured wall. The spherules are large, varying from 20 to 80 μm in diameter, and contain tiny endospores (sporangiospores). These endospores burst through the cell wall propagating the fungus.

Mycotic infections that appear as hyphae in the lungs are most often caused by *Aspergillus fumigatus* **(Fig. 7.36)**, which can be identified in smears stained with H & E or with the Papanicolaou technique. These organisms are characterized by septate hyphae that dichotomously branch at 45° angles. The hyphae measure 30–35 μm in width, as opposed to the larger nonseptate hyphae of mucormycosis, which measure about 50 μm in width.

Pulmonary lesions caused by the protozoan *Pneumocystis carinii* have been increasingly encountered in recent years.[44] This organism occurs chiefly in patients with impaired immunity. The infection manifests radiologically as a diffuse pulmonary infiltrative process. Needle aspiration provides a relatively simple means of diagnosis.[45] Organisms are not visualized on routinely stained material. The smear shows a mass of honeycombed, eosinophilic material. In such a situation, one should decolorize the slide and restain with methenamine silver. The silver stain will stain the organisms as cysts about 6–8 μm in diameter **(Fig. 7.37)**. Sometimes, a small dark-staining globoid structure can be seen within the cyst. Cysts may be spherical, cup-shaped, or crescentic, and usually form small clumps.

References

1. Jamieson WRE, Suen KC, Hicken P, Martin AL, Burr LH, Munro AI. Reliability of percutaneous needle aspiration biopsy for diagnosis of bronchogenic carcinoma. Cancer Detect Prev 1981;4:331–336.
2. Simpson RW, Johnson DA, Wold LE, Goellner JR. Transthoracic needle aspiration biopsy. Review of 233 cases. Acta Cytol 1988;32:101–104.
3. Young GP, Young I, Cowan DF, Blei RL. The reliability of fine needle aspiration biopsy in the diagnosis of deep lesions of the lung and mediastinum. Diagn Cytopathol 1987;3:1–7.
4. Pilotti S, Rilke F, Gribaudi G, Damascelli B, Ravasi G: Transthoracic fine needle aspiration biopsy in pulmonary lesions; updated results. Acta Cytol 1984;28:225–232.
5. Michel RP, Lushpihan A, Ahmed MN. Pathologic findings of transthoracic needle aspiration in the diagnosis of localized pulmonary lesions. Cancer 1983;51:1663–1672.
6. Sinner WN. Complications of percutaneous transthoracic needle aspiration biopsy. Acta Radiol Diagn 1976;17:813–828.
7. Garret M. Cellular atypias in sputum and bronchial secretions associated with tuberculosis and bronchiectasis. Am J Clin Pathol 1960;34:237–246.
8. Kern WH. Cytology of hyperplastic and neoplastic lesions of terminal bronchioles and alveoli. Acta Cytol 1965;9:372–380.
9. Johnston WW, Frable WJ. Diagnostic respiratory cytopathology. New York: Masson Publishing, 1979:69–73.
10. Vincent RG, Pickren JW, Lane WW, et al. The changing histopathology of lung cancer: A review of 1,682 cases. Cancer 1977;39:1647–1655.
11. World Health Organization. The World Health Organization histological typing of lung tumours, 2nd ed. Am J Clin Pathol 1982;77:123–136.
12. Manning JT Jr, Spjut HJ, Tschen JA. Bronchioloalveolar carcinoma: The significance of two histologic types. Cancer 1984;54:525–534.
13. Tao LC, Delarue HC, Sanders D, Weisbrod G. Bronchiolo-alveolar carcinoma. A correlative clinical and cytologic study. Cancer 1978;42:2759–2767.
14. Sterrett G, Whitaker D, Glancy J. Fine needle aspiration of lung, mediastinum, and chest wall. Pathol Annu 1982;17(part 2):197–228.
15. Silverman JF, Finley JL, Park HK, Strausbauch P, Unverferth M, Carney M. Fine needle aspiration cytology of bronchioloalveolar cell carcinoma of the lung. Acta Cytol 1985;29:887–894.
16. Jarrett DD, Betsill WL Jr. A Problem-oriented approach regarding the fine needle aspiration cytology diagnosis of bronchioloalveolar carcinoma of the lung: A comparison of diagnostic criteria with benign lesions mimicking carcinoma. Acta Cytol 1987;31:684–685.
17. Finkle HI. Type 1 bronchioloalveolar carcinoma in a fine needle aspirate. Acta Cytol 1988;32:733–735.
18. Carney DN, Matthews M, Ihde DC, et al. Influence of histologic subtype of small cell carcinoma of the lung on clinical presentation response to therapy and survival. J Natl Cancer Inst 1980;65:1225–1230.
19. McDowell EM. Lung carcinomas. Edinburgh: Churchill Livingstone, 1987:270–276.
20. Churg A. The fine structure of large cell undifferentiated carcinoma of the lung. Evidence of its relation to squamous cell carcinomas and adenocarcinomas. Hum Pathol 1978;9:143–156.
21. Johnston WW, Frable WJ. Diagnostic respiratory cytopathology. New York: Masson Publishing, 1979:175.
22. Pearse AGE. The cytochemistry and ultrastructure of polypeptide hormone-producing cells of the APUD series and the embryologic, physiologic and pathologic implications of the concept. J Histochem Cytochem 1969;17:303–313.
23. Churg A. Large spindle cell variant of peripheral bronchial carcinoid tumor. Arch Pathol Lab Med 1977;101:216–218.
24. Lozowski W, Hajdu SI, Melamed MR. Cytomorphology of carcinoid tumors. Acta Cytol 1979;23:360–365.
25. Gephardt GN, Belovich DM. Cytology of pulmonary carcinoid tumors. Acta Cytol 1982;26:434–438.
26. Kyriakos M, Rockoff SD. Brush biopsy of bronchial carcinoid—a source of cytologic error. Acta Cytol 1972;16:261–268.
27. Koss LG. Diagnostic cytology and its histopathologic bases, 3rd ed. Philadelphia: JB Lippincott, 1979:666.
28. Frierson HF Jr, Covell JL, Mills SE. Fine needle aspiration cytology of atypical carcinoid of the lung. Acta Cytol 1987;31:471–475.
29. Jordan AG, Predmore L, Sullivan MM, Memoli VA. The cytodiagnosis of well-differentiated neuroendocrine carcinoma. Acta Cytol 1987;31:464–470.
30. Szyfelbein WM, Ross JS. Carcinoids, atypical carcinoids, and small-cell carcinomas of the lung: Differential diagnosis of fine needle aspiration biopsy specimens. Diagn Cytopathol 1988;4:1–8.
31. Spencer H. Pathology of the lung, 3rd ed. Oxford: Pergamon Press, 1977.
32. Koss MN, Hochholzer L, Nichols PW, Wehunt WD, Lazarus AA. Primary non-Hodgkin's lymphoma and pseudolymphoma of lung. Hum Pathol 1983;14:1024–1038.
33. Habein HC Jr, Clagett OT, McDonald JR. Pulmonary resection for metastatic tumors. Arch Surg 1959;78:716–723.

34. Barrett RJ II, Davos I, Leuchter RS, Lagasse LD. Neuroendocrine features in poorly differentiated and undifferentiated carcinomas of the cervix. Cancer 1987;60:2325–2330.

35. Sargent EN, Turner AF, Gordonson J, Schwinn CP, Pashley O. Percutaneous pulmonary needle biopsy. Report of 350 patients. Am J Roentgenol 1974;122:758–764.

36. Dahlgren SE, Ekström P. Aspiration cytology in the diagnosis of pulmonary tuberculosis. Scand J Resp Dis 1972:53;196–201.

37. Jackson R, Coffin L, DeMeules J, et al. Percutaneous needle biopsy of pulmonary lesions. Am J Surg 1980;139:586–590.

38. Suen KC, Quenville NF. Fine needle aspiration cytology of uncommon thoracic lesions. Am J Clin Pathol 1981;75:803–809.

39. Dahlgren S. Needle biopsy of intrapulmonary hamartoma. Scand J Resp Dis 1966;47:187–194.

40. Ramzy I. Pulmonary hamartomas: Cytologic appearances of fine needle aspiration biopsy. Acta Cytol 1976;20:15–18.

41. Tomashefski JF, Cramer SF, Abramowsky C, Cohen AM, Horak G. Needle biopsy of solitary amyloid nodule of the lung. Acta Cytol 1980;23:224–227.

42. Bailey TM, Akhtar M, Ali MA. Fine needle aspiration biopsy in the diagnosis of tuberculosis. Acta Cytol 1985;29:732–736.

43. Tani EM, Schmitt FCL, Oliveira MLS, Gobetti SMP, Decarlis RMST. Pulmonary cytology in tuberculosis. Acta Cytol 1987;31:460–463.

44. Gottlieb MS, Schroft R, Schanker HM, et al. Pneumocystis carinii pneumonia and mucosa candidiasis in previously healthy homosexual men. Evidence of a new acquired cellular immunodeficiency. N Engl J Med 1981;305:1425–1431.

45. Bhatt ON, Miller MSR, LeRiche J, King EG. Aspiration biopsy in pulmonary opportunistic infections. Acta Cytol 1977;21:206–209.

8

Mediastinum and Pleura

The mediastinum is the irregular space within the chest lying between the two pleural sacs and is generally divided into four anatomic compartments: superior, anterior, middle, and posterior. The superior mediastinum extends above a line drawn from the manubrium of the sternum through the lower border of the fourth thoracic vertebral body. The anterior mediastinum lies below the superior mediastinum, between the sternum and pericardium. The middle mediastinum contains the heart and major blood vessels. The posterior mediastinum is the space located behind the pericardium. To facilitate cytologic interpretation of mediastinal lesions, it is crucial that the cytopathologist be aware of the exact location of the lesions. Each tumor type has a predilection for a certain part of the mediastinum (**Table 8.1** and **Fig. 8.1**). Although this chapter concerns itself solely with primary mediastinal lesions, one must not forget that metastases to mediastinal lymph nodes are common and cytologic interpretation of mediastinal tumors necessitates differential diagnosis between primary and metastatic neoplasms. Suffice it to say that the majority of metastases to the mediastinum are from the lung, breast, esophagus, and stomach.

THYMIC NEOPLASMS
Thymoma

Thymomas are epithelial neoplasms of the thymic gland, typically occurring in the anterior mediastinum and, less frequently, in the superior mediastinum.[1] About 30% of thymomas are associated with myasthenia gravis. Most thymomas are benign and encapsulated; about 20% show direct invasion into the adjoining tissues and are, therefore, classified as malignant. Most malignant thymomas show the same histologic picture as the benign counterpart; an occasional malignant thymoma may exhibit obvious cytologic atypia.[2] The histology of thymomas is basically composed of two cell types, the epithelial cell and the small lymphocyte. There is considerable variation in the appearance of the epithelial cells and in the proportion of the epithelial cells to lymphocytes. Correct diagnosis of thymoma by fine needle aspiration biopsy is possible and has been reported by many workers.[3–10] Tao et al.[3] reported 37 cases of thymomas diagnosed by FNAB; all were verified histologically, with no false-positive results. Finley et al.[4] diagnosed a case of malignant thymoma and a case of thymic carcinoma by FNAB and demonstrated the value of immunocytochemistry and ultrastructural studies in confirming the diagnoses. Dahlgren et al.[5] studied 23 cases of anterior mediastinal tumors, in which 12 cases were cytologically diagnosed as thymoma. Spahr and Frable[6] described the exfoliative cytology of an invasive thymoma that penetrated a bronchus.

Table 8.1. Primary Tumors of the Mediastinum

Thymic tumors (anterior mediastinum)[a]
  Thymoma
  Thymic carcinoma
  Carcinoid and oat cell carcinoma
Lymphomas (anterior and middle mediastinum)
  Hodgkin's disease
  Non-Hodgkin's lymphoma
Germ cell tumors (anterior mediastinum)
  Teratoma
  Seminoma
  Embryonal carcinoma
  Yolk sac tumor
  Choriocarcinoma
  Mixed germ cell tumor
Thyroid tumors (superior mediastinum)
  Nodular goiter
  Thyroid neoplasm
Benign cysts (middle mediastinum)
  Pericardial
  Bronchogenic
Neurogenic tumors (posterior mediastinum)

[a]Parentheses indicate the locations in which the tumors are usually found.

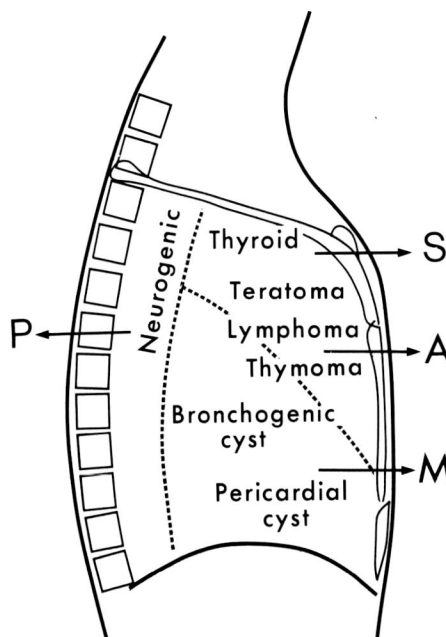

Figure 8.1. Anatomic compartments of the mediastinum and topographic distribution of some common mediastinal lesions. S, A, M, P = superior, anterior, middle, and posterior mediastinum, respectively.

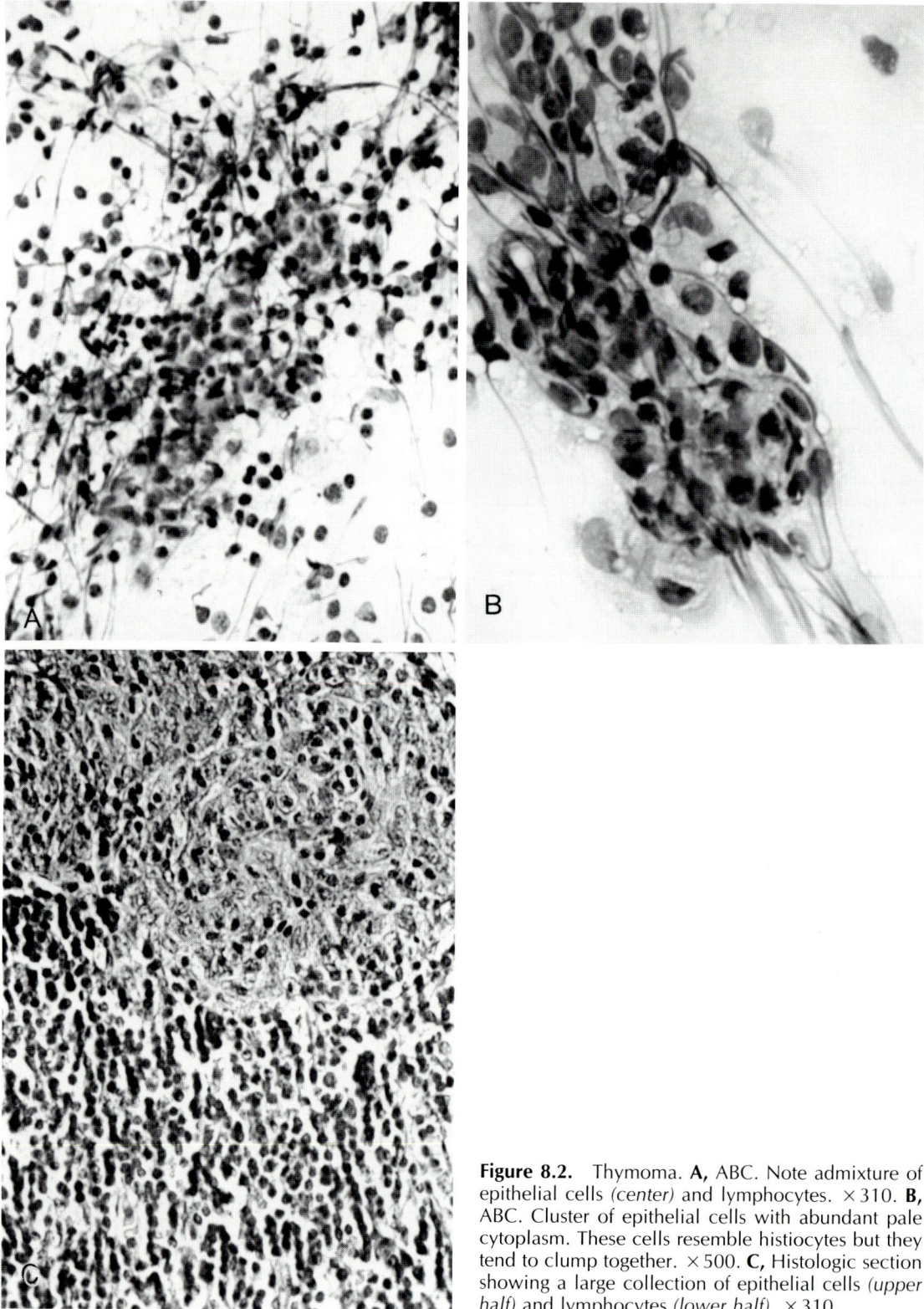

Figure 8.2.   Thymoma. **A,** ABC. Note admixture of epithelial cells *(center)* and lymphocytes. ×310. **B,** ABC. Cluster of epithelial cells with abundant pale cytoplasm. These cells resemble histiocytes but they tend to clump together. ×500. **C,** Histologic section showing a large collection of epithelial cells *(upper half)* and lymphocytes *(lower half).* ×310.

Aspiration Cytology

Cellular Pattern.   Aspirates are cellular, and a biphasic pattern is typical. The relative proportions of epithelial cells and lymphocytes vary considerably from case to case. The epithelial cells form cohesive cell groups, while the lymphocytes are scattered throughout the smear as single cells **(Fig. 8.2)**. In the lymphocyte-predominant variant, the epithelial cells may be so few that their presence may be obscured by lymphocytes that dominate the smear **(Fig. 8.3)**.

Cell Morphology.   The neoplastic cells are the epithelial cells, which in most cases are histiocyte-like, and three or four times as large as the lymphocytes. These cells are polygonal or oval in shape and have a moderately abundant, clear or pale staining cytoplasm. The vesicular nuclei are round, occasionally indented or lobulated, and show inconspicuous nucleoli. The epithelial cells occur frequently in groups **(Fig. 8.2)**, but if they are isolated **(Fig. 8.3)**, it may be impossible to differentiate them from histiocytes, although the absence of nuclear debris in the cytoplasm should provide the first clue. In some cases **(Fig. 8.4)**, the epithelial cells are spindle-shaped with elongated nuclei (spindle cell thymoma). In rare cases **(Fig. 8.5)**, the epithelial cells exhibit malignant cytologic features (thymic carcinoma).[2,4]

The second cell type is the lymphocyte. The lymphocytes do not show cytologic atypia; most are mature, with a small dark nucleus and a scant or invisible cytoplasm. Others are stimulated lymphocytes, characterized by a larger nucleus, a more open chromatin pattern, and a visible nucleolus.

Diagnostic Pitfalls.   Thymomas with a predominance of lymphocytes must be distinguished from malignant lymphomas. The lymphocytes in thymomas are small and benign-appearing, while those in lymphomas are generally cytologically atypical. Immunoperoxi-dase studies demonstrate the polyclonal nature of the thymic lymphocytes and positive staining for thymocyte antigen (Leu-6).[4] In addition, it is important to be familiar with the appearance of the epithelial cells from studying those thymomas in which they predominate; otherwise their presence in predominantly lymphocytic thymomas may be mistaken for histiocytes. The epithelial cells, however, react with antibodies to cytokeratin, while histiocytes do not.

Thymomas with predominantly spindle cells may be confused with neuroma or sarcoma.[5] The identification of lymphocytes in the smear background and the immunocytochemical demonstration of cytokeratin reactivity in the tumor cells aid in the identification of spindle cell thymoma.

In most cases, preoperative cytologic evaluation of a thymoma cannot determine whether the tumor is benign or malignant. The diagnosis of malignancy is dependent on the radiologic or intraoperative demonstration of tumor invasion into adjoining tissues; hence, the importance of team approach cannot be overemphasized.

Only a small number of malignant thymomas show obvious cellular pleomorphism.[2] When they do, they are referred to as thymic carcinoma. In these instances, one must rule out a metastatic poorly differentiated carcinoma from the lung or elsewhere. Some thymic carcinomas show considerable epidermoid features, indistinguishable from squamous cell carcinoma.

Thymic Neuroendocrine Tumors

Thymic carcinoids are derived from neuroendocrine cells with biochemical characteristics of APUD (amine precursor uptake and decarboxylation) cells. The ABC is similar to that described for pulmonary carcinoids (see Chapter 7). The cells are oval to round with amphophilic, finely granular cytoplasm, uniform nuclei, stippled

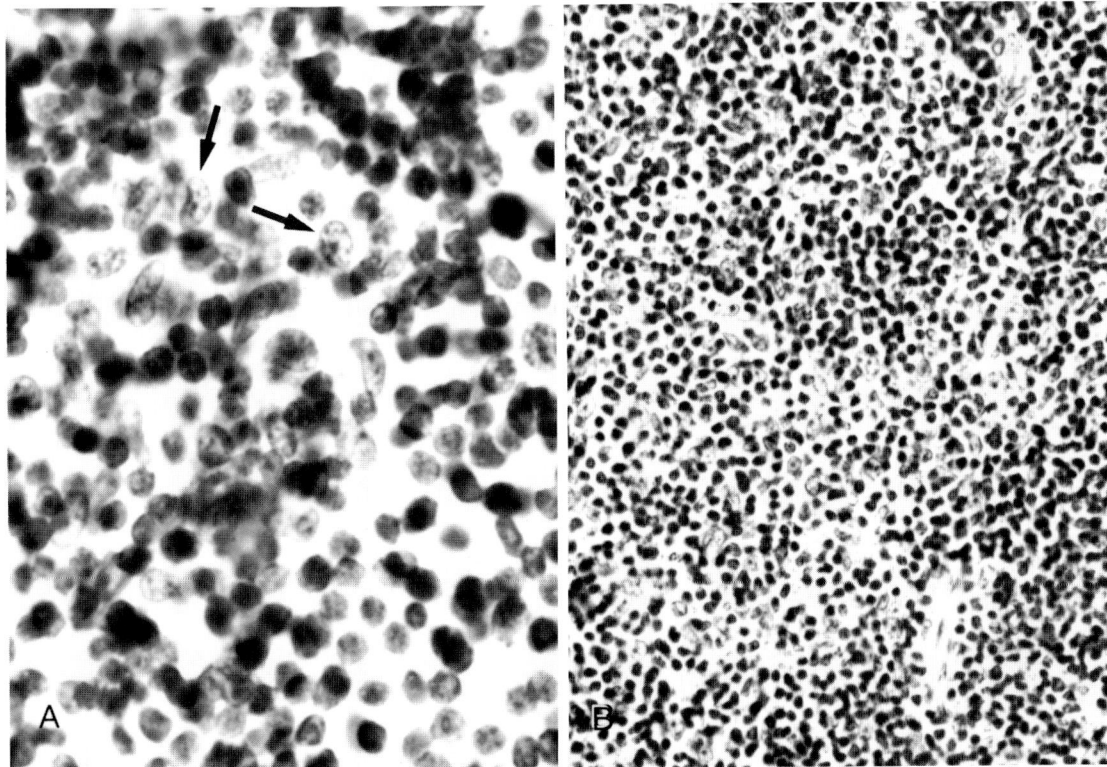

Figure 8.3.   Thymoma, predominantly lymphoid type. **A,** ABC. Note numerous small lymphocytes and few epithelial cells. The latter *(arrows)* are large cells with vesicular nuclei and clear cytoplasm. ×500. **B,** Histology. Note similarity between cytologic and histologic appearance. ×160.

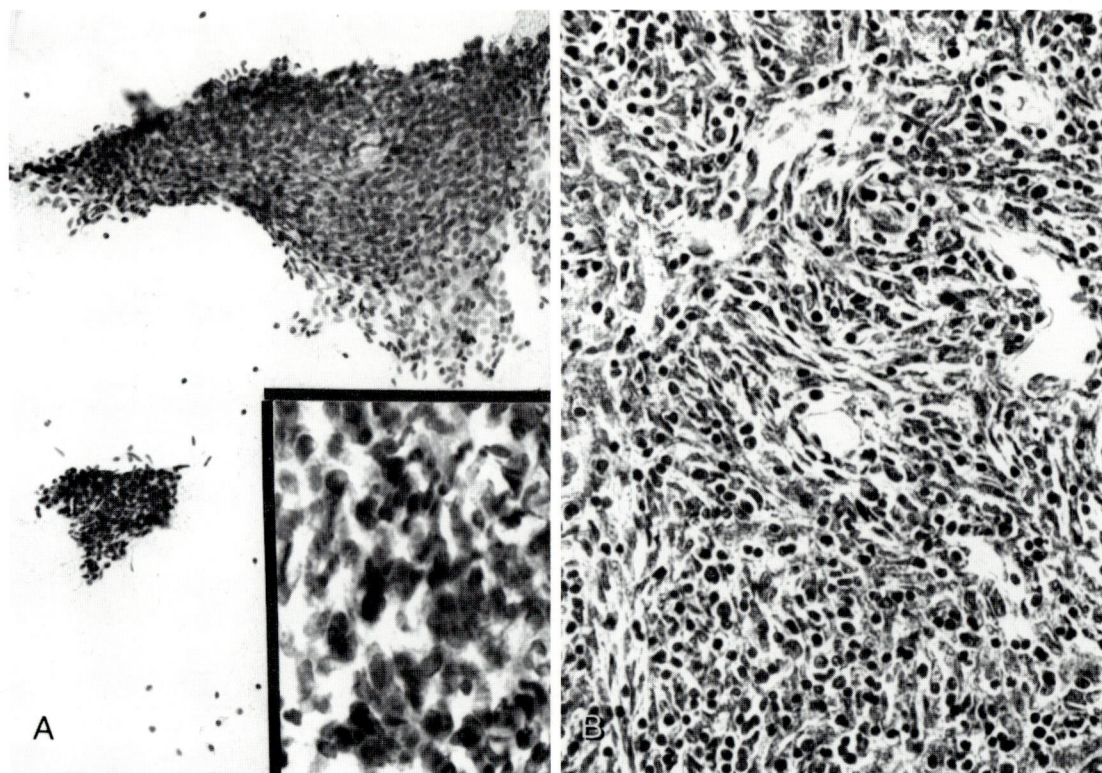

Figure 8.4. Thymoma, spindle cell type. **A,** ABC. Note two tissue fragments composed of cohesive spindle cells and a few lymphocytes scattering in the background. ×125. *Inset* shows spindle cells at higher magnification. ×500. **B,** Histologic section showing intimate admixture of spindle cells and lymphocytes. ×125.

chromatin pattern, and inconspicuous nucleoli. We have encountered two cases of thymic carcinoid on FNAB. One of the two was an atypical carcinoid. The patient had Cushing's syndrome, and the tumor was composed of pleomorphic carcinoid cells arranged in pseudorosettes, with mitoses and extensive necrosis.

We have also seen a case of oat cell carcinoma of the thymus, which was morphologically identical to small cell anaplastic carcinoma of the lung, but no primary lung tumor was found at autopsy. Other authors have observed differentiated areas of carcinoid tumor in oat cell carcinomas of the thymus.[11,12] In other words, the whole spectrum of neuroendocrine tumor can be seen in the thymus as it is in the lung (see Chapter 7).[13]

GERM CELL TUMORS

Mediastinal germ cell tumors have identical histologic appearances to their gonadal counterparts. Indeed, before the tumor is considered to be primary in the mediastinum, it is always necessary to rule out the presence of a small occult gonadal neoplasm.[14,15] Luna[16] studied 20 autopsy cases of clinical extragonadal germ cell tumors arising in the anterior mediastinum. All the patients were male, and all but three were in the third decade of life. Testicular disease was found in only two patients: an occult tumor in a case of embryonal carcinoma and a testicular scar in a patient with choriocarcinoma. Both patients had retroperitoneal metastases. These findings support the premise that the majority of mediastinal germ cell tumors have a primary extragonadal origin.

Teratoma

Of all the germ cell tumors in the mediastinum, teratomas are the most common and are composed of tissues derived from two or three of the embryonic layers (ectoderm, endoderm, and mesoderm). Teratomas are subdivided into mature, immature, and carcinomatous.

Mature teratomas are the most common of all mediastinal germ cell tumors, accounting for up to 75% of the cases.[17,18] Although they are benign, life-threatening hemoptysis or recurrent pericarditis have been described.[19] The gross appearace of most mature teratomas is cystic. Histologically, the cyst is lined by mature stratified squamous epithelium and containing various other mature tissues in its wall such as sebaceous glands, adipose tissue, intestinal or bronchial epithelia, neural tissue, bone, and cartilage. **Figure 8.6A** is an example of the ABC of mature cystic teratoma, featuring groups of benign squamous cells and adipose tissue fragments. **Figure 8.6B** shows the corresponding histology of the resected tumor.

Immature teratoma and teratocarcinoma are seldom encountered in the mediastinum and both are malignant. The former is characterized by the presence of various incompletely differentiated tissues that are readily recognizable as embryonic tissue, while the latter contains, in addition to the normal components of teratoma, elements of seminoma, embryonal carcinoma, or choriocarcinoma, alone or in various combinations.

Other Germ Cell Tumors

Besides teratomas, other types of germ cell tumors that are found in the testes or ovaries can also be found in the mediastinum, including seminoma (germinoma), embryonal carcinoma, yolk sac tumor, and choriocarcinoma.[14,15,20] The ABC of these tumors is discussed in detail in Chapter 14.

Diagnostic Problems in Germ Cell Tumors

Germ cell tumors arising in the anterior mediastinum may be mistaken for metastatic poorly differentiated carcinomas of somatic

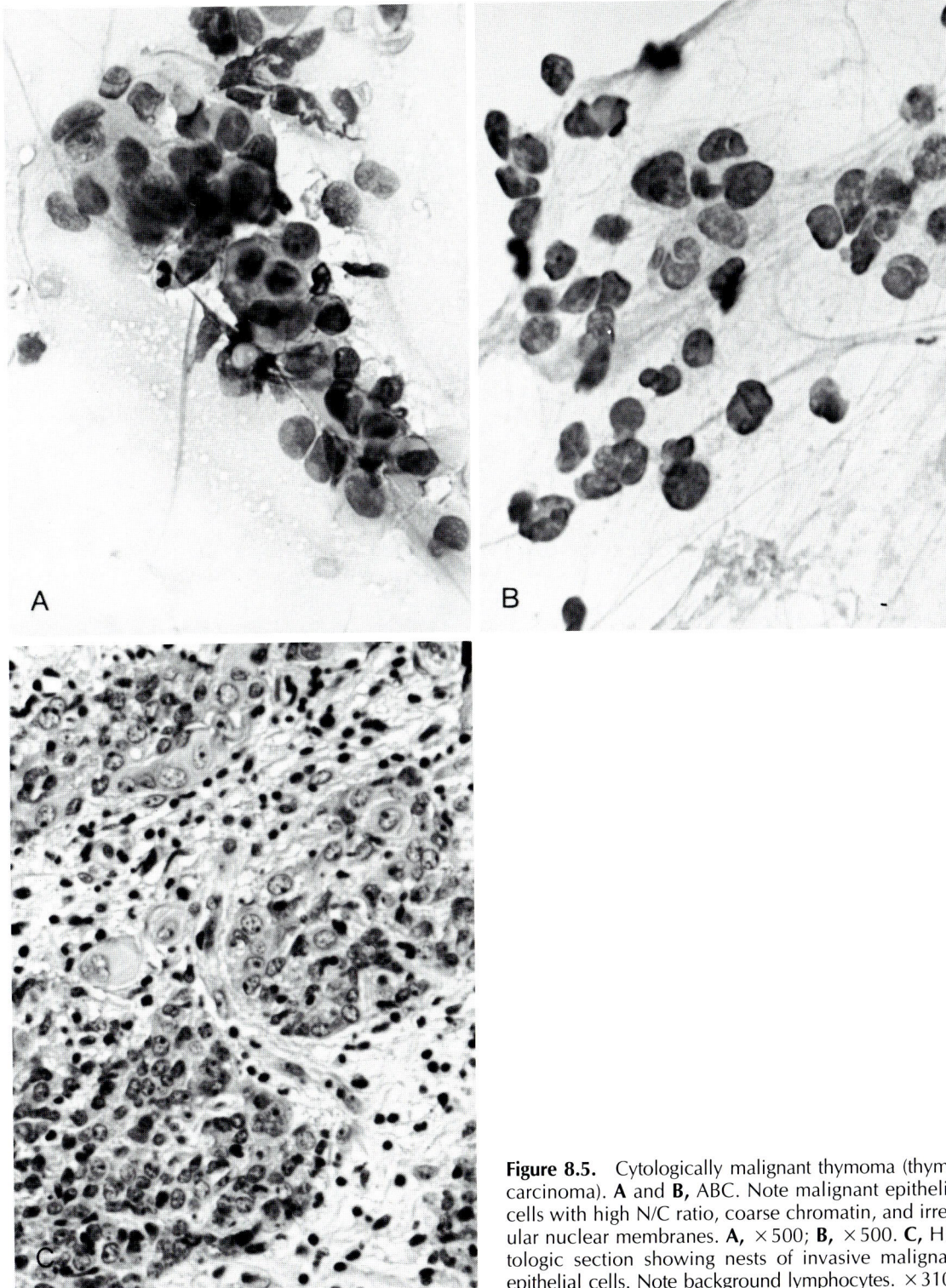

Figure 8.5. Cytologically malignant thymoma (thymic carcinoma). **A** and **B,** ABC. Note malignant epithelial cells with high N/C ratio, coarse chromatin, and irregular nuclear membranes. **A,** ×500; **B,** ×500. **C,** Histologic section showing nests of invasive malignant epithelial cells. Note background lymphocytes. ×310.

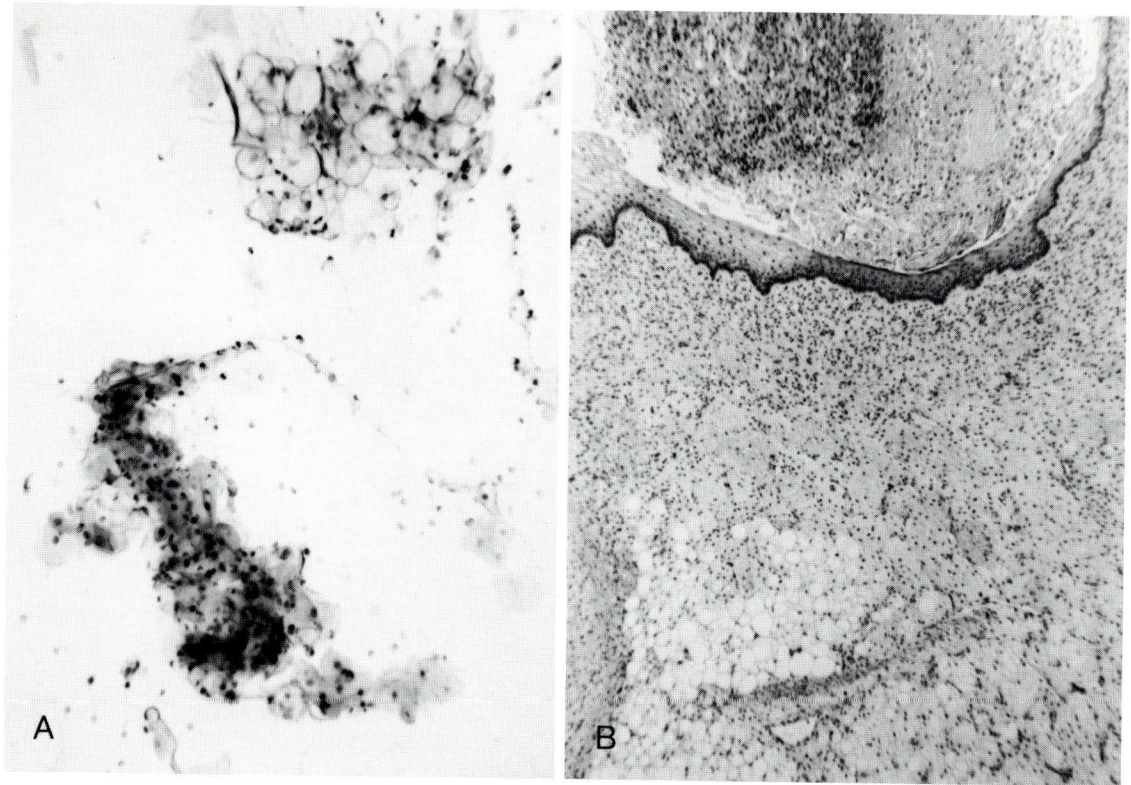

Figure 8.6.

Figure 8.6. Mature teratoma of anterior mediastinum. **A,** ABC. Note benign adipose tissue and squamous cell fragments. ×125. **B,** Histologic section showing a cystic space lined by mature stratified squamous epithelium, and inflammed fibrofatty connective tissue in the wall. ×125.

Figure 8.7. Embryonal carcinoma of anterior mediastinum, Cytospin, ABC. A syncytial cluster of cells simulating adenocarcinoma in arrangement. The cells have pleomorphic nuclei, with irregular macronucleoli and extremely coarse chromatin. ×310.

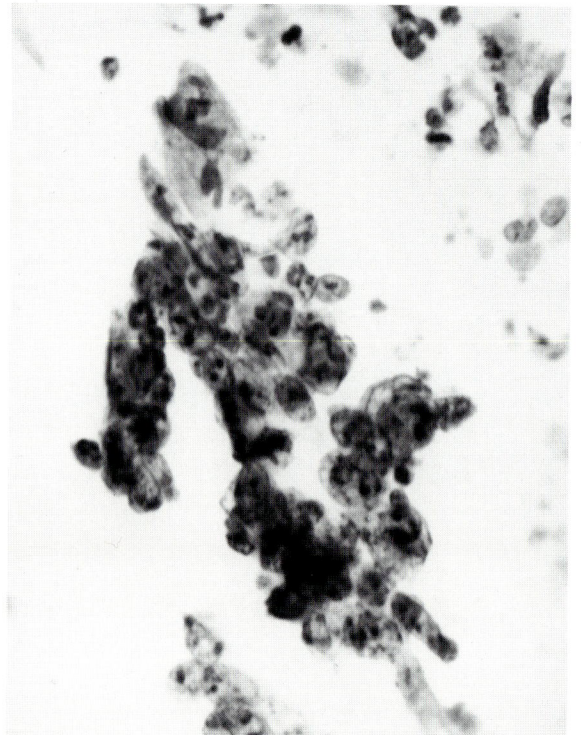

Figure 8.7.

origin. Embryonal carcinoma with its papillary or glandular structures may mimic adenocarcinoma, whereas choriocarcinoma with bizarre giant cells may cause confusion with giant cell carcinoma. In general, compared with carcinoma, cells in germ cell tumors are more pleomorphic and have larger irregular nucleoli (Fig. 8.7).[20,21] The cytopathologist should always consider germ cell tumor in the differential diagnosis of a poorly differentiated anterior mediastinal tumor in a young patient with no evidence of a lung primary or other neoplasm. The aspirated material should be studied with immunoperoxidase technique (see Chapter 16) for the detection of α-fetoprotein and human chorionic gonadotropin.[20,21]

The responsibility to establish that the germ cell tumor is primary in the mediastinum rests on the clinician, as there are no histologic or cytologic features that will enable the cytopathologist to differentiate a gonadal from a mediastinal germ cell tumor.

LYMPHOMAS

Lymphomas are the most frequent malignant neoplasms of the anterior mediastinum. In a large series of mediastinal lymphomas, about 50–60% were Hodgkin's disease, and the remainder were non-Hodgkin's lymphomas.[22] Hodgkin's disease shows a polymorphic cellular population containing lymphocytes, histiocytes, plasma cells, eosinophils, large mononuclear cells with prominent nucleoli, and variable numbers of Reed-Sternberg cells (Fig. 8.8). The latter establish the diagnosis of Hodgkin's disease.

Non-Hodgkin's lymphomas usually consist of a monomorphic population of atypical lymphoid cells (see Chapter 4). Thymomas of lymphocyte predominance are distinguished from non-Hodgkin's lymphoma by the biphasic cell population and the mature uniform appearance of the lymphocytes.

NEUROGENIC TUMORS

Intrathoracic neurogenic tumors occur most frequently in the posterior mediastinum. Most are benign, with an overall incidence of malignancy ranging from 3 to 19%.[23] They can be classified into tumors of peripheral nerves, autonomic ganglia, and paraganglia (Table 8.2). Over 70% of the mediastinal neurogenic tumors are of peripheral nerve origin, with schwannomas being the most common.[23] Dahlgren and Ovenfors[24] were able to diagnose neural tumors of the posterior mediastinum in 11 of 16 cases by observing groups of spindled-shaped cells with monomorphic nuclei. They were unable to classify the tumors further into schwannomas, neurofibromas, or ganglioneuromas, since the bland, spindle-shaped cells are common to all these tumors. Fig. 8.9A depicts the ABC of a large ganglioneuroma, which we have encountered recently. The tissue fragments are composed of fascicles of spindle cells showing point-ended, serpentine nuclei, embedded in a fibrillar matrix. The serpentine nuclei are characteristic of cells of neural origin. The cytologic

Table 8.2.   Neurogenic Tumors of the Mediastinum

Tumors of peripheral nerves
    Schwannoma
    Neurofibroma
    Neurogenic sarcoma (malignant schwannoma)
Tumors of autonomic ganglia
    Ganglioneuroma
    Ganglioneuroblastoma
    Neuroblastoma
Tumors of paraganglia
    Paraganglioma (extraadrenal pheochromocytoma)

picture along with the posterior mediastinal location of the lesion provides sufficient evidence to render the diagnosis of a neoplasm of neurogenic origin. Ganglion cells, which are large cells having prominent nucleoli and abundant cytoplasm, are not present in the aspirate but are present in the histologic section of the resected tumor (Fig. 7.9B).

MESOTHELIOMA

Mesotheliomas are neoplasms that originate from the mesothelial cells lining the coelomic cavities. There are two main types of mesothelioma based on gross appearance: the localized fibrous type and the diffuse malignant type. Accurate and pertinent clinical data are the most important accompaniment to the cytologic examination in cases of suspected mesothelioma. Examination of the chest roentgenograms and consultation with the radiologist to determine the location and extent of the disease is vital. The adjacent lung tissue may be invaded, but when invasion is present, it tends to remain superficial. In 18 cases of mesothelioma studied by FNAB, correct diagnosis was made in eight cases; the findings were consistent with or suggestive of mesothelioma in four cases; accurate distinction from other neoplasms was not possible in four; and in two, the diagnosis of adenocarcinoma was suggested.[25]

Localized Fibrous Mesothelioma

Localized fibrous mesotheliomas are well-circumscribed tumors with no invasive characteristics and are often asymptomatic. The tumor may be found attached to the pleura by a broad base or a stalk. The current trend tends to exclude them from the mesothelioma category and consider them as fibromas. Histologically they consist of hyalinized fibrous connective tissue, and the cellularity varies greatly from case to case. The ABC shows scattered benign-appearing spindle cells (Fig. 8.10). If attention is paid to the lack of nuclear aberrations and the rarity or absence of mitoses, confusion with a fibrosarcoma is unlikely.

Diffuse Mesothelioma

Diffuse mesotheliomas are almost always malignant. They frequently produce pleural effusion and show encasement and compression of the subjacent lung at the time of presentation. On histologic examination, most tumors show both epithelial and fibrous (spindle cell) components, with the former predominating. The epithelial cells form solid sheets, tubules and papillae, resembling bronchioloalveolar adenocarcinoma (Fig. 8.11A). On the other hand, a dominant spindle cell pattern may resemble a high-grade sarcoma (Fig. 8.11B).

Aspiration Cytology

Cellular Pattern. The aspirates usually contain large numbers of tumor cells, which may be lying singly but are often arranged in large aggregates resulting in formation of cell sheets, papillae, and balls (Figs. 8.12–8.14). The component cells within the mosaic sheets have flattened apposing cell borders, separated by prominent intercellular gaps (Fig. 8.15). The latter are presumably produced by the long microvilli on the cell surfaces, clearly visible on electron microscopic examination.

Cell Morphology. The neoplastic mesothelial cells generally retain the configuration and staining characteristic of normal mesothelial cells, but are larger and exhibit prominent anisocytosis. The cells are cuboidal or polygonal in shape, having a centrally placed nucleus and a frequently prominent nucleolus. The well-defined cytoplasm is moderate in amount and optically dense, with a ruffled cell border or foaminess at the periphery, corresponding to the nu-

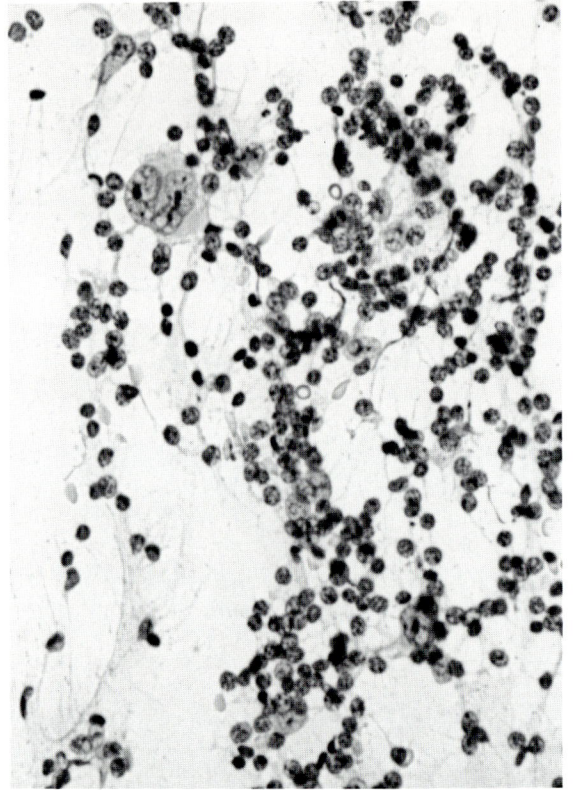

Figure 8.8. Hodgkin's disease, ABC. Note numerous mature lymphocytes, few plasma cells and a Reed-Sternberg cell, characterized by large cell size, binucleation, and prominent nucleoli. ×310.

Figure 8.9. Ganglioneuroma, posterior mediastinum. **A,** ABC. Note tissue fragment composed of spindle cells with delicate serpentine nuclei. ×310. **B,** Histologic section. Note many spindle cells, a large ganglion cell, and a fibrillary matrix. ×500.

Figure 8.8.

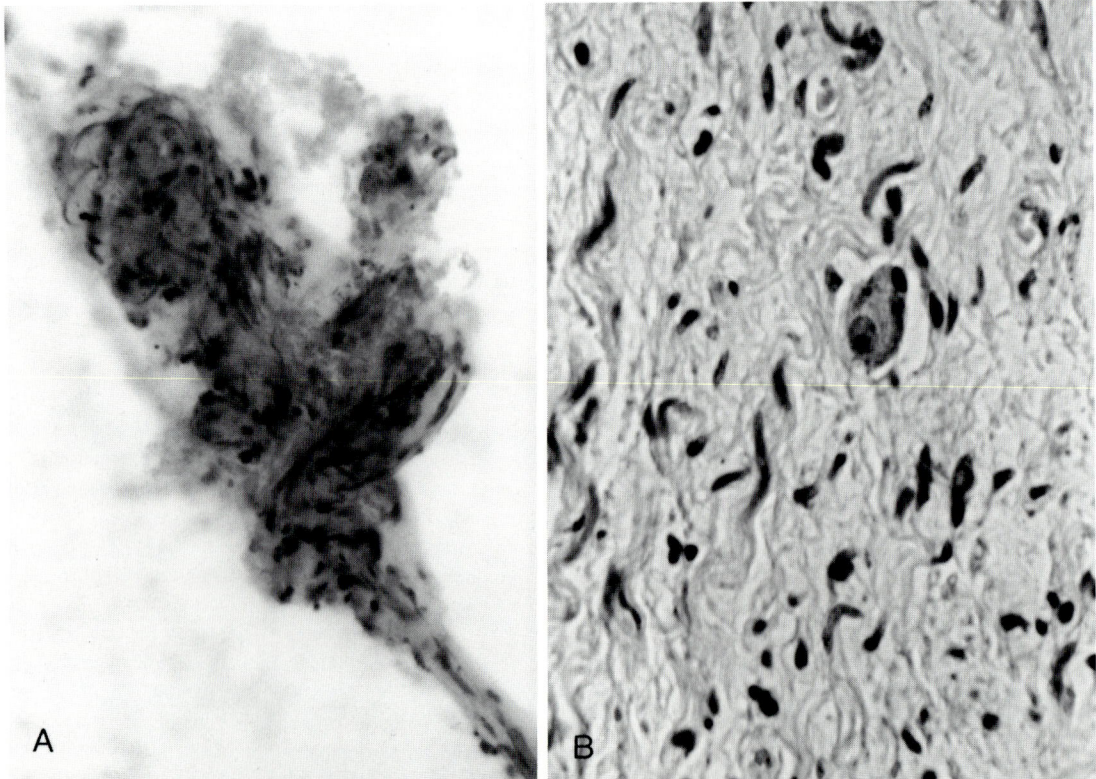

A

B

Figure 8.9.

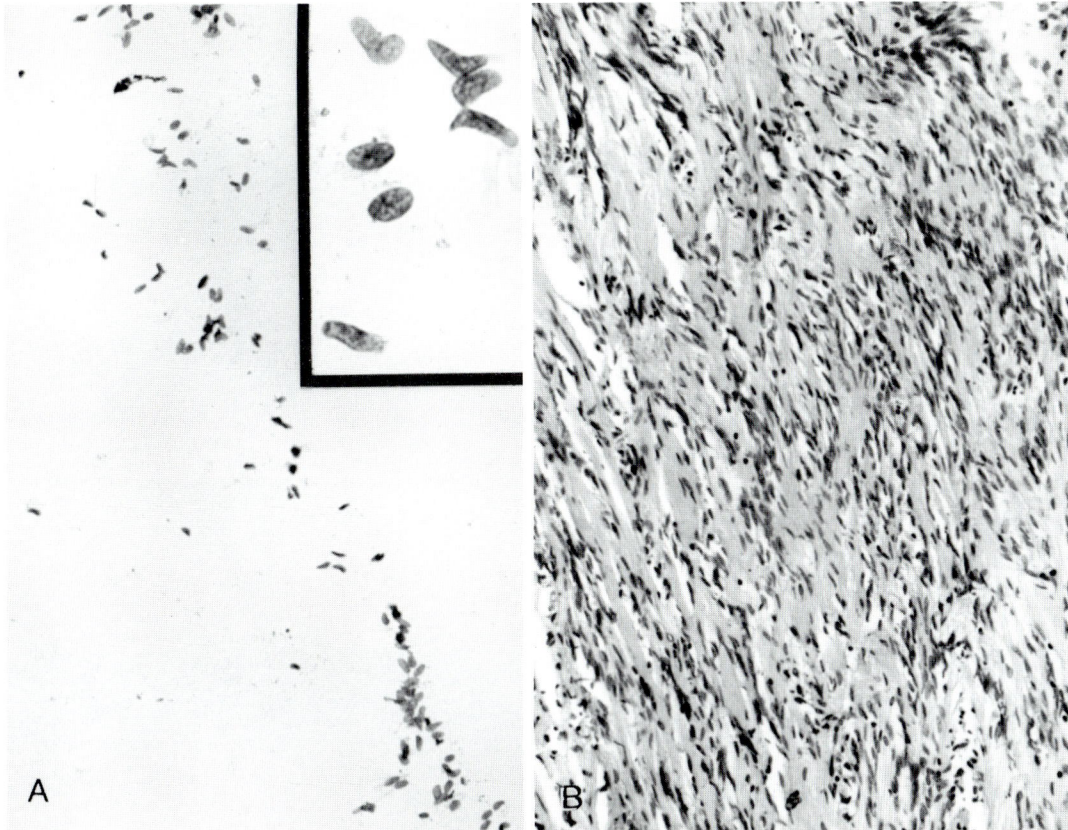

Figure 8.10. Benign, localized, fibrous mesothelioma (fibroma). **A,** ABC. Note benign fibroblast-like spindle cells. ×125; *inset,* ×500. **B,** Histology. Note spindle cells and hyalinized fibrous stroma. ×125.

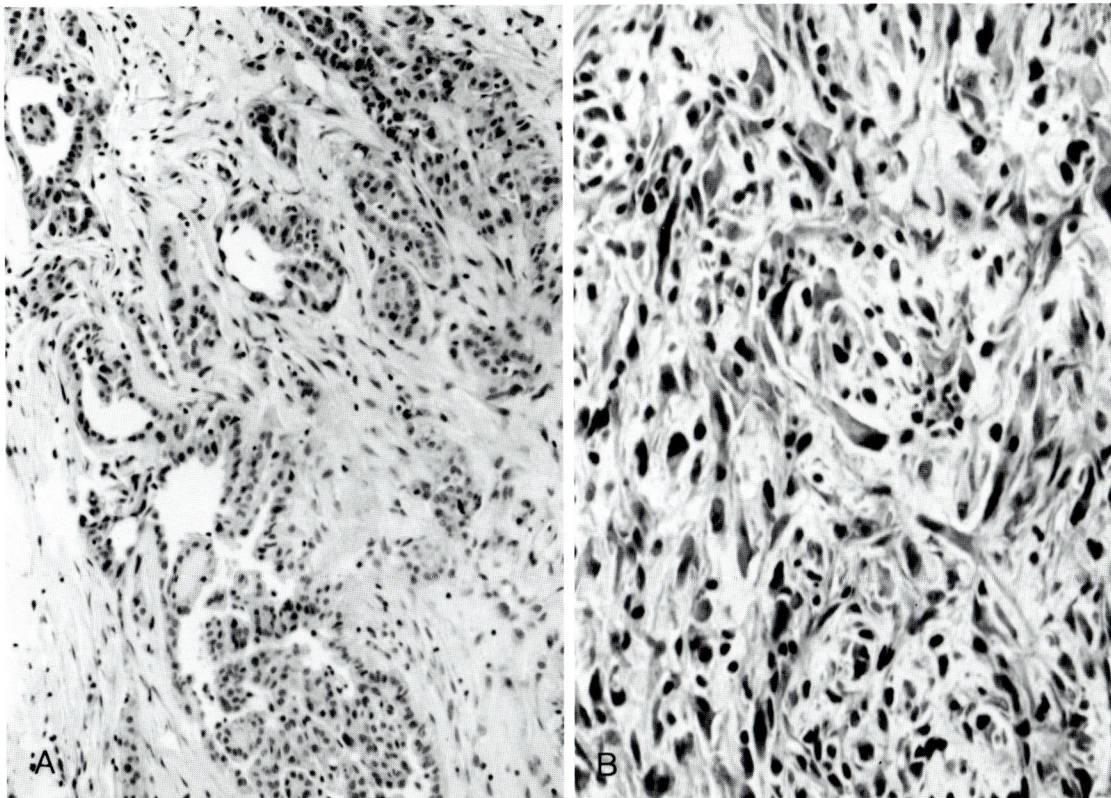

Figure 8.11. Histologic spectrum of diffuse malignant mesothelioma. **A,** Epithelial cell type. Note epithelial cells with a papillo-tubular growth pattern. ×125. **B,** Spindle cell type. Note malignant spindle cells. ×310.

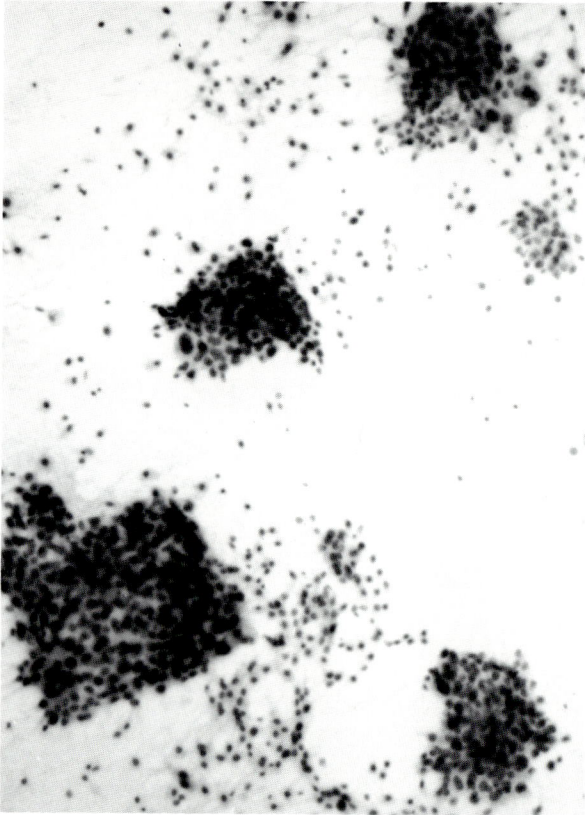

Figure 8.12.

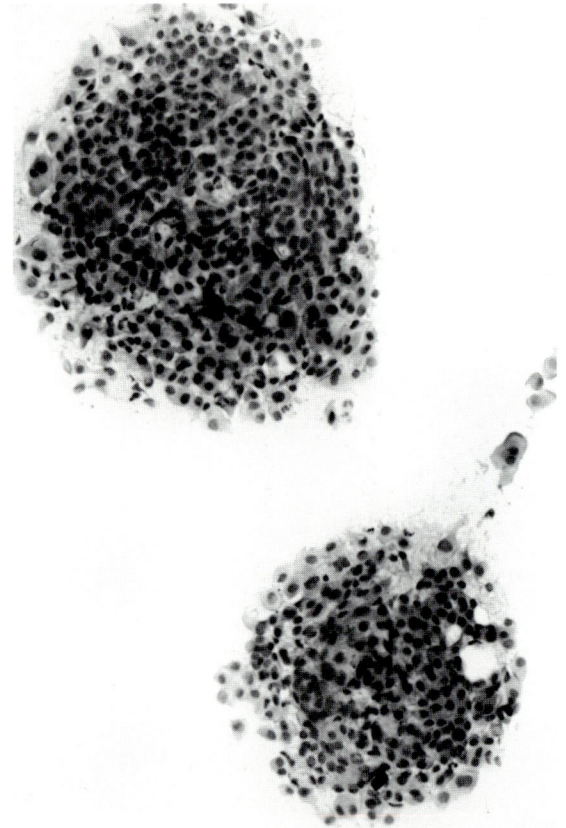

Figure 8.13.

Figure 8.12. Malignant mesothelioma, ABC. This is a characteristic field showing many single cells as well as multilayered tissue fragments. ×125.

Figure 8.13. Malignant mesothelioma, ABC. Two large cell balls typical of mesothelioma. It is worth noting that reactive mesothelial proliferations seldom produce more than 15–20 cells in a cell ball. ×125.

Figure 8.14. Malignant mesothelioma, ABC, cell block preparation. Malignant mesothelial cells in smaller clusters. This pattern is not exclusive for mesothelioma but can be seen in other adenocarcinomas, especially breast carcinoma. ×310.

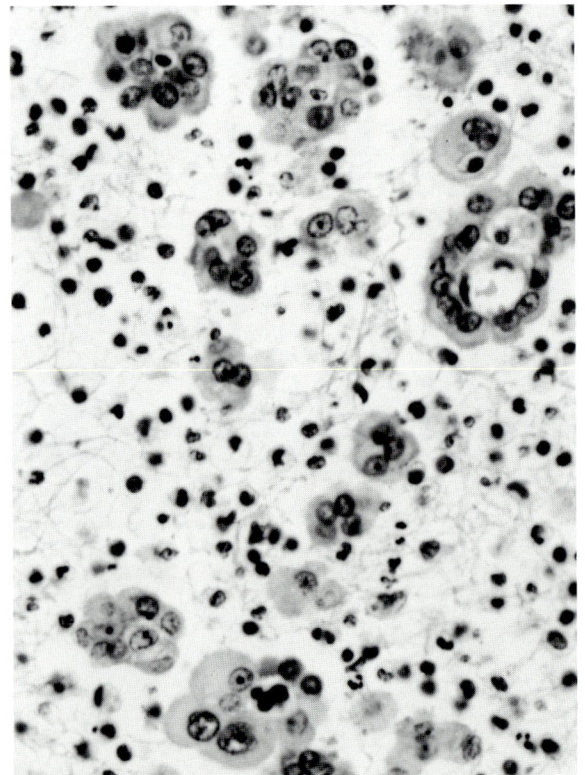

Figure 8.14.

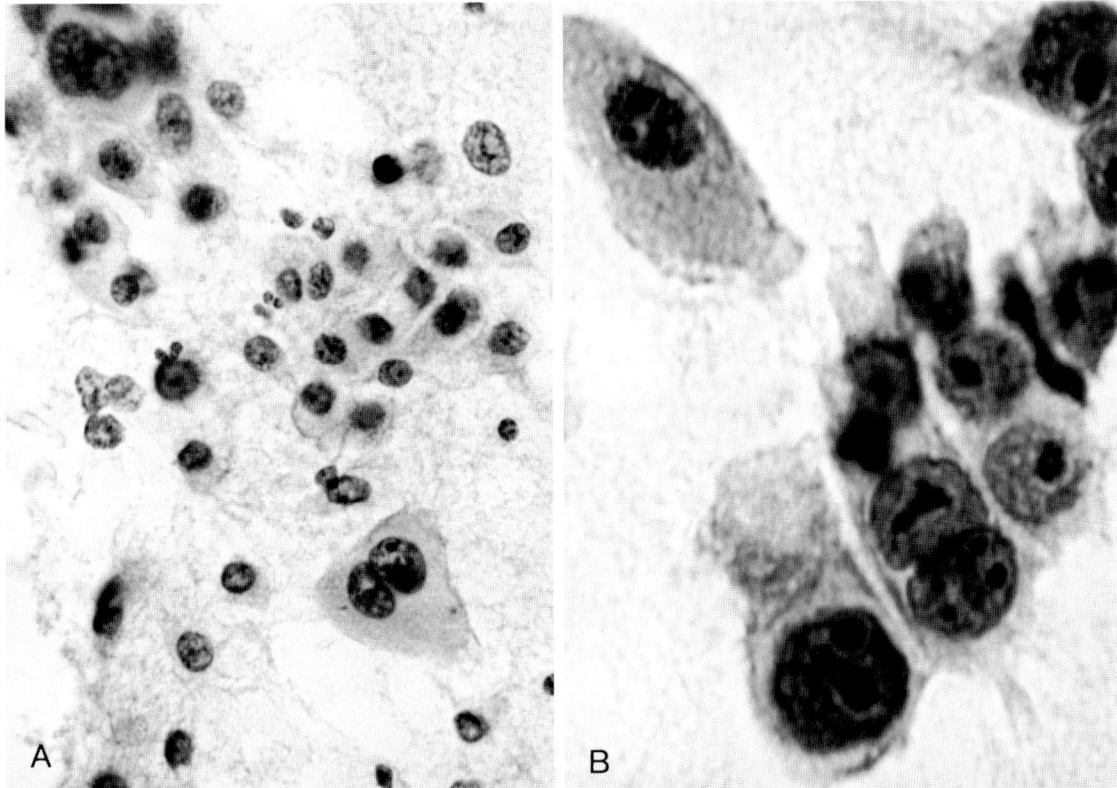

Figure 8.15. Malignant mesothelioma, ABC. **A,** The polyhedral malignant cells retain mesothelial cell features, and there is considerable anisocytosis and binucleation. ×500. **B,** Higher magnification view. The nuclei show prominent nucleoli. The sharply defined, clear areas between cells are characteristic for cells of mesothelial origin. Also note ruffled cell borders. ×1250.

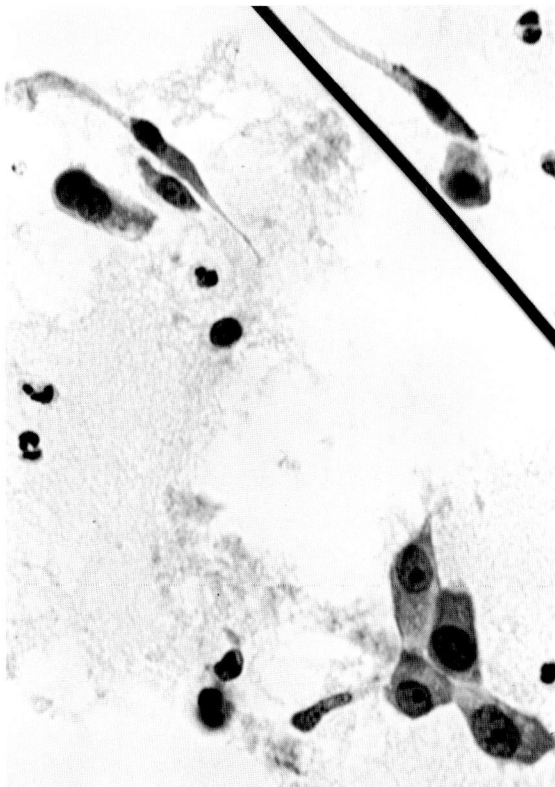

Figure 8.16. Malignant mesothelioma, ABC, showing admixture of polyhedral cells and spindle cells. Note apposition of cell borders, separated by clear spaces *(lower right field)*. ×500.

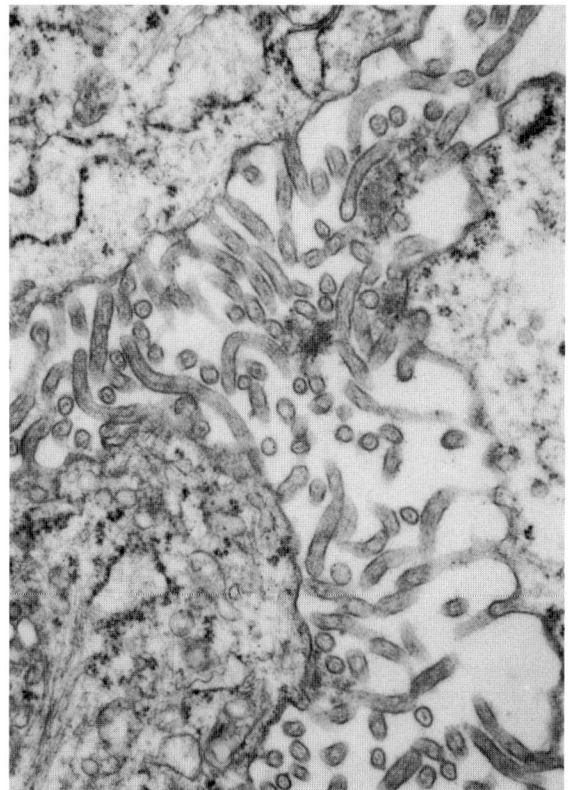

Figure 8.17. Ultrastructure of mesothelioma. Note characteristic long microvilli occupying the intercellular space. Uranyl acetate and lead citrate preparation. ×25,000.

merous long microvilli present on the cell surfaces **(Fig. 8.15)**. In some cases, one may notice a transition from normal-appearing to pleomorphic mesothelial cells.

The spindle tumor cells show varying degrees of nuclear pleomorphism and often are admixed with the epithelial cells **(Fig. 8.16)**. Infrequently, the spindle cell component predominates, mimicking a sarcoma.

Special Stains. A positive staining of tumor cells with diastase-resistant periodic acid-Schiff (PAS) or mucicarmine tends to rule out mesothelioma in favor of adenocarcinoma, while positive staining with alcian blue that becomes negative after treatment with hyaluronidase is strongly suggestive of mesothelioma.[26,27]

In recent years conventional cytochemistry has been largely replaced by immunocytochemistry. Mesotheliomas show negative or only weakly positive results for carcinoembryonic antigen (CEA), while many adenocarcinomas show results that are strongly CEA-positive.[28] Although these results are useful, they are not entirely specific, since up to 20–35% of adenocarcinomas may be CEA-negative,[29] and occasional mesotheliomas are weakly CEA-positive. More recently, Battifora and Kopinski[29] have showed 100% positive staining results of breast, lung, and ovarian adenocarcinomas with a monoclonal antibody (anti-HMFG2) to an epithelial marker derived from milk fat globule membranes. This monoclonal antibody consistently fails to stain normal, reactive, and neoplastic mesothelial cells. Because of its greater sensitivity and specificity, this antibody is believed to be superior to anti-CEA.

Spindle cell mesotheliomas can be distinguished from sarcomas by demonstrating both vimentin and cytokeratin in the former, while sarcomas are vimentin-positive and cytokeratin-negative.[30]

Diagnostic Pitfalls. Since mesothelioma is regarded as an occupation-related cancer due to asbestos exposure, it is recommended that interpretation of this neoplasm be approached cautiously because of legal implications.[31]

Reactive mesothelial cells may closely resemble malignant mesothelial cells. The former are generally single, but when hyperplastic, may stick together in small groups. Malignant mesothelial cells are distinguished by their cellularity, formation of large tissue fragments, increased cell and nuclear size, anisocytosis, and macronucleoli **(Table 8.3)**.[25–27]

Cytologic features that distinguish between mesothelioma and adenocarcinoma are listed in **Table 8.4**. When the distinction is not clear, the use of histochemical and immunocytochemical techniques as discussed previously may offer great help. Electron microscopy is another useful tool for confirming the diagnosis of mesothelioma. Mesothelial cells show numerous bushy, long microvilli, which are the most distinctive ultrastructural features, and bundles of cytoplasmic tonofilaments **(Fig. 8.17)**.

Table 8.3. ABC of Malignant Mesothelioma

Hypercellularity with large tissue fragments or cell balls
Epithelial cells showing mesothelial cell characteristics
Nuclei showing subtle malignant features: irregular chromatin pattern, macronucleoli, anisonucleosis
Combination of epithelial and spindle cells

Table 8.4. Distinguishing Features of Malignant Mesothelioma and Adenocarcinoma

	Malignant Mesothelioma	Adenocarcinoma
Asbestos exposure	Yes	No
X-ray findings	Pleural-based tumor	Not pleural-based
Cytology		
Tumor cells	Mesothelial-like and some spindle cells	Glandular cells Vacuolated or foamy cytoplasm
	Flattened apposing cell surfaces separated by intercellular gaps	
Nuclei	Low-grade malignant	More pleomorphic
Cell arrangement	Cell sheets and balls	Gland and acinar formations
PAS with diastase	Negative	Usually positive
Alcian blue	May be positive	Positive or negative
Alcian blue with hyaluronidase	Negative	Unchanged
Immunostaining for CEA	Negative or weakly positive	Often strongly positive
Electron microscopy	Long microvilli (1–3 μm) and tonofilaments	Short microvilli (<1 μm)

References

1. Rosai J, Levine GD. Tumors of the thymus. Atlas of tumor pathology, 2nd Series, Fascicle 13. Washington, D.C.: Armed Forces Institute of Pathology, 1976.
2. Minkowitz S, Solomon L, Nicastri AD. Cytologically malignant thymoma with distant metastasis. Cancer 1968;21:426–433.
3. Tao LC, Pearson FG, Cooper JD, Sanders DE, Weisbrod, Donat EE. Cytopathology of thymoma. Acta Cytol 1984;28:165–170.
4. Finley JL, Silverman JF, Strausbach PH, et al. Malignant thymic neoplasms: Diagnosis by fine-needle aspiration biopsy with histologic, immunocytochemical and ultrastructural confirmation. Diagn Cytopathol 1986;2:118–125.
5. Dahlgren S, Sandstedt B, Sundstrom C. Fine needle aspiration cytology of thymic tumors. Acta Cytol 1983;27:1–6.
6. Spahr J, Frable WJ. Pulmonary cytopathology of an invasive thymoma. Acta Cytol 1981;25:163–166.
7. Millar J, Allen R, Wakefield JSJ, Buchanan AJ, Gupta RJ. Diagnosis of thymoma by fine-needle aspiration cytology: A light and electron microscopic study of a case. Diagn Cytopathol 1987;3:166–169.
8. Suen KC, Quenville NF. Fine needle aspiration cytology of uncommon thoracic lesions. Am J Clin Pathol 1981;75:803–809.
9. Pak HY, Yokota SB, Friedberg HA. Thymoma diagnosed by transthoracic fine needle aspiration. Acta Cytol 1982;26:210–216.
10. Sajjad SM, Lukeman JM, Llamas FT. Needle biopsy diagnosis of thymoma. A case report. Acta Cytol 1982;26:503–506.
11. Wick MR, Scheithauer BW. Oat cell carcinoma of the thymus. Cancer 1982;49:1652–1657.
12. Salyer WR, Salyer DC, Eggleston JC. Carcinoid tumors of the thymus. Cancer 1976;37:958–973.
13. Rosai J, Levine G, Weber WR, Higa E. Carcinoid tumors and oat cell carcinomas of the thymus. Pathol Annu 1976;11:201–226.

14. Cox JD. Primary malignant germinal tumors of the mediastinum: A study of 24 cases. Cancer 1975;36:1162–1168.

15. Martini N, Golbey RB, Hajdu SI, et al. Primary mediastinal germ cell tumors. Cancer 1974;33:763–769.

16. Luna M. Germ-cell tumors of the mediastinum. Postmortem findings. Am J Clin Pathol 1976;65:264.

17. Marchevsky AM, Kaneko M. Surgical pathology of the mediastinum. New York: Raven Press, 1984:129.

18. Pugsley WS, Carleton RL. Germinal nature of teratoid tumors of the thymus. Arch Pathol 1953;56:341–347.

19. Robertson JM, Fee HJ, Mulder DG. Mediastinal teratoma causing life-threatening hemoptysis. Its occurrence in an infant. Am J Dis Child 1981;135:148–150.

20. Sangalli G, Livraghi T, Giordano F, Tavani E, Schiaffino E. Primary mediastinal embryonal carcinoma and choriocarcinoma. A case report. Acta Cytol 1986;30:543–546.

21. Kapila K, Hajdu SI, Whitmore WF, Golbey RB, Beattie EJ. Cytologic diagnosis of metastatic germ cell tumors. Acta Cytol 1983;27:245–251.

22. Benjamin SP, McCormack LJ, Effler DB, et al. Primary lymphatic tumors of the mediastinum. Cancer 1972;30:708–712.

23. Marchevsky AM, Kaneko M. Surgical pathology of the mediastinum. New York: Raven Press, 1984:256.

24. Dahlgren SE, Ovenfors CO. Aspiration biopsy diagnosis of neurogeneous mediastinal tumours. Acta Radiol Diagn 1970;10:289–298.

25. Sterrett GF, Whitaker D, Shilkin KB, Walters MNI. Fine needle aspiration cytology of malignant mesothelioma. Acta Cytol 1987;31:185–193.

26. Triol JH, Conston AS, Chandler SV. Malignant mesothelioma. Cytopathology of 75 cases seen in a New Jersey community hospital. Acta Cytol 1984;28:37–45.

27. Ehya H. The cytologic diagnosis of mesothelioma. Semin Diagn Pathol 1986;3:196–203.

28. Walts AE, Said JW, Banks-Schlegel S. Keratin and carcinoembryonic antigen in exfoliated mesothelial and malignant cells: An immunoperoxidase study. Am J Clin Pathol 1983;80:671–676.

29. Battifora H, Kopinski MI. Distinction of mesothelioma from adenocarcinoma, an immunohistochemical approach. Cancer 1985;55:1679–1685.

30. Lucas JG, Tuttle SE. Diagnostic histochemical and immunohistochemical studies in malignant mesothelioma. J Surg Oncol 1987;35:30–34.

31. Kline TS. Handbook of fine needle biopsy cytology, 2nd ed. New York: Churchill Livingstone, 1988:280.

9

Liver

In the past decade, fine needle aspiration biopsy (FNAB) has largely replaced conventional, large-bore needle biopsy as an accurate means of making the diagnosis of neoplastic hepatic lesions.[1-16] On the other hand, the use of FNAB in the evaluation of nonneoplastic parenchymal liver diseases has been somewhat controversial, despite its advocacy by many Scandinavian workers.[17-19] We feel, as do most pathologists in North America,[11,20-23] that although FNAB may yield useful information, the large-bore needle biopsy is still the procedure of choice in evaluating parenchymal diseases of the liver, since detailed examination of tissue architecture is often necessary.

FNAB of the liver can be performed at the bedside or in the radiology department under direct visualization, using modern imaging techniques such as ultrasonography and computed tomography. A 22–gauge needle measuring 80–150 mm long is the standard needle used at our institution. The biopsy is performed percutaneously, after local anesthesia, through the lower thoracic or abdominal wall. In addition to direct smearing, any macroscopically visible tissue fragments are collected, fixed in Bouin's fixative, and processed for histological examination as cell blocks. Some workers[4,24] prefer heparinized syringes for this form of tissue collection, but others,[10,13] including ourselves, have not found heparinization necessary.

Because of its longer length and relative atraumatic nature, a fine needle can virtually reach all regions of the liver, including the deep sites and the left lobe, which are generally beyond the reach of the conventional thick needle. While the number of passes with a thick needle is limited because of its potential complications, FNAB allows multiple punctures and multidirectional sampling. In necrotic tumors, a thick needle may fail to obtain viable tissue while multiple aspirations with a fine needle increases the chance of obtaining nonnecrotic cells for diagnosis.[25]

Significant complications are rare if fine needles of 21–23 gauge are used. Wasastjerna[19] reported no complications in a series of 1500 patients. Bleeding diathesis is a relative contraindication. Hemorrhage occurring after FNAB of the liver resulted in one fatality,[26] and one patient required blood tranfusion.[27] Schulz[28] reported one case of bile peritonitis, which necessitated laparotomy. Considering the large number of fine needle aspirations that have been performed, the complication rate is acceptable.

Diagnostic Accuracy

Series of hepatic aspirates, mostly from patients with metastatic neoplasms, have shown the sensitivity of the technique to be ranging from 81 to 96%.[1-9] Tao and associates[21] reported that detection of hepatic tumors increased from 72% with a single puncture to 95% with at least three punctures. Bell and associates[10] reported the accuracies of cytologic diagnoses and histologic diagnoses (based on cell blocks) to be 73 and 67%, respectively, but the combined accuracy of cytologic and histologic studies was 85%. The accuracy of diagnosing primary hepatic neoplasms is more variable, depending on the experience of the pathologist and whether or not primary hepatic tumors are commonly encountered at the locale of practice. Lundquist[18] reported 1748 cases of liver aspirates, in which there were 10 cases of hepatocellular carcinoma (HCC), but only five had been diagnosed by cytology. Johansen and Svendsen[1] described briefly the cytologic features of nine cases of HCC but conceded that a specific diagnosis generally requires histologic evaluation. More recently, papers have been published that stress the useful role of FNAB in the diagnosis of HCC.[29-34] Tao et al.[30] diagnosed 12 cases of hepatocellular carcinoma by FNAB, and on follow-up, all were proven to be correct. In our series,[32] 30 cases were diagnosed as "hepatocellular carcinoma," of which 28 (93.3%) were proven correct. The remaining two cases (6.7%) were metastatic adenocarcinomas that were mistaken for HCC. The largest series has been reported by Ajdukiewicz and associates.[31] In their series, a correct positive cytologic diagnosis was given in 117 (88%) of 133 patients with HCC. There was one false-positive finding among the 177 cases, which gave a predictive value of positive diagnosis of 99.1%. There were 10 false benign reports, making the predictive value of a benign report 64.3%.

NORMAL CYTOLOGY

Normal hepatocytes, measuring 15–20 μm in diameter, are polygonal cells with distinct cytoplasmic borders (**Fig. 9.1**). The cells have ample granular cytoplasm, which stains eosinophilic with hematoxylin and eosin, and orange brown with the Papanicolaou stain. The nuclei are round and central. The chromatin is finely granular and evenly distributed; the nucleoli are small but distinct. Intracytoplasmic pigment in the form of fine to coarse granules can sometimes be seen. The pigment stains brown with H & E and is probably lipofuscin. Normal hepatocytes occur in small monolayered sheets or larger sheets within which the cells are orderly arranged in cords one to two cells thick (**Fig. 9.2**). Mild to moderate anisonucleosis and binucleation are not infrequent (**Fig. 9.3**).

Biliary epithelial cells (**Fig. 9.4**) are generally arranged in clusters or palisades. These cells are smaller than hepatocytes and are cuboidal or low columnar in shape. The nuclei are small and basal; the scant cytoplasm is basophilic.

MALIGNANT HEPATIC NEOPLASMS

The possibility of primary or metastatic cancer in the liver should be considered in all patients who have hepatomegaly. Hepa-

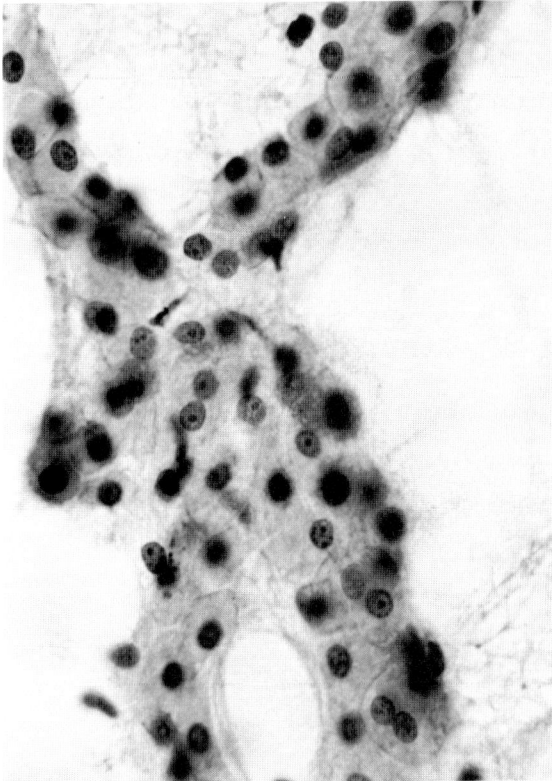

Figure 9.1. Normal hepatocytes, ABC. The liver cells are arranged in thin cords one to two cells thick. ×500.

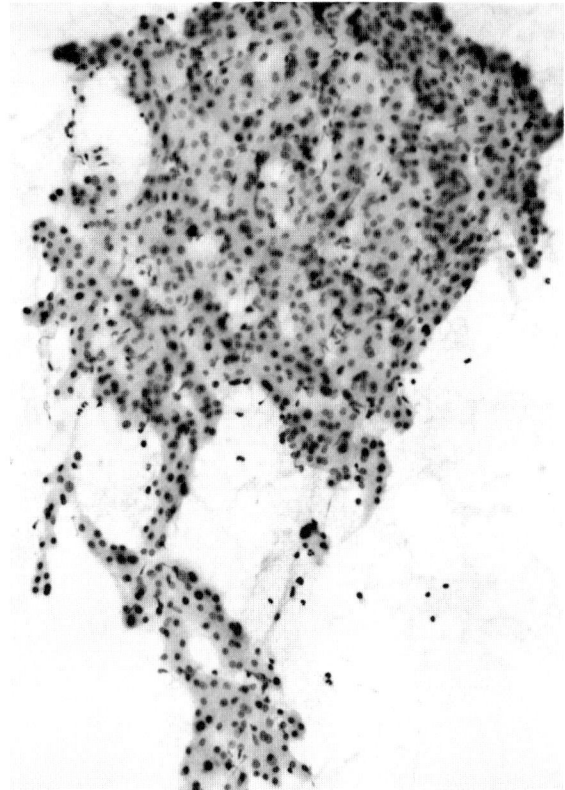

Figure 9.2. Normal hepatocytes, ABC. Note large, two-dimensional cell sheet composed of thin liver cords, many of which are covered by a single layer of endothelial cells. ×125.

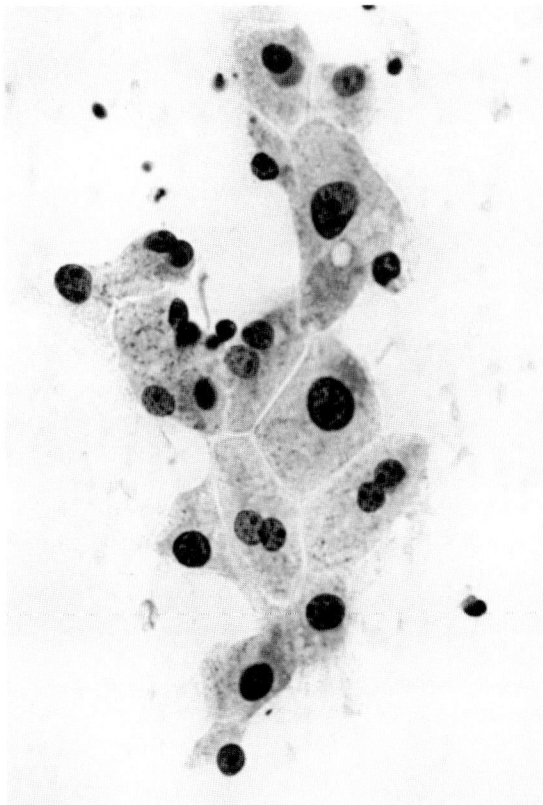

Figure 9.3. Reactive hepatocytes, ABC. Note cellular enlargement, anisocytosis, binucleation, and increased pigment granules in cytoplasm. ×500.

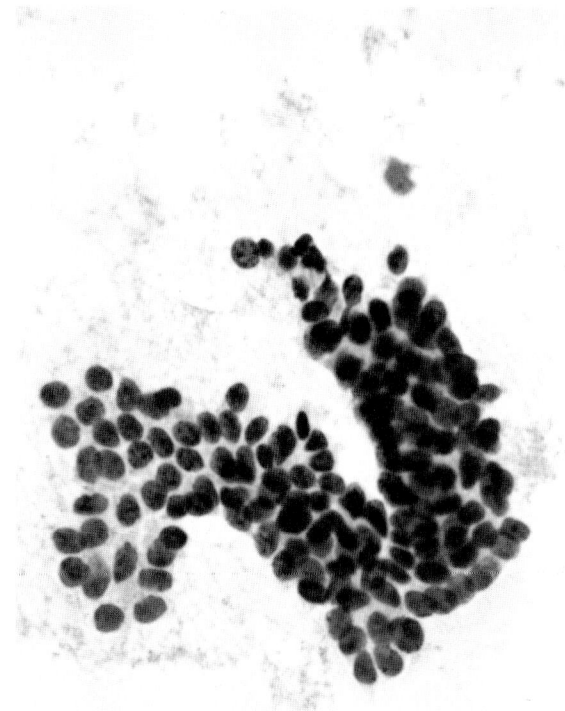

Figure 9.4. Biliary duct cells, ABC. The duct cells are smaller than hepatocytes and display a tubular or palisading arrangement. ×500.

tocellular carcinomas (HCCs) frequently develop in association with cirrhosis; conversely, metastatic liver carcinomas are rarely manifested together with cirrhosis. An important biochemical differentiation between HCC and metastatic liver cancer should be the presence of α-fetoprotein (AFP) at diagnostically high levels in the sera of the patients with HCC.[35,36] If ABC suggests, but is not diagnostic of, hepatocellular carcinoma, an immunoassay of AFP in the patient's serum may help to confirm the diagnosis. In HCC, AFP is usually greater than 1000 ng/ml, as opposed to 100 ng/ml or less in metastatic liver cancer. It must be remembered, however, that a normal AFP level does not eliminate the possibility of HCC. The average frequency with which AFP is detected in the sera of patients with HCC is about 60%. Using the history and physical examination with biochemical data, modern imaging and FNAB will allow a specific diagnosis of HCC in most instances[29,30,32,33] and will direct resectable cases promptly to surgery. The final diagnosis of HCC in those patients who are clinically operative candidates should be obtained at surgery where exploration will determine the ultimate resectability of the primary liver cancer.

Hepatocellular Carcinoma

Hepatocellular carcinoma is one of the most prevalent human cancers.[37] Although it is less frequently seen in western countries, HCC is the most common cancer in parts of Asia and Africa, responsible for as many as 30–40% of all cancer deaths.[38] The prognosis is dismal; the average survival rate is 4.3 months from onset of symptoms.[39] From 80 to 90% of hepatocellular carcinomas occur in cirrhotic livers.[40] The hepatitis B virus is the most important putative etiologic factor in the majority of HCCs in Asian and African populations.[41] In the western world, alcoholic liver cirrhosis is considered the main cause of primary liver cancer.[42,43] The role of oral contraceptives in liver carcinogenesis has been studied for many years, although its relationship still remains speculative. In general, it seems that long-term use of oral contraceptives are more often associated with the development of hepatic adenoma and much less often with hepatocellular carcinoma.[44,45]

Aspiration Cytology

Cell Morphology. Depending on the degree of differentiation of the tumor, the malignant hepatocytes resemble to a variable extent the benign hepatocytes, but are usually larger and the N/C ratio is increased. The morphologic characteristics of the cells (**Fig. 9.5**) are as follows. (*a*) The tumor cells retain a polygonal or polyhedral shape. (*b*) The nuclei are oval to round, centrally located, with finely to coarsely granular chromatin and thickened nuclear membranes. Prominent, eosinophilic nucleoli are observed in about 80% of our cases. Intranuclear cytoplasmic inclusions, similar to those seen in papillary thyroid cancer, are seen in about 40% of the cases (**Fig. 9.5A**, *inset*). (*c*) The cytoplasm is finely granular and typically stains eosinophilic with the hematoxylin and eosin technique. Depending on the content of fat, which is a variable feature, the cytoplasm may be vacuolated (**Fig. 9.6**). Cytoplasmic PAS-positive hyaline globules and bile pigment are present in about 15% of our cases (**Fig. 9.7**). Cytoplasmic glycogen as indicated by PAS-diastase labile reaction was described by Gupta and associates[46] in 80% of their cases.

As the tumor becomes less differentiated, the cells appear more anaplastic and the resemblance to hepatocytes is less apparent. Pleomorphic and multinucleated giant cells may be seen. In occasional cases, there may be spindle cells, which can mimic a sarcoma (**Fig. 9.8**).[29]

Cellular Pattern. The aspirates from HCCs are highly cellular. The following growth patterns are characteristic: trabecular, adenomatoid, anaplastic, and dispersed cell. The trabecular pattern is the most common, observed in 75% of our cases. The tumor cells are arranged in well-defined, thick, often anastomosing trabeculae, invested by an incomplete layer of flattened endothelial cells (**Fig. 9.9**). The trabeculae are separated from one another by empty spaces, corresponding to the sinusoidal spaces on histologic sections. Trabeculae of varying lengths are usually seen in the same aspirate. The short, broad trabeculae may have a pseudopapillary configuration (**Fig. 9.10**).

The adenomatoid or alveolar pattern is present in about 15 to 20% of the cases, and often it is seen together with the trabecular pattern. The tumor cells are arranged loosely around variably sized spaces (**Fig. 9.11**). Many of the metastatic adenocarcinomas also exhibit this pattern, but the cells in HCC have the characteristics of liver cells.

The anaplastic pattern is present in about 10% of the cases. The anaplastic cells are arranged in small dyshesive groups or in multilayered unstructured tissue fragments.

A dispersed cell pattern (**Fig. 9.12**) is present in many of the aspirates, but is almost always seen in combination with another cell pattern. In some cases, there may be many malignant stripped nuclei lying singly. In the absence of the granular eosinophilic cytoplasm, the macronucleoli may be the only clue to the hepatic origin of such tumor cells.

Diagnostic Pitfalls. It has been said that our ability to accurately diagnose HCC is based upon the odd rule that "the neoplastic cells should resemble hepatocytes but not too closely."[47] This axiom highlights the two main problems encountered in the cytologic diagnosis of HCC: (*a*) to distinguish cells of hepatocellular carcinoma from cells of other malignancies, particularly metastastic adenocarcinomas, and (*b*) to distinguish malignant hepatocytes from nonmalignant reactive liver cells, particularly from cirrhotic livers.

To distinguish HCC from other malignancies, the cytopathologist should look for the cytologic features of HCC: (*a*) resemblance to liver cells, (*b*) trabecular structures with endothelial sheathes, (*c*) bile production by the malignant cells, (*d*) PAS-positive cytoplasmic hyaline globules, (*e*) characteristic immunostaining of bile canaliculi with polyclonal anticarcinoembryonic antigen.[47a] (In contrast, carcinomas from other sites in the gastrointestinal tract show a diffuse cytoplasmic immunostaining pattern.) The cytologic features of the common metastatic tumors of the liver are discussed later in this chapter (see "Metastatic Tumors").

Many reports in the literature have also warned of the difficulties in distinguishing well-differentiated hepatocellular carcinomas from reactive or regenerative processes of the liver on FNAB. Cirrhosis,[18,48] viral hepatitis,[49] and drug-induced hepatitis[22] have all been mistaken for HCC. Careful study of the individual cell morphology and the pattern of cellular arrangement is crucial to correct diagnosis. In difficult cases, it would be advisable to obtain aspirates from the mass as well as from the uninvolved area so that a comparative evaluation can be made. The aspirates from HCCs generally reveal only a single population of cells. The morphologic changes (in terms of nuclear, nucleolar, and cytoplasmic characteristics) are rather constant from cell to cell, producing a rather monomorphic cellular picture. Bile duct epithelium and normal liver cells are conspicuous by their absence. Thick trabeculae are characteristic, and other patterns may also be seen, alone or in combination with the trabecular pattern. On the other hand, in reactive conditions the cytologic atypia, when present, does not affect the liver cells in a uniform fashion. Within a tissue fragment, transitions from normal to mildly atypical to markedly atypical hepatocytes can often be seen. A mixed popu-

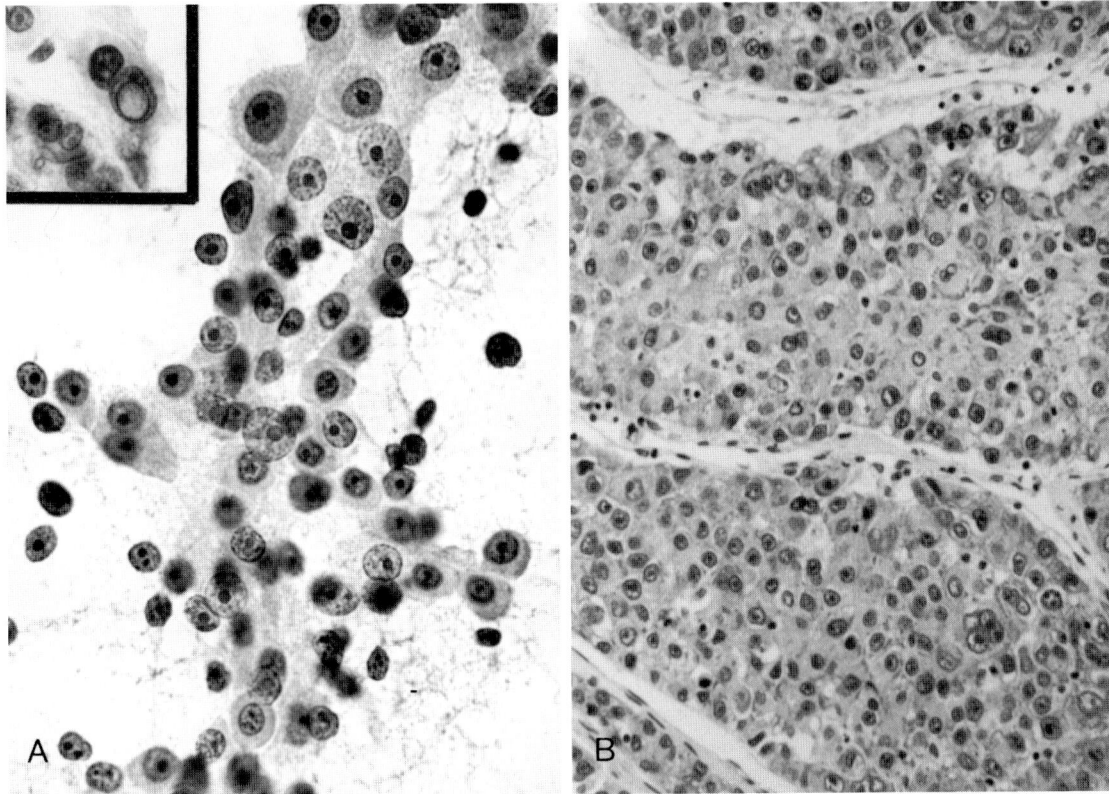

Figure 9.5. Hepatocellular carcinoma. **A,** ABC. Prototypic polygonal cells with eosinophilic granular cytoplasm, resembling normal hepatocytes. Note prominent nucleoli and increased N/C ratio. *Inset* shows an intranuclear cytoplasmic inclusion. ×500. **B,** Histologic section of hepatocellular carcinoma. ×310.

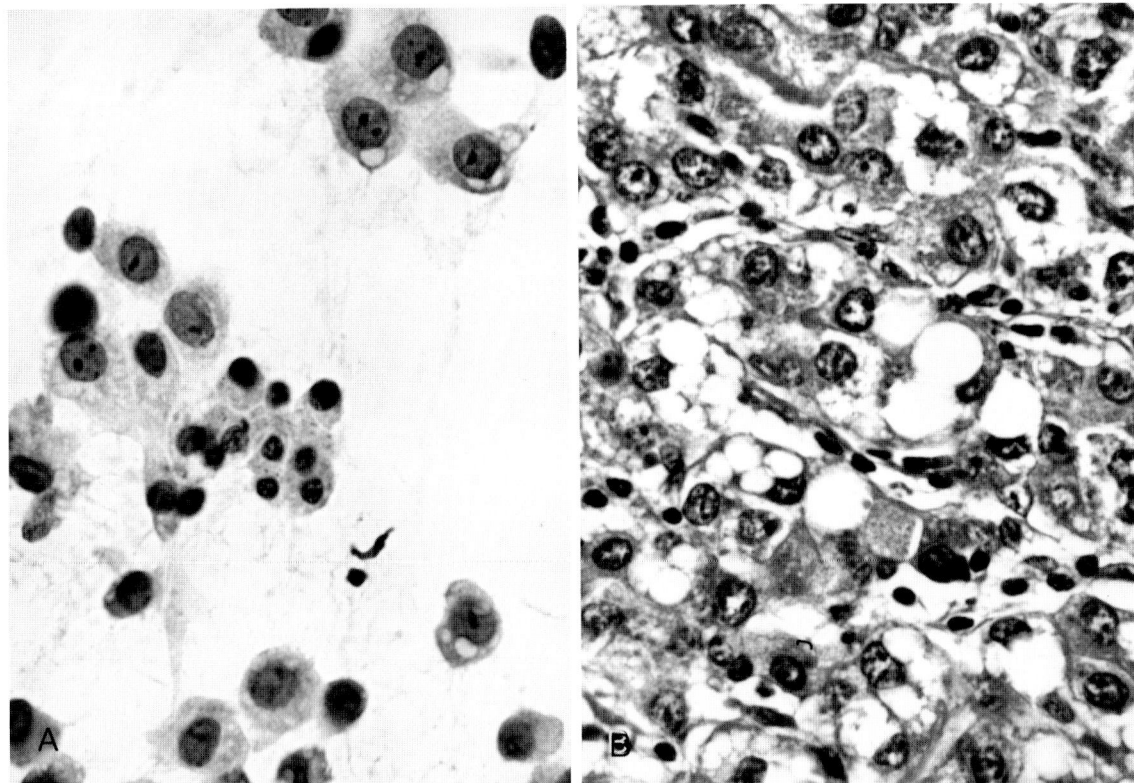

Figure 9.6. Hepatocellular carcinoma. **A,** ABC. Malignant hepatocytes with intracytoplasmic fat globules. ×500. **B,** Histologic section revealing extensive fatty change in the tumor cells. ×500.

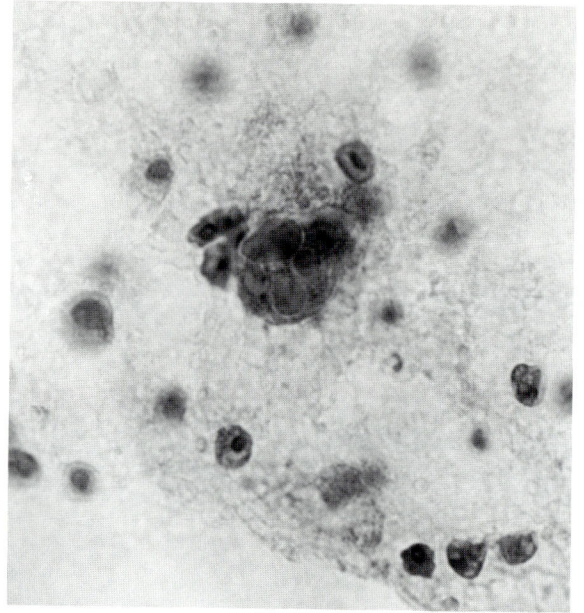

Figure 9.7. Hepatocellular carcinoma, ABC. Note a malignant hepatocyte containing multiple, PAS-positive, eosinophilic hyaline globules. Periodic acid-Schiff stain; ×500.

Figure 9.8. Hepatocellular carcinoma. **A,** ABC. Note spindle-shaped malignant cells. ×500. **B,** Histologic section showing the spindle cell variant of HCC. ×310.

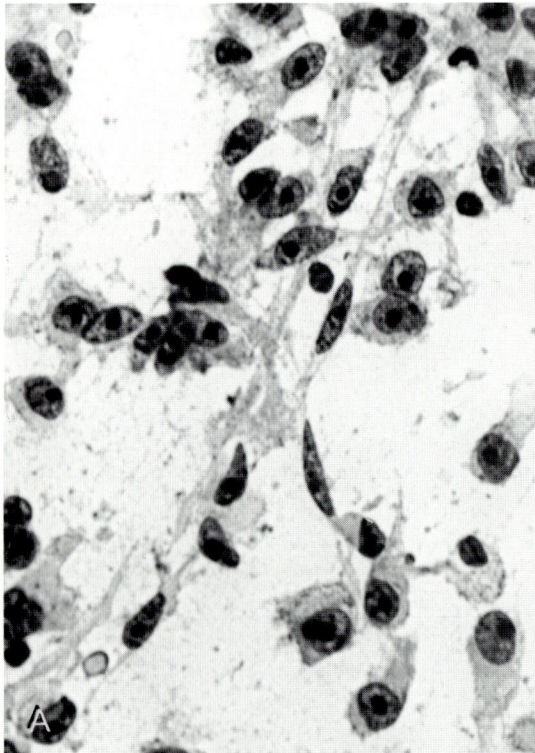

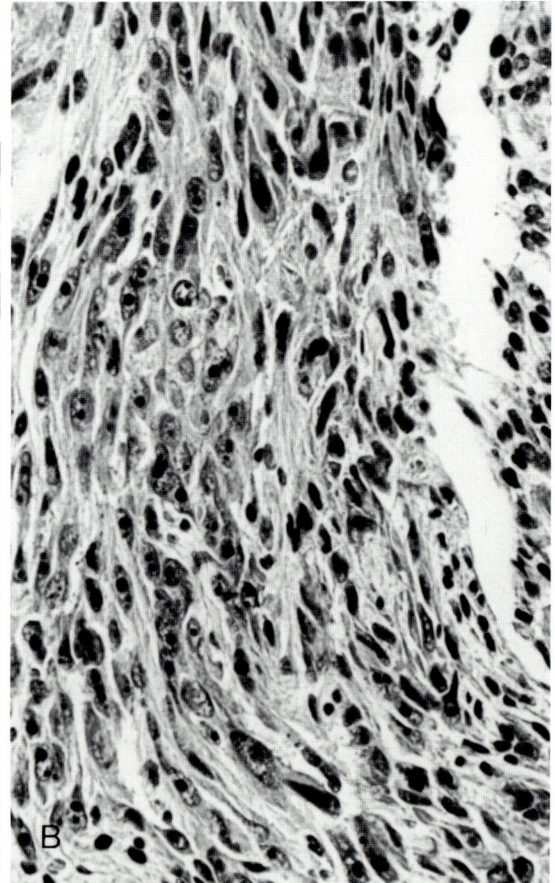

Figure 9.7.

Figure 9.8.

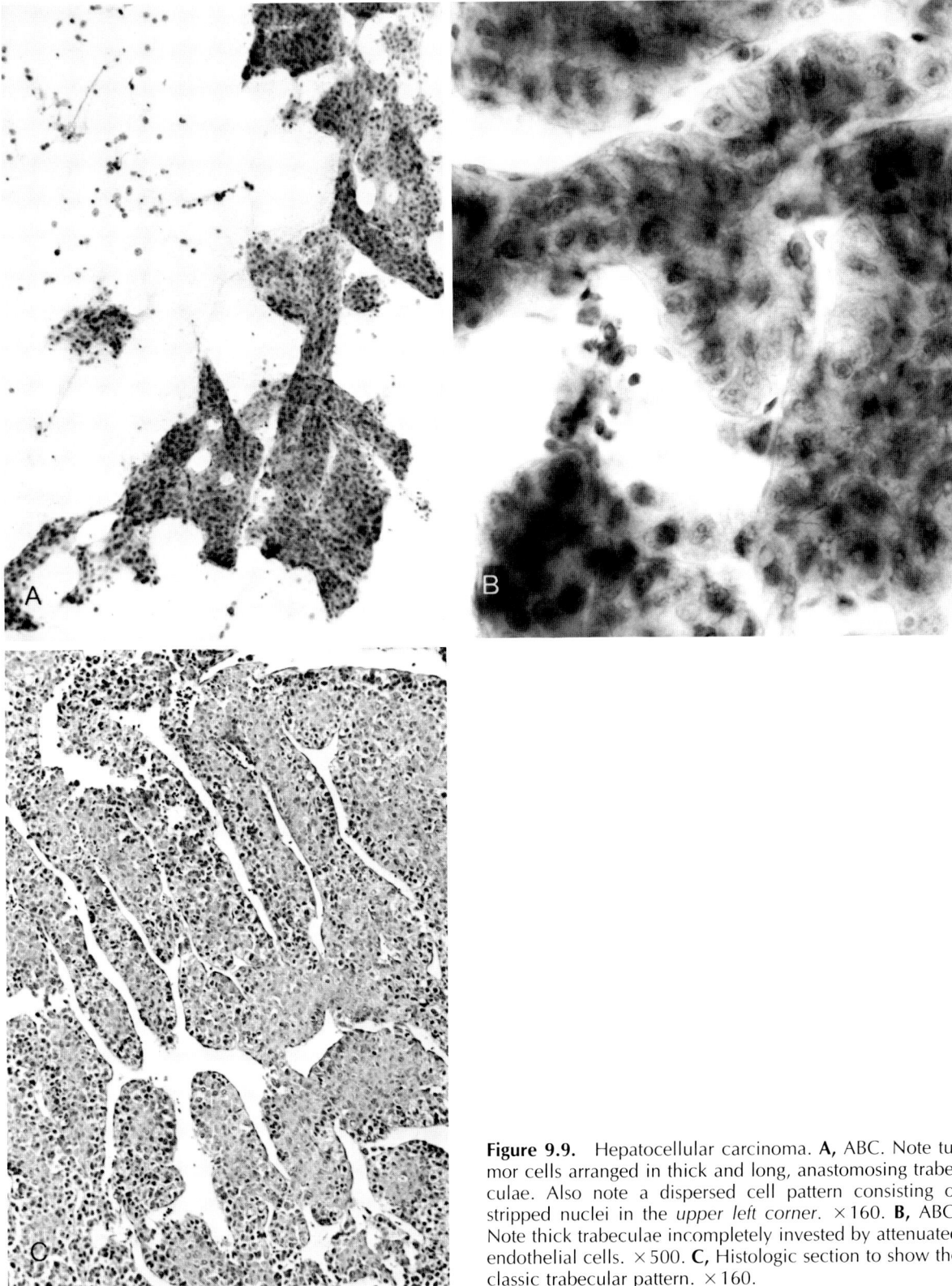

Figure 9.9. Hepatocellular carcinoma. **A,** ABC. Note tumor cells arranged in thick and long, anastomosing trabeculae. Also note a dispersed cell pattern consisting of stripped nuclei in the *upper left corner*. ×160. **B,** ABC. Note thick trabeculae incompletely invested by attenuated endothelial cells. ×500. **C,** Histologic section to show the classic trabecular pattern. ×160.

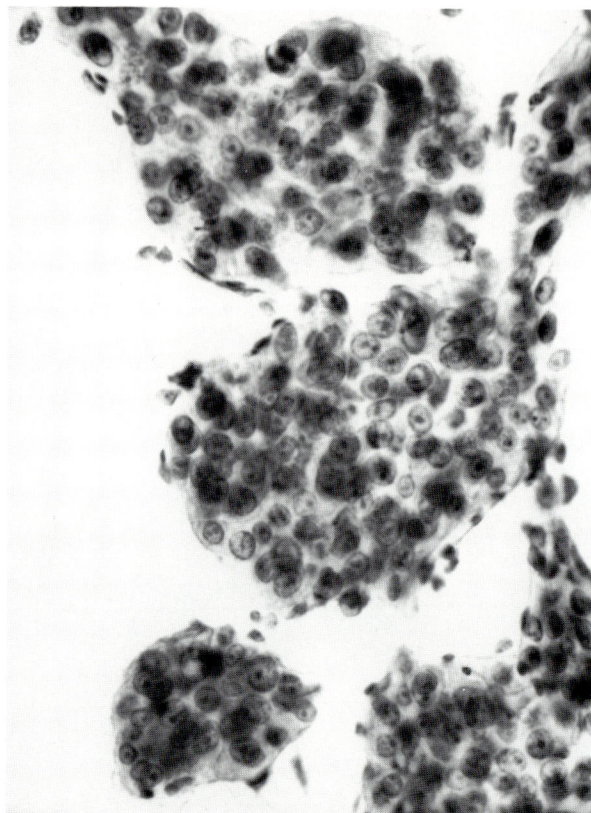

Figure 9.10. Hepatocellular carcinoma, ABC. Short, broad trabeculae mimicking papillae. Note endothelial cell covering. × 500.

lation of atypical cells and normal liver cells favors the diagnosis of a benign process. Other cell types such as bile ductular cells, inflammatory cells, and fibroblastic cells in the case of cirrhosis, are present. Tissue fragments, both large and small, can be found in benign reactive conditions, but the constituent cells are arranged in thin cords of 1–2 cells thick, in contrast to the thick trabecular arrangement seen in HCC.

Fibrolamellar Hepatocellular Carcinoma

Fibrolamellar hepatocellular carcinoma is a distinct variant of HCC that has a much better prognosis than the ordinary HCC. It is typically seen in younger patients with noncirrhotic livers.[50–52] Histologically, the tumor is characterized by large, polygonal cells having prominent eosinophilic nucleoli and wide lamellar bands of fibrous tissue separating the tumor cells into nodules of variable size **(Fig. 9.13)**.

Aspiration Cytology

Cellular Pattern. The aspirates are highly cellular. While some tumor cells may be arranged in trabeculae, most of the cells are loosely grouped or lying singly. Characteristically, parallel rows of benign-appearing fibrocytes are seen intermingled with the tumor cells or dividing the tumor cells into small nests **(Fig. 9.14)**.

Cell Morphology. The tumor cells **(Fig. 9.15)** bear a resemblance to normal liver cells but are at least three to four times larger. The cells are polyhedral, with abundant, deeply eosinophilic cytoplasm and distinct cytoplasmic membranes. The nuclei are uniform, large and oval, with peripheral margination of chromatin. Each nu-

cleus contains an extremely prominent nucleolus. Intranuclear cytoplasmic inclusions are readily seen. Well-defined, intracytoplasmic *pale bodies,* as previously described by Craig,[50] are present.

Differential Diagnosis. It is important to distinguish fibrolamellar HCC from ordinary HCC since the former has a much better prognosis. An aggressive surgical approach is especially warranted because the tumor usually afflicts a young patient with a noncirrhotic liver; hence, postoperative liver failure is less likely. To distinguish fibrolamellar HCC from ordinary HCC, besides the clinical data, the following cytologic features can be sought.[33] (*a*) The tumor cells are much larger than those from ordinary HCC. (*b*) The tumor cells have abundant oncocytic granular cytoplasm and very large solitary nucleoli. (*c*) Intracytoplasmic *pale bodies* are often seen. (*d*) Lamellar fibrosis is present. It is worthy of note that ordinary HCC is a cellular neoplasm that has little connective tissue stroma. The finding of abundant fibrous bands should arouse the suspicion of fibrolamellar HCC or a rare desmoplastic HCC. (To distinguish from cirrhosis, the fibrous bands must be found within the neoplastic tissue fragments.)

Hepatoblastoma

Hepatoblastoma usually occurs before the age of 3 years, an age at which HCC is rare.[53] Occasional examples of hepatoblastoma may be seen in older children when it may be difficult to decide whether the tumor is a late-appearing hepatoblastoma or an early-appearing adult HCC. Since hepatoblastoma is rare, there are few publications describing the ABC of this neoplasm. The first ABC account was reported simultaneously by Suen[32] and Bhatia and

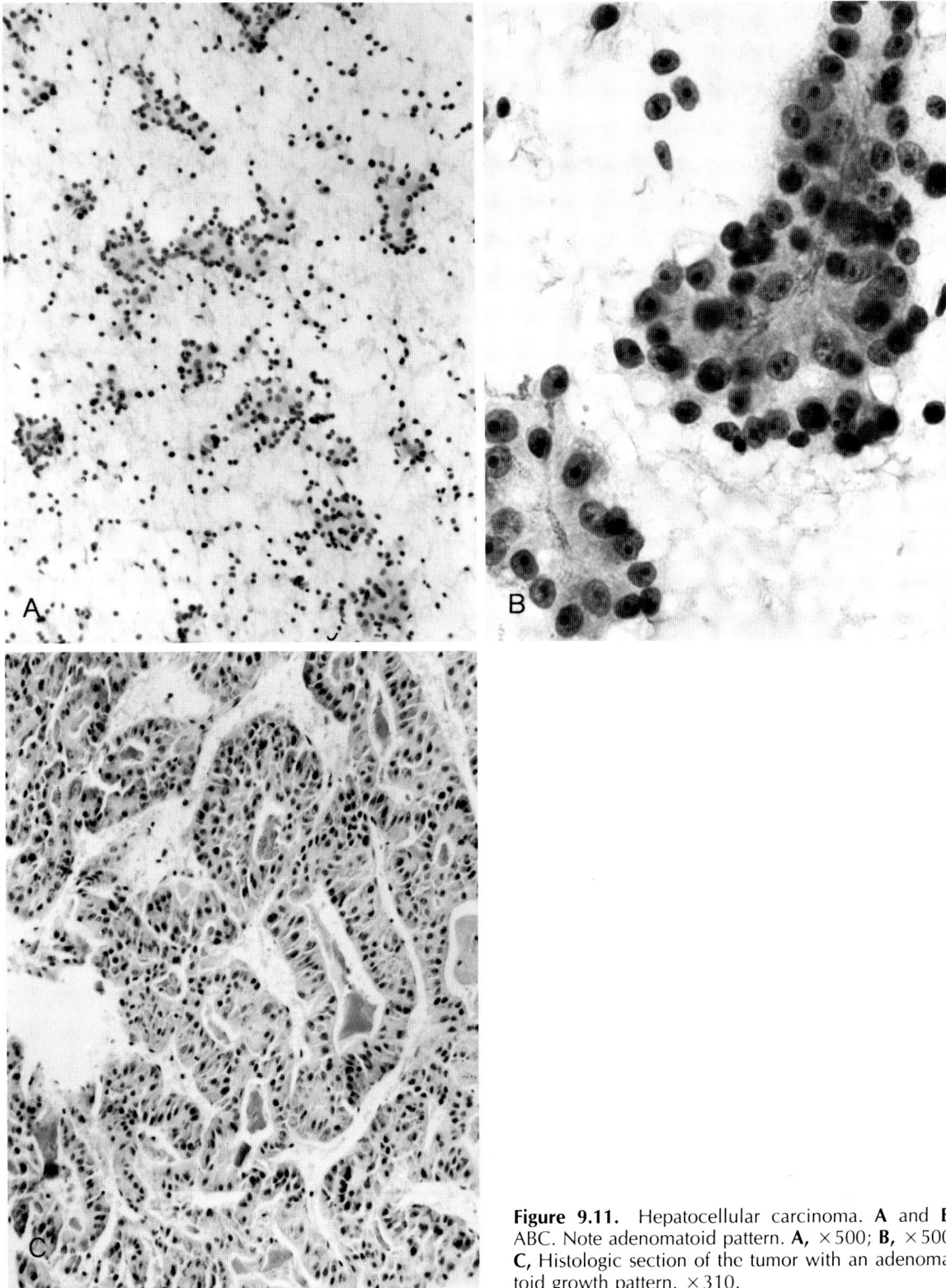

Figure 9.11. Hepatocellular carcinoma. A and B, ABC. Note adenomatoid pattern. A, ×500; B, ×500. C, Histologic section of the tumor with an adenomatoid growth pattern. ×310.

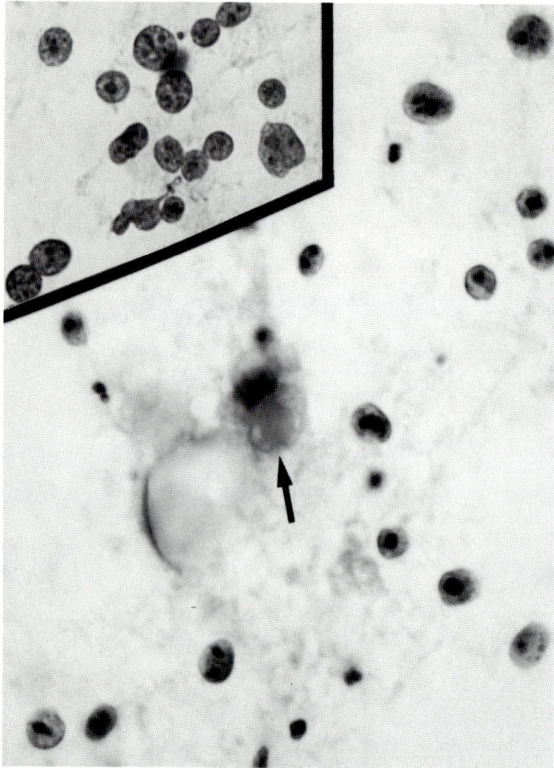

Figure 9.12.

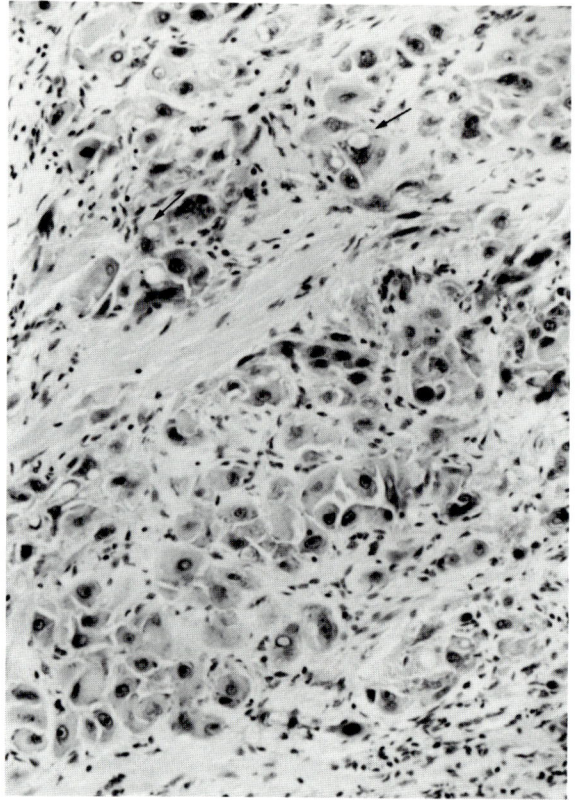

Figure 9.13.

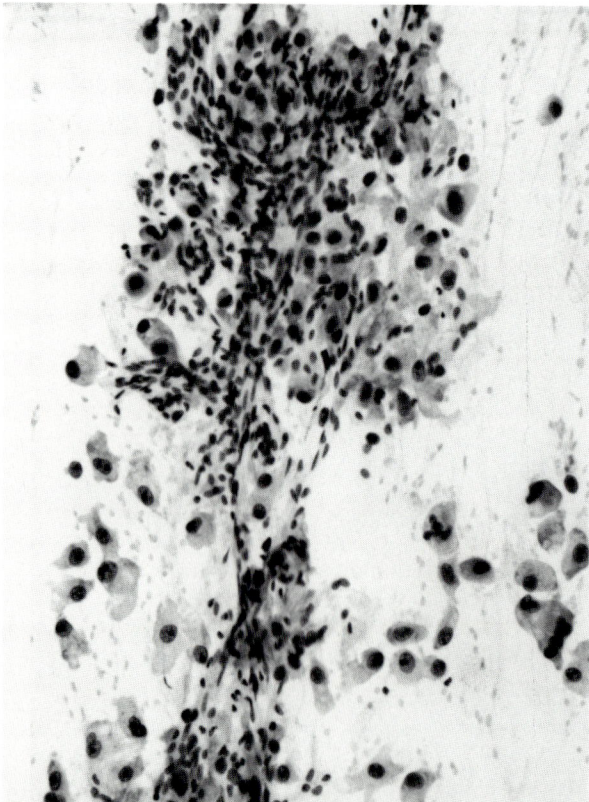

Figure 9.14.

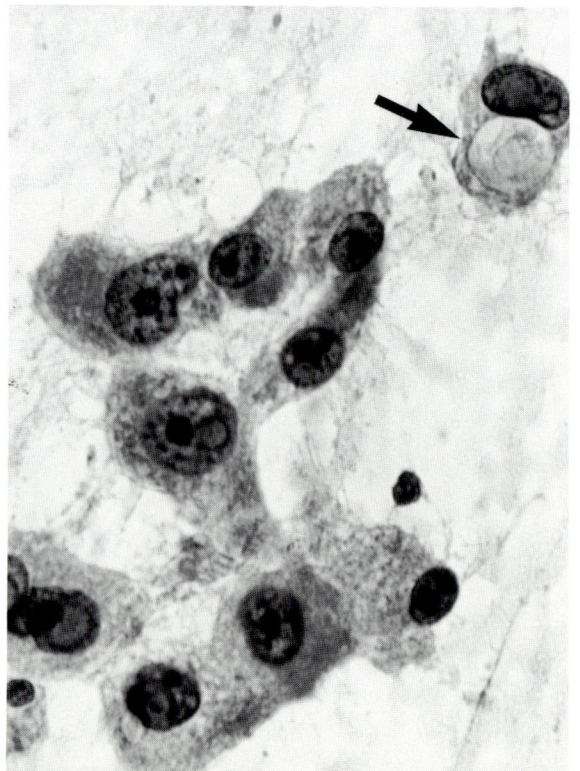

Figure 9.15.

Mehrotra.[54] More recently, Dekmezian et al.[55] have reported two additional cases.

Aspiration Cytology

Cellular Pattern. The epithelial cells are arranged in branching ribbons or thin trabeculae, producing a gyriform pattern **(Fig. 9.16A)**.[32] Rosette structures are also common **(Fig. 9.16B)**.

Cell Morphology. The tumor cells are immature, resembling embryonal or fetal liver cells. The embryonal type cells are small, oval, and exhibit a high N/C ratio. The nuclei are round and hyperchromatic, with a distinct nucleolus. The more mature fetal type cells are larger, but still smaller than adult hepatocytes **(Fig. 9.16)**. Pleomorphism is generally negligible. However, in one reported case considerable pleomorphism was observed.[55]

In addition to the epithelial cells, extramedullary hematopoiesis, primitive spindle cells, and metaplastic elements (chondroid and osteoid tissues) have been observed by others.[54,55]

Differential Diagnosis. Hepatoblastoma can be differentiated from hepatocellular carcinoma by the younger age at which the tumor occurs, the presence of small uniform cells and extramedullary hematopoiesis, and the absence of cirrhotic changes. Metaplastic components, e.g., osteoid-like material, if identified, are also a very helpful clue to the diagnosis of hepatoblastoma.[55]

Cholangiocarcinoma

Cholangiocarcinomas are malignant neoplasms arising from the bile duct epithelium. The tumor is known to develop following *Clonorchis sinensis* infestation, Thorotrast injection, hemochromatosis, and duct ectasia disease.[56] Grossly, the tumor may be solitary, multinodular, or diffuse. It is not commonly associated with cirrhosis, but there is often considerable desmoplasia within the tumor. α-Fetoprotein is not elevated in the serum of patients with cholangiocarcinoma.

Aspiration Cytology

Cholangiocarcinomas are adenocarcinomas, and cells derived from these tumors show conventional malignant cytologic criteria **(Fig. 9.17)**. The tumor cells are cuboidal to columnar, with vesicular eccentric nuclei, and frequently, prominent nucleoli. The cytoplasm is lightly stained and may be vacuolated. Intracytoplasmic mucin is common, whereas bile production is never seen. The cells are arranged in gland-like or palisading clusters. For the most part, it is not difficult to distinguish cholangiocarcinoma from HCC. But it is virtually impossible to separate cholangiocarcinoma from metastatic adenocarcinoma, especially those of the pancreas and gall bladder, on purely morphologic grounds. Clinical data are required to determine the origin of such adenocarcinomas.

Primary Hepatic Sarcomas

Primary sarcoma of the liver is extremely rare. The term *malignant mesenchymoma* has been applied to undifferentiated hepatic sarcomas in children,[57] even though only a few of the cases fit Stout's definition of a mesenchymal neoplasm, i.e., a neoplasm consisting of two or more unrelated mesenchymal elements, such as liposarcoma and rhabdomyosarcoma.[58] Most of the liver sarcomas occur in young adults and the term *undifferentiated sarcoma* seems more appropriate. The cytologic features are those of an anaplastic spindle cell sarcoma.[32,59]

Angiosarcoma of the liver is a malignant tumor of the endothelial cells or Kupffer cells. Its development has been associated with exposure to certain carcinogens, such as Thorotrast, vinyl chloride, and arsenic.[60] The ABC **(Fig. 9.18)** consists of anaplastic endothelial cells, which are elongated and have faintly eosinophilic cytoplasm and ill-defined cell borders. The nuclei are hyperchromatic, ovoid or elongated, and have small nucleoli.[61] There is a variable degree of nuclear pleomorphism in different tumors and in different parts of the same tumor.

Since primary hepatic sarcomas are so uncommon, it is essential that a metastatic sarcoma must always be ruled out on clinical history and findings. A rare anaplastic HCC with spindle cells may also simulate a sarcoma. Multiple aspirated samples obtained from different areas of the lesion may show typical foci of HCC.

Metastatic Tumors

Metastatic cancer is the most common malignancy of the liver.[62] Unlike hepatocellular carcinomas, such cases rarely occur on the background of a cirrhotic liver. Metastatic cancer may manifest itself as a liver mass occurring some months or years after the resection of the primary tumor. Therefore, the clinical history is important in ruling out previous cancers that may have metastasized to the liver. Whenever feasible, the previous histologic slides should be reviewed and compared with the current aspirate specimen. In about 12–20% of cases, the site of the primary cancer may not be known.[63] Primary organ sites of liver metastases of obscure origin include lung, colon, breast, ovary, esophagus, pancreas, and stomach. If the pathologist cannot suggest a possible primary site on FNAB, search for a primary source may be worthwhile in selective cases.[64] For instance, carcinomas of the breast and ovary would be treated with a somewhat better prognosis and therefore should be evaluated. For other primary tumors, such as gastrointestinal tract, current therapy is less successful and elaborate evaluation is usually not indicated in the absence of a clincial clue.

Aspiration Cytology

The cytopathologist should strongly suspect the presence of a metastatic tumor if cells foreign to the liver are seen on the smear.[65]

Figure 9.12. Hepatocellular carcinoma with a dispersed cell pattern, ABC. Note many stripped nuclei with prominent nucleoli. The tumor cell at the center contains an eosinophilic hyaline globule *(arrow)*. ×500; *inset,* ×500.

Figure 9.13. Fibrolamellar hepatocellular carcinoma, histology. Note tumor nodules separated by lamellar fibrosis. Many tumor cells show a well-defined pale body *(arrows)* in the cytoplasm. ×125.

Figure 9.14. Fibrolamellar hepatocellular carcinoma, ABC. Note nests of tumor cells separated by bands of fibrocytes. ×125.

Figure 9.15. Fibrolamellar hepatocellular carcinoma, ABC. Close-up view of the tumor cells. Note large size, polyhedral shape, prominent nucleoli, granular oncocytic cytoplasm, and a so-called pale body *(arrow)* in the cytoplasm of a tumor cell. ×500.

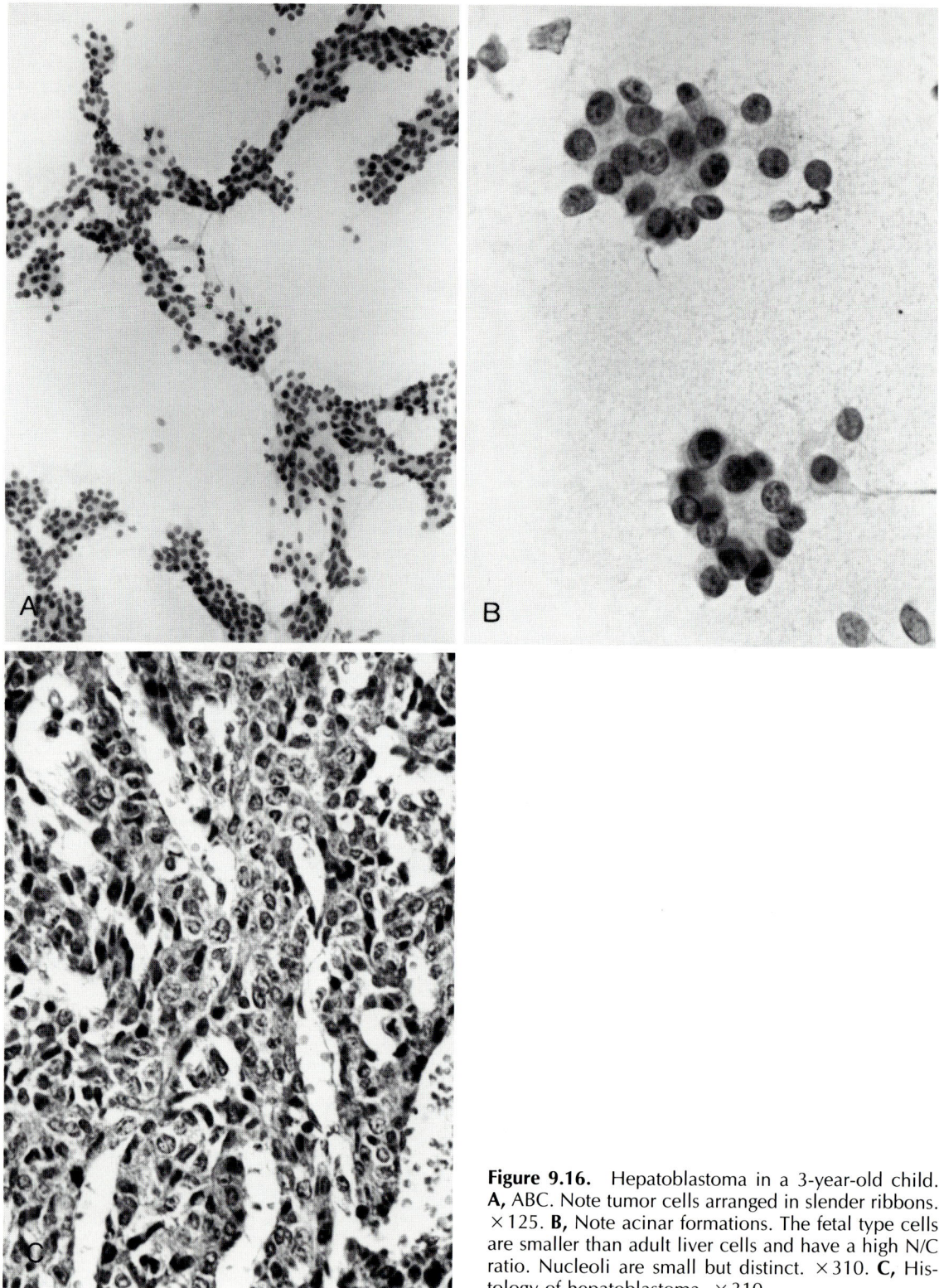

Figure 9.16. Hepatoblastoma in a 3-year-old child. **A,** ABC. Note tumor cells arranged in slender ribbons. ×125. **B,** Note acinar formations. The fetal type cells are smaller than adult liver cells and have a high N/C ratio. Nucleoli are small but distinct. ×310. **C,** Histology of hepatoblastoma. ×310.

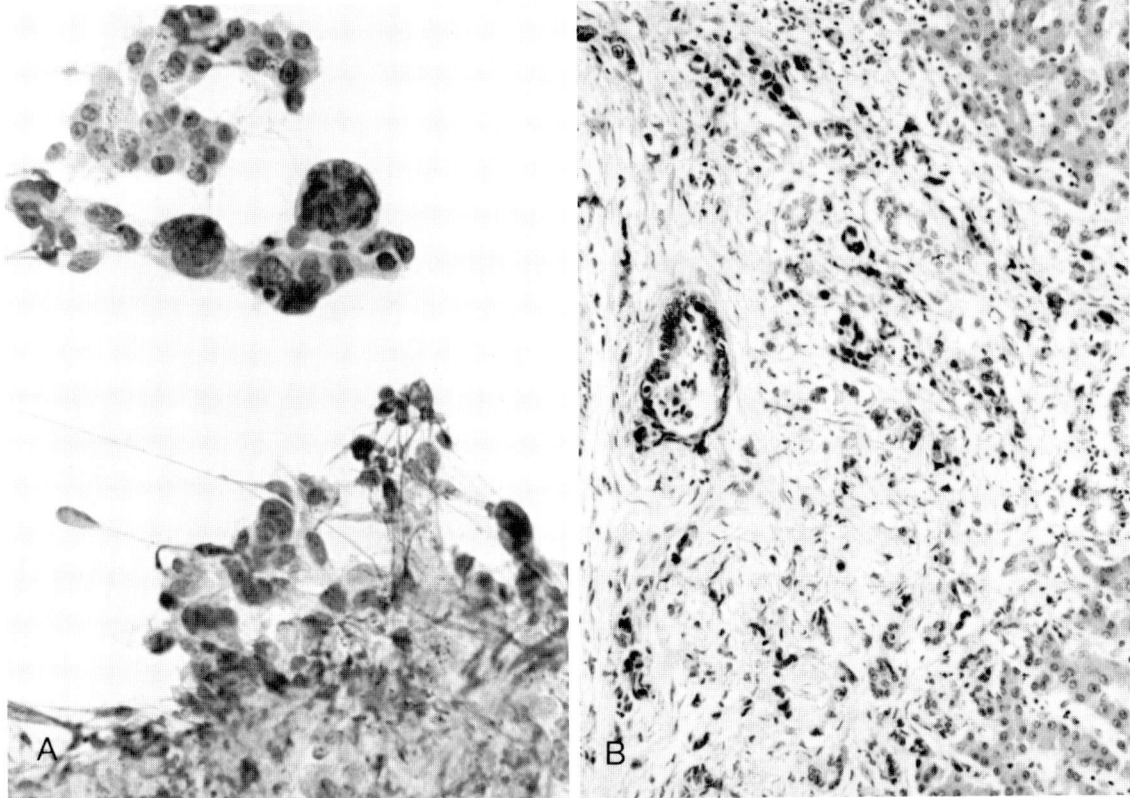

Figure 9.17. Cholangiocarcinoma. **A,** ABC. Note malignant cells intimately admixed with normal liver cells containing pigment granules *(top)* and fibrous tissue *(bottom).* This mixed pattern is common in cholangiocarcinoma and metastatic cancer but sel-dom seen in hepatocellular carcinoma. ×310. **B,** Histologic section. A carcinomatous nodule is surrounded by benign liver pa-renchyma. Also note desmoplasia within the tumor nodule. ×125.

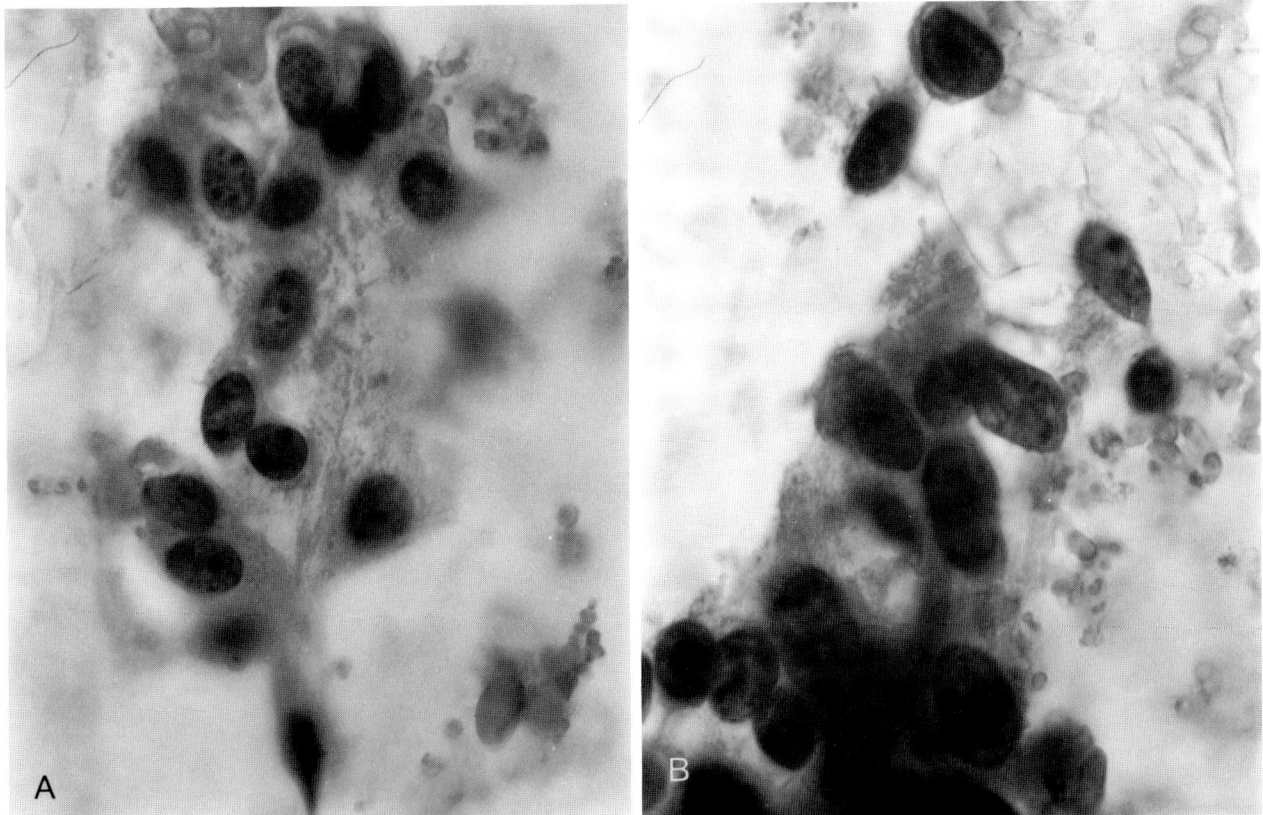

Figure 9.18. Angiosarcoma, ABC. **A** and **B,** Note malignant, oval to elongated nuclei and pale eosinophilic cytoplasm. ×1000. (Reproduced by permission. Nguyen GK, McHattie JD, Jeannot A. Cytomorphologic aspects of hepatic angiosarcoma: Fine-needle aspiration biopsy of a case. Acta Cytol 1982;26:527–531.)

Table 9.1. Comparison of Cytologic Features of Reactive Hepatocytes, Hepatocellular Carcinoma, and Other Tumors

	Reactive Hepatocytes	HCC	Adenocarcinoma	Carcinoid	Melanoma
Cell form	Polygonal	Polygonal	Columnar, cuboidal, pleomorphic	Round to oval	Oval, plasmacy-toid, spindly
Cytoplasm	Eosinophilic, granu-lar, lipofuscin +	Eosinophilic, granular	Clear, foamy, vacu-olated	Finely granulated	Finely granulated
N/C ratio	Low to moderate	Moderate to high	Moderate to high	Low to moderate	High
Nucleolar prominence	+ to + +	+ + +	+ + +	− / +	+ + +
Growth patterns	Small cords, mono-layers	Trabeculae, acini, single cells, striped nuclei	Glands, acini, pali-sades	Mosaic, acini, thin cords	Dispersed cells
Cellular composition	Normal hepatocytes + atypical hepa-tocytes + biliary epithelial cells	Monomorphous population of malignant hepatocytes	Tumor cells ± be-nign hepatocytes	Tumor cells ± benign hepa-tocytes	Tumor cells ± benign hepa-tocytes
Special stains		Bile, PAS, AFP, pCEA[a]	Epithelial mucins	Grimelius	Melanin, S100 protein

[a]The abbreviations used are: PAS, periodic acid-Schiff; AFP, anti-α-fetoprotein; pCEA, polyclonal anticarcinoembryonic antigen.

If differentiation is good, cell type can be readily determined. **Table 9.1** compares the cytologic features of atypical reactive hepatocytes, HCC, and some common metastatic tumors of the liver.

Cytologic diagnosis of metastatic squamous cell carcinoma and oat cell carcinoma generally should not present any problem (see Chapter 7 for cytologic features). Immunostaining for lymphocyte markers aids in separating malignant lymphoma from oat cell carcinoma.

Metastatic melanoma cells with macronucleoli may simulate cells of HCC. Dispersed, single cells are present in both conditions, but melanoma cells do not form trabeculae. The cytoplasm of HCC cells are acidophilic, whereas melanoma cell cytoplasm is cyano-philic, with or without melanin pigment (see Chapter 4). The mela-noma cells are immunoreactive for S100 protein.

Metastatic carcinoid tumor may exhibit acinar structures and ribbons, superficially resembling the patterns seen in HCC. But the cells are small and relatively uniform, and macronucleoli are not seen. The Grimelius stain is positive in carcinoid tumors (see Chap-ters 7 and 11). An elevated amount of 5–hydroxyindoleacetic acid may be found in the urine of patients with a carcinoid tumor.

Metastatic adenocarcinomas are distinguished from HCC by the presence of clusters of cuboidal to columnar shaped (rather than polyhedral) cells, with single or multiple nucleoli. The cytoplasm is foamy or vacuolated (rather than granular and eosinophilic) and may contain mucicarmine-positive secretory vacuoles. With some excep-tions, identification of the primary site of a metastatic adenocarci-noma is often difficult, unless adequate clinical data are given or previous histologic sections are available for comparison. Well-dif-ferentiated colonic adenocarcinoma displays a rather distinctive pat-tern, characterized by uniform, columnar cells forming glandular structures or showing nuclear palisading (see Chapter 11).[21,29] Ad-enocarcinomas with papillary formations most frequently arise from the ampulla of Vater, colon, and ovary. Signet-ring cell adenocar-cinoma most often originates from the stomach. Prostatic adenocar-cinoma frequently shows small regular cells in sheets with a micro-acinar pattern (see Chapter 14).[12,21] Immunoperoxidase staining of the tumor cells for prostate-specific antigen or acid phosphatase aids

in separating prostatic adenocarcinoma from nonprostatic adenocar-cinomas.

BENIGN HEPATIC NEOPLASMS
Hepatocellular Adenoma and Focal Nodular Hyperplasia

Hepatocellular adenoma (HA) and focal nodular hyperplasia (FNH) are benign focal lesions that usually occur in women during the reproductive years and, particularly HA, are thought to be asso-ciated with long-term use of steroid contraceptives.[44,45]

Aspiration Cytology

Hepatocellular adenomas **(Fig. 9.19)** are composed of hepa-tocytes that quite closely resemble normal liver cells. The cells are arranged in cords one to three cells thick. Occasionally an acinar pattern is observed. The neoplastic cells, as well as their nuclei and nucleoli, tend to be slightly larger than normal hepatocytes, and their cytoplasm frequently is rather pale because of increased fat or gly-cogen content. Cytoplasmic eosinophilic globules, which are PAS-positive, diastase resistant, and identifiable histochemically as α_1-antitrypsin, have been reported to be present in some lesions.[66] Ne-crosis and hemorrhage are not uncommon and do not indicate malig-nancy.

The hepatocytes in focal nodular hyperplasia, like those in he-patocellular adenoma, are morphologically similar to normal liver cells. In an occasional case, cytologic atypia may be present and even severe enough for a diagnosis of hepatocellular carcinoma.[67] In tissue sections, FNH differs from HA in having wide collagenous septa radiating from a central scar. The septa contain blood vessels and bile ductules. Unlike HA, necrosis and hemorrhage are infre-quently encountered in FNH.

Diagnostic Pitfalls. It must not be assumed that HA and FNH can be readily diagnosed on FNAB. The aspirates are often reported as showing benign or reactive hepatocytes.[32] But in the presence of a demonstrable hepatic mass lesion, and in the appropriate clinical setting and with an assurance from an experienced radiologist of the

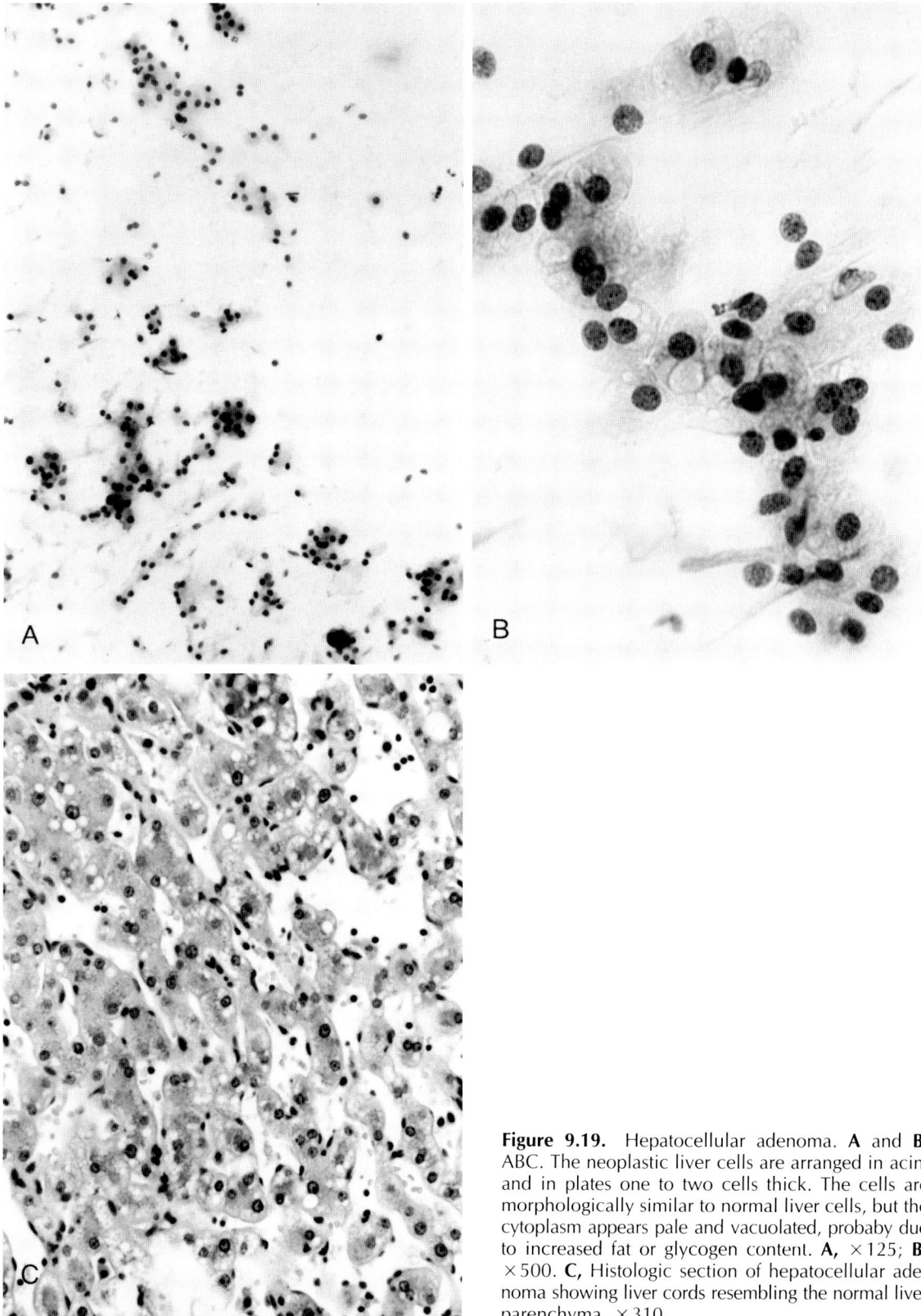

Figure 9.19. Hepatocellular adenoma. **A** and **B,** ABC. The neoplastic liver cells are arranged in acini and in plates one to two cells thick. The cells are morphologically similar to normal liver cells, but the cytoplasm appears pale and vacuolated, probaby due to increased fat or glycogen content. **A,** ×125; **B,** ×500. **C,** Histologic section of hepatocellular adenoma showing liver cords resembling the normal liver parenchyma. ×310.

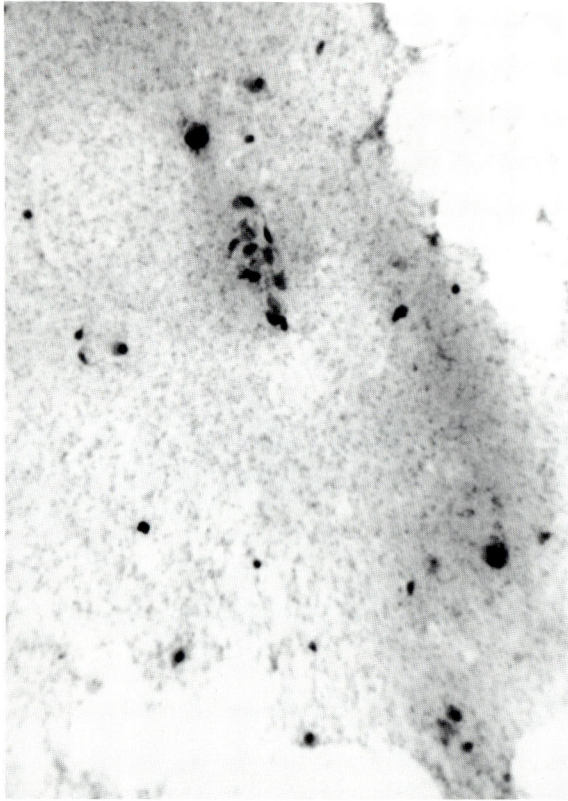

Figure 9.20.   Cavernous hemangioma, ABC. Note hypocellular smear with a small number of spindle cells, some hemosiderin-laden macrophages, and a bloody background. ×125.

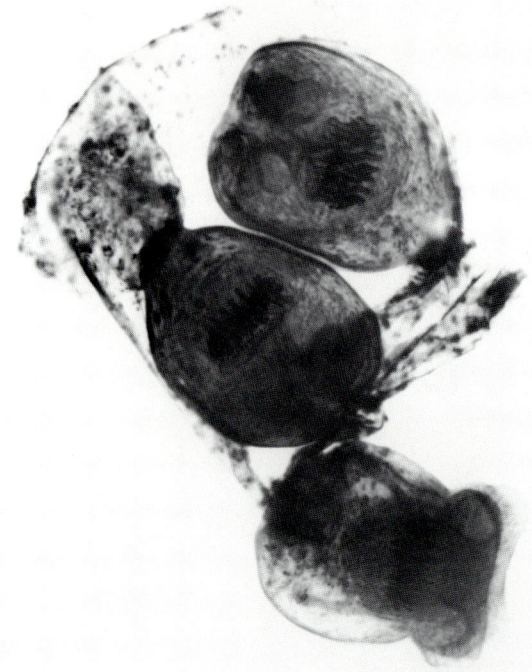

Figure 9.21.   Echinococcus cyst, ABC. Note scolices with hook-lets. ×125.

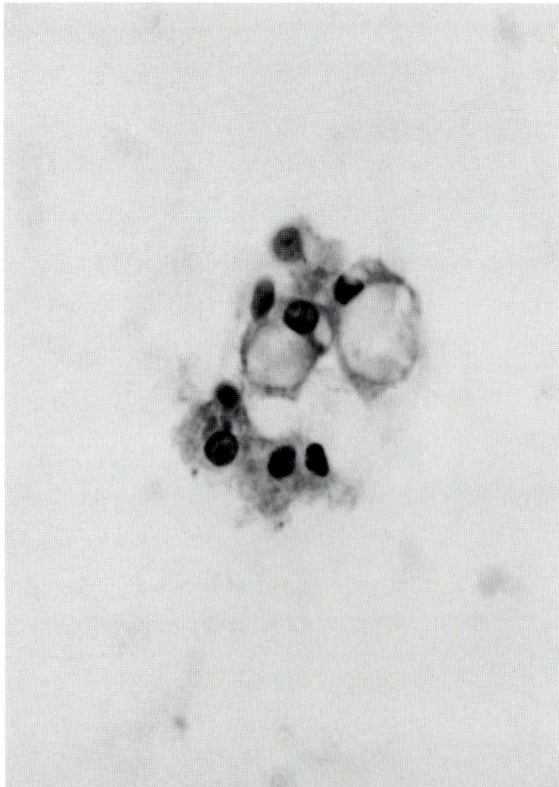

Figure 9.22.   Hepatocytes showing fatty change, ABC. Note cytoplasmic vacuoles distending the liver cells. ×500.

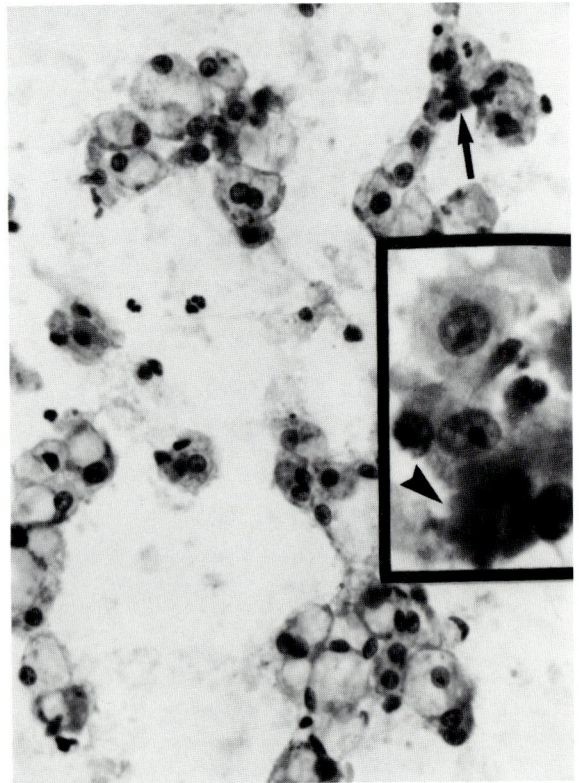

Figure 9.23.   Alcoholic hepatitis, ABC. Note degenerated and reactive hepatocytes containing fat globules, Mallory bodies (arrow), and scattered polymorphonuclear leukocytes. Inset shows reactive hepatocytes with prominent nucleoli and a Mallory body (arrowhead). ×310; inset, ×600.

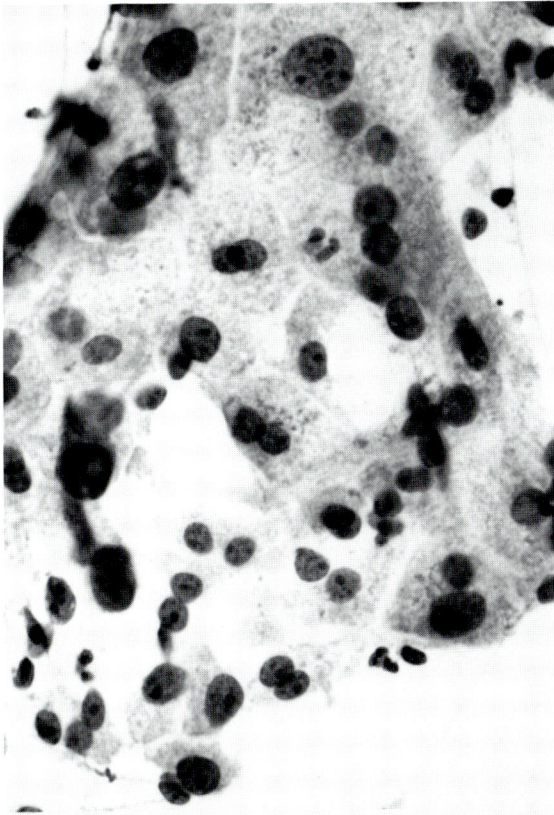

Figure 9.24. Cirrhosis, ABC. Note large atypical hepatocytes admixed with small normal hepatocytes. There is increased cytoplasmic pigment. ×500.

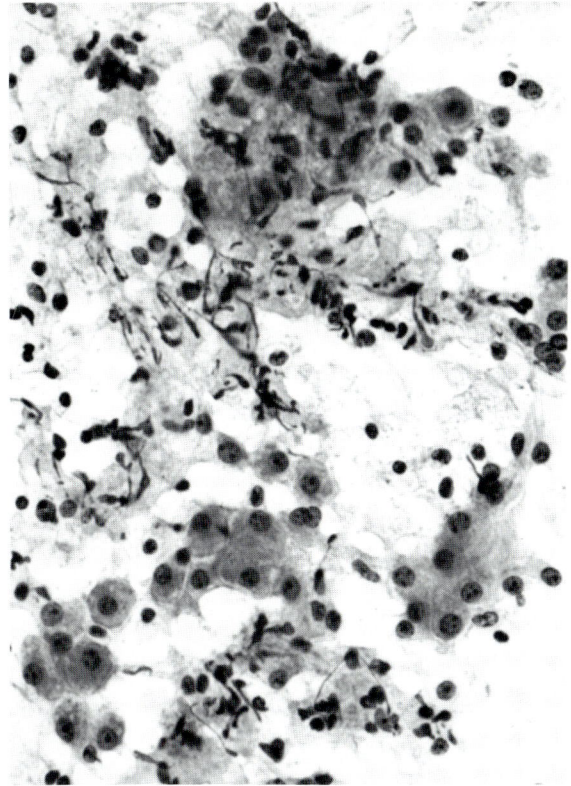

Figure 9.25. Cirrhosis, ABC. Note fibrocytes and scattered lymphocytes. ×310.

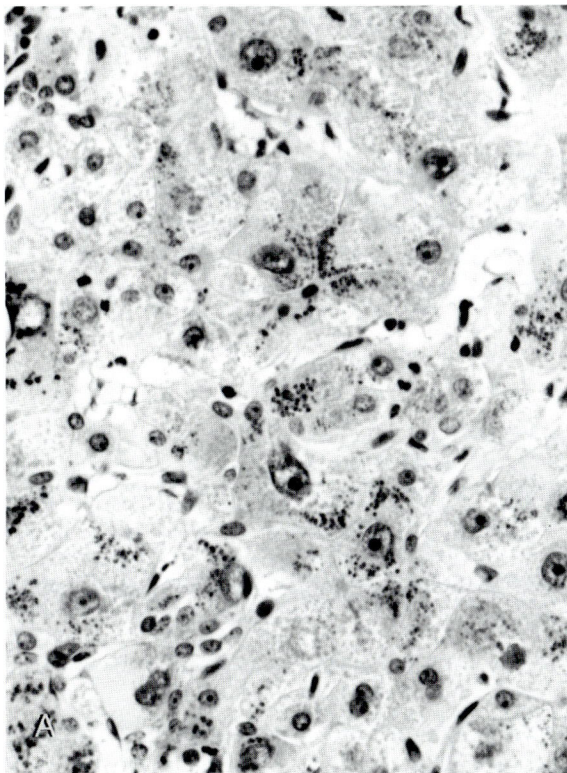

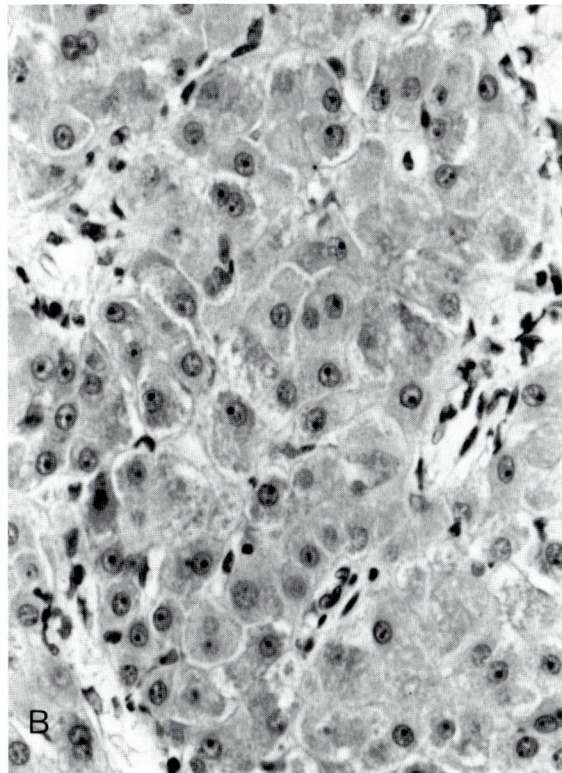

Figure 9.26. Contrasting cirrhosis and hepatocellular carcinoma, histologic sections. This patient had hepatitis B antigenemia, cirrhosis, and hepatocellular carcinoma. **A,** Cirrhotic nodule showing a spectrum of polymorphous changes. ×310. **B,** Hepatocellular carcinoma showing morphologic purity. ×310.

correct placement of the needle, the possibility of HA or FNH should be seriously considered.

Hemangioma

The hemangioma is the most common benign tumor of the liver and can be seen in up to 8% of autopsies.[68] Most are small (a few millimeters in size), asymptomatic, and are discovered incidentally at laparotomy or at autopsy. They are histologically cavernous in type. Recent refinements of computed tomography and magnetic resonance imaging have facilitated the identification of hepatic hemangiomas, which show a typical appearance in most instances.[69,70] But a few cases may not be radiologically diagnostic and may require further investigation. Needle biopsies of cavernous hemangiomas with needles larger 1 mm in external diameter (20 gauge) has resulted in reports of hemorrhage and even death.[70] More recent studies have documented the safety of fine needle biopsy (20–22 gauge) in the investigation of cavernous hemangioma.[71] Hemangiomas that are sufficiently large to be symptomatic should be resected or treated with hepatic artery ligation, because of the potential danger of intraperitoneal hemorrhage.[72]

The aspirate (**Fig. 9.20**) consists of blood, with only a few clumps of benign spindle cells, which may be derived from the endothelium or from the fibrous stroma. In one series of 33 cases, blood only was aspirated in 24 cases; blood was accompanied by endothelial cells in five cases and by capillaries in four.[73] The cytologic features in most cases are therefore not specific; the role of the pathologist is to confirm that there are no malignant cells present.

NONNEOPLASTIC LESIONS
Benign Tumor-like Lesions

It is important to separate the curable tumor-like lesions from malignant liver tumors that are generally not curable. The conditions that are most likely to be clinically confused with hepatic neoplasms are cysts, abscesses, and tuberculomas.

An aspirate from a simple cyst consists of clear or thin yellow fluid. The smears are hypocellular, with only a few benign epithelial cells and some macrophages. The fluid from an echinococcus, or hydatid, cyst may contain white membranous tissue fragments and the diagnosis rests on the identification of scolices and/or hooklets (**Fig. 9.21**).[32,74] It is generally not advisable to aspirate a suspected echinococcus cyst because of the potential risk of anaphylactic shock if spillage of cyst content should occur.

In the case of a liver abscess, FNAB yields purulent material. The smears show many polymorphonuclear leukocytes and necrotic debris. In addition to submitting the aspirate for microbiological culture, it is important to search cytologically for malignant cells because a hepatic neoplasm may become secondarily infected and undergo cystic degeneration.[75]

The cytologic features of hepatic granulomas are similar to those seen in other sites (see Chapters 4 and 7). In a series of seven patients with hepatic granulomas, ABC revealed epithelioid cells in all cases and multinucleated giant cells in one.[76]

Parenchymal Liver Disease

As stated in the beginning of this chapter, we do not attempt to make a specific diagnosis in parenchymal liver disease, instead we report the cytologic findings descriptively. Fatty changes of hepatocytes are characterized by the presence of multiple intracytoplasmic vacuoles of variable sizes and eccentrically placed nuclei (**Fig. 9.22**). Mild degrees of fatty change are frequent and occur focally in the livers of patients with chronic debilitating diseases. Severe fatty changes are often seen in our practice in chronic alcoholic patients.

The presence of hepatitis is suggested by the decreased cohesion of hepatocytes, with many single cells.[77] The degenerated hepatocytes are swollen and the cytoplasm stains unevenly and is paler than usual. In severe cases, necrotic or pyknotic liver cells are discernible.[17–19] In viral hepatitis, scattered lymphocytes and mononuclear phagocytes are present. In alcoholic hepatitis (**Fig. 9.23**), in addition to the degenerated hepatocytes described above, there are hepatocytes with marked fatty change, Mallory hyalin bodies, and many scattered polymorphonuclear leukocytes. The Mallory bodies are observed in the cytoplasm of hepatocytes as ropy eosinophilic strands that appear to condense to become irregular but discrete masses of waxy, amorphous material.

In cirrhosis, there is an increase in the number of hepatocytes that exhibit binucleation, megakaryosis, and prominent nucleoli. These features are indicative of liver cell regeneration. At times, some hepatocytes may be so atypical that they may be mistaken for cells of hepatocellular carcinoma.[48] Nevertheless, even though the individual cell morphology may mimic malignancy, the cellular composition and the growth pattern differ from those of HCC (see ''Diagnostic Pitfalls'' under ''Hepatocellular Carcinoma''). In cirrhosis (**Figs. 9.24–9.26**) the cellular composition is polymorphous; there is a cytologic continuum of normal, mildly atypical and severely atypical hepatocytes. The biliary epithelial cells are increased in number, and fascicles of fibroblastic cells, which are not observed on normal smears, are seen in cirrhosis.

References

1. Johansen P, Svendsen KN. Scan-guided fine needle aspiration biopsy in malignant hepatic disease. Acta Cytol 1978;22;292–296.
2. Zornoza J, Wallace S, Ordonez N, Lukeman J. Fine-needle aspiration biopsy of the liver. AJR 1980;143:331–334.
3. Ho CS, McLoughin MJ, Tao LC, Blendis L, Evans WK. Guided percutaneous fine-needle biopsy of the liver. Cancer 1981;47:1781–1785.
4. Schwerk WB, Schmitz-Moormann P. Ultrasonically guided fine-needle biopsies in neoplastic liver disease: Cytohistologic diagnoses and echo pattern of lesions. Cancer 1981;48:1469–1477.
5. Rosenblatt R, Kutcher R, Moussouris HF, Schrieber K, Koss LG. Sonographically guided fine-needle aspiration of liver lesions. JAMA 1982;248:1639–1641.
6. Montali G, Solbiati L, Croce F, Ierace T, Ravetto C. Fine-needle aspiration biopsy of liver focal lesions ultrasonically guided with a real-time probe. Report on 126 cases. Br J Radiol 1982;55:717–723.
7. Pagani JJ. Biopsy of focal hepatic lesions. Comparison of 18 and 22 gauge needles. Radiology 1983;147:673–675.
8. Alspaugh JP, Bernardino ME, Sewell CW, et al. CT directed hepatic biopsies: Increased diagnostic accuracy with low patient risk. J Compt Assist Tomogr 1983;7:1012–1017.
9. Whitlach S, Nunez C, Pitlik DA. Fine needle aspiration of the liver. A study of 102 consecutive cases. Acta Cytol 1984;28:719–725.
10. Bell DA, Carr CP, Szyfelbein WM. Fine needle aspiration cytology of focal liver lesions; results obtained with examination of both

cytologic and histologic preparations. Acta Cytol 1986;30:397–402.

11. Hajdu SI, D'Ambrosio FG, Fields V, Lightdale CJ. Aspiration and brush cytology of the liver. Semin Diagn Pathol 1986;3:227–238.
12. Nguyen GK. Fine-needle aspiration biopsy cytology of hepatic tumors in adults. Pathol Annu 1986;21(Part 1):321–349.
13. Pinto MM, Avila NA, Heller CI, Criscuolo EM. Fine needle aspiration of the liver. Acta Cytol 1988;32:15–21.
14. Pilotti S, Rilke F, Claren R, Milella M, Lombardi L. Conclusive diagnosis of hepatic and pancreatic malignancies by fine needle aspiration. Acta Cytol 1988;32:27–38.
15. Bognel C, Rougier P, Leclere J, Duvillard P, Charpentier P, Prade M. Fine needle aspiration of the liver and pancreas with ultrasound guidance. Acta Cytol 1988;32:22–26.
16. Jacobsen GK, Gammelgaard J, Fugl M. Coarse needle biopsy versus fine needle aspiration in the diagnosis of focal lesions of the liver: Ultrasonically guided needle biopsy in suspected hepatic malignancy. Acta Cytol 1983;27:152–156.
17. Johansen S, Myren J. Fine needle aspiration biopsy smears in the diagnosis of liver diseases. Scand J Gastroenterol 1971;6:583–588.
18. Lundquist A. Fine needle aspiration biopsy of the liver. Acta Med Scand Suppl 1971;520:5–28.
19. Wasastjerna C. Liver. In Zajicek J. Aspiration biopsy cytology, Part II. Cytology of infradiaphragmatic organs. Basel: S Karger, 1979.
20. Carney CN. Clinical cytology of the liver. Acta Cytol 1975;19:244–250.
21. Tao LC, Donat EE, Ho CS, McLoughlin MJ. Percutaneous fine needle aspiration biopsy of the liver. Acta Cytol 1979;23:287–291.
22. Frable WJ. Thin-needle aspiration biopsy. Philadelphia: WB Saunders, 1983:232–235.
23. Perry MD, Johnston WW. Needle biopsy of the liver for the diagnosis of non-neoplastic liver diseases. Acta Cytol 1985;29:385–390.
24. Tatsuta M, Yamamoto R, Kasugai H, et al. Cytohistologic diagnosis of neoplasms of the liver by ultrasonically guided fine needle aspiration biopsy. Cancer 1984;54:1682–1686.
25. Innes DJ Jr, Feldman PS. Comparison of diagnostic results obtained by fine needle aspiration cytology and Tru-cut or open biopsies. Acta Cytol 1983;27:350–354.
26. Riska H, Friman C. Fatality after fine-needle aspiration biopsy of liver. Br Med J 1975;1:517.
27. Civardi G, Fornari F, Cavanna L, et al. Ultrasonically guided fine needle aspiration biopsy (UG-FNAB): A useful technique for the diagnosis of abdominal malignancies. Eur J Cancer Clin Oncol 1986;22:225–227.
28. Schulz TB. Fine-needle biopsy of the liver complicated with bile peritonitis. Acta Med Scand 1976;199:141–142.
29. Greene CA, Suen KC. Some cytologic features of hepatocellular carcinoma as seen in fine needle aspirates. Acta Cytol 1984;28:713–718.
30. Tao LC, Ho CS, McLoughlin MJ, Evans WK, Donat EE. Cytologic diagnosis of hepatocellular carcinoma by fine needle aspiration biopsy. Cancer 1984;53:547–552.
31. Ajdukiewicz A, Crowden A, Hudson E, Pyne C. Liver aspiration in the diagnosis of hepatocellular carcinoma in Gambia. J Clin Pathol 1985;38:185–192.
32. Suen KC. Diagnosis of primary hepatic neoplasms by fine needle aspiration cytology. Diagn Cytopathol 1986;2:99–109.
33. Suen KC, Magee F, Halparin L, Chan NH, Greene CA. Fine needle aspiration cytology of fibrolamellar hepatocellular carcinoma. Acta Cytol 1985;29:867–872.
34. Noguchi S, Yamamoto R, Tatsuta M, Kasugai H, Okuda S, Wada A, Tamura H. Cell features and patterns in fine-needle aspirates of hepatocellular carcinoma. Cancer 1986;58:321–328.
35. Johnson PJ, Portmann B, Williams R. Alpha-fetoprotein concentra-

tions measured by radioimmunoassay in diagnosing and excluding hepatocellular carcinoma. Br Med J 1978;2:661–663.
36. Masseyeff RF. Factors influencing alpha-fetoprotein biosynthesis in patients with primary liver cancer and other diseases. In Hirai H, Miyaji T. Alpha fetoprotein and hepatoma. Gaan monograph on cancer research, No. 14, Tokyo: University of Tokyo Press, 1973.
37. Maltz C, Lightdale CJ, Winawer SJ. Hepatocellular carcinoma. Am J Gastroenterol 1980;74:361–365.
38. Sumithran E, Prathap K. Hepatocellular carcinoma in the Malaysian Orang Asli. Cancer 1976;37:2263–2266.
39. Geddes EW, Falkson G. Malignant hepatoma in the Bantu. Cancer 1970;25:1271–1278.
40. Edmondson HA, Steiner PE. Primary carcinoma of the liver: An autopsy study of 100 cases among 48,900 necropsies. Cancer 1954;7:462–502.
41. Kew MC, Desmyter J, Bradburne AF, Macnab GM. Hepatitis B virus infection in southern African blacks with hepatocellular cancer. J Natl Cancer Inst 1979;62:517–520.
42. Purtilo DT, Gottlieb LS. Cirrhosis and hepatoma occurring at Boston City Hospital (1917–1968). Cancer 1973;32:458–462.
43. Lehmann FG, Wegener T. Etiology of human liver cancer: Controlled prospective study in liver cirrhosis. J Toxicol Environ Health 1979;5:281–299.
44. Baum J, Bookstein JJ, Holtz F, Klein WE. Possible association between benign hepatomas and oral contraceptives. Lancet 1973;2:926–929.
45. Christopherson WM, Mays ET, Barrows GH. Liver tumors in young women: A clinical pathologic study of 201 cases in the Louisville registry. In Feneglio CM, Wolff M. Progress in surgical pathology. New York: Masson Publishing, 1980:187–205.
46. Gupta SK, Das DK, Rajwanshi A, et al. Cytology of hepatocellular carcinoma. Diagn Cytopathol 1986;2:290–294.
47. Becker FF. Hepatoma—Nature's model tumor. Am J Pathol 1974;74:179–200.
47a. Christensen WN, Boitnott JK, Kuhajda FP. Immunoperoxidase staining as a diagnostic aid for hepatocellular carcinoma. Mod Pathol 1989;2:8–12.
48. Berman JJ, McNeill RE. Cirrhosis with atypia. A potential pitfall in the interpretation of liver aspirates. Acta Cytol 1988;32:11–14.
49. Atterbury CE, Enriquez RE, Desutonagy GI, Conn HO. Comparison of the histologic and cytologic diagnosis of liver biopsies in hepatic cancer. Gastroenterology 1979;76:1352–1357.
50. Craig JR, Peters RL, Edmondson HA, Omata M. Fibrolamellar carcinoma of the liver: A tumor of adolescents and young adults with distinctive clinico-pathologic features. Cancer 1980;46:372–379.
51. Berman MM, Libbey NP, Foster JF. Hepatocellular carcinoma: Polygonal cell type with fibrous stroma. An atypical variant with a favorable prognosis. Cancer 1980;46:1448–1455.
52. Farhi DC, Shikes RH, Silverberg SG. Ultrastructure of fibrolamella oncocytic hepatoma. Cancer 1982;50:702–709.
53. Ishak KG, Glunz PR. Hepatoblastoma and hepatocarcinoma in infancy and childhood. Report of 47 cases. Cancer 1967;20:396–422.
54. Bhatia A, Mehrotra P. Fine needle aspiration cytology in a case of hepatoblastoma. Acta Cytol 1986;30:439–441.
55. Dekmezian R, Sneige N, Popok S, Ordonez NG. Fine needle aspiration cytology of pediatric patients with primary hepatic tumors: A comparative study of two hepatoblastomas and a liver cell carcinoma. Diagn Cytopathol 1988;4:162–168.
56. Edmondson HA, Peters RL. Liver. In Kissane JM. Anderson's pathology, Vol. 2. St. Louis: CV Mosby, 1985:1194.
57. Dehner LP. Hepatic tumors in the pediatric age group. A distinctive clinicopathologic spectrum. In Rosenberg HS, Bolande RP. Pediatric pathology, Vol. 4. Chicago: Year Book Medical Publishers, 1978:217.
58. Stout AP. Tumors of soft tissues. Atlas of tumor pathology. Washington D.C.: Armed Forces Institute of Pathology, 1953:118.

59. Pieterse AS, Smith M, Smith LA, Smith P. Embryonal (undifferentiated) sarcoma of the liver. Fine-needle aspiration cytology and ultrastructural findings. Arch Pathol Lab Med 1985;109:677–680.

60. Popper H, Thomas LB, Telles NC, Falk H, Selikoff IJ. Development of hepatic angiosarcoma in man induced by vinyl chloride, Thorotrast, and arsenic. Am J Pathol 1978;92:349–369.

61. Nguyen GK, McHattie JD, Jeannot A. Cytomorphologic aspects of hepatic angiosarcoma: Fine-needle aspiration biopsy of a case. Acta Cytol 1982;26:527–531.

62. Bloustein PA. Surgical diseases of the liver. In Silverberg SG. Principles and practice of surgical pathology, Vol. 2. New York: John Wiley & Sons, 1983:995–1015.

63. Didolkar MS, Fanous N, Elias EG, et al. Metastatic carcinomas from occult primary tumors. A study of 254 patients. Ann Surg 1977;186:625–630.

64. Osteen RT, Kopf G, Wilson RE. In pursuit of the unknown primary. Am J Surg 1978;135:494–498.

65. Carney CN. Cytology and liver biopsy [Correspondence]. Gastroenterology 1980;78:1119.

66. Palmer PE, Christopherson WM, Wolfe HJ. Alpha-1–antitrypsin, protein marker in oral contraceptive-associated hepatic tumors. Am J Clin Pathol 1977;68:736–739.

67. Wetzel WJ, Alexander RW. Focal nodular hyperplasia of the liver with alcoholic hyalin bodies and cytologic atypia. Cancer 1979;44:1322–1326.

68. Ishak KG, Rabin L. Benign tumors of the liver. Med Clin N Am 1975;59:995–1013.

69. Itai Y, Ohtomo K, Araki T, et al. Computed tomography and sonography of cavernous hemangioma of the liver. Am J Roentgenol 1983;141:315–320.

70. Brant WE, Floyd JL, Jackson DE, Gilliland JD. The radiological evaluation of hepatic cavernous hemangioma. JAMA 1987;257:2471–2474.

71. Taavitsainew M, Kivisaari L. Is fine needle biopsy of liver hemangioma hazardous? AJR 1987;148:231–232.

72. Takagi H, Kido C, Morimoto T, et al. Surgical treatment of hepatic cavernous hemangioma. J Surg Oncol 1984;26:91–99.

73. Solbiati L, Livraghi T, DePra L, et al. Fine-needle biopsy of hepatic hemangioma with sonographic guidance. AJR 1985;144:471–474.

74. Vercelli-Retta J, Manana G, Reissenweber NJ. The cytologic diagnosis of hydatid disease. Acta Cytol 1982;26:159–164.

75. Dent GA, Feldman JM. Pseudocystic liver metastases in patients with carcinoid tumors: Reports of three cases. Am J Clin Pathol 1984;82:275–279.

76. Stormby N, Akerman M. Aspiration cytology in the diagnosis of granulomatous liver lesions. Acta Cytol 1973;17:200–204.

77. Orell SR, Sterrett GF, Walters MNI, Whitaker D. Manual and atlas of fine needle aspiration cytology. Edinburgh: Churchill Livingstone, 1986:171

10

Pancreas

Cancer of the pancreas is now the fourth most common cause of cancer deaths in men and the fifth most common in women, and its incidence is increasing.[1,2] Ultrasonography and computed tomography (CT) are currently the most sensitive noninvasive tests for investigating patients suspected of having a pancreatic tumor. Ultrasonography is preferable to CT as the first line of investigation because the former does not entail ionizing radiation and is less costly and less time consuming. Once a pancreatic mass is visualized by one of the imaging techniques, a preoperative morphologic diagnosis can be obtained by a percutaneous fine needle aspiration biopsy. Similarly, enlarged peripancreatic lymph nodes can be targeted and aspirated without much difficulty. Intraoperative FNAB[3-5] can also replace intraoperative surgical biopsy, which carries a higher risk of complications, such as pancreatitis, thrombosis, and fistula formation.[6,7]

Reported sensitivity of FNAB for the detection of pancreatic cancer ranges from 64 to 100%, with an average of 80.5%.[3-5,8-12b] Increased operator experience improves sensitivity.[13] Hajdu et al.[12] have reported the largest series, consisting of 126 cases, in which the sensitivity was 97%, specificity 100%, and predictive value 100%. When cytologic examination was combined with carcinoembryonic antigen assay of the aspirated material, the diagnostic accuracy rate reached 100%.[14]

NORMAL CYTOLOGY

Ductal epithelial cells are columnar or cuboidal in shape. The nuclei are round, bland, and basal, with small or inconspicuous nucleoli. The cytoplasm is pale and finely vacuolated. The cells are typically arranged in monolayer sheets of various sizes, which exhibit a regular honeycomb appearance when seen en face and a palisade arrangement when seen from the side (**Fig. 10.1**).

The acinar cells are small, oval to round cells, and arranged in well-defined cohesive acinar groups (**Fig. 10.2**). The uniform nuclei are slightly eccentric, and the cytoplasm is cyanophilic and granulated.

Islet cells are similar in size to acinar cells and are usually not identifiable in smears. Special staining technique may be used to enhance their identification. When stained with the periodic acid-Schiff (PAS)-Trichrome technique,[15] the β cells appear pale yellow-green with yellow-orange granules, the δ cells exhibit translucent green cytoplasm, and the α cells have a deep orange cytoplasm.

Mesothelial cells and hepatocytes may be seen and their morphologies are described in Chapters 7 and 9, respectively.

NEOPLASMS OF DUCT AND DUCTULE CELLS
Adenocarcinoma

The most common pancreatic malignancy is an adenocarcinoma arising from the epithelial cells of the pancreatic ducts. It constitutes about 75–80% of all pancreatic malignancies. The prognosis is poor; the 5–year mortality is greater than 90%.[16] Histologically, most adenocarcinomas are well to moderately differentiated and the neoplastic cells resemble to a variable extent the duct or ductule epithelial cells (**Fig. 10.3**). The malignant cells lining the ducts show considerable stratification, nuclear atypia, and loss of nuclear polarity. The following growth patterns are common: glandular, papillary, and solid.

Aspiration Cytology

Cellular Pattern. The aspirates are usually hypercellular, except when the tumor is desmoplastic, in which case tumor cells may not be easily aspirated. In well-differentiated adenocarcinomas (**Figs. 10.4** and **10.5**), glandular or papillary tissue fragments are readily apparent. In less differentiated tumors (**Fig. 10.6**), there are more architectural disorganization and more dissociated cells. Necrotic debris may be conspicuous in the background.

Cell Morphology. The tumor cells vary from tall columnar to cuboidal. The cytoplasm varies from pale or mucin-secreting to densely eosinophilic. Cells from well-differentiated adenocarcinoma (**Figs. 10.4** and **10.5**) may exhibit only minimal atypia, but there is a notable increase in cell and nuclear size, cell crowding, and architectural disarray. In less-differentiated adenocarcinomas (**Fig. 10.6**), macronucleoli, marked anisocytosis, nuclear membrane irregularity, and chromatin clumping are commonly seen.

Diagnostic Pitfalls. Well-differentiated adenocarcinoma and reactive ductal hyperplasia may resemble each other on FNAB. Most of the diagnostic errors are false-negative diagnoses, which occur because: *(a)* a well-differentiated adenocarcinoma was misinterpreted as a reactive process, *(b)* material from chronic pancreatitis adjacent to the tumor is aspirated, or *(c)* the needle is deflected by a desmoplastic tumor. If malignancy is suspected, several samples from different areas of the lesion must be obtained in order to minimize the likelihood of a false-negative result. On the other hand, to avoid overcalling reactive ductal cells as adenocarcinoma, one must be familiar with the cytologic criteria for adenocarcinoma. According to Mitchell and Carney,[9] the most useful criteria for diagnosing pancreatic adenocarcinoma are irregular nuclear contour, extreme nuclear enlargement, and disoriented or crowded cells in three-dimensional groups (**Table 10 .1**).

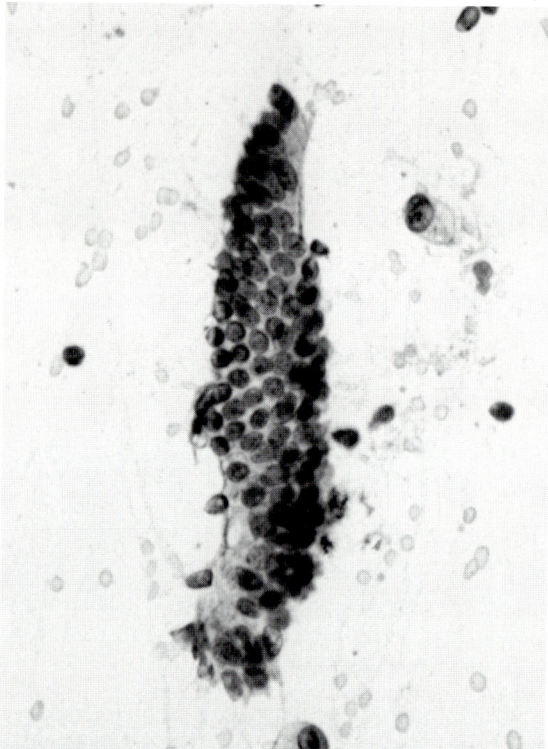

Figure 10.1. Normal pancreatic ductal epithelium, ABC. En face cells have a cobblestone arrangement, and peripheral cells seen from the side have columnar configuration and palisade arrangement. ×310.

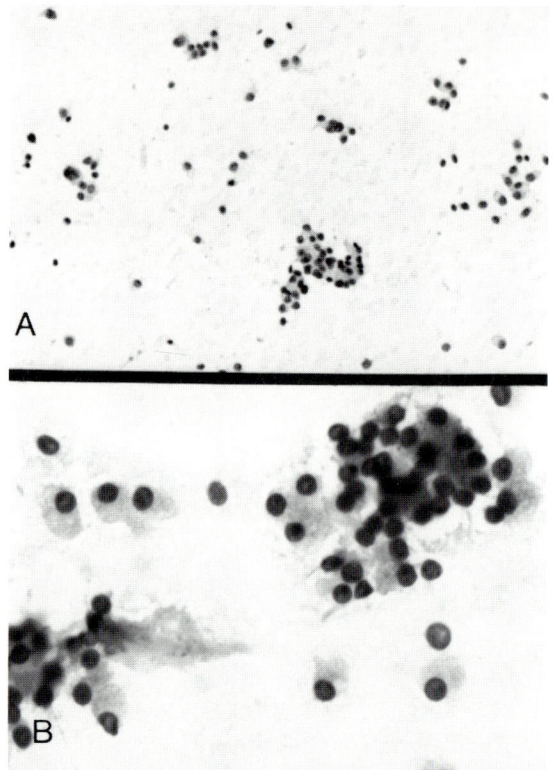

Figure 10.2. Normal acinar cells, ABC. **A** and **B,** Note single cells and acinar units. The cells have small, uniform, polar nuclei and granular cytoplasm. **A,** ×125; **B,** ×310.

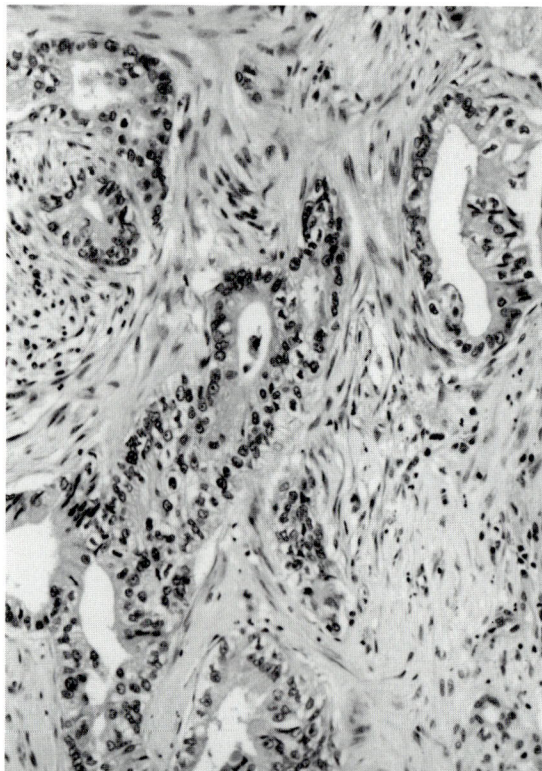

Figure 10.3. Histology of well-differentiated adenocarcinoma of the pancreas, with desmoplasia. ×310.

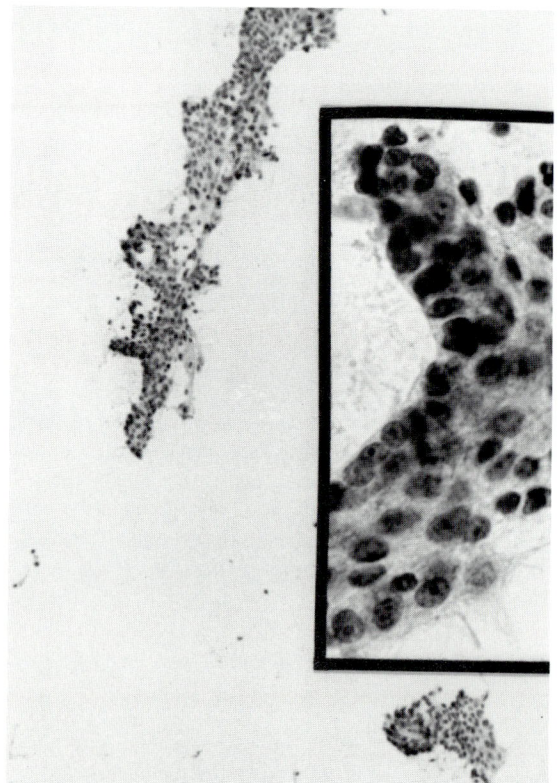

Figure 10.4. Well-differentiated adenocarcinoma, ABC. Low-power view showing two tissue fragments with a glandular pattern. *Inset* shows the close-up view of the columnar cells with nuclear palisading and crowding. (Compare **Figure 10.1.**) ×125; *inset,* ×500.

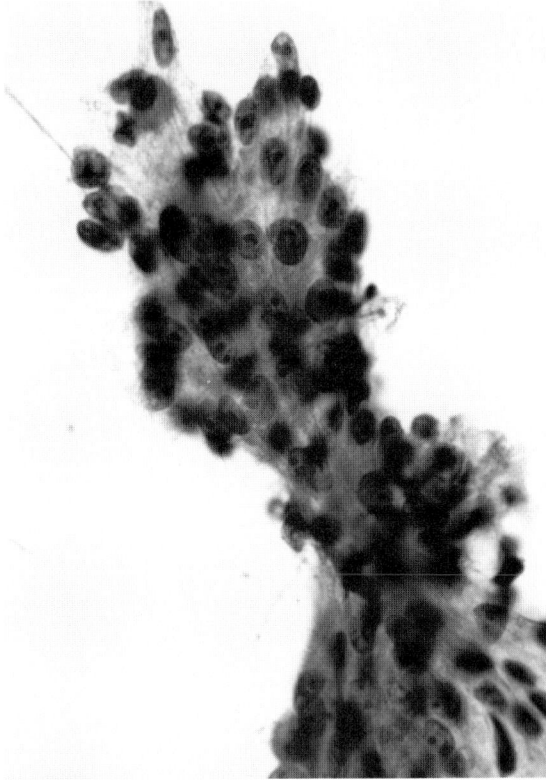

Figure 10.5. Well-differentiated adenocarcinoma, ABC. Note enlarged tumor cells in three-dimensional acinar arrangement, and prominent nucleoli. ×500.

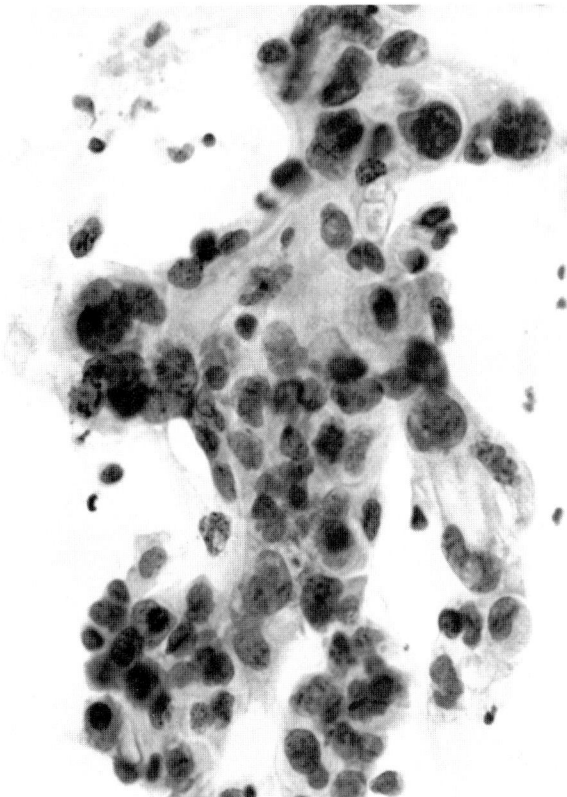

Figure 10.6. Moderately differentiated adenocarcinoma, ABC. Note nuclear enlargement with increased nuclear pleomorphism, and disorganized acinar structures. ×500.

TABLE 10.1.   ABC Criteria for Pancreatic Adenocarcinoma[a]

(Listed in order of importance)
Disoriented or crowded cells in three-dimensional groups
Extreme nuclear enlargement with nuclear contour irregularity
Extreme nuclear enlargement
Nuclear contour irregularity
Uneven chromatin distribution
Anisonucleosis
Increased nuclear cytoplasmic ratio
Nucleolar prominence

[a] Proposed by Mitchell ML, Carney CN. Cytologic criteria for the diagnosis of pancreatic carcinoma. Am J Clin Pathol 1985;83:171–176.

Giant Cell Carcinoma

Giant cell carcinoma is an uncommon, highly malignant variant of ductal adenocarcinoma.[17,18] Most patients die with widespread metastases within weeks to a few months after diagnosis.

Aspirates are composed of malignant multinucleated giant cells with relatively dense cytoplasm, smaller polyhedral bizarre cells, and spindle cells (**Fig. 10.7**). Prominent tumor diathesis and neutrophilic infiltrate in the background are common.

There is also a very rare form of giant cell carcinoma in which osteoclast-like giant cells are observed.[19]

Diagnostic Pitfalls.   A retroperitoneal sarcoma is often included in the differential diagnosis of giant cell carcinoma of the pancreas. The problem may be solved if tumor cells with glandular differentiation or tissue fragments with a glandular pattern are identified; otherwise, immunoperoxidase studies to demonstrate cytoplasmic keratin and electron microscopy to demonstrate the epithelial nature of the tumor are helpful.[20]

Cystic Neoplasms of the Pancreas

Within the group of uncommon cystic neoplasms of the pancreas, two types can be distinguished: a microcystic type, which shows multiple small cysts lined by low cuboidal serous epithelium, and a macrocystic type, which shows larger mucus-filled cysts lined by tall columnar mucus-secreting cells, resembling cells of pancreatic duct epithelium or intestinal epithelium. The microcystic type (also known as serous cystadenoma or microcystic adenoma) is invariably benign, while the mucinous cystic neoplasm can be benign or malignant.[21,22] In all cases of mucinous cystadenoma, multiple histologic sections must be taken to exclude a focus of malignant change, which has been estimated to exist in as many as 42% of cases.[23] Since one cannot rule out a focus of adenocarcinoma until the entire mucinous cystic tumor is excised and examined, it is advisable to designate these tumors noncommittally on biopsy material as "mucinous cystic neoplasm." Separating mucinous and serous cystic neoplasms is important because mucinous cystic neoplasms need to be totally excised, whether or not malignant cells are identified in the aspirates. Serous cystadenomas, on the other hand, have no capacity for malignant transformation. They probably can be treated by internal drainage or marsupialization, especially in elderly persons who constitute a majority of those affected.[21] Furthermore, it is important to distinguish mucinous cystadenocarcinoma from the ordinary ductal adenocarcinoma, as the former represents one of the few surgically curable malignancies of the pancreas.[22] If FNAB incorrectly reports mucinous cystadenocarcinoma as duct adenocarcinoma, the dismal prognosis associated with the latter may discourage the surgeon to carry out an aggressive curative operation.

Aspiration Cytology

The ABC of each of the two types of cystic neoplasms of the pancreas is quite distinctive.[24–27] Aspirates of microcystic adenomas (**Fig. 10.8**) show scattered small groups of uniform cuboidal or polygonal cells with clear cytoplasm, which contain glycogen but little or no mucin. The nuclei are dark staining but do not show an atypical chromatin pattern. The smear background is clean or watery and devoid of mucin.

Aspirates of mucinous cystic neoplasms characteristically show a large amount of mucus, observed both macroscopically when the smears are spread, and microscopically, where it can be seen within the cells as well as extracellularly in the background.[25] There are many tall columnar mucin-secreting cells, arranged in sheets, gland-like clusters, or papillae. The morphology of the tumor cells varies from benign-appearing cells with bland basal nuclei in cystadenoma (**Fig. 10.9**) to malignant glandular cells in cystadenocarcinoma (**Fig. 10.10**).

Diagnostic Pitfalls.   The diagnostic challenges confronting the cytopathologist are (a) to differentiate the neoplastic epithelium from normal epithelium of the bowel and pancreatic ducts, and (b) to differentiate cystic neoplasms from the more common pseudocysts.

Since the neoplastic cells from many cystic neoplasms of the pancreas are benign-appearing, they must be distinguished from normal pancreatic duct epithelium or bowel epithelium. Atypical or overtly malignant cells, if seen, indicate that there is a dysplastic or malignant lesion and essentially rule out normal mucosal epithelium. A complex papillogandular pattern or presence of micropapillae is consistent with neoplasm even though the individual cells may resemble normal epithelium.[24] Problems arise, however, when the aspirate consists of a small number of benign epithelial cells and no papillary structures are seen. Under such circumstances, the radiographic demonstration of a pancreatic cyst and the assurance by an experienced radiologist that the aspiration is taken from the lesion, combined with the cytologic observation, should alert the pathologist to the possibility of a cystic neoplasm.

Another diagnostic problem is the separation of cystic neoplasms from the more common inflammatory pseudocyst. The latter is nonneoplastic and a true epithelial lining is lacking. A history of pancreatitis may be elicited from the patient. Aspirates show acute inflammatory cells and granulation tissue (see "Pancreatic Pseudocysts").

NEOPLASMS OF ACINAR CELL ORIGIN
Acinar Cell Carcinoma

Acinar cell carcinoma is an uncommon cancer, accounting for no more than 1–2% of pancreatic cancers. It typically occurs in elderly people, with no sex predilection.[16] Histologically, the tumor shows a well-differentiated acinic pattern, but undifferentiated solid areas can also be seen.[28]

The aspirates are cellular. The tumor cells resemble pancreatic acinar cells, having polar nuclei and faintly granular cytoplasm. There are varying degrees of nuclear atypia and prominent nucleoli in some cells. The cells occur in disorganized clusters and acinar groups (**Fig. 10.11**). Differential diagnosis must include tumors from the islet cell-carcinoid spectrum.[29,29a] The uniform nuclei and the evenly distributed nuclear chromatin of the islet cell-carcinoid group tumors are helpful features that distinguish them from acinar cell carcinoma, whose nuclei are more pleomorphic. In practice, some islet cell and carcinoid tumors also show less than uniform nuclei; therefore, light microscopic differentiation of these tumors from acinic cell carcinoma may be difficult. The use of special stains, immunocytochem-

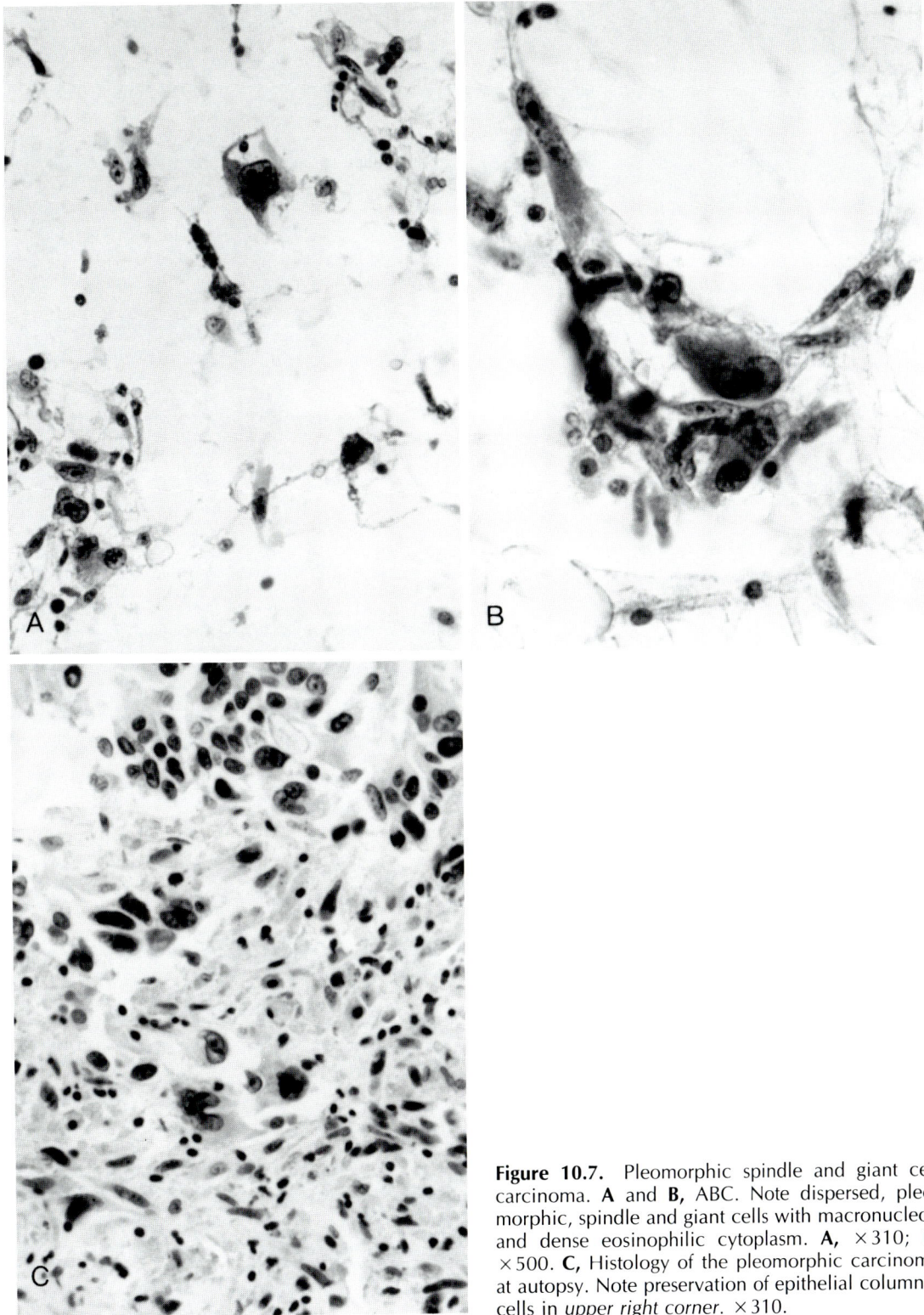

Figure 10.7. Pleomorphic spindle and giant cell carcinoma. **A** and **B,** ABC. Note dispersed, pleomorphic, spindle and giant cells with macronucleoli and dense eosinophilic cytoplasm. **A,** ×310; **B,** ×500. **C,** Histology of the pleomorphic carcinoma at autopsy. Note preservation of epithelial columnar cells in *upper right corner.* ×310.

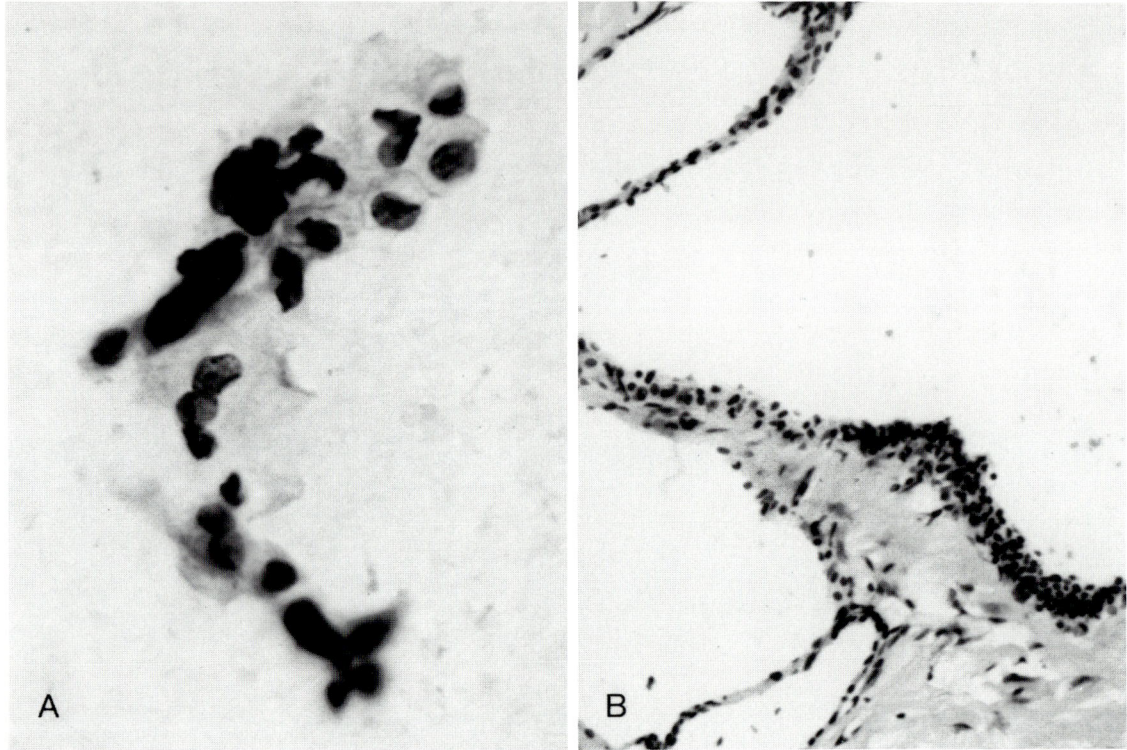

Figure 10.8.

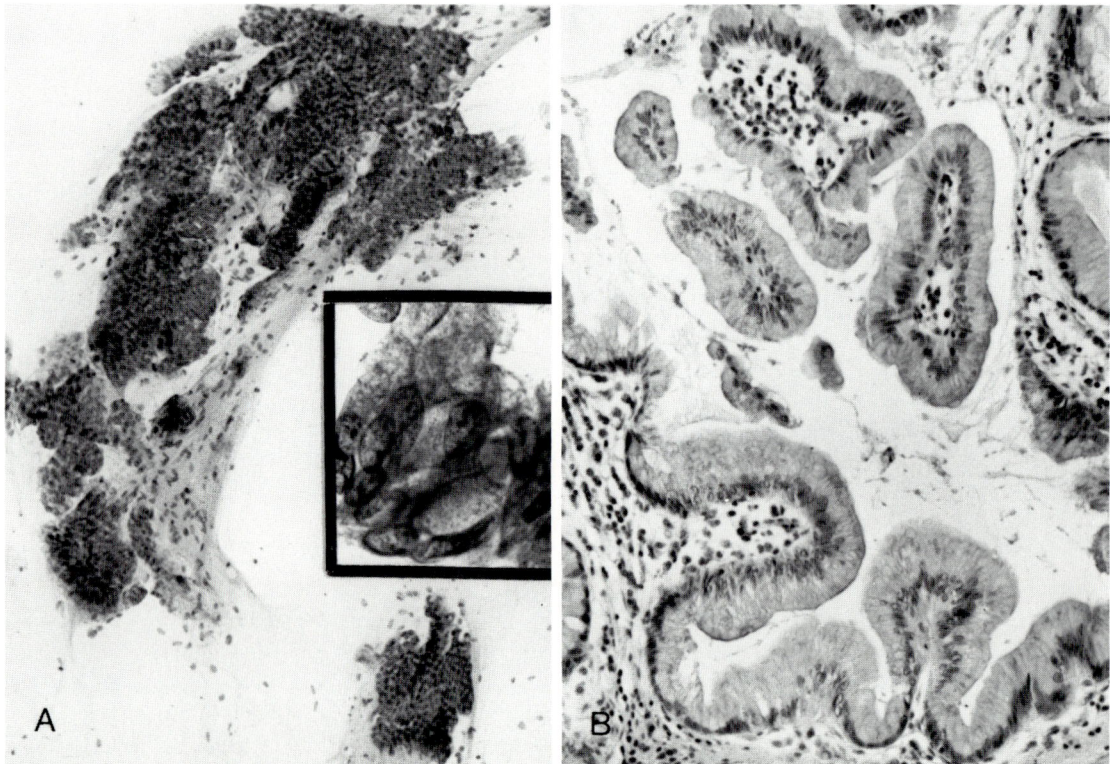

Figure 10.9.

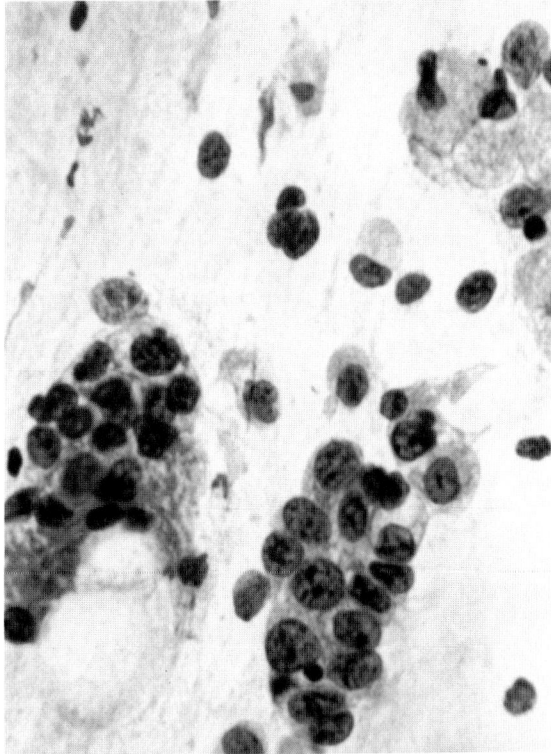

Figure 10.10. Malignant mucinous cystic neoplasm (cystaden-ocarcinoma), ABC. Note mucinous columnar cells of cytologically low-grade malignancy. Also note extracellular mucin in background. ×500.

Figure 10.8. Microcystic adenoma. **A,** ABC. Note a ribbon of cohesive cuboidal cells with clear cytoplasm, corresponding to the epithelial lining cells of the microcysts. Also note clean background. ×500. **B,** Histology of microcystic adenoma. Note similarity of the cells in the aspirate and the cells lining the microcysts. ×310.

Figure 10.9. Mucinous cystic neoplasm, benign. **A,** ABC. Large tissue fragments with a complex papilloglandular pattern. *Inset,* Detail of the benign columnar cells with bland, basal nuclei. Note intracellular and extracellular mucin. ×125; *inset,* ×500. **B,** Histologic section of the mucinous cystic neoplasm showing similar benign columnar epithelium. ×310.

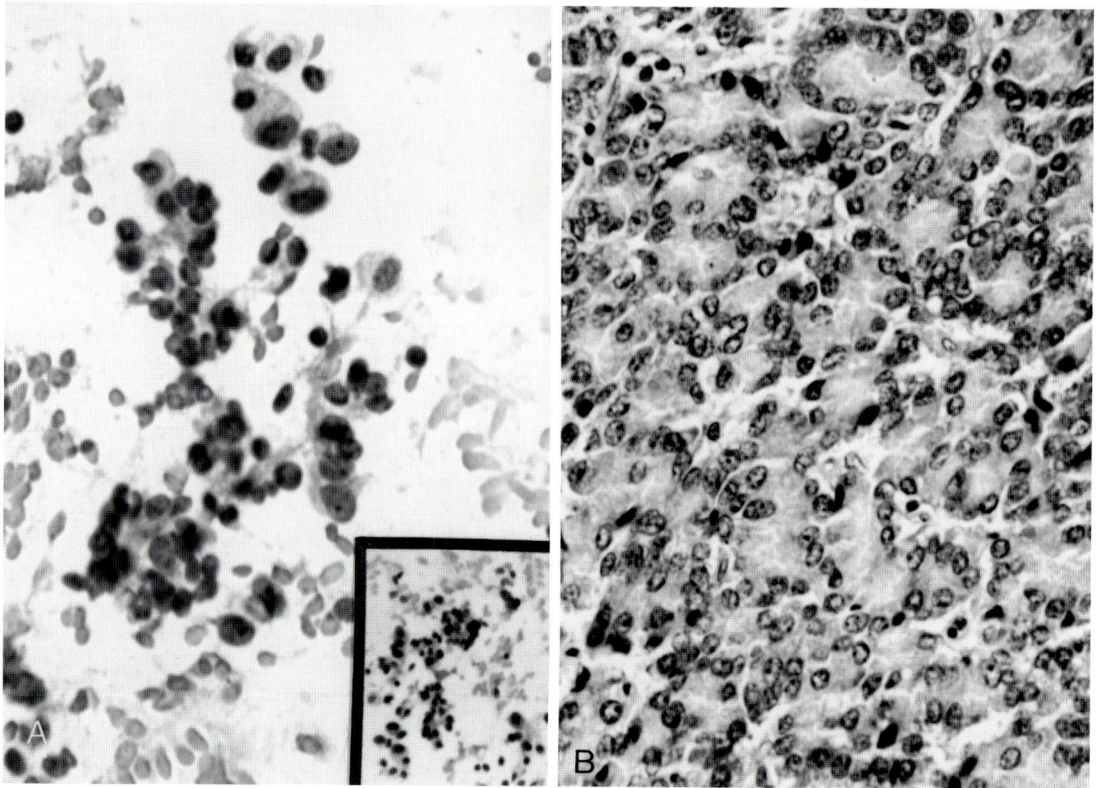

Figure 10.11. Acinar cell carcinoma. **A,** ABC. Tumor cells are arranged in abortive acini. Note polar nuclei, slight to moderate nuclear pleomorphism, and distinct nucleoli. ×500; *inset,* ×125. **B,** Histology of acinar cell carcinoma. Note nuclear pleomorphism. ×310. (Courtesy of Sudha R. Kini, M.D., Henry Ford Hospital, Detroit.)

Figure 10.12. Histology of papillary-cystic neoplasm of the pancreas. Note microcystic spaces, pseudorosettes, and resemblance to carcinoid tumor. However, electron microscopic examination of this tumor shows neither zymogen nor neurosecretory granules. ×125.

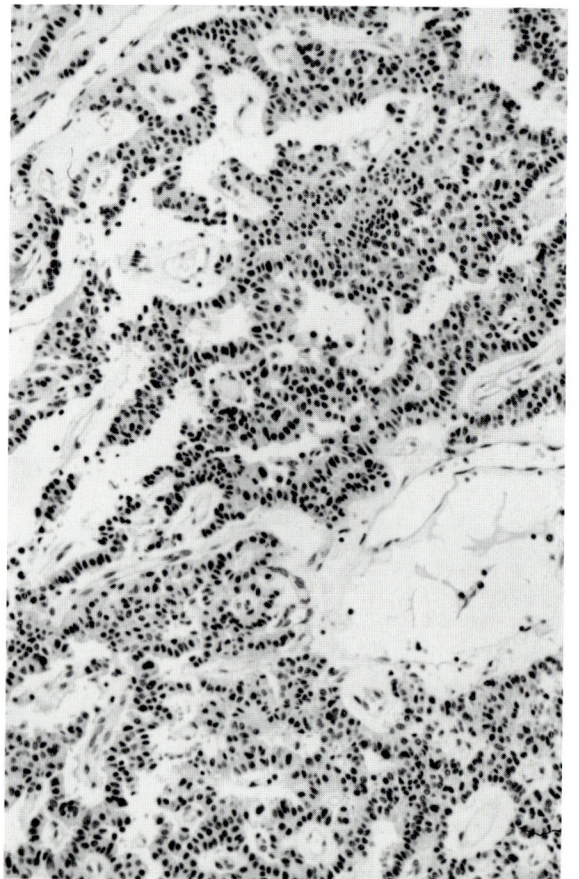

Figure 10.12.

istry, and/or electron microscopy facilitates the diagnosis (see "Islet Cell Tumor").

Papillary-Cystic Neoplasm

Papillary-cystic neoplasm (PCN) is an uncommon, interesting tumor that occurs mostly in adolescent and young adult females.[16] It is a low-grade carcinoma with a favorable prognosis if completely resected. The histogenesis of this tumor remains controversial. Ultrastructural studies show rudimentary acinar formation and zymogen-like granules in some cases,[30] while demonstration of somatostatin immunoreactivity in other cases suggests a relation to islet cells.[31] It seems probable that these tumors may represent neoplasms of intermediate cells capable of both acinar and endocrine differentiation.[32]

The histology of PCN (Fig. 10.12) somewhat resembles islet cell tumor (discussed below). The tumor cells are arranged in psuedorosettes around delicate fibrovascular stalks. Numerous small blood vessels traverse the neoplasm. Degeneration of those areas farthest away from the blood vessels appears to result in formation of microcystic spaces and papillae.

Aspiration Cytology

Cell Morphology.   The aspirates (Fig. 10.13) show a monomorphic population of small, oval cells with a variable amount of pale, eosinophilic cytoplasm. The round nuclei have uniform nuclear membranes and one or two small but rather conspicuous nucleoli. Nuclear chromatin is finely dispersed.

Cellular Pattern.   The ABC exhibits a high cellularity. Pseudorosette formations and clusters of cells grouped like bunches of grapes are evident (Fig. 10.13A). Another characteristic pattern is papillary clusters of cells arranged around a vascular core (Fig. 10.13B).

Diagnostic Pitfalls.   Although papillary-cystic neoplasms of the pancreas have been diagnosed by FNAB,[33–35] the cytohistologic features of PCN, acinar cell carcinoma, and islet cell tumor are remarkably similar. In FNAB, papillary and grape-like clusters with blood vessels traversing the tumor seem to distinguish PCN from the two other neoplasms.[33,34] Yet even on frozen section examination, PCN has been diagnosed erroneously as endocrine tumor.[30]

Kini[29] has realistically pointed out that even though absolute classification of these neoplasms may not be possible on FNAB, a presumptive diagnosis of neoplasm is feasible and useful differential diagnosis can be given. Clinically, PCN occurs in young women and tends to be localized; acinar cell carcinoma occurs in the elderly and often metastasizes by the time of diagnosis; islet cell tumor may be hormonally active.

NEOPLASMS OF ENDOCRINE PANCREAS
Islet Cell Tumor

Islet cell tumors are relatively rare neoplasms compared to pancreatic adenocarcinomas. They may be hormonally active or inactive, and belong to the group of APUD (amine precursor uptake and decarboxylation) tumors capable of producing a variety of polypeptide hormones and certain amines. Depending on the type of hormones secreted, islet cell tumors may have diverse clinical presentations, such as Zollinger-Ellison syndrome in the case of gastrinoma, hypoglycemia in insulinoma, and hyperglycemia in glucagonoma. However, the morphologic features of islet cell tumors arising from different functional cell types are similar and are identical to those of carcinoid tumor. The ABC of islet cell tumor has been reported by various authors.[36–38]

Aspiration Cytology

Cell Morphology.   The smears are cellular, with a monomorphic cell population. The tumor cells (Fig. 10.14) are small to medium in size, with rounded regular nuclei and finely granular chromatin. Nucleoli may be present but small. The cytoplasm is moderately abundant and pale to finely granular. Single, larger cells with hyperchromatic nuclei may sometimes occur among the smaller cells.

Cellular Pattern.   The tumor cells are dispersed singly as well as arranged in various patterns characteristic of neuroendocrine tumors: mosaic, insular, ribbon, and acinar (Fig. 10.14). These patterns are illustrated in detail elsewhere (see Chapters 7 and 11).

Special Procedures.   Great advances have been made in recent years in the precise diagnosis of islet cell tumors. The traditional Grimelius silver impregnation stain,[39] which demonstrates cytoplasmic neuroendocrine granules (see Fig. 11.14B, inset), is now only part of a panel of studies used, which also include immunocytochemistry and electron microscopy. Sensitive and specific monoclonal antibodies are used to stain tumor cells for various specific peptides, such as insulin, glucagon, somatostatin, and gastrin.[36] An antibody against neuron-specific enolase (NSE), a sensitive, but nonspecific, marker of the neuroendocrine system, can also be used.[36] Despite NSE nonspecificity, it is a reliable test if it is judiciously interpreted along with the clinical and light microscopic findings. Finally, electron microscopy can be used to demonstrate the presence of membrane-bound, dense-core neurosecretory granules (see Fig. 13.12).

Diagnostic Pitfalls.   Like carcinoid tumors in other sites, it is difficult to predict the biologic behavior of an islet cell tumor on morphologic grounds. Malignant potential is suggested by atypical mitoses, nuclear pleomorphism, macronucleoli, and necrosis. Generally, small tumors (<2 cm) that are surgically resectable have a favorable prognosis, whereas the larger ones are more likely to be malignant.[40]

As already discussed, islet cell tumor, acinar cell carcinoma, and papillary-cystic neoplasm of the pancreas may not be distinguishable on purely cytologic grounds, but a diagnosis of neoplasm can be rendered and aids the clinicians in planning surgery.[29]

Due to the small cell size and the uniformity of the cell population, islet cell tumor may be mistaken for normal acinar cells of the pancreas and vice versa. Normal acinar cells occur in regular, cohesive acini (Fig. 10.2); whereas islet cell tumor yields many loose aggregates of cells and disorganized acini.

INFLAMMATORY LESIONS
Pancreatitis

Acute pancreatitis, characterized by upper abdominal pain, shock, and metabolic disturbances, is a debilitating illness and the diagnosis is usually suspected on clinical grounds and comfirmed by a marked elevation of serum amylase. Percutaneous FNAB is therefore seldom carried out. Aspirates from such cases show acute inflammatory cells, macrophages, lipophages, reactive ductal epithelial cells, and calcified debris from fat necrosis.[41]

Chronic pancreatitis is the end result of recurrent attacks of acute inflammation. The disease is frequently associated with alcoholism or biliary tract disease. The pancreas becomes firm and nodular, and a mass simulating carcinoma may develop as a result of fibroblastic proliferation and repair reaction. FNAB is useful in separating pancreatic neoplasm from pancreatitis. The aspirates of chronic pancreatitis, unlike those obtained from carcinomas, are generally cell-poor. There are scattered inflammatory cells, consisting mainly

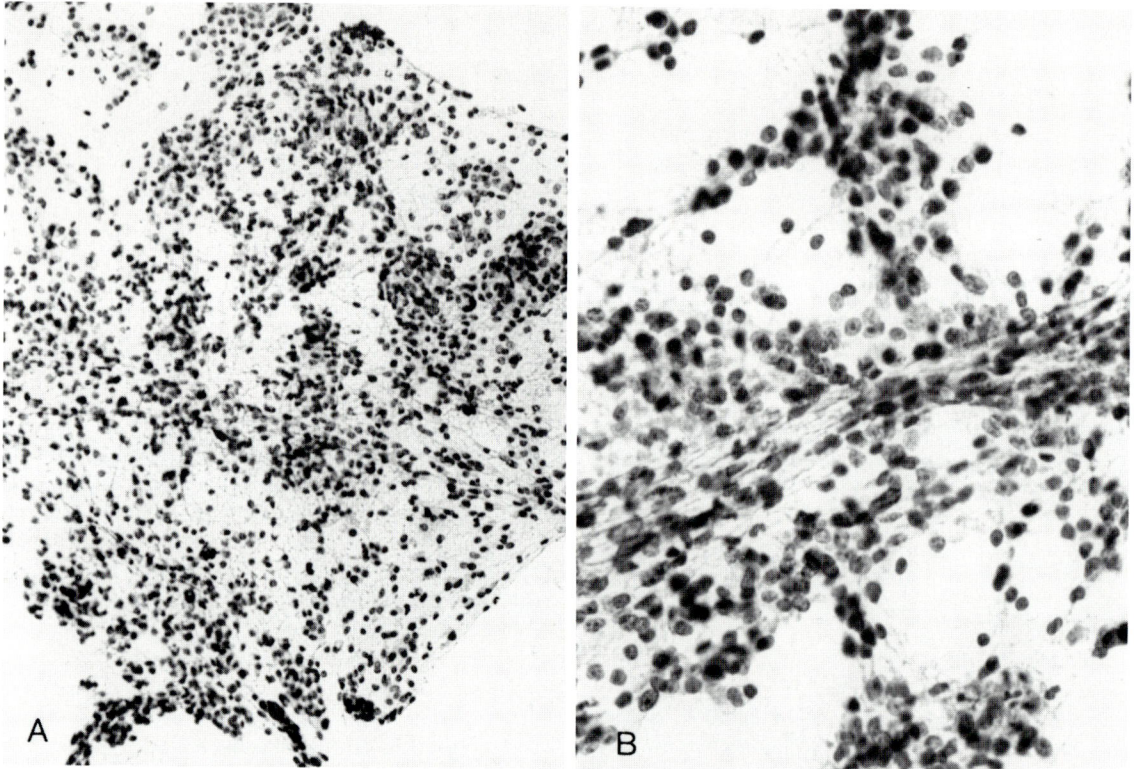

Figure 10.13.   Papillary-cystic neoplasm, ABC. **A,** Note pronounced cellularity and the uniform round cells arranged like bunches of grapes.   ×125. **B,** Papillary clusters and pseudorosettes around a central blood vessel (running across the *middle* of the photomicrograph).   ×310.

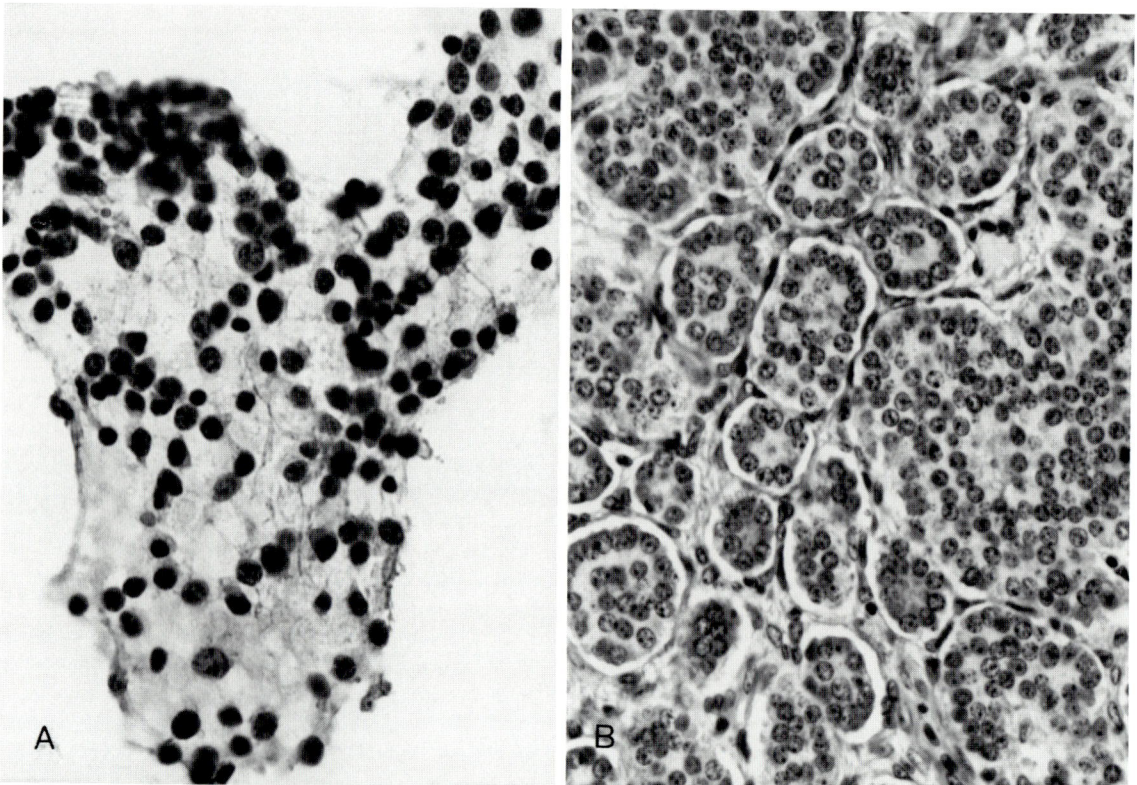

Figure 10.14.   Islet cell tumor. **A,** ABC. Note uniform cells in acinar arrangement. There are occasional larger atypical cells.   ×500. **B,** Histology of islet cell tumor showing an acinar pattern of uniform, round to oval cells.   ×310.

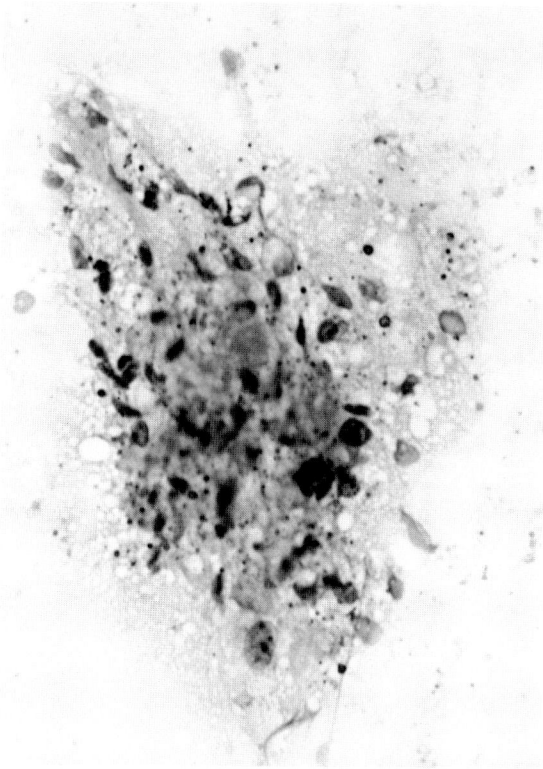

Figure 10.15. Pseudocyst, ABC. Fragment of granulation tissue composed of fibroblastic cells and macrophages. The numerous scattered pigment granules are hemosiderin. × 310.

of lymphocytes, plasma cells, and macrophages. In acute exacerbation, neutrophils are also present. To make certain that a carcinoma is not missed, representative aspirates from different areas of the lesion must be obtained.

Pancreatic Pseudocyst

A pancreatic pseudocyst is not a true epithelium-lined cyst, but a collection of necrotic debris, enzyme-rich fluid, and blood, confined by fibrous connective tissue and granulation tissue. Pseudocysts develop as a late complication of acute pancreatitis or develop in acute exacerbation of chronic pancreatitis. Occasionally, a pseudocyst may be a sequela to blunt trauma to the abdomen. Because pseudocysts of the pancreas present as a mass, they are considered in the differential diagnosis of pancreatic neoplasms, especially the cystic neoplasms.

Aspiration Cytology

The fluid aspirated from these cysts varies in amount, ranging from a few milliliters to several liters. It may be clear, turbid, or hemorrhagic. The ABC reveals amorphous debris, calcified particles, a few inflammatory cells, reactive fibrocytes, and macrophages **(Fig. 10.15)**.

Diagnostic Pitfalls. The pseudocyst must be differentiated from the microcystic adenoma and mucinous cystic neoplasm. One expects to see groups of cuboidal epithelial cells with clear cytoplasm in microcystic adenomas and mucin-producing columnar cells in mucinous cystic neoplasm. Since the wall of a pseudocyst has no epithelial lining, the finding of epithelial cells in the aspirate should, in theory, rule out a pseudocyst.[26] However, problems arise when reactive ductal epithelium from areas adjacent to the pseudocyst are also included in the aspirates. In general, inflammatory cells should be the dominating cellular elements in pseudocyst aspirates, and a history of pancreatitis can often be elicited from the patient.

Amylase and carcinoembryonic antigen (CEA) assays of the aspirated fluid aid in differentiating neoplastic cyst from pseudocyst. An elevated fluid CEA over 60 ng/ml is specific for cystic neoplasm, while an elevated amylase (of up to 421,000 units/liter) and negative CEA (<0.5 ng/ml) suggests pseudocyst.[42]

References

1. Wynder E, Mabuchi K, Maruchi N, Fortner JG. Epidemiology of cancer of the pancreas. J Natl Cancer Inst 1973;50:647–667.

2. Hermann RE, Cooperman AM. Current concepts in cancer: Cancer of the pancreas. N Engl J Med 1979;301:482–485.

3. Arnesjo B, Stormby N, Akerman M. Cytodiagnosis of pancreatic lesions by means of fine needle biopsy during operation. Acta Chir Scand 1972;138;363–369.

4. Kline TS, Abramson J, Goldstein F, Neal HS. Needle aspiration biopsy of the pancreas at laparotomy. Am J Gastroenterol 1977;68:30–33.

5. An-Foraker SH, Fong-Mui KK. Cytodiagnosis of lesions of the pancreas and related areas. Acta Cytol 1982;26:814–818.

6. Lightwood R, Reber HA, Way LW. The risk and accuracy of pancreatic biopsy. Am J Surg 1976;132:189–194.

7. Schultz NJ, Sanders RJ. Evaluation of pancreatic biopsy. Ann Surg 1963;158:1053–1057.

8. Yamamoto R, Tatauta M, Noguchi S, et al. Histocytologic diagnosis of pancreatic cancer by percutaneous aspiration biopsy under ultrasonic guidance. Am J Clin Pathol 1985;83:1985.

9. Mitchell ML, Carney CN. Cytologic criteria for the diagnosis of pancreatic carcinoma. Am J Clin Pathol 1985;83:171–176.

10. Bret PM, Nicolet V, Michel L. Percutaneous fine needle aspiration biopsy of the pancreas. Diagn Cytopathol 1986;2:221–227.

11. Grant EG, Richardson JD, Smirniotopoulos JG, Jacobs NM. Fine needle biopsy directed by real-time sonography; technique and accuracy. AJR 1983;141:29–32.

12. Hajdu EO, Kumari-Subaiya S, Phillips G: Ultrasonically guided percutaneous aspiration biopsy of the pancreas. Semin Diagn Pathol 3:166–175, 1986.

12a. Mitchell ML, Bittner CA, Wills JS, Parker FP. Fine needle aspiration cytology of the pancreas. A retrospective study of 73 cases. Acta Cytol 1988;32:447–451.

12b. Al-Kaisi N, Siegler EE. Fine needle aspiration cytology of the pancreas. Acta Cytol 1989;33:145–152.

13. Goldstein H, Zornoza J. Percutaneous transperitoneal aspiration biopsy of pancreatic masses. Dig Dis 1978;23:840–843.

14. Tatsuta M, Yamamoto R, Yamamura H, Okuda S, Tamura H. Cytologic examination and CEA measurement in aspirated pancreatic material collected by percutaneous fine needle aspiration biopsy under guidance for the diagnosis of pancreatic carcinoma. Cancer 1983;52:693–698.

15. Hidvegi D, Nieman HL, DeMay RM, Jones W. Percutaneous transperitoneal aspiration of pancreas guided by ultrasound: Morphologic and cytochemical appearance of normal and malignant cells. Acta Cytol 1979;23:181–184.

16. Cubilla AL, Fitzgerald PJ. Cancer of the exocrine pancreas; the pathologic aspects. CA 1985;35:2–18.

17. Pinto MM, Monteiro NL, Tizol DM. Fine needle aspiration of pleomorphic giant-cell carcinoma of the pancreas. Acta Cytol 1986;30:430–433.

18. Silverman JF, Dabbs DJ, Finley JL, Geisinger KR. Fine needle aspiration biopsy of anaplastic (pleomorphic) malignant tumors of the pancreas: Cytologic, immunocytochemical and ultrastructural findings. Acta Cytol 1987;31:663–664.

19. Manci EA, Gardner LL, Pollock WJ, Dowling EA. Osteoclastic giant cell tumor of the pancreas. Aspiration cytology, light microscopy, and ultrastructure with review of the literature. Diagn Cytopathol 1985;1:105–110.

20. Cubilla AL, Fitzgerald PJ. Tumors of the exocrine pancreas. Atlas of tumor pathology, 2nd Series, Fascicle 19. Washington D.C.: Armed Forces Institute of Pathology, 1984:158–159.

21. Compagno J, Oertel JE. Microcystic adenomas of the pancreas (glycogen-rich cystadenomas). Am J Clin Pathol 1978;69:289–298.

22. Compagno J, Oertel JE. Mucinous cystic neoplasms of the pancreas with overt and latent malignancy (cystadenocarcinoma and cystadenoma). Am J Clin Pathol 1978;69:573–580.

23. Moossa AR, Dawson PJ, Franklin WA, Udekwu AO, Lavella-Jones M. Tumors of the pancreas. In Moossa AR, Robson MC, Schimpff SC. Comprehensive textbook of oncology. Baltimore: Williams & Wilkins, 1986:1107.

24. Jones EC, Suen KC, Grant DR, Chan NH. Fine-needle aspiration cytology of neoplastic cysts of the pancreas. Diagn Cytopathol 1987;3:238–243.

25. Vellet D, Leiman G, Mair S, Bilchik A. Fine needle aspiration cytology of mucinous cystadenocarcinoma of the pancreas. Acta Cytol 1988;32:43–48.

26. Emmert GM, Bewtra C. Fine-needle aspiration biopsy of mucinous cystic neoplasm of the pancreas: A case study. Diagn Cytopathol 1986;2:69–71.

27. Stormby N. Pancreas. In Zajicek J. Aspiration biopsy cytology. Part 2. Cytology of infradiaphragmatic organs. Basel: S Karger, 1979:206.

28. Rosai J. Ackerman's surgical pathology, 6th ed. St. Louis: CV Mosby, 1981:688

29. Kini SR. Aspiration biopsy cytology of unusual lesions of the pancreas. Am Soc Clin Pathol Check Sample 1984;12:4.

29a. Ishihara A, Sanda T, Takanari H, Yatani R, Liu PI. Elastase-1–secreting acinar cell carcinoma of the pancreas. Acta Cytol 1989;33:157–163.

30. Ladanyi M, Mulay S, Arseneau J, Bettez P. Estrogen and progesterone receptor determination in the papillary cystic neoplasms of the pancreas. Cancer 1987;60:1604–1611.

31. Mietinen M, Partanen S, Fraki O, Kivilaakso E. Papillary cystic tumor of the pancreas. An analysis of cellular differentiation by electron microscopy and immunohistochemistry. Am J Surg Pathol 1987;11:855–865.

32. Oertel JE, Mendelsohn G, Compagno J. Solid and papillary epithelial neoplasms of the pancreas. In Humphrey GB, Grindey GB, Dehner LP, Acton RT, Pysher TJ. Pancreatic tumors in children. The Hague: Martinus Nijhoff, 1982:167–171.

33. Foote A, Simpson JS, Stewart RJ, Wakefield JSJ, Buchanan A, Gupta RJ. Diagnosis of the rare solid and papillary epithelial neoplasm of the pancreas by fine needle aspiration cytology. Acta Cytol 1986;30:519–522.

34. Chen KTK, Workman DD, Efird TA, Cheng AC. Fine needle aspiration cytology diagnosis of papillary tumor of the pancreas. Acta Cytol 1986;30:523–527.

35. Bondeson L, Bondeson AG, Genell S, Lindholm K, Thorstenson S. Aspiration cytology of a rare solid and papillary epithelial neoplasm of the pancreas. Acta Cytol 1984;28:605–609.

36. Sneige N, Ordonez NG, Veanattukalathil S, Samaan NA. Fine needle aspiration cytology in pancreatic endocrine tumors. Diagn Cytol 1987;3:35–40.

37. Bell DA. Cytologic features of islet-cell tumors. Acta Cytol 1987;31:485–492.

38. Hsiu JG, D'Amato NA, Sperling MH, Greenspan M, Jaffe AH, Smith R III, DeLaTorre R. Malignant islet-cell tumor of the pancreas diagnosed by fine needle aspiration biopsy. A case report. Acta Cytol 1985;29:576–579.

39. Ascoli V, Newman GA, Kline TS. Grimelius stain for cytodiagnosis of carcinoid tumor. Diagn Cytopathol 1986;2:157–159.

40. Bloodworth JMB Jr, Greider MH. The endocrine pancreas and diabetes mellitus. In Bloodworth JMB Jr. Endocrine pathology, 2nd ed. Baltimore: Williams & Wilkins, 1982:586.

41. Hastrup J, Thommesen P, Frederiksen P. Pancreatitis and pancreatic carcinoma diagnosed by peroperative fine needle aspiration biopsy. Acta Cytol 1978;21:731–734.

42. Pinto MM, Avila NA, Criscuolo EM. Fine needle aspiration of the pancreas. Acta Cytol 1988;32:39–42.

11

Gastrointestinal Tract and Retroperitoneum

GASTROINTESTINAL TRACT

Fine needle aspiration biopsy has been successfully used in diagnosing metastatic carcinomas from the gastrointestinal tract. Diagnosis of primary neoplasms, on the other hand, are traditionally made by direct-vision endoscopic bite biopsy and brush cytology. Unfortunately, the present endoscopic techniques may fail to detect intramural tumors without mucosal invasion or ulcerated necrotic tumors with an overlying fibrin coat. Not infrequently the diagnosis of malignancy is made only at laparotomy. More recently, there are a number of reports documenting the usefulness of percutaneous as well as endoscopically directed fine needle aspiration biopsies in the diagnosis of gastrointestinal tract tumors, especially when the lesions are inaccessible by endoscopic bite biopsies or brush cytology.[1–5]

Using FNAB, Torp-Pedersen et al.[2] successfully diagnosed 50 of 61 gastrointestinal malignancies that were visualized ultrasonically, with no false-positive results. In 5 of the 18 gastric malignancies, endoscopic bite biopsy failed to provide sufficient material, despite repeated attempts in two cases. Of the 40 cancers of the colon, 7 were not disclosed by barium enema studies. Likewise, using FNAB Solbiati et al.[3] were able to diagnose correctly 24 of 24 bowel lesions that could be imaged on sonogram. At our institution, analysis of the results of 27 primary gastrointestinal lesions that were aspirated under ultrasound guidance showed correct or suggestive diagnosis in 23 cases, false-negative diagnosis in 4 cases, and no false-positive diagnosis.[4]

Histologically, neoplastic lesions of the alimentary tract show a diverse spectrum. Carcinomas make up the majority of the malignant tumors; smooth muscle (stromal) tumors, carcinoids, and lymphomas make up the bulk of the rest. In some parts of the world (e.g., the Middle East and Mediterranean), the incidence of lymphomas of the bowel is significantly increased.[6]

Squamous Cell Carcinoma

The oral cavity, esophagus and anus are the sites of the gastrointestinal tract in which squamous cell carcinomas commonly arise. The diagnosis is easily made by direct bite biopsy or endoscopic biopsy. Rarely, they may first manifest as metastatic disease (e.g., to the supraclavicular lymph nodes in the case of esophageal carcinoma, and to the inguinal lymph nodes in the case of anal carcinoma.)

Aspiration Cytology

The cytologic features of the well-differentiated (keratinizing) and poorly differentiated squamous carcinomas of the digestive tract differ little from those of squamous cell carcinomas in other sites of the body and will not be repeated here (see Chapters 4 and 7). One uncommon, peculiar subtype, i.e., the spindle cell variant, is seen more often in the esophagus, laryngopharynx, and oral cavity than in any other body sites.[7,8] Unless the cytopathologist is familiar with this unusual tumor, an erroneous diagnosis of sarcoma may be made. The ABC consists of both isolated cells and cell aggregates. In the large aggregates, a swirling pattern is sometimes evident.[9] The cells vary from polygonal to spindle shaped, with marked cellular pleomorphism (**Fig. 11.1**). The spindle cells usually predominate. Chromatin is coarse and nucleoli are prominent. The cytoplasm is eosinophilic and rather fibrillar in appearance. Squamous cells should be carefully sought among the spindle cells. If squamous cells are not found, the use of immunoperoxidase stain to demonstrate cytokeratin and/or electron microscopy to identify desmosomes is helpful for diagnosis.[9]

Adenocarcinoma

Adenocarcinoma is the most common gastrointestinal tract malignancy. It is frequently found in the colon and stomach, and less frequently in the lower part of the esophagus and small intestine. Adenocarcinomas show marked variation in histology, ranging from well-differentiated with well-formed glands and papillae to poorly differentiated with solid sheets of cells and little or no gland formation. A special variant of adenocarcinoma is the signet-ring cell carcinoma, in which the tumor cells become so distended with mucus that the nucleus is compressed against the cell membrane. The stomach is a common site from which signet-ring cell carcinoma develops and the tumor is notorious for its poor prognosis.

Aspiration Cytology

Well-differentiated Adenocarcinoma. Well-differentiated adenocarcinoma of the bowel is an example, par excellence, of tumors that recapitulate faithfully the normal architecture of the tissue of origin. Normal mucosal cells of the stomach and bowel appear in ABC as tall columnar cells with elongated, vesicular, basally situated nuclei. The cytoplasm is pale and delicate and has a lacy appearance. Typically, these cells form glands of varying sizes. A well-developed gland is represented by a cell cluster formed by cells arranged radially around a lumen, with the nuclei lying at the basal end opposite from the luminal surface (**Fig. 11.2**). Not uncommonly, long strips of columnar cells with palisading basal nuclei are aspirated, representing part of a gland or the surface epithelium of the intestinal mucosa (**Fig. 11.3**). In malignant glands, the basic architectural pattern is preserved but there is a varying degree of architectural disarray with cell crowding and loss of nuclear polarity (**Figs. 11.4** and **11.5**). Additionally, the individual tumor cell shows cytologic criteria of malignancy, such as anisokaryosis, uneven

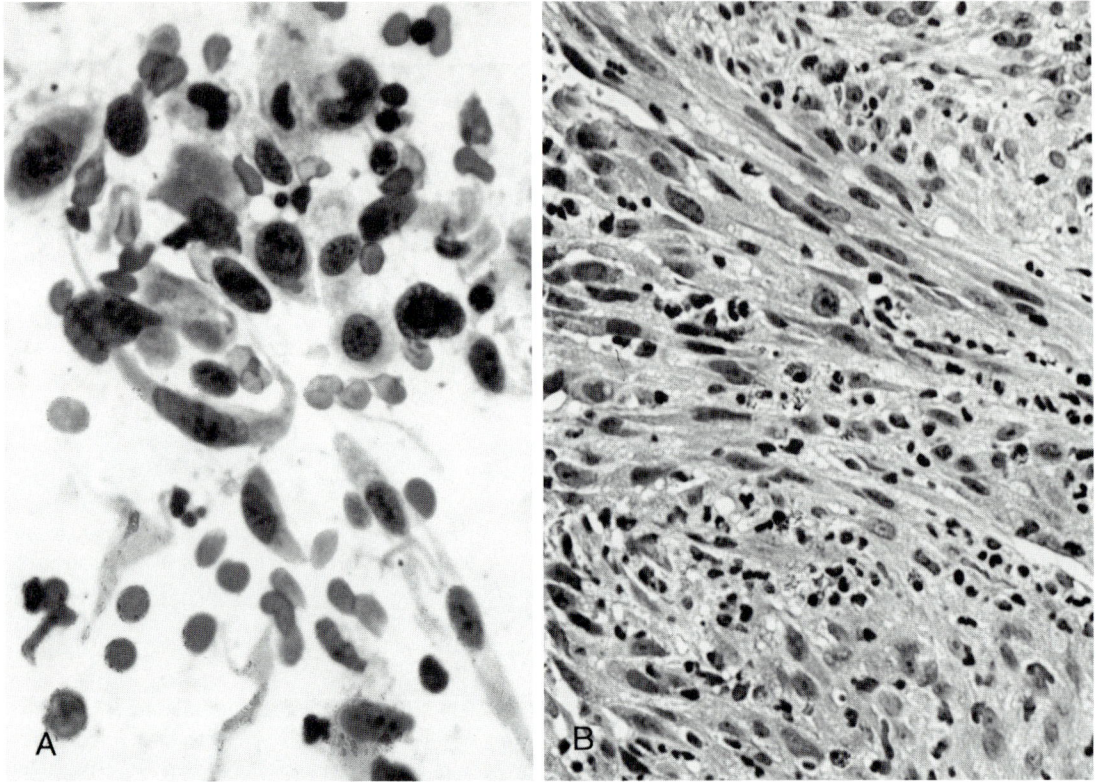

Figure 11.1.

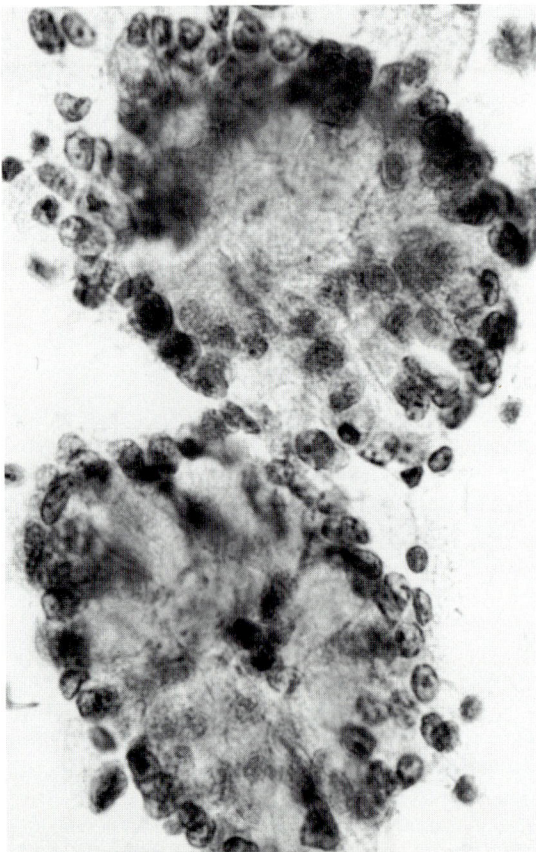

Figure 11.2.

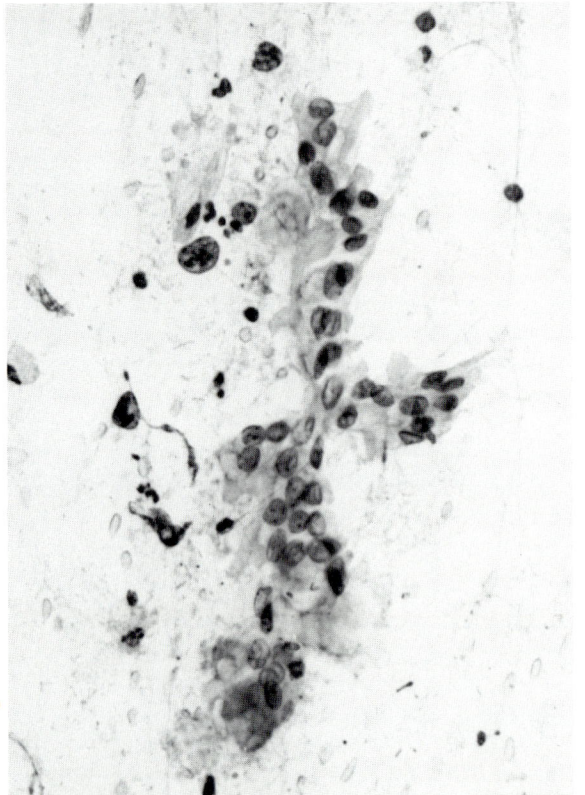

Figure 11.3.

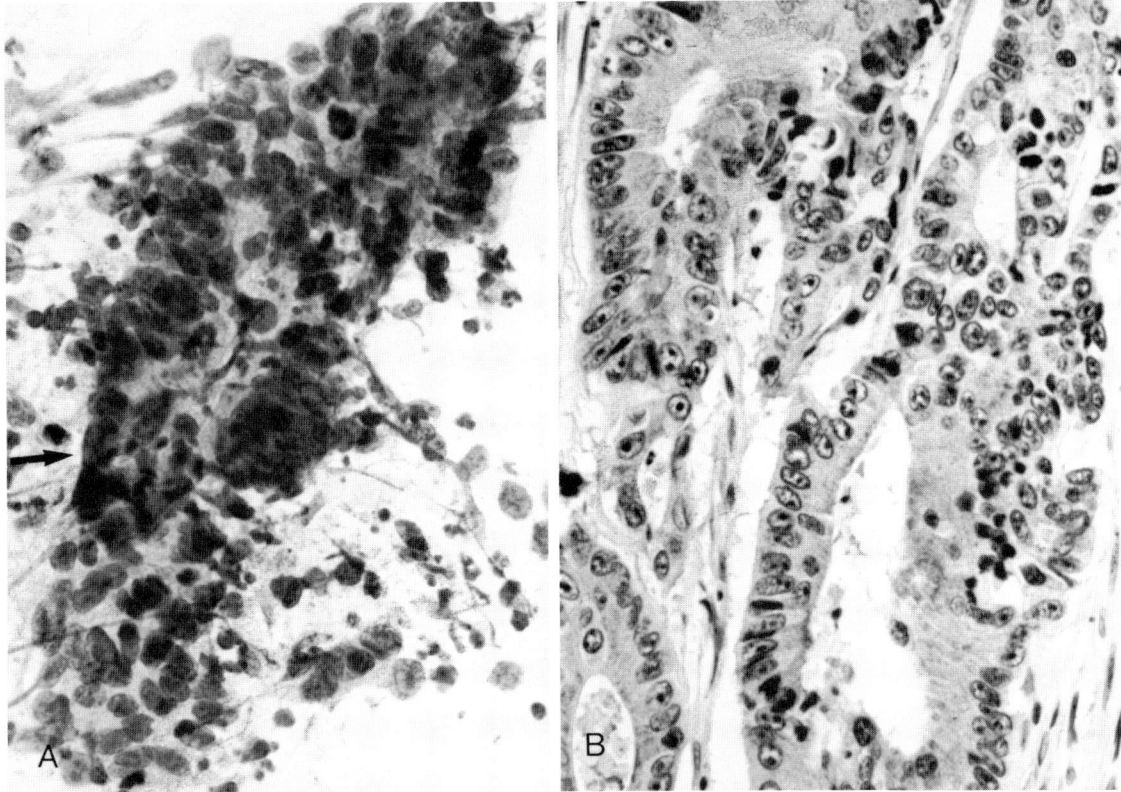

Figure 11.4.

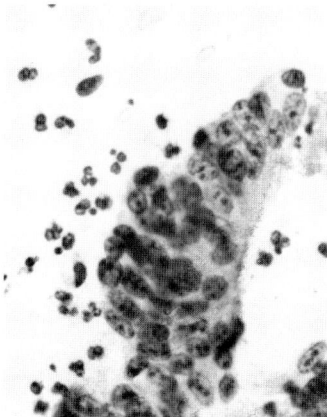

Figure 11.5.

Figure 11.4. Well-differentiated adenocarcinoma of the bowel. **A,** ABC. A glandular tissue fragment showing nuclear palisading and crowding. Note central lumina and smooth outer border *(arrow).* ×310. **B,** Histology of the resected adenocarcinoma. Note architectural similarity between the histologic section and the smear. The elongated nuclei are situated at the basal end opposite from the luminal edge. ×310.

Figure 11.5. Well-differentiated adenocarcinoma of the bowel, ABC. Note strip of cohesive columnar cells in fence-like arrangement. This strip represents part of a large gland wall. ×500.

Figure 11.1. Squamous cell carcinoma of the esophagus, spindle cell variant. Aspirate of metastasis in a supraclavicular lymph node. **A,** ABC. Note admixture of spindle and round cells, with hyperchromatic nuclei and eosinophilic cytoplasm. ×500. **B,** Histology of the primary esophageal carcinoma. Note morphologic similarity between histologic section and smear. ×310.

Figure 11.2. Benign mucosal glands of the bowel. Normal glands formed by columnar cells whose nuclei are situated peripherally away from the central luminal surface. ×480.

Figure 11.3. Strips of benign mucosal epithelium of the bowel. Note "fence-like" arrangement of the nuclei. Two or three malignant cells with bare nuclei are also present. ×310.

TABLE 11.1.   Comparison of Glandular and Papillary Tissue Fragments

Glandular Tissue Fragment	Papillary Tissue Fragment
Two- or three-dimensional	Three-dimensional
Inner luminal surface	Inner fibrous stroma (outer luminal surface)
Polarization of epithelial cell nuclei toward periphery	Polarization of epithelial cell nuclei toward center
Well-demarcated outer border	Well-demarcated outer border

chromatin distribution, increased N/C ratio, and nucleolar prominence.[10,11]

A papillary pattern together with the glandular pattern may be observed in well-differentiated adenocarcinomas. In ABC, papillary structures (**Figs. 11.6** and **11.7**) are represented by solid, finger-like, three-dimensional cell clusters or tissue fragments, which can be conceptualized as having the lumen on the surface.[12] The nuclei, lying at the end opposite the luminal edge, therefore are polarized toward the center of the fragments, where a fibrovascular tissue core is present. The latter, however, is not always readily discernible as in tissue sections because the papillae are completely aspirated rather than being sectioned. **Table 11.1** compares the morphologic appearances of glandular and papillary tissue fragments.

Poorly Differentiated Adenocarcinoma. While the glandular structure is a marker for well-differentiated adenocarinomas, aspirates from poorly differentiated adenocarcinomas show predominately dyshesive cells, with a few small abortive acinous groups and cellular cords.[11,13] A necrotic cellular background is common. Many tumor cells (**Fig. 11.8**) have lost their columnar shape and are somewhat round. The nuclei are hyperchromatic, and the nucleoli are usually large, single, and central. The amount of cytoplasm is variable. If it is scanty, the cells may resemble large lymphoid cells. More often, the cytoplasm contains numerous small mucin vacuoles. In the signet-ring type adenocarcinoma, the cytoplasm of the rounded neoplastic cells is distended by a large mucin (mucicarmine-positive) vacuole, which in turn displaces the nucleus to one side of the cell (**Fig. 11.9**).

Diagnostic Pitfalls. Cells from well-differentiated adenocarcinomas and those from reparative or reactive mucosa may look similar. Conditions such as peptic ulceration, gastritis, ulcerative colitis, and Crohn's disease may give rise to cells that may mimic adenocarcinomas in brush cytology.[11] Fortunately, these conditions seldom present as mass lesions on ultrasound or CT and therefore are seldom subjected to FNAB. Although regenerative mucosal cells have enlarged nuclei with single or multiple prominent nucleoli, the nuclear membranes are smooth. The chromatin content may be increased but is evenly distributed. Cells are arranged in an orderly fashion (**Fig. 11.10**).

Adenomatous polyp and villous adenoma must enter into the differential diagnosis of a well-differentiated adenocarcinoma. Generally they are not targets for percutaneous FNAB: the material in our file has come from endoscopic brush specimens (**Figs. 11.11** and **11.12**). Cells from adenomas retain the columnar configuration and have hyperchromatic nuclei with coarse chromatin without prominent nucleoli and chromatin clearing. The nuclear membranes are thickened but smooth. Anisonucleosis and nuclear enlargement are not as pronounced as in adenocarcinomas. Cellular necrosis and dyshesive cells are conspicuously absent.

Pseudomyxoma Peritonei

Pseudomyxoma peritonei is a rare disease, caused by a ruptured, low-grade, mucin-producing adenocarcinoma within the abdominal cavity.[14] The primary tumor usually arises from the appendix or ovary. Although at the time of initial surgical exploration the lesion's gross appearance may give an erroneous impression that the tumor is at a far advanced incurable stage, the disease usually runs a prolonged indolent course. The abdomen is distended with several liters of gelatinous mucoid material. The ABC (**Fig. 11.13**) consists of a large pool of mucus with clusters of free-floating tumor cells. The latter are mucin-producing, columnar cells, whose nuclei appear deceptively bland.[15]

Carcinoid Tumor

Carcinoid tumor, an endocrine tumor with a low malignant potential, can be found anywhere throughout the gastrointestinal tract, particularly in the small bowel. It is the second most common malignancy of the small bowel, next only to adenocarcinoma. Morphologically identical tumors may arise in the pancreas and the bronchial and tracheal mucosa, and occasionally they are found in the hepatobiliary tract, breast, prostate, ovary, uterine cervix, and testis.[16,17] Most gastrointestinal carcinoids produce serotonin, which is inactivated by the liver. However, when liver metastases are present, the release of serotonin to the general circulation results in the carcinoid syndrome, consisting of diarrhea, vasomotor flushing, asthma, and triscupid endocardial fibrosis. Some carcinoid tumors can also produce adrenocorticotropic hormone (ACTH), antidiuretic hormone, gastrin, or insulin.

Aspiration Cytology

The ABC is cellular and consists of rather small, uniform polygonal cells. The nuclei are oval, the chromatin is evenly distributed and granular, and the nuclear membranes are smooth. The nucleoli are usually present but small. The cytoplasm is moderate in amount, pale or finely granular. The tumor cells are arranged in anastomosing cords, acini, and solid large nests (see **Figs. 7.20–7.23** and **Fig. 10.14**).

Diagnostic Pitfalls. In an occasional carcinoid tumor, the cells can be quite small and exhibit a fair degree of nuclear pleomorphism (**Fig. 11.14**), thus mimicking small cell undifferentiated carcinoma. This diagnostic dilemma most often arises in specimens obtained from the lung where small cell undifferentiated carcinomas are common; it is an uncommon occurrence in the setting of a bowel-wall tumor. In general, small cell undifferentiated carcinomas have a necrotic background, and the nuclei have a "salt and pepper" appearance and no visible nucleoli. Nuclear molding is a common feature.

Aspirates of carcinoid tumors that contain acinar structures may be mistaken for adenocarcinomas. Acini from carcinoid tumors are formed by orderly, small, round cells, whereas acini from adenocarcinomas have larger, irregular lumina lined by large, atypical cells with disorderly crowding. Intracytoplasmic endocrine granules in a carcinoid tumor can be demonstrated with a silver-impregnation technique, e.g., Grimelius stain (**Fig. 11.14B**).

Neoplasms of Smooth Muscle

With the exception of the uterus, the alimentary tract gives rise to more tumors of smooth muscle than any other organ or organ system of the body.[18] Although these tumors may grow into the gut lumen, they often project primarily from the serosa and grow to a large size without producing gastrointestinal symptoms. Because of

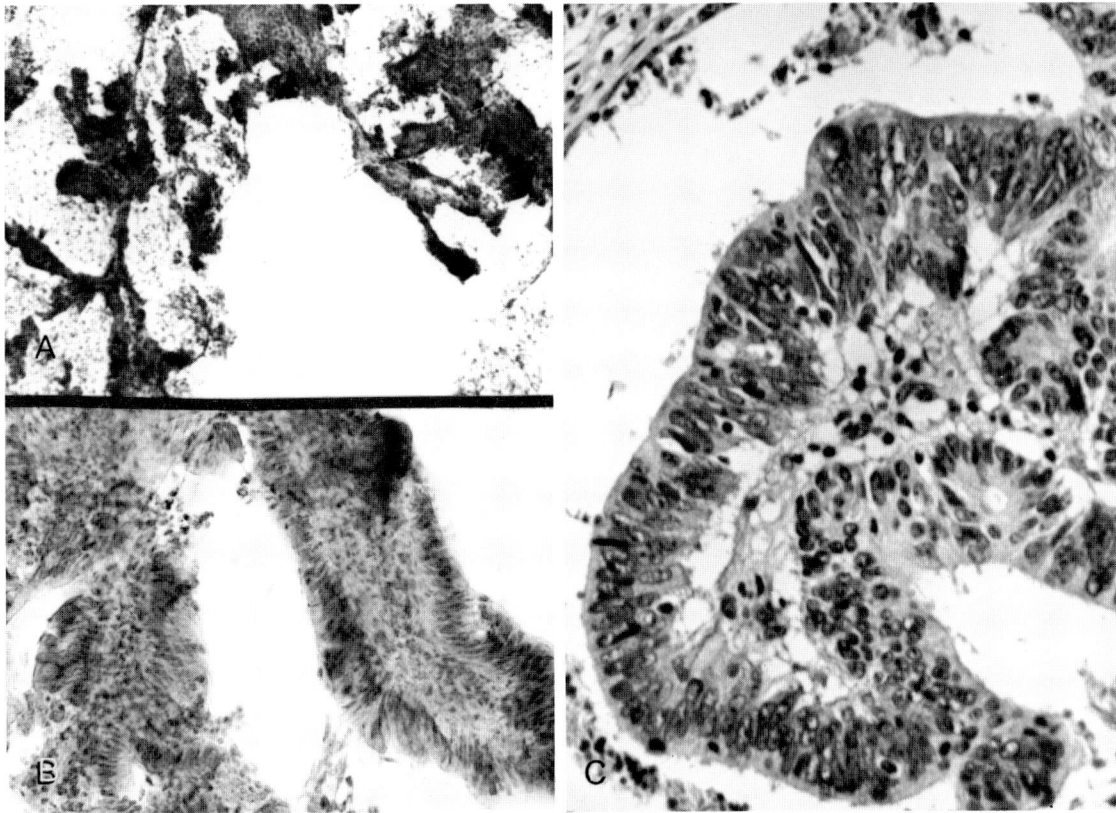

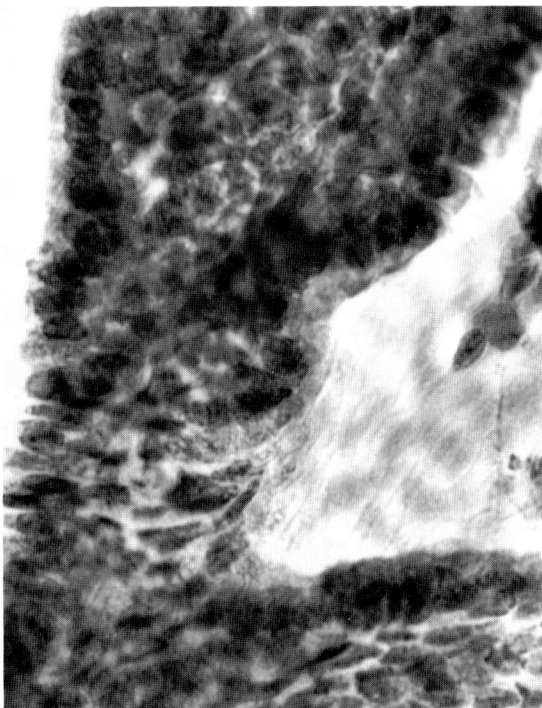

Figure 11.6. Well-differentiated papillary adenocarcinoma of the bowel, ABC. **A,** Note numerous three-dimensional branching papillary structures. ×60. **B,** Papillary fronds. Note central fibrous stroma rimmed by palisading tumor cells. Nuclei of the tumor cells are polarized toward the center of the papillae. ×125. **C,** Histologic section to show a papillary frond. Note central stroma and an external luminal space. ×310.

Figure 11.7. Well-differentiated papillary adenocarcinoma of the bowel, ABC. The nuclei at the periphery of the thick papillary tissue fragment are located toward the center. The central fibrous core is not visible, but instead, en face tumor cells are seen. ×500.

Figure 11.7.

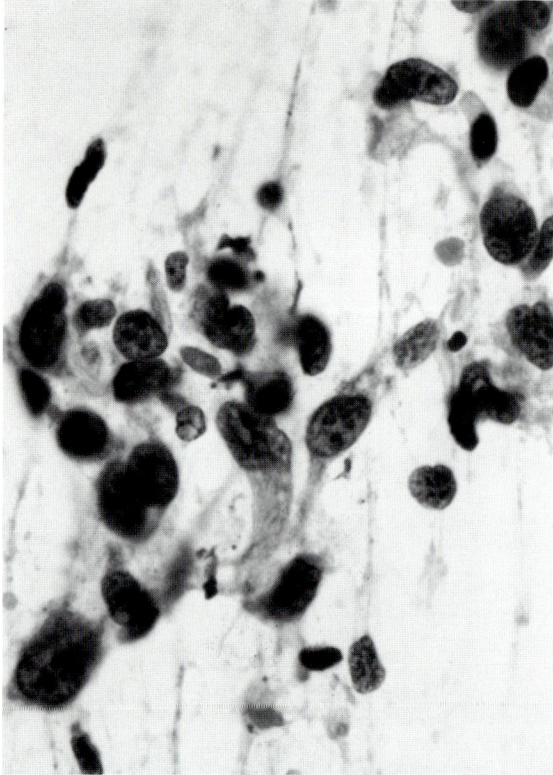

Figure 11.8.

Figure 11.8. Poorly differentiated adenocarcinoma of the bowel. ABC. Note marked cellular dyshesion and pleomorphism. Some cells still retain a columnar shape. ×500.

Figure 11.9. Poorly differentiated adenocarcinoma of the stomach, signet-ring cell type. **A,** ABC. There are many round tumor cells, two of which have a signet-ring appearance. ×500. **B,** Histology of the signet-ring cell adenocarcinoma. ×310.

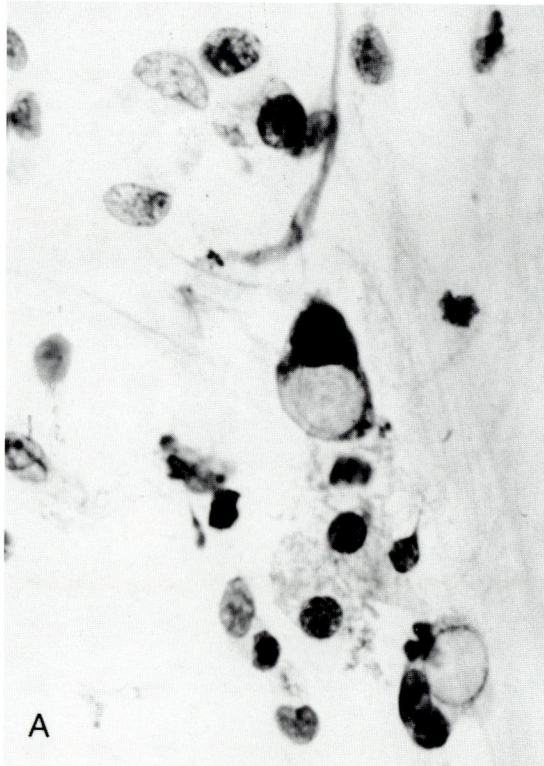

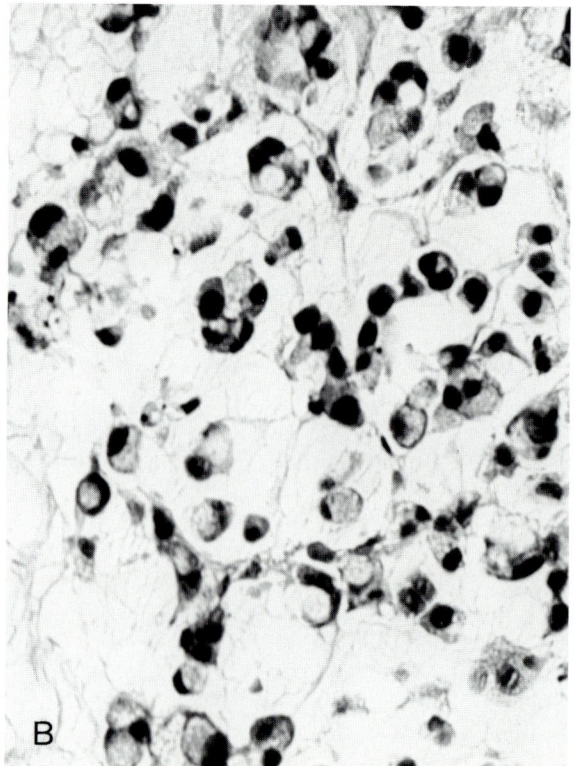

Figure 11.9.

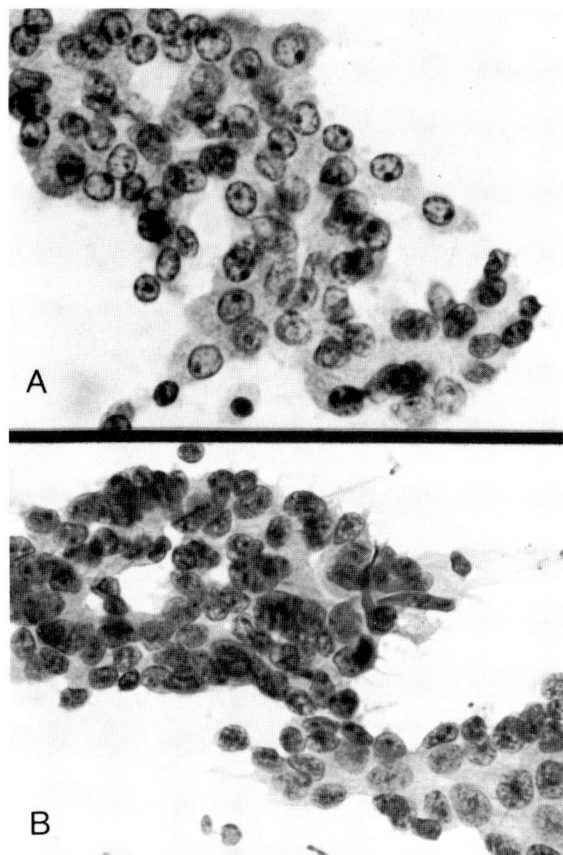

Figure 11.10.

Figure 11.10. Contrasting chronic gastritis and adenocarcinoma. **A,** Chronic gastritis presenting as thickening of stomach wall on CT. ABC shows atypical mucosal cells, with prominent nucleoli but smooth nuclear membranes. Also note general uniformity. ×400. **B,** Gastric adenocarcinoma. Note cellular disarray and crowding, irregular chromatin distribution, irregular nucleoli and loss of nuclear membrane smoothness. ×400.

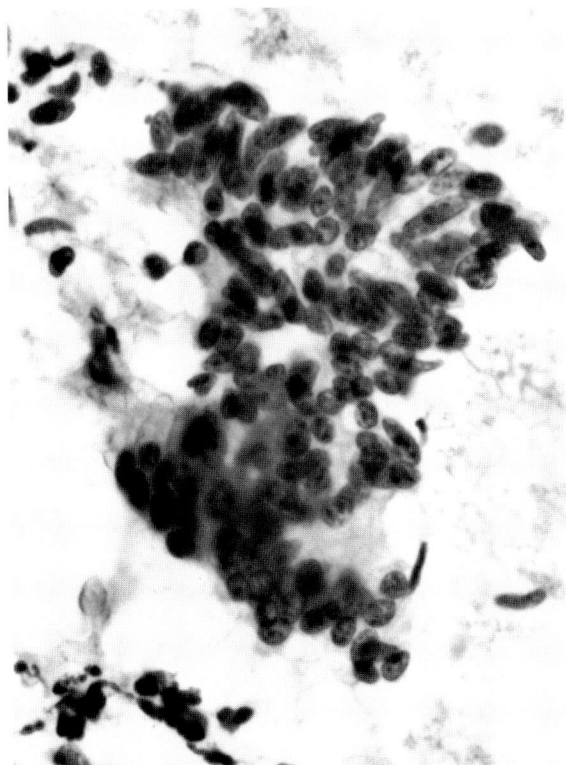

Figure 11.11.

Figure 11.11. Villous adenoma of the colon, endoscopic brush specimen. Note columnar cells in palisade. The cells are regular and smaller than those of adenocarcinoma. ×500.

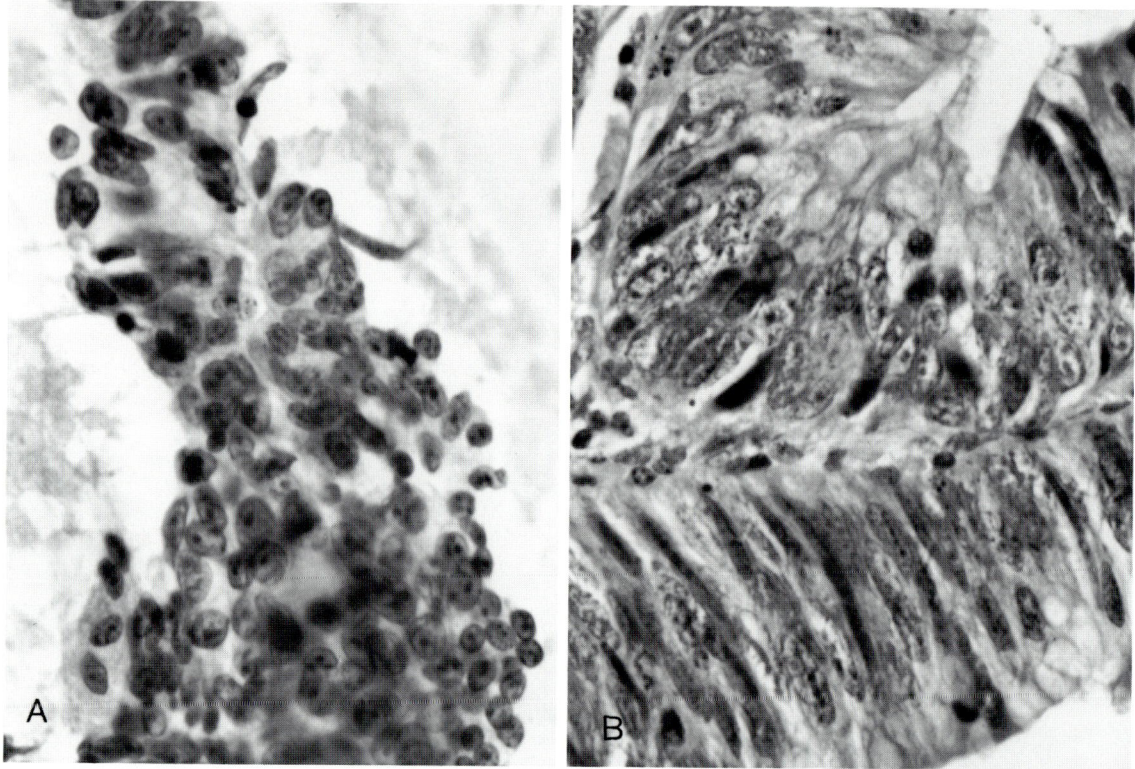

Figure 11.12.

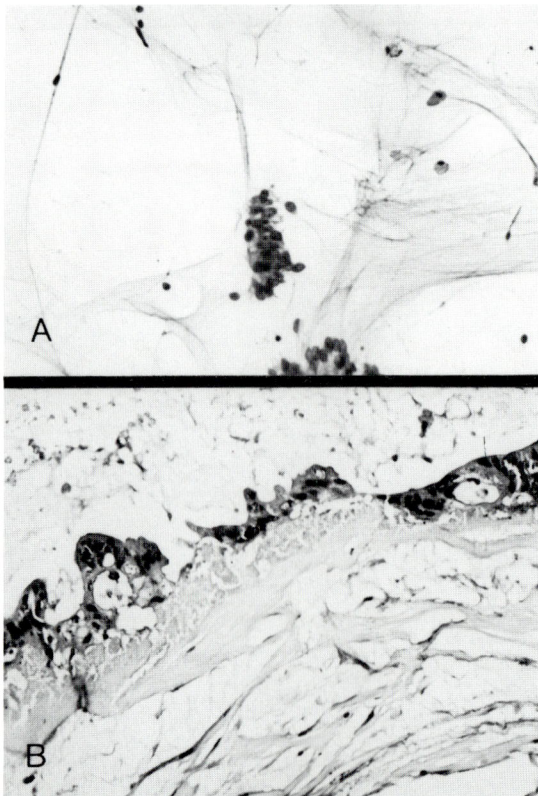

Figure 11.12. Villous adenoma with dysplasia. **A,** Endoscopic brush specimen. Note nuclear enlargement and marked atypia, but the changes are still below the level of carcinoma. Also note completely benign-appearing epithelial cells in the *right lower corner*. This combination of atypical and benign cells within the same tissue fragment is not a feature of adenocarcinoma. ×500. **B,** Histologic section of the dysplastic villous adenoma. ×500.

Figure 11.13. Pseudomyxoma peritonei. **A,** ABC. Note clusters of bland columnar cells in a mucous background. ×125. **B,** Histology of the low-grade adenocarcinoma of the appendix. ×125. (From Suen KC. Guides to clinical aspiration biopsy. Retroperitoneum and intestine. New York, Igaku Shoin, 1987).

Figure 11.13.

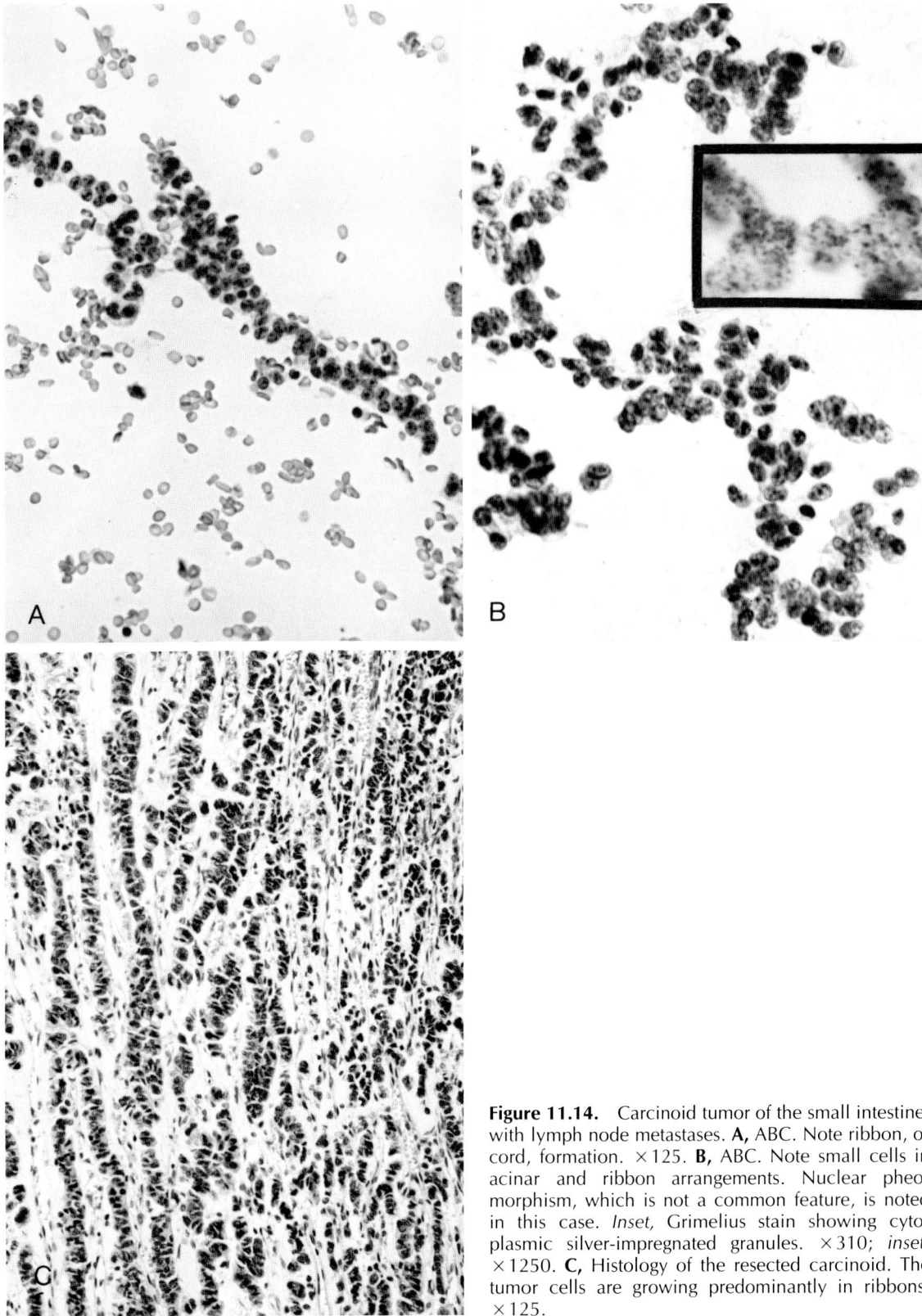

Figure 11.14. Carcinoid tumor of the small intestine, with lymph node metastases. **A,** ABC. Note ribbon, or cord, formation. ×125. **B,** ABC. Note small cells in acinar and ribbon arrangements. Nuclear pheomorphism, which is not a common feature, is noted in this case. *Inset,* Grimelius stain showing cytoplasmic silver-impregnated granules. ×310; *inset,* ×1250. **C,** Histology of the resected carcinoid. The tumor cells are growing predominantly in ribbons. ×125.

the submucosal or exoenteric location, endoscopic biopsy often results in a false-negative diagnosis. In our experience, transabdominal FNAB can frequently provide a diagnosis, especially when the tumor is bulky.[4] Histologically, smooth muscle tumors of the gut show features similar to those arising in other locations. On immunohistochemical and ultrastructural examinations, however, not all tumors show smooth muscle differentiation. Schwann cell differentiation has been shown to be present in some cases and total lack of differentiation in still others.[19–21]

Aspiration Cytology

In poorly differentiated leiomyosarcomas, the cytologic picture is that of a spindle cell sarcoma and the diagnosis is quite easy. The cellular ABC consists of many dyshesive malignant-appearing spindle cells with mitoses. Necrosis is not uncommon. On the other hand, differentiation between low-grade leiomyosarcoma and cellular leiomyoma may be difficult. Cellular atypia in the former may be subtle, characterized by uneven distribution of chromatin and by nuclear membrane irregularity. Nucleoli may or may not be prominent (**Fig. 11.15**). In leiomyomas, the smears show relatively poor cellularity compared with their malignant counterparts. The spindle tumor cells (**Fig. 11.16**) are mitotically inactive and are uniform in appearance.[22] Chromatin is evenly distributed; nuclear membrane irregularity and nucleoli are absent.

Diagnostic Pitfalls. Low-grade leiomyosarcomas and cellular leiomyomas may be morphologically indistinguishable until recurrence or metastases occur.[23–25] In general, leiomyosarcomas are larger than leiomyomas. Fifty percent of leiomyosarcomas are more than 10 cm in diameter, whereas only 19% of the benign lesions are of that size.[24] Tumors that are mitotically active are more likely to be malignant (5 or more mitoses per 10 high-power fields in tissue sections). Unfortunately, tumors with a maximal mitotic rate as low as 1 mitosis/10 high-power fields have also known to metastasize.[25]

Epithelioid Variant

The epithelioid variant is a special morphologic type of smooth muscle tumor that occurs with increased frequency in the gastrointestinal tract, especially in the stomach. They can be benign (epithelioid leiomyoma) or malignant (epithelioid leiomyosarcoma). Ultrastructural and immunohistochemical studies indicate that these tumors do not differ from their more spindled conterparts.[26] Histologically the tumor consists of round rather than spindle cells, with central nuclei and abundant somewhat clear cytoplasm. In our experience with four FNAB cases, spindle-shaped cells were also found in the smears from each case when deligently searched for. Some tumor cells have vacuolated clear cytoplasm, and others show eosinophilic cytoplasm. The nuclei are oval, with finely granular chromatin and micronucleoli (**Fig. 11.17**). In the two cases reported by Nguyen,[27] the tumor cells were pleomorphic and both rounded and spindled cells were identified. The cytologic findings suggested malignant mesenchymal tumor.

The epithelioid variant may be difficult to distinguish from poorly differentiated carcinoma, sarcomatoid carcinoma, or other types of sarcoma.[26] Clinical correlation, ultrastructural studies, and immunostaining of tumor cells for cytokeratin, vimentin, and various muscle antigens aid in interpretation (see Chapter 16).

Lymphoma

The single most common site for primary extranodal lymphomas to occur is the gastrointestinal tract, within which stomach involvement accounts for about 50% of cases, and the small bowel, 30%.[28] In the past, the diagnosis of primary gut lymphoma was usu-

ally made at laparotomy. With advent of flexible endoscopic biopsy and percutaneous FNAB, the diagnosis is made more frequently before surgery. Any type of lymphoma can be found in the alimentary tract. The most common is the diffuse large cell type of non-Hodgkin's lymphoma, present in nearly two-thirds of cases. On the other hand, no instance of Hodgkin's lymphoma primary in the stomach, small bowel, or large bowel could be confirmed in one large series.[29] In our experience and those of others,[11] cytology is more rewarding than endoscopic bite biopsy in the diagnosis of gastrointestinal lymphomas. The bite biopsy usually gives rise to crush artifact that may render the distinction between a lymphoma and an anaplastic carcinoma impossible. For a detailed description of malignant lymphomas in fine needle aspirates, the readers are referred to Chapter 4.

RETROPERITONEUM

By *retroperitoneum* we refer to the tissues remaining on the posterior abdominal wall after the large viscera, including pancreas, kidneys, and adrenals, are excluded. Traditionally, the term *retroperitoneal tumor* does not include metastatic malignancies secondary to tumors elsewhere in the body or direct spread from nearby organs. Therefore, retroperitoneal tumors are uncommon, representing only 0.3% of all neoplasms. Sarcomas account for approximately 55% of all retroperitoneal tumors, lymphomas account for 30%, and benign tumors account for the remainder.[30]

Sarcomas

Liposarcoma is the most common sarcoma in the retroperitoneum, making up 47% of the cases in one recent series.[31] It often arises in the adipose tissue in the perirenal area, sometimes necessitating removal of the kidney. The myxoid and well-differentiated types are most commonly encountered.

Leiomyosarcoma, second in frequency to the liposarcoma, can frequently be shown on exploratory laparotomy to arise from the gastrointestinal tract or uterus and grows retroperitoneally.

The third most common sarcoma is the category of pleomorphic sarcomas, most of which are malignant fibrous histiocytomas, rarely pleomorphic liposarcomas or rhabdomyosarcomas.

See Chapter 5 for cytologic descriptions of sarcomas.

Lymphoma

The majority of retroperitoneal lymphomas are non-Hodgkin's lymphomas; Hodgkin's disease presenting as a primary retroperitoneal mass is rare. A diagnosis of lymphoma by transabdominal FNAB should prompt the clinician to initiate a workup for lymphoma. The cytologic diagnosis can often be supported by a minor procedure such as a bone marrow biopsy or liver biopsy. Since 28–80% of non-Hodgkin's lymphomas (depending on the subtype) have disseminated disease, stage III or IV, at the time of initial presentation,[32,33] it is not uncommon that careful examination of the patient may show peripheral lymphadenopathy, which lends itself readily to surgical biopsy.

Other Primary Tumors

Retroperitoneum is a favorite site for neural tumors, which may attain a large size. Ganglioneuromas, ganglioneuroblastomas, and neuroblastomas identical to those seen in the adrenal may be found arising in the sympathetic ganglia of the retroperitoneum proper. Cellular schwannoma has been mistaken for spindle cell sarcoma on FNAB.[4] Paraganglioma has a wide range of cytologic appearance.[34,35] At one end of the spectrum, the tumor may contain bizarre giant cells like pheochromocytoma, and at the other end the tumor

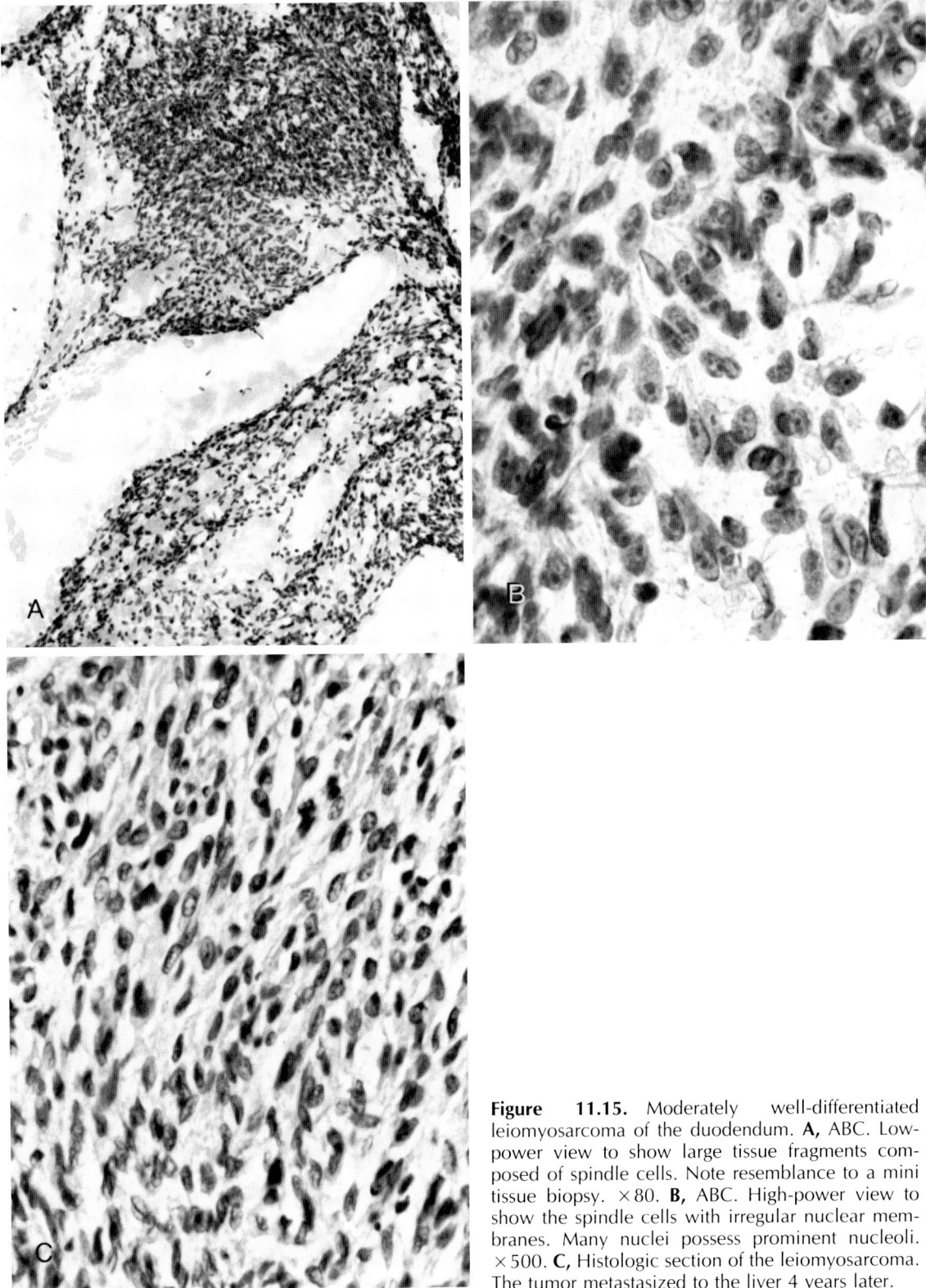

Figure 11.15. Moderately well-differentiated leiomyosarcoma of the duodendum. **A,** ABC. Low-power view to show large tissue fragments composed of spindle cells. Note resemblance to a mini tissue biopsy. ×80. **B,** ABC. High-power view to show the spindle cells with irregular nuclear membranes. Many nuclei possess prominent nucleoli. ×500. **C,** Histologic section of the leiomyosarcoma. The tumor metastasized to the liver 4 years later.

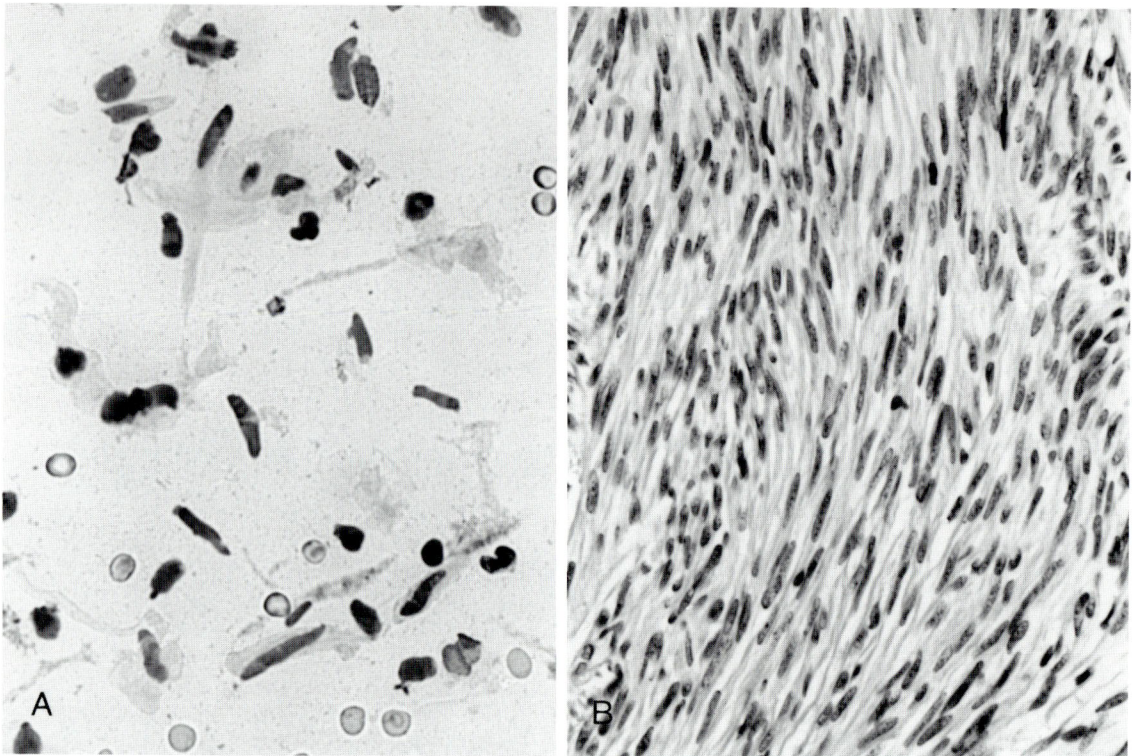

Figure 11.16. Leiomyoma of the stomach. ABC. **A,** Note benign, regular, spindle cells. Also note poor cellularity. ×500. **B,** Histology of leiomyoma. ×310.

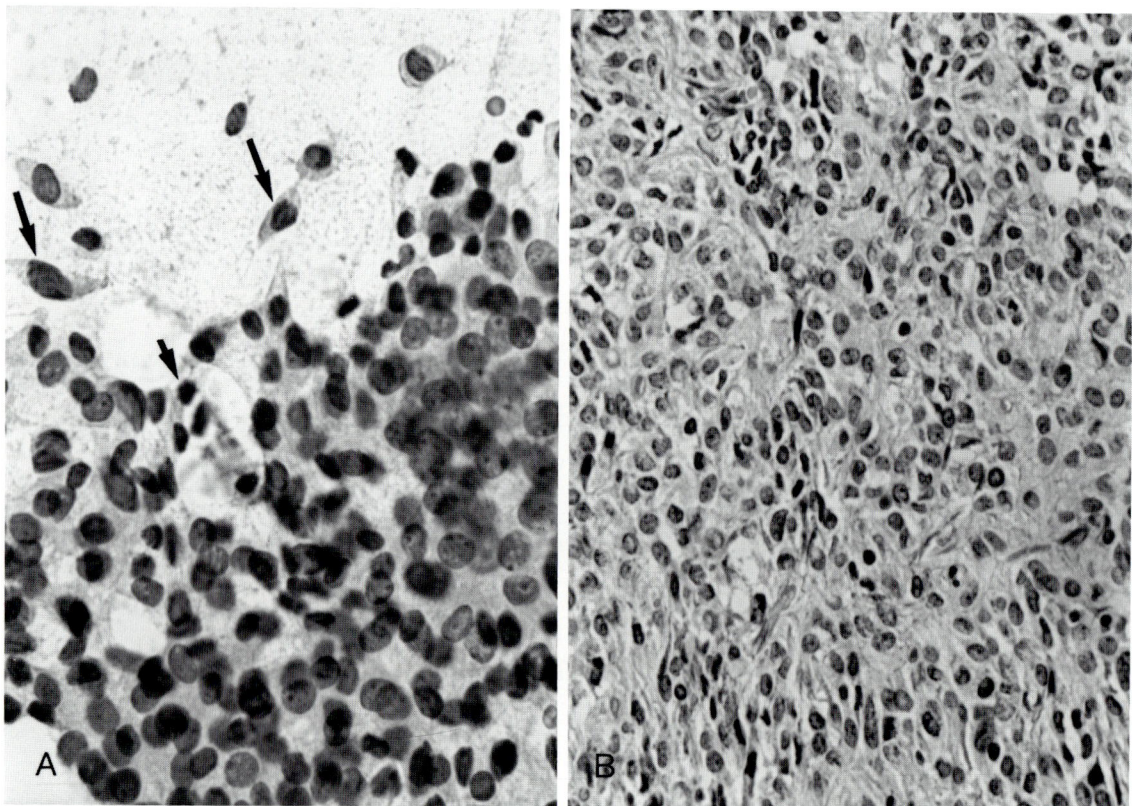

Figure 11.17. Low-grade epithelioid leiomyosarcoma of the stomach. **A,** ABC. Note predominance of rounded cells in sheets, with few elongated cells (long arrows). Cytoplasm is either clear or eosinophilic. Short arrow indicates a mitotic figure. ×500. **B,** Histology showing epithelioid appearance of the tumor. ×310.

cells may be regular and monomorphic, so that carcinoid and islet cell tumors may have to be excluded from the differential diagnosis. As a rule, the predominant cells are the medium-sized polygonal cells, with round nuclei and abundant eosinophilic, finely granular cytoplasm (see Chapter 13, ''Pheochromocytoma'').

Besides schwannomas and ganglioneuromas, other benign tumors occur in the retroperitoneum. Leiomyomas are much less common than leiomyosarcomas. Most are derived from the gastrointestinal tract or uterus. Lipomas can arise in the retroperitoneal fatty tissue. Some attain tremendous size and may not be distinguishable from liposarcomas. In fact, many cases originally diagnosed as retroperitoneal lipoma proved to be well-differentiated liposarcoma.[36,37]

Tumor-like lesions in the retroperitoneum that have been aspirated by us and others include tuberculous granuloma,[4] hematoma,[38] abscess,[38] and cysts.[39]

Metastatic Tumors

The incidence of metastatic tumors to the retroperitoneum is quite variable, depending on how vigorous are the investigations carried out for their detection and whether the statistics are derived from surgical or autopsy series. Understandably, the incidence is much higher in autopsy series, but with widespread use of modern imaging techniques and FNAB, more retroperitoneal metastases will be uncovered during life. Adenocarcinomas are most frequently encountered, and the ovary, colon, stomach, and breast are the common primary sites.

An important function of FNAB is in assessing the stage of the malignant disease and aiding in planning therapy. Lymphangiography can be used to opacify the retroperitoneal lymph nodes so that they can be imaged and aspirated. This technique has been useful in evaluating patients with urinary tract cancers and prostatic, gynecologic, and testicular cancers.[40-42]

References

1. Carrera GF, Mastcatello VJ, Holm HH, Berger M, Smith EH. Ultrasonically guided percutaneous biopsy of gastric lesions. Wis Med J 1979;78:28–29.
2. Torp-Pedersen S, Gronvall S, Holm HH. Ultrasonically guided fine-needle aspiration biopsy of gastrointestinal mass lesions. J Ultrasound Med 1984;3:65–68.
3. Solbiati L, Montali G, Croce F, Ravetto C, Livraghi T. Fine needle aspiration biopsy of bowel lesions under ultrasound guidance: Indications and results. Gastrointest Radiol 1986;11:172–176.
4. Suen KC. Guides to clinical aspiration biopsy. Retroperitoneum and intestine. New York: Igaku Shoin, 1987.
5. Iishi H, Yamamoto R, Tatsuta M, Okuda S. Evaluation of fine needle aspiration biopsy under direct vision gastrofiberscopy in diagnosis of diffusely infiltrative carcinoma of the stomach. Cancer 1986;57:1365–1369.
6. Isaacson P, Al-Dewachi HS, Mason DY. Middle Eastern intestinal lymphoma: A morphological and immunohistochemical study. J Clin Pathol 1983;36:489–498.
7. Fraser GM, Kinley CE. Pseudosarcoma with carcinoma of the esophagus. Arch Pathol 1968;85:325–330.
8. Battifora H. Spindle cell carcinoma. Ultrastructural evidence of squamous origin and collagen production by the tumor cells. Cancer 1976;37:2275–2282.
9. Schantz HD, Ramzy I, Tio FO, Buhaug J. Metastatic spindle-cell carcinoma. Cytologic features and differential diagnosis. Acta Cytol 1985;29:435–441.
10. Pilotti S, Rilke F, Clemente C, Alasio L, Grigioni M. The cytologic diagnosis of gastric carcinoma related to histologic type. Acta Cytol 1977;21:48–59.
11. Hajdu SI. Cytopathology of human gastrointestinal cancers. In Lipkin M, Good RA. Gastrointestinal tract cancer. New York: Plenum, 1978:489–508.
12. Frost JK. The cell in health and disease, 2nd ed. Basel: S Karger, 1986:96.
13. Hall TE, Manalo P. Cytologic findings in signet-ring adenocarcinoma of the large bowel. A case report. Acta Cytol 1985;29:616–619.
14. Rosai J. Ackerman's surgical pathology, 6th ed. St. Louis: CV Mosby, 1981:1487.
15. Rammou-Kinia R, Sirmakechian-Karra T. Pseudomyxoma peritonei and malignant mucocele of the appendix. Acta Cytol 1986;30:169–172.
16. Albores-Saavedra J, Larraza O, Poucell S, Rodriguez HA. Carcinoid of the uterine cervix. Additional observations on a new tumor entity. Cancer 1976;38:2328–2342.
17. Weitzman S, Robison JR. Primary carcinoid of testis. J Urol 1976;116:821–822.
18. Fine G, Ma CK. Alimentary Tract. In Kissane JM. Anderson's pathology, Vol. 2. St. Louis: CV Mosby, 1985:1088.
19. Mazur MT, Clark HB. Gastric stromal tumors. Reappraisal of histogenesis. Am J Surg Pathol 1983;7:507–519.
20. Miettinen M. Gastrointestinal stromal tumors. An immunohistochemical study of cellular differentiation. Am J Clin Pathol 1988;89:601–610.
21. Mackay B, Ro J, Floyd C, Ordonez NG. Ultrastructural observations on smooth muscle tumors. Ultrastruct Pathol 1987;11:593–607.
22. Appelman H, Helwig EB. Cellular leiomyomas of the stomach in 49 patients. Arch Pathol Lab Med 1977;101:373–377.
23. Evans HL. Smooth muscle tumors of the gastrointestinal tract. A study of 56 cases followed for a minimum of 10 years. Cancer 1985;56:2242–2250.
24. Ranchod M, Kempson RL. Smooth muscle tumors of the gastrointestinal tract and retroperitoneum. Cancer 1977;39:255–262.
25. Sagi A, Feuchtwanger MM, Yanai-Inbar I, Walfisch S. Smooth muscle tumors of the small bowel: A case report and review of the literature. J Surg Oncol 1985;30:120–123.
26. Appelman HD, Helwig EB. Gastric epithelioid leiomyoma and leiomyosarcomas (leiomyoblastoma). Cancer 1976;38:708–728.
27. Nguyen GK. Cytopathologic aspects of leiomyoblastoma in fine needle aspiration biopsy. Report of two cases. Acta Cytol 1983;27:173–177.
28. Green MR, Kroener JF. Hodgkin's disease and the non-Hodgkin's lymphomas. In Pilch YH. Surgical oncology. New York: McGraw-Hill, 1984:923.
29. Weingrad DN, DeCosse JJ, Sherlock P, Straus DJ, Lieberman PH. Lymphomas of the gut. In DeCosse JJ, Sherlock P. Gastrointestinal cancer 1. The Hague: Martinus Nijhoff, 1981:311–341.
30. Storm FK, Sondak VK, Economou JS. Sarcomas of the retroperitoneum. In Eilber FR, Morton DL, Sondak VK, Economou JS. The soft tissue sarcomas. Orlando: Grune & Stratton, 1987:239.
31. Harrison LB, Gutierrez E, Fischer JJ. Retroperitoneal sarcoma. The Yale experience and a review of the literature. J Surg Oncol 1986;32:159–164.
32. Chabner BA, Fisher RI, Young RC, DeVita VT. Staging of non-Hodgkin's lymphoma. Semin Oncol 1980;7:285–291.
33. Chabner BA, Johnson RE, Young RC, et al. Sequential nonsurgical and surgical staging of non-Hodgkin's lymphoma. Ann Intern Med 1976;85:149–154.
34. Hood IC, Qizilbash AH, Young JEM, Archibald SD. Fine needle as-

piration biopsy cytology of paragangliomas. Acta Cytol 1983;27:651–657.

35. Gonazlez-Campora R, Otal-Salaverri C, Panea-Flores P, Lerma-Puertas E, Galera-Davidson H. Fine needle aspiration cytology of paraganglionic tumors. Acta Cytol 1988;32:386–390.

36. DeWeerd JH, Dockerty MB. Lipomatous retroperitoneal tumors. Am J Surg 1952;84:397–407.

37. Braasch JW, Mon AB. Primary retroperitoneal tumors. Surg Clin North Am 1967;47:663–678.

38. Haaga JR, Weinstein AJ. CT-guided percutaneous aspiration and drainage of abscesses. AJR 1980;135:1187–1194.

39. Sarno RC, Carter BL, Bankoff MS. Cystic lymphangiomas: CT diagnosis and thin needle aspiration. Br J Radiol 1984;57:424–426.

40. Bonfiglio TA, MacIntosh PK, Patten SF Jr, Cafer DJ, Woodworth FE, Kim CW. Fine needle aspiration cytopathology of retroperitoneal lymph nodes in the evaluation of metastatic disease. Acta Cytol 1979;23:126–130.

41. Wajsman Z, Gamarra M, Park JJ, Beckley SA, Pontes JE, Murphy GP. Fine needle aspiration of metastatic lesions and regional lymph nodes in genitourinary cancer. Urology 1982,19:356–360.

42. Piscioli F, Scappini P, Luciani L. Aspiration cytology in staging of urologic cancer. Cancer 1985;56:1173–1180.

12

Kidney and Urinary Tract

Until recently in North America, needle aspirations of the kidney were used mostly for identification and evacuation of renal cysts. The demonstration of a solid renal mass by ultrasound or CT scan has been considered sufficient indication for an open renal operation. On the other hand, FNAB of solid renal lesions has been practiced successfully in Europe, especially in the Scandinavian countries. In addition to its being used for the diagnosis of primary renal tumors by the Scandinavians, FNAB is useful in the following circumstances: (a) confirming a recurrent renal cancer in the renal fossa after nephrectomy, (b) evaluating bilateral renal masses, (c) evaluating a renal mass in a patient with a known primary cancer elsewhere (to distinguish cancer metastatic to the kidney from primary renal cancer), (d) diagnosing a simple renal cyst, (e) in cases in which operation is not contemplated, and (f) diagnosing metastatic renal cancer at extrarenal sites.[1-7]

The approach to most renal masses is retroperitoneal. For bulky masses, a transperitoneal anterior route may be used. Complications are uncommon and include occasional pyrexia, hematuria, hematomas, and local infections.[8-10] Gibsons et al.[11] reported a case of tumor seeding following FNAB. Von Screeb et al.[12] found no difference in survival rate between those cases that had preoperative aspirations and those that did not.

Diagnostic Accuracy

The diagnostic accuracy of FNAB in patients with renal lesions has ranged from 82 to 95%.[13] In 301 cases of utrasonically guided FNAB, Juul et al.[3] obtained a 95% retrieval rate of material satisfactory for interpretation. The predictive value of a benign aspirate was 71%, that of a malignant aspirate, 93%, and the overall accuracy, 82%. Nosher et al.[14] reported a diagnostic accuracy of 95% in 21 cases, with no false-negative results. We analyzed the results in 96 cases, comprising 38 renal cysts, 44 solid renal masses, and 14 renal cancers at metastatic sites. The overall diagnostic accuracy was 92%, sensitivity of detecting malignancy, 88%, and predictive value of malignancy, 100%.[15]

Normal Cytology

The normal ABC of the kidney is sparsely cellular. The epithelial cells of the proximal convoluted tubules (**Fig. 12.1A**) are represented by small monolayered sheets of large polygonal cells with abundant granular eosinophilic cytoplasm. The nuclei are round, with evenly distributed coarse chromatin and small nucleoli. The cells of the distal convoluted tubules (**Fig. 12.1B**) are smaller and cuboidal, with compact nuclei and pale or clear cytoplasm. The cells of the collecting tubules are similar to those of the distal convoluted tubules, and the cell borders are well-defined. The glomeruli (**Fig.**

12.2) are seldom aspirated. When present, they appear as large, lobulated, ball-like structures containing an admixture of endothelial cells and mesangial cells.

MALIGNANT NEOPLASMS
Renal Cell Carcinoma

Renal cell carcinoma (clear cell carcinoma, renal adenocarcinoma, and hypernephroma) is the most common primary renal neoplasm in adults, constituting about 2–3% of all adult cancers.[16,17] At the time of initial diagnosis, about one-third of the patients already have distant metastases. In some cases the metastases may precede the clinical manifestation of the primary tumor or appear several decades after the primary tumor has been removed.[18] Histogenetically, renal cell carcinomas are derived from the epithelial cells of the proximal convoluted tubules. On microscopic examination, two cell types, the clear cells and the granular cells, characterize this tumor. Although the majority of the tumors consists of both cell types in varying proportions, about 30% are composed of clear cells alone and 12% are composed of principally granular cells.[19] The clear cells are rich in lipid and glycogen, and the granular cells contain many mitochondria that produce the effect of a granular, eosinophilic cytoplasm. Occasionally a tumor may contain spindle cells, giant cells, or pleomorphic ''rhabdoid'' cells, mimicking a sarcoma. The growth patterns of renal cell carcinoma are many and varied, including solid, cystic, alveolar, lace-like, trabecular, and papillary.

Aspiration Cytology

Cellular Pattern. The aspirates are generally cellular, unless there is excessive hemorrhage, which may dilute the cell concentration. The smears consist of dispersed single cells, irregular cell clusters, and cell sheets of various sizes. If one has an opportunity to study a large number of cases, one will frequently encounter tumor cells arranged in the following patterns, alone or in combination: lace-like, acinar, trabecular, and papillary (**Figs. 12.3** and **12.4**).

Cell Morphology. The tumor cells (**Figs. 12.4–12.7**) are large and polygonal, with fairly distinct cell borders. The nuclei are round and more or less centrally located. The chromatin is finely granular with some clumping under the nuclear membrane, and the nucleoli are prominent (but not in grade 1 tumors). Cytoplasm is ample. It is vacuolated or clear in the clear cells and granular and eosinophilic in the granular cells. Some cells have a filmy, ground-glass rather than clear cytoplasm (**Fig. 12.5A**). In histologic sections, these cells will probably appear as clear cells as a result of paraffin embedding process.

Based on nuclear features, renal cell carcinomas are classified into four grades.[20] In grade 1 tumors, the cells have small, regular,

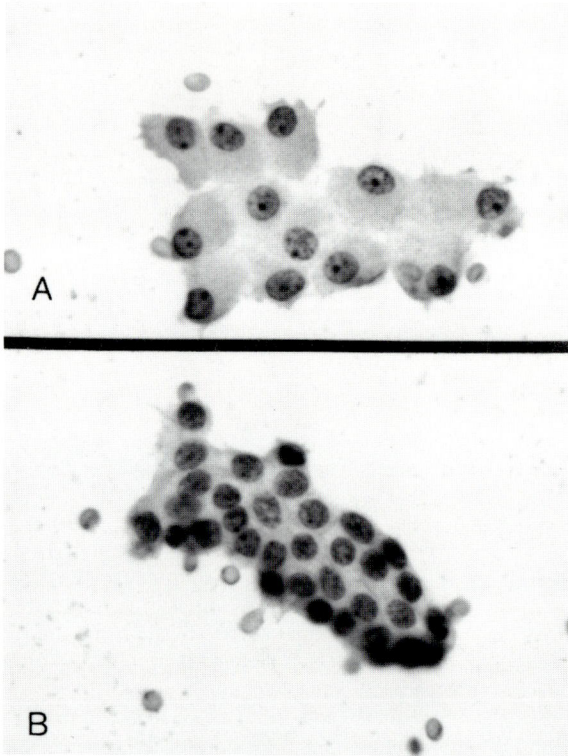

Figure 12.1.

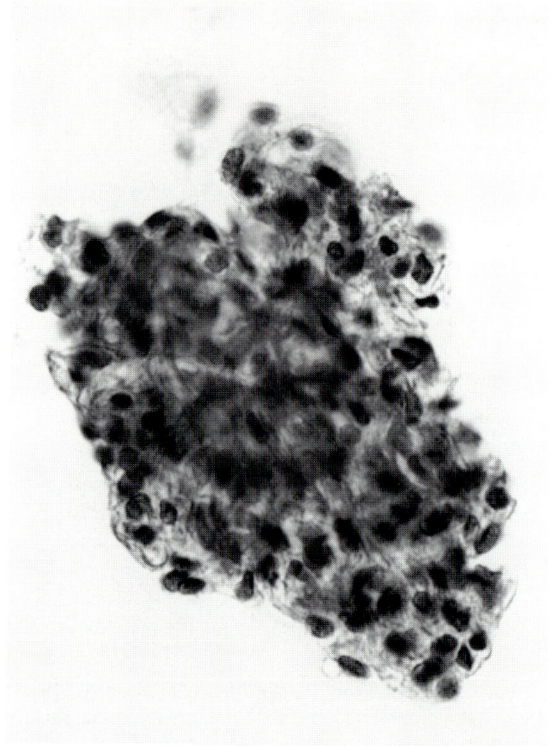

Figure 12.2.

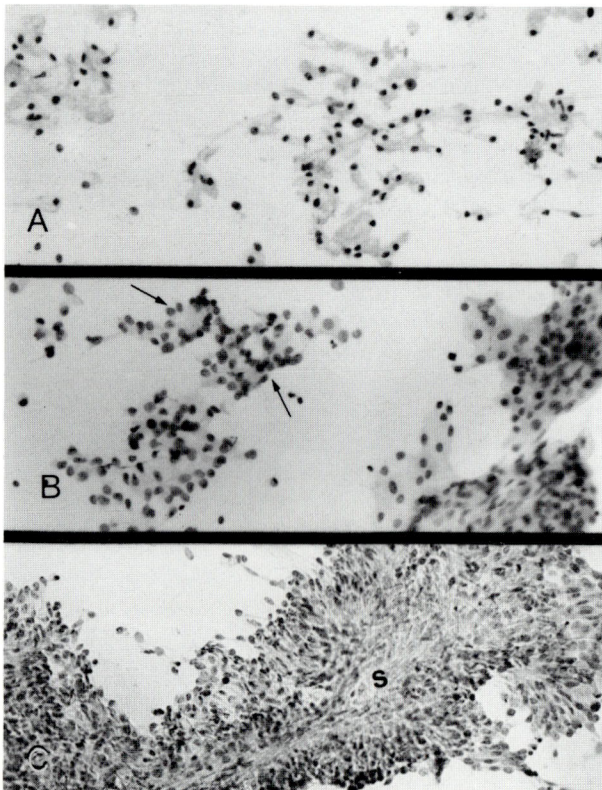

Figure 12.3.

Figure 12.1. Normal kidney, ABC. **A,** Epithelial cells of the proximal tubule. Note large polygonal cells with abundant granular eosinophilic cytoplasm. ×500. **B,** Epithelial cells of the distal tubule. Note cohesive, smaller cells with pale cytoplasm. ×500.

Figure 12.2. Normal kidney, ABC. A normal glomerulus, characterized by a large lobular structure containing endothelial and mesangial cells. ×310.

Figure 12.3. Renal cell carcinoma, ABC. **A,** Tumor cells lying singly and in lace-like arrangement. ×125. **B,** Tumor cells arranged in tubules or acini *(arrows)* and in thick tissue fragments. ×125. **C,** Tumor cells forming papillary tissue fragment. Note central fibrous stroma *(S)*. ×125. (Reproduced with permission. Suen KC. Guides to clinical aspiration biopsy. Retroperitoneum and intestine. New York: Igaku Shoin, 1987.)

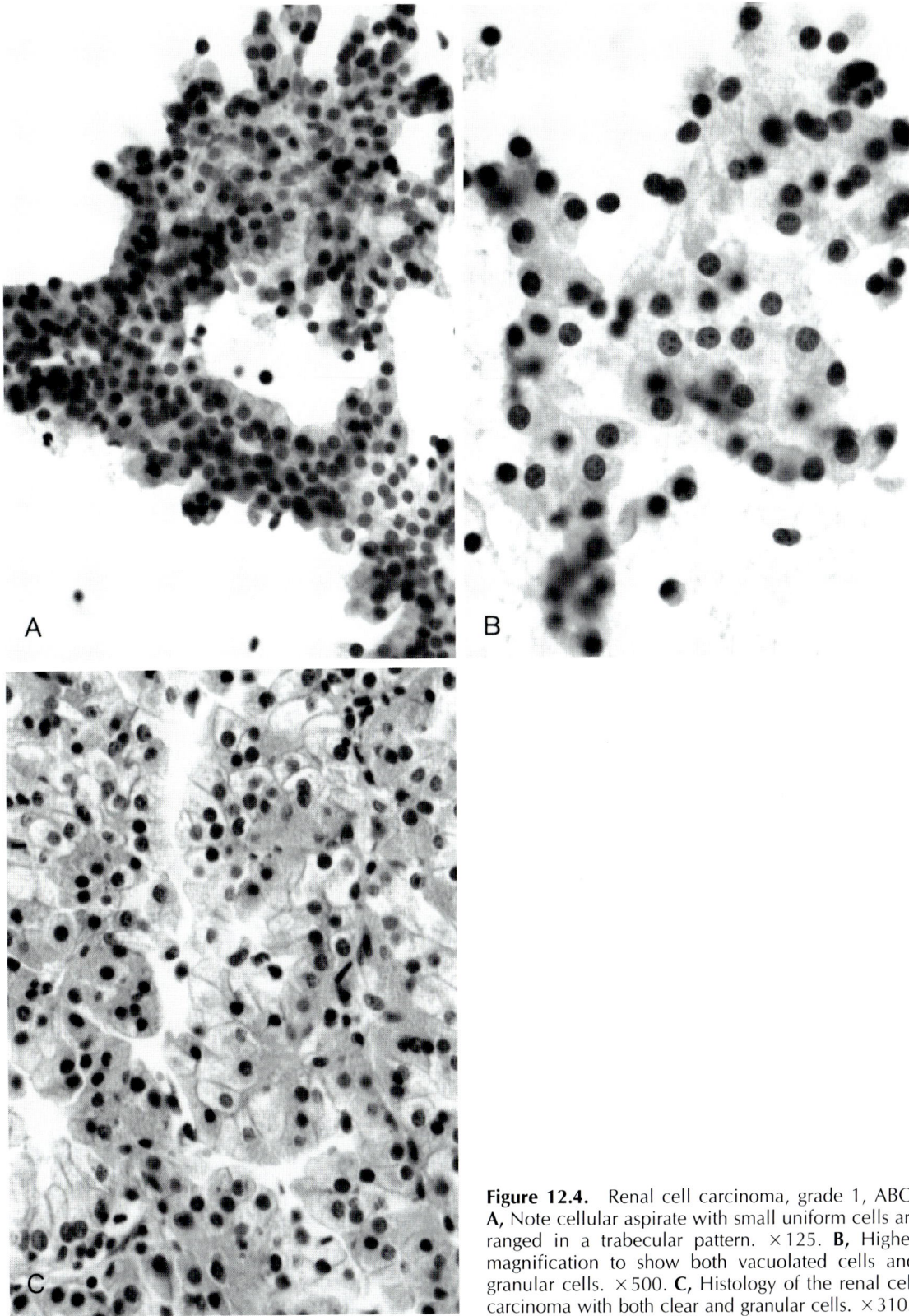

Figure 12.4. Renal cell carcinoma, grade 1, ABC.
A, Note cellular aspirate with small uniform cells arranged in a trabecular pattern. ×125. **B,** Higher magnification to show both vacuolated cells and granular cells. ×500. **C,** Histology of the renal cell carcinoma with both clear and granular cells. ×310.

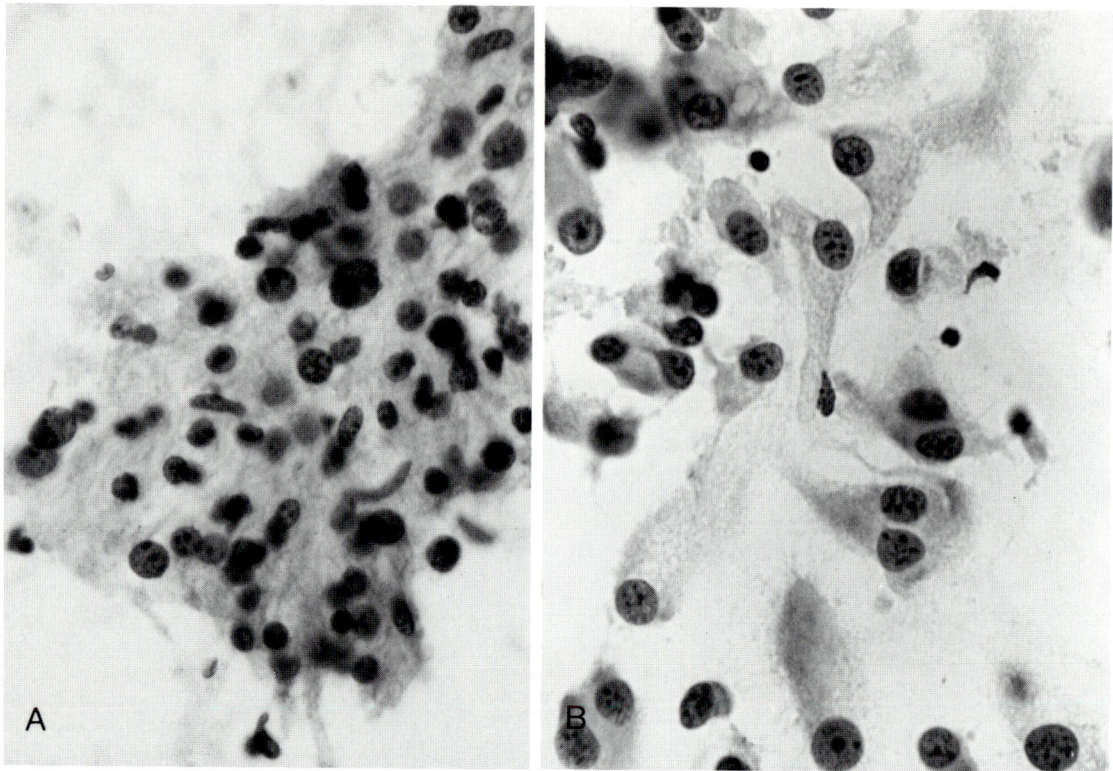

Figure 12.5.   Renal cell carcinoma, grade 2, ABC. **A,** Cell sheet. ×500. **B,** Single cells, both vacuolated and granular types are present. Note prominent nucleoli. ×500.

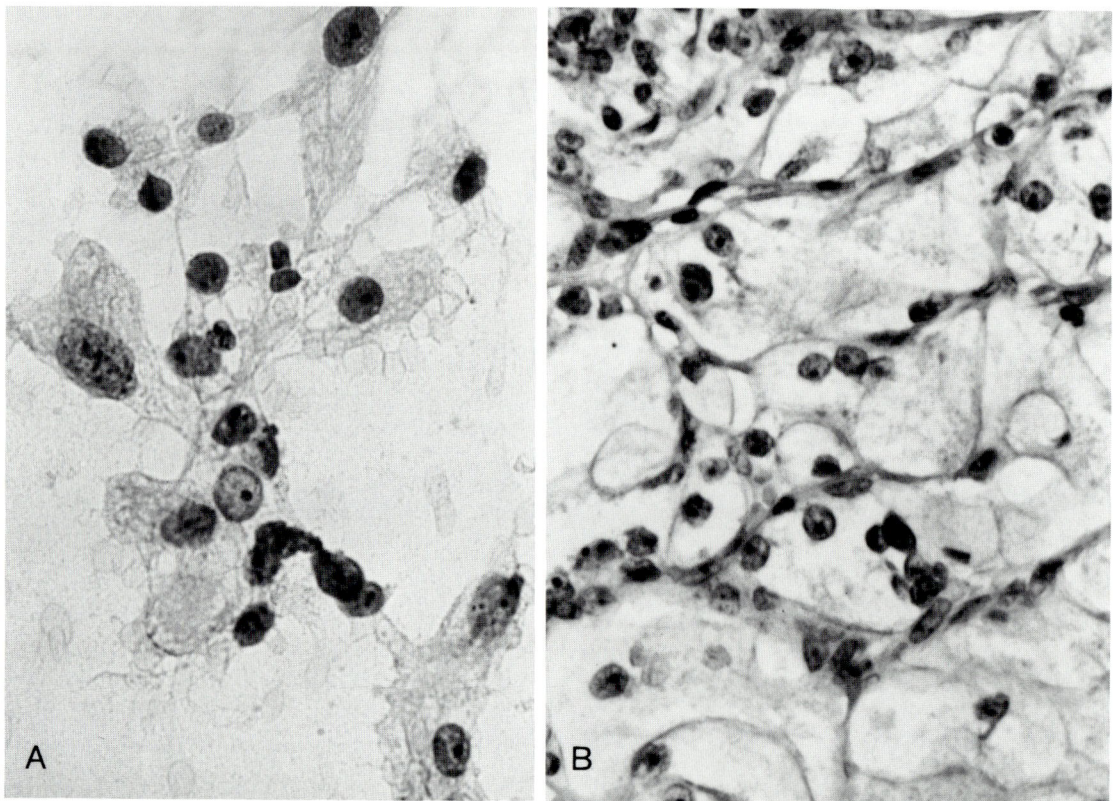

Figure 12.6.   Renal cell carcinoma, grade 3. **A,** ABC. Note clear cells showing anisonucleosis and prominent nucleoli. ×500. **B,** Histologic section showing pleomorphic clear cells with prominent nucleoli. ×500.

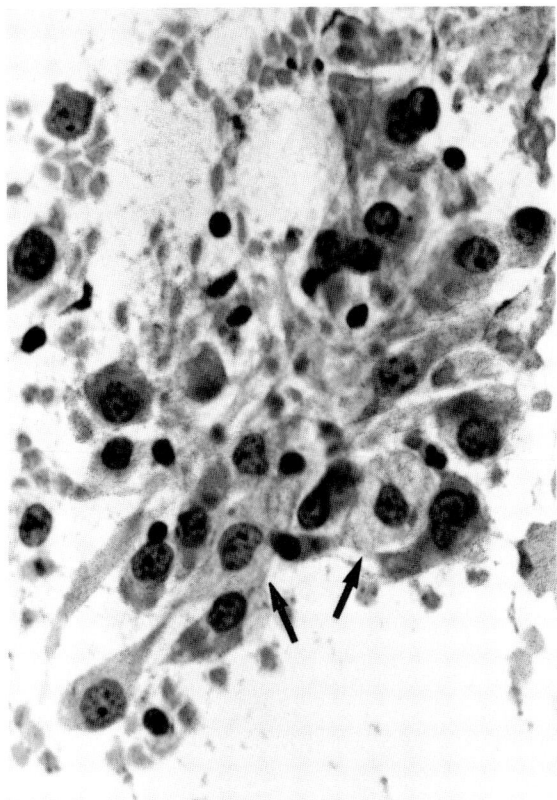

Figure 12.7.

Figure 12.7. Renal cell carcinoma, grade 3, ABC. Note pronounced nuclear atypia. *Arrows* indicate vacuolated tumor cells. ×500.

Figure 12.8. Renal cell carcinoma, grade 4. **A,** ABC. Note pleomorphic giant cells and spindle cells. ×500. **B,** Histologic section of the spindle and giant cell carcinoma. ×310.

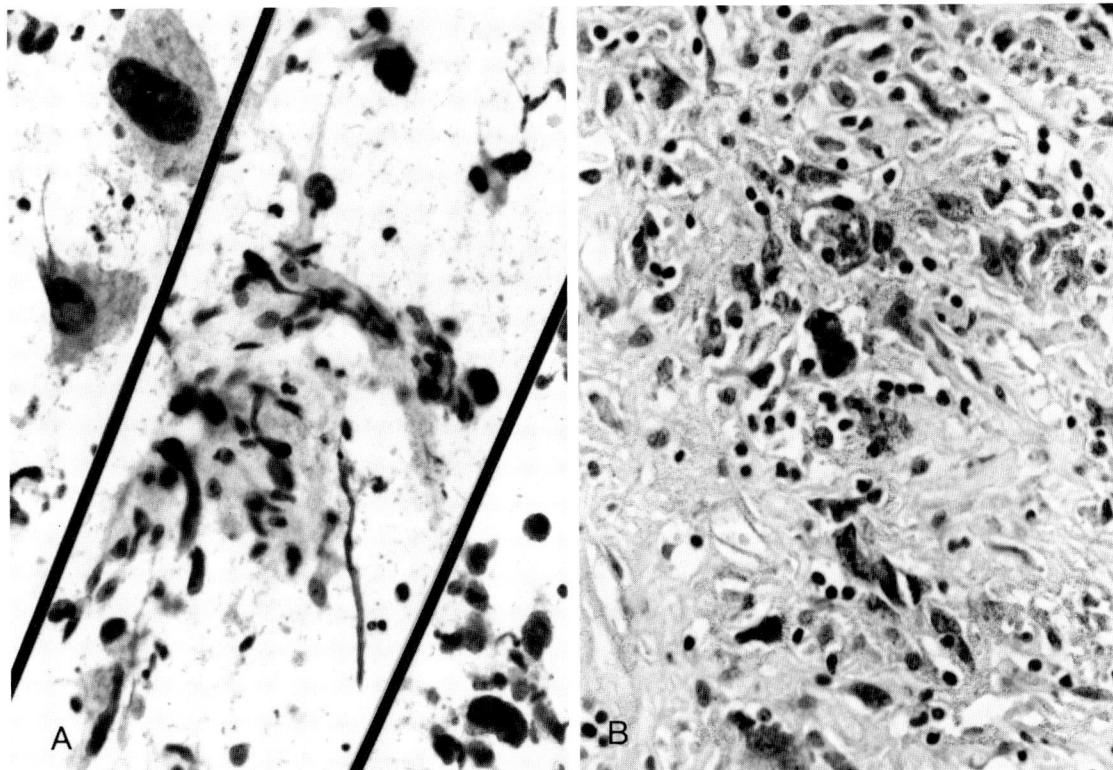

Figure 12.8.

round nuclei and inconspicuous or absent nucleoli. In grade 2 tumors, the cells have larger nuclei, which show membrane irregularities and nucleoli when examined under high ($\times 400$) power. Grade 3 tumors have even larger nuclei, which exhibit anisonucleosis, abnormal chromatin pattern, and large irregular nucleoli. In grade 4 tumors, the nuclear alternations are more marked than those of grade 3 tumors. Grade 4 tumors may contain bizarre giant cells, rhabdoid cells, or spindle cells **(Fig. 12.8),** simulating a sarcoma. Many studies have attested to the excellent correlation between tumor grade and patients' survival.[19,20] Nevertheless, it is important to remember that in about 15% of the cases, multiple grades coexist within the same tumor.[20] Multiple samples are necessary for accurate assessment.[21]

Diagnostic Pitfalls.   False-negative diagnoses may occur in the following circumstances:

1. In the absence of clinical and radiologic data, it is not possible to separate cytologically grade 1 renal cell carcinoma from renal cell adenoma (see ''Problems in Diagnosing Renal Adenoma'').
2. The clear cells from renal cell carcinoma may be mistaken for histiocytes and vice versa (see below).
3. The granular cells from renal cell carcinoma may mimic those from renal oncocytoma (see ''Renal Oncocytoma'').
4. The granular cancer cells may be mistaken for benign epithelial cells of the proximal convoluted tubules. The high cellularity and larger tissue fragments are features in favor of renal cell carcinoma.
5. The granular cancer cells may mimic benign hepatocytes. The latter usually contain yellow-brown pigment granules in the cytoplasm and are arranged in characteristic cords, resembling normal liver parenchyma.

False-positive reports may occur in the following circumstances:

1. Aspirates from renal cysts may on occasion contain atypical epithelial cells that simulate malignancy.[22,23] The ABC, however, is generally scant in cells that do not form large tissue fragments. Ultrasound will show a cystic lesion, and the double-contrast study will demonstrate a smooth lining of the cyst.
2. Foamy histiocytes may simulate the clear cells from renal cell carcinoma. A case of chronic xanthogranulomatous pyelonephritis is shown in **Fig. 12.9,** consisting of many foamy histiocytes and fibrocytes. Diagnosis of renal cell carcinoma should be based on cells in clusters rather than single cells, as is generally the case with histiocytes.[2] Moreover, prominent nucleoli are a reliable marker for clear cell carcinoma and are absent in histiocytes.
3. Benign renal tubular cells, hepatocytes, and oncocytes from oncocytomas are all potential sources of false-positive diagnoses.

At times, there are difficulties in identifying a tumor as being of renal origin. Renal cell carcinomas that exhibit spindle cells may be mistaken for sarcoma. The demonstration of coexpression of keratin and vimentin in the tumor cells by the immunoperoxidase technique substantiates the diagnosis of renal cell carcinoma, whereas sarcomas are keratin-negative. Ultrastructural studies may be helpful in those sarcomatoid renal cell carcinomas that retain epithelial characteristics, such as desmosomes, intracytoplasmic lumina with brush borders, and/or basement membrane formation. Another diagnostic problem is in excluding an adrenocortical carcinoma, which also can produce vacuolated and granular cells. Uroradiographic and angiographic studies may clarify the relationship of the mass to the kidney. The majority of adrenocortical carcinomas are functional endocrine tumors, hence examination of serum and urine for elevation of adrenocortical hormones and their metabolites is diagnostically

useful. The immunoperoxidase technique can also be used in the differential diagnosis of renal versus adrenal carcinomas. Adrenocortical carcinomas are uniformly nonreactive for keratin and epithelial membrane antigen; positive immunoreactivity for either keratin or epithelial membrane antigen supports a renal derivation.[24]

Problems in Diagnosing Renal Adenoma

Much controversy exists concerning the diagnostic criteria used to separate renal cell carcinoma from adenoma. On histologic examination, grade 1 carcinomas and adenomas are indistinguishable. Traditionally, tumors that are larger than 3 cm in diameter are considered malignant and those less than 3 cm are considered benign. However, there are cases of small tumors (<3 cm) producing widespread metastases, and large tumors remaining localized.[25,26] Mostofi and Davis[27] suggested that tumors that produce clinical symptoms and those with cellular anaplasia or evidence of invasion or aggressive behavior should be regarded as malignant. On the other hand, a tumor incidentally found in a kidney removed for other reasons or at autopsy should be classified as benign, unless there is cellular anaplasia or invasion.

Bennington[28] demonstrated a linear relationship between the tumor size and the propensity to metastasize, thus providing evidence that renal cell adenoma and carcinoma are different stages of the same tumor, whose metastatic potential increases proportionally with tumor size.

Wilms' Tumor

Wilms' tumor (nephroblastoma) is the most common renal malignancy of infancy and childhood. Of all malignant neoplasms in patients under the age of 15 years, 6% are Wilms' tumors.[29] It is a malignant embryonic neoplasm that develops from the metanephrogenic blastema. Besides giving rise to the primitive nephrogenic epithelia, blastema also produces mesoblastic stroma. Hence, a classical Wilms' tumor, which in essence is a primitive adenosarcoma, consists of the following three elements, in varying proportions: (a) the undifferentiated blastemic cells, (b) the epithelial cells, and (c) a mesenchymal stromal component. The blastemic component consists of closely packed, small, oval cells with dark nuclei and scanty cytoplasm. Differentiation of the epithelial elements embraces a rather broad spectrum. On the one hand, very immature epithelial differentiations may be present in the form of rosettes, and on the other hand, formation of well-developed tubules and glomeruloid structures may be seen. The stromal component consists of fibroblastic and myxoid tissues, and less frequently, muscle, cartilage, or bone.

In the past, primary Wilms' tumors were seldom investigated by FNAB. A more recent study[30] has shown that FNAB can assume a pivotal role in the preoperative diagnosis of Wilms' tumor. In the context of a classical clinical presentation, the correct cytologic diagnosis will increase the attractiveness of preoperative radiation and chemotherapy in those patients with bulky tumors or significant vascular invasion. FNAB can also be used effectively in documenting tumor recurrence and metastases.[15]

Aspiration Cytology

The smears are cellular and faithfully mirror the histologic appearance of the tumor **(Figs. 12.10 and 12.11).** In general, the predominant cell type is the undifferentiated blastemic cells, characterized by dyshesive, small, oval to fusiform-shaped cells, with hyperchromatic nuclei and scanty cytoplasm. The epithelial cells are small and cohesive, forming nests, rosettes, and tubules. The mesenchymal cells are most often represented by elongated fibroblastic cells. In one of the cases the author examined, the tumor for the

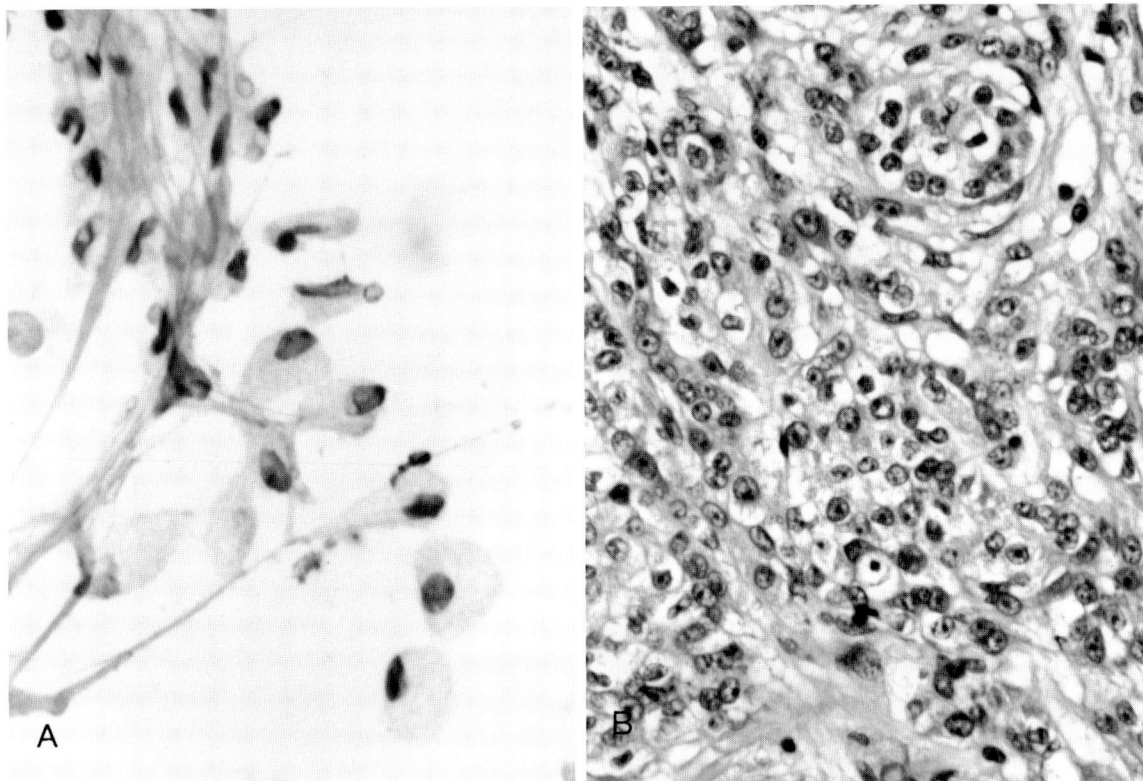

Figure 12.9.   Chronic xanthogranulomatous pyelonephritis. **A,** ABC. Note foamy histiocytes (xanthomatous cells) and elongated fibroblasts. ×500. **B,** Histologic section showing xanthomatous cells and fibroblasts. ×310.

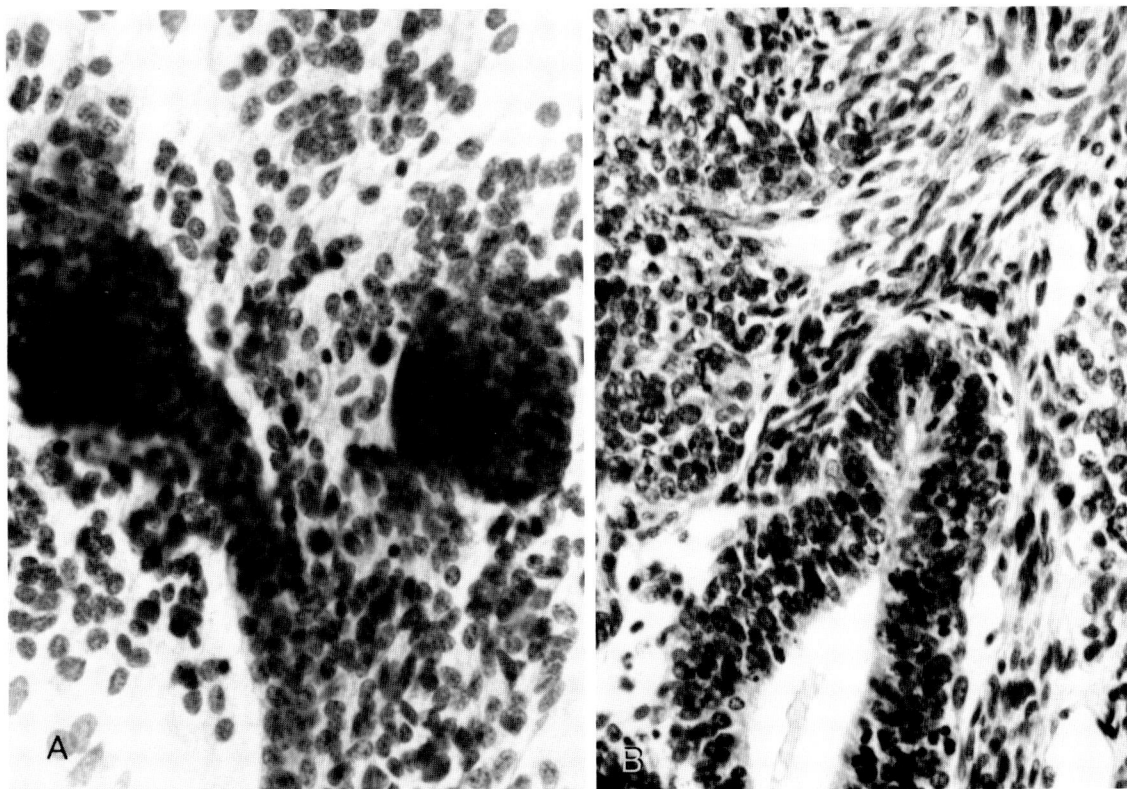

Figure 12.10.   Wilms' tumor. **A,** ABC. Note scattered small blastemic cells and two tubular structures with sharply defined borders (basement membranes). ×500. **B,** Histology of Wilms' tumor. Note classical triphasic pattern of blastemic cells, spindle stromal cells and epithelial tubules. ×310.

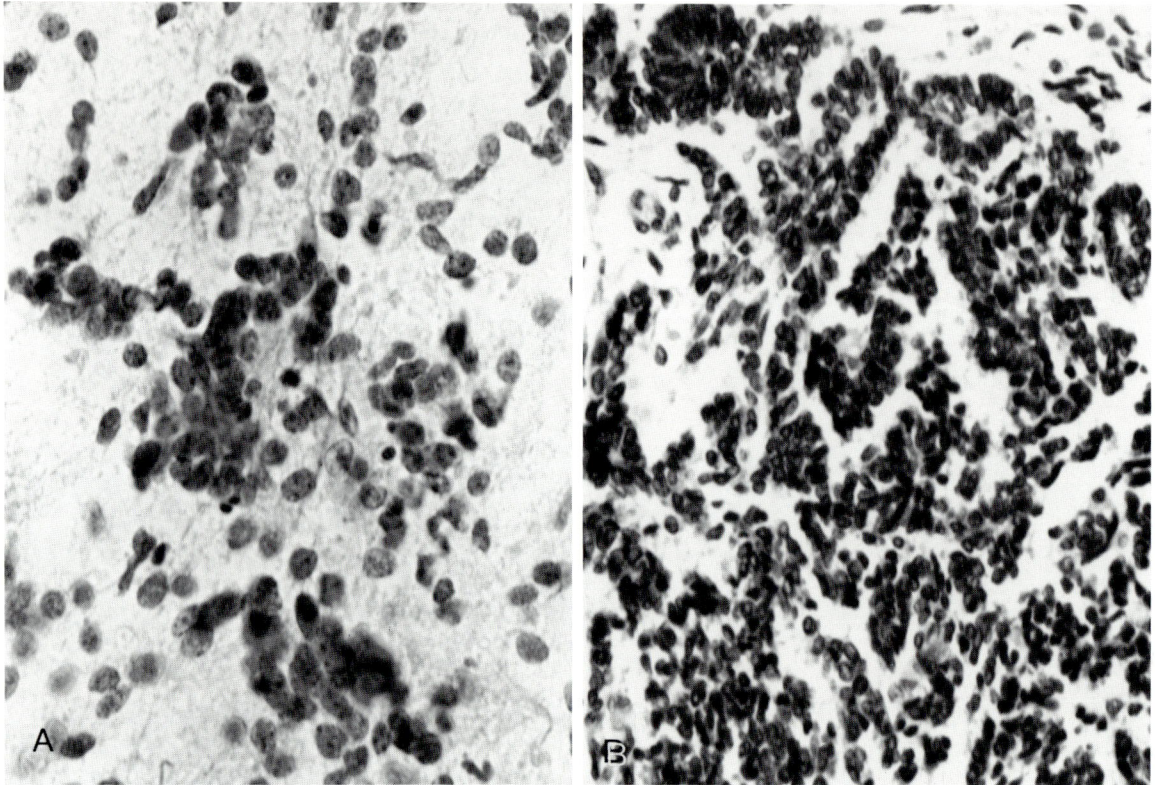

Figure 12.11.

Figure 12.11. Wilms' tumor. **A,** ABC. The blastemic cells are isolated and the epithelial cells are in rosettes and in abortive tubular formation. ×500. **B,** Histology of Wilms' tumor to show rosettes and primitive tubules. ×310.

Figure 12.12. Rhabdomyomatous Wilms' tumor. **A,** ABC. Note a group of fetal striated muscle cells. ×500. **B,** Histologic section showing the rhabdomyomatous area of the Wilms' tumor. ×310.

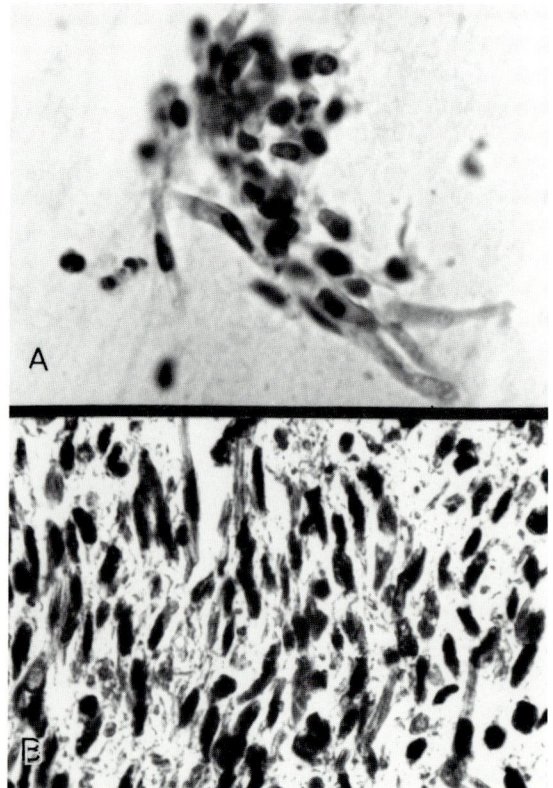

Figure 12.12.

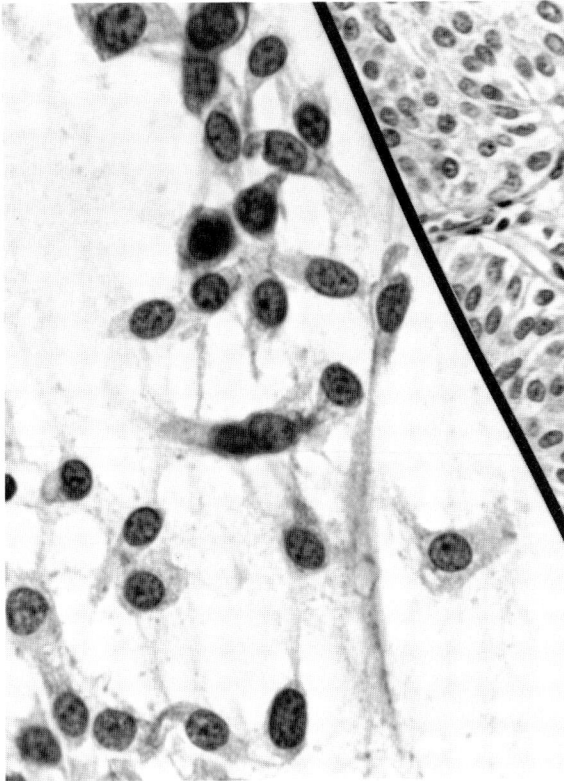

Figure 12.13.

Figure 12.13. Low-grade transitional cell carcinoma, recurrent in the retroperitoneum, ABC. The tumor cells are fairly uniform, with central or eccentric nuclei. Also note cytoplasmic elongation comparable to that seen in the histologic section. *Inset* shows the histology of the original transitional cell carcinoma of the ureter. ×500; *inset,* ×125.

Figure 12.14. Recurrent high-grade transitional cell carcinoma of the bladder, infiltrating to prostate gland. **A,** Transrectal aspiration showing pleomorphic carcinoma cells with prominent nucleoli and abundant cytoplasm ×500. **B,** Histology of the transitional cell carcinoma. ×310.

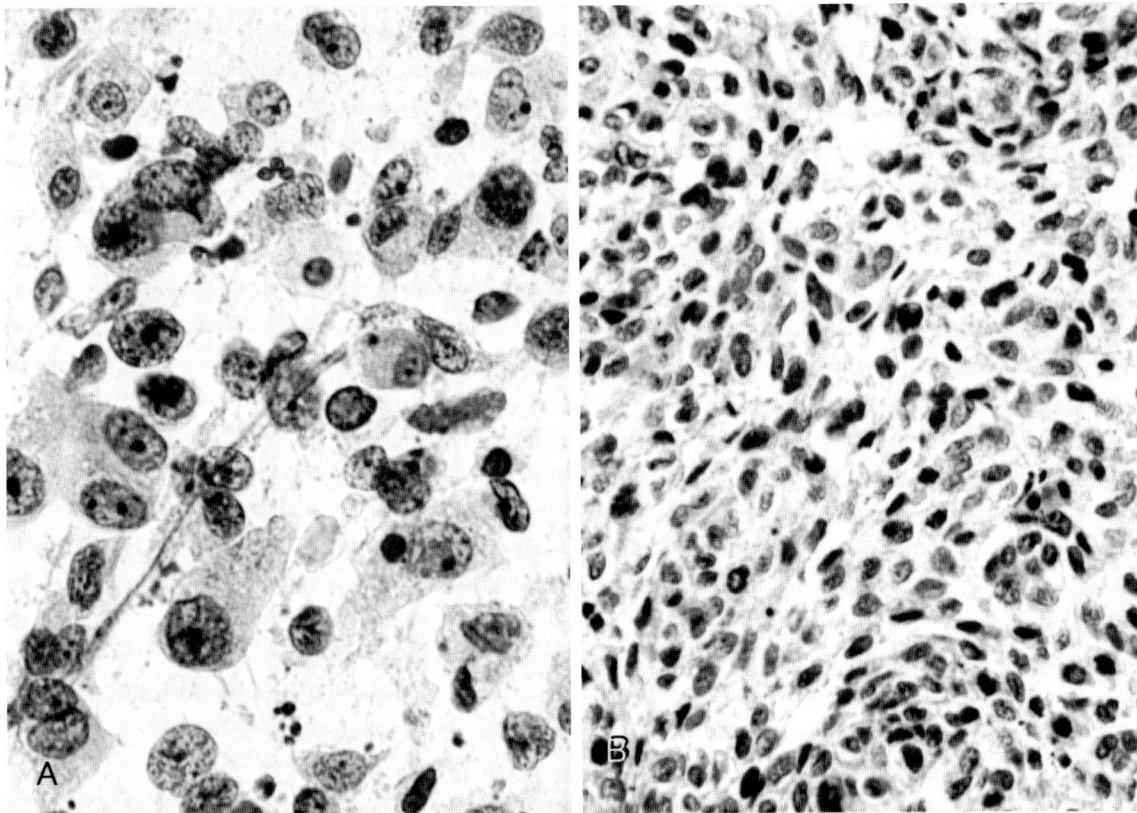

Figure 12.14.

most part was made up of myogenous cells. The aspirate clearly showed groups of fetal striated muscle cells, which had an elongated shape, a centrally placed nucleus, and intensely eosinophilic striated cytoplasm (**Fig. 12.12**).

Diagnostic Pitfalls. The small, dark blastemic cells must be distinguished from cells derived from other small cell tumors of childhood, such as neuroblastoma, Ewing's sarcoma, lymphoma, and embryonal rhabdomyosarcoma. The presence of both small dark cells and tubular structures is diagnostic of Wilms' tumor.[30a] The rosettes are not specific, since they are found also in neuroblastomas (see Chapter 13). The use of anti-neuron-specific enolase to distinguish between neuroblastoma and Wilms' tumor has been discredited since cells from both tumors show positive reactivity.[31] For further discussion on the differential diagnosis of small cell tumors see **Table 5.4**.

Epithelial Tumors of the Renal Pelvis, Ureter, and Bladder

Epithelial tumors of the renal pelvis, ureter, and bladder have the same histologic spectrum since they all arise from urothelial cells. The ratio of tumors of the bladder, renal pelvis, and ureter is estimated to be 51:3:1.[32] The vast majority of these neoplasms are transitional cell carcinomas; squamous cell carcinoma constitutes only 8–10% and adenocarcinoma less than 1% of urinary tract tumors.[16] The last two types of epithelial tumors are usually associated with chronic urinary tract infection or stones.

Primary urothelial tumors are unlikely targets for fine needle aspiration biopsy, since these tumors are usually symptomatic before they attain a large size and are diagnosed by urologic endoscopic procedures. On the other hand, recurrent tumors in the pelvis and retroperitoneum are easy targets for percutaneous FNAB. The following ABC account deals with transitional cell neoplasms only. The cytologic features of squamous cell carcinoma and adenocarcinoma are the same as those arising elsewhere and will not be repeated here.

Aspiration Cytology

The aspirates of transitional cell carcinomas are generally rich in dispersed single cells, which are either polygonal or columnar, with well-defined cell borders. The nuclei may be central or eccentric; the eccentricity may impart a plasmacytoid appearance. Based on the degree of nuclear anaplasia, transitional cell carcinomas are divided into grades 1, 2, and 3. Low-grade carcinomas are generally smaller and noninvasive and hence are unlikely targets for aspiration biopsy. A case of low-grade transitional cell carcinoma of the ureter recurring in the retroperitoneum is shown in **Figure 12.13**. The neoplastic cells, with only slight nuclear atypia, closely resemble the normal urothelial cells, which are polygonal or columnar. In contrast, high-grade transitional cell carcinomas (**Fig. 12.14**) are aggressive tumors capable of widespread metastases. Tumor cells are dispersed, vary considerably in size and shape, and show obvious malignant cytologic features. The nuclei are hyperchromatic with coarse granular chromatin and large nucleoli. The high-grade tumor cells have no specific features, and differentiation from other anaplastic carcinomas may be impossible. Differential diagnosis requires a team approach.

Sarcomas

Sarcomas of the urinary tract are rare; most are embryonal rhabdomyosarcomas arising in the bladders of children. In the kidney, leiomyosarcoma is believed to be the most common, based on a study by Farrow et al.[33]

Before a renal sarcoma is diagnosed, one must be certain that the lesion is not, in fact, a pseudosarcomatous renal cell carcinoma containing spindle and pleomorphic giant cells.[15]

Metastatic Tumors

Metastatic carcinoma can involve the kidney as a part of a disseminated process. The metastatic spread is mostly hematogenous and therefore sometimes bilateral. Multifocal growth is not uncommon. The diagnosis should be suspected in patients who have a documented history of a nonrenal malignancy and who present with sudden onset of hematuria and have radiologic findings consistent with metastatic neoplasm. On the other hand, the development of renal cell carcinoma in patients with a nonrenal primary is not a rare occurrence and must be considered. FNAB is a useful tool in discriminating renal cell carcinoma from metastatic tumors to the kidney. The most common metastases derive from small cell carcinoma of the lung, adenocarcinoma of the breast, and malignant melanoma.[34] When the metastasis in the kidney is diagnosed, the tumor is already at an advanced stage and generally only palliative treatment is used.

BENIGN NEOPLASMS AND TUMOR-LIKE LESIONS
Renal Oncocytoma

Renal oncocytoma is a benign neoplasm composed of uniform, polygonal cells with characteristic abundant eosinophilic granular cytoplasm, small nuclei without prominent nucleoli, and without mitoses.[35] Interestingly, there are occasional cases that showed malignant behavior in this otherwise benign group of neoplasms. A reasonable explanation for this is that oncocytomas and other adenomas probably represent the benign side of a spectrum of renal cell neoplasms, with renal cell carcinoma being at the other extreme. If this "spectrum" concept is correct, then an overlap in clinical and histologic characteristics of these benign and malignant tumors is to be expected.[36] In fact, this has been the experience of some investigators, who were able to identify grade 2 nuclei in oncocytomas that subsequently metastasized.[37–39]

Aspiration Cytology

The cellular ABC (**Fig. 12.15**) consists of large polygonal cells with ample granular eosinophilic cytoplasm. The nuclei are round and uniform and either centrally or eccentrically situated. The chromatin is finely granular and uniformly distributed, and nucleoli are readily discernible but are small. The cells are lying singly or arranged in monolayered groups.[15,40–42]

Diagnostic Pitfalls. The neoplastic oncocytes and the epithelial cells of the proximal convoluted tubules are similar in appearance. Two important features serve to separate them. First, the aspirates from renal oncocytomas are much more cellular than those obtained from normal renal parenchyma. Second, the cellular composition in the former is monotypic, being composed of one type of cells (i.e., the neoplastic oncocytes), whereas in the latter a mixture of proximal, distal, and connecting tubular cells and glomeruli can often be seen.

The differential diagnosis of renal oncocytoma should also include renal cell carcinoma of the granular cell type.[35] Caution should be exercised in making a diagnosis of oncocytoma if the oncocytes exhibit nuclear atypia and prominent nucleoli. Multiple samples are necessary to rule out a renal cell carcinoma.

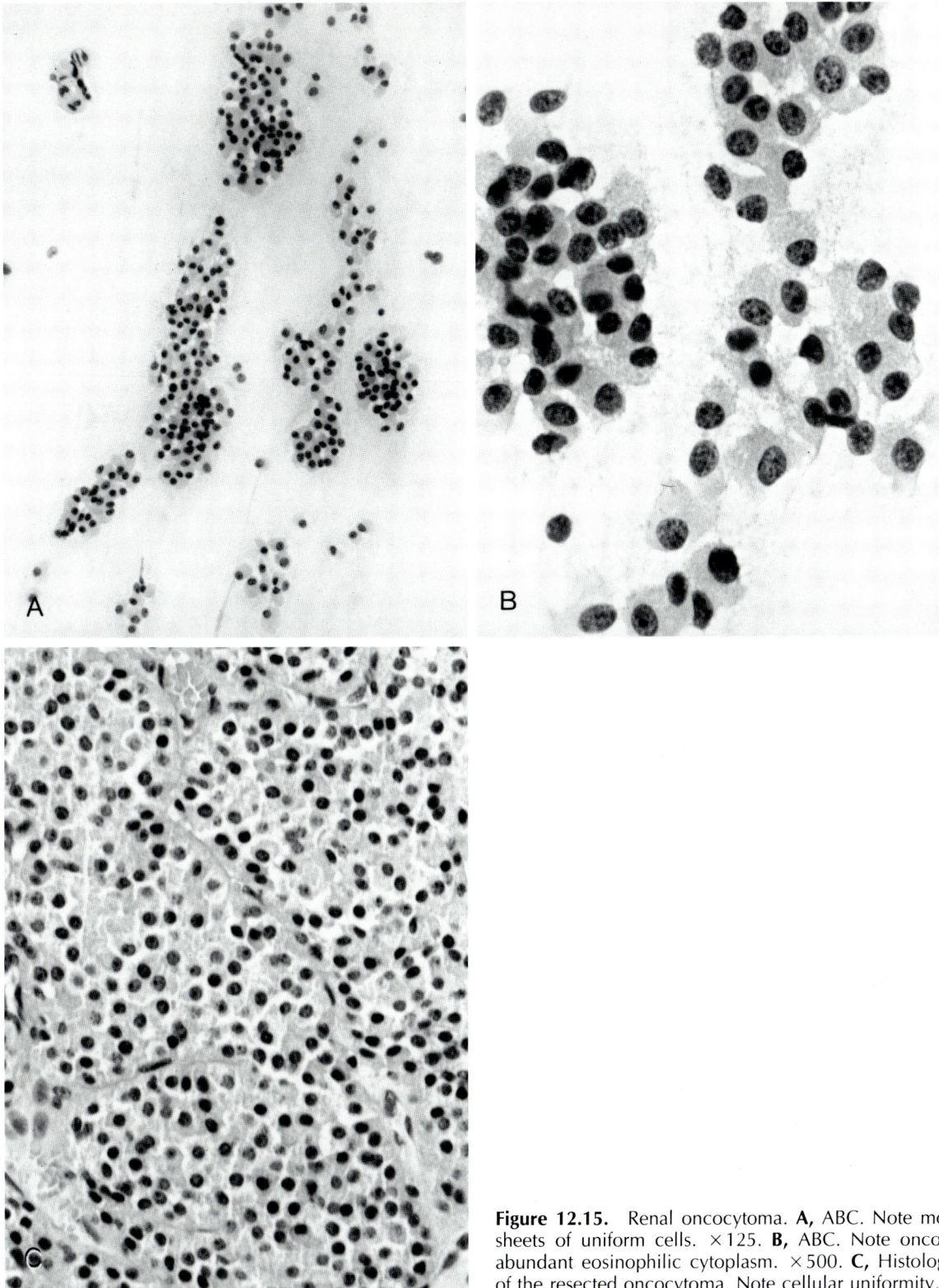

Figure 12.15. Renal oncocytoma. **A,** ABC. Note monolayered sheets of uniform cells. ×125. **B,** ABC. Note oncocytes with abundant eosinophilic cytoplasm. ×500. **C,** Histologic section of the resected oncocytoma. Note cellular uniformity. ×310.

Angiomyolipoma

Renal angiomyolipoma is a hamartomatous lesion with no malignant potential. About 80% of patients with angiomyolipoma have tuberous sclerosis. The converse, however, is not true. A considerable number of patients with angiomyolipomas do not have tuberous sclerosis. A relatively specific diagnosis can now be made with computed tomography (CT), due to the low tissue density of the fat content in the tumor.[43] The use of FNAB in the diagnosis of this tumor has also been reported.[44,45] A preoperative diagnosis of suspected angiomyolipoma made by CT and aspiration cytology may prompt exploration of the renal mass and frozen section. A partial, instead of total, nephrectomy may then be performed.[46]

Aspiration Cytology

The smears show variable cellularity and consist of at least two components, the smooth muscle cells and fat cells (Fig. 12.16). The smooth muscle cells are elongated and often arranged in parallel rows within varying-sized tissue fragments. The nuclei are cigar-shaped, with uniform, finely to coarsely granular chromatin. The nucleoli are usually small, but may be prominent. The moderately abundant cytoplasm is pale and eosinophilic, sometimes fibrillary, and shows ill-defined cytoplasmic borders. The fat cells are of the mature type and appear as large polygonal cells with small eccentric nuclei and completely clear cytoplasm. They frequently intermingle with the smooth muscle cells. Glenthoj and Partoft[45] identified thick vessel wall lined with endothelial cells in their two cases.

Diagnostic Pitfalls. It is important to be familiar with the cytologic features of angiomyolipomas because the literature indicates that the morphology of these benign lesions can be at times confused with that of a number of malignancies such as leiomyosarcoma, liposarcoma, or malignant mesenchymoma.[46,47]

Renal Cysts

The increased use of ultrasound and CT has undoubtedly demonstrated many more cysts than were identified on excretory urograms. Cystic renal masses are common; benign simple cysts occur in about 50% of the patients over the age of 55 years.[48] If a renal mass is discovered radiographically by intravenous urography or nephrotomography, it can be further characterized by ultrasound to determine whether it is cystic or solid. A benign simple cyst on ultrasound examination will show smooth, sharply defined walls, absence of internal echogenicity, and acoustic enhancement beyond the posterior wall. If these sonographic criteria for simple cysts are fulfilled, some authorities indicate that no further investigation or treatment is necessary.[49] If these criteria are not met or a cyst occurs in the clinical setting of hematuria or pain, additional evaluation is required. Percutaneous aspiration of a benign renal cyst is both a diagnostic and a therapeutic tool. The aspirated fluid is clear or straw-colored, and is low in fat and protein.[50] Microscopic examination shows foamy histiocytes and some scattered groups of benign epithelial cells with bland nuclei. If the aspirate is bloody, one must carefully rule out a malignancy. On the other hand, clear fluid is not necessarily always indicative of a benign process.

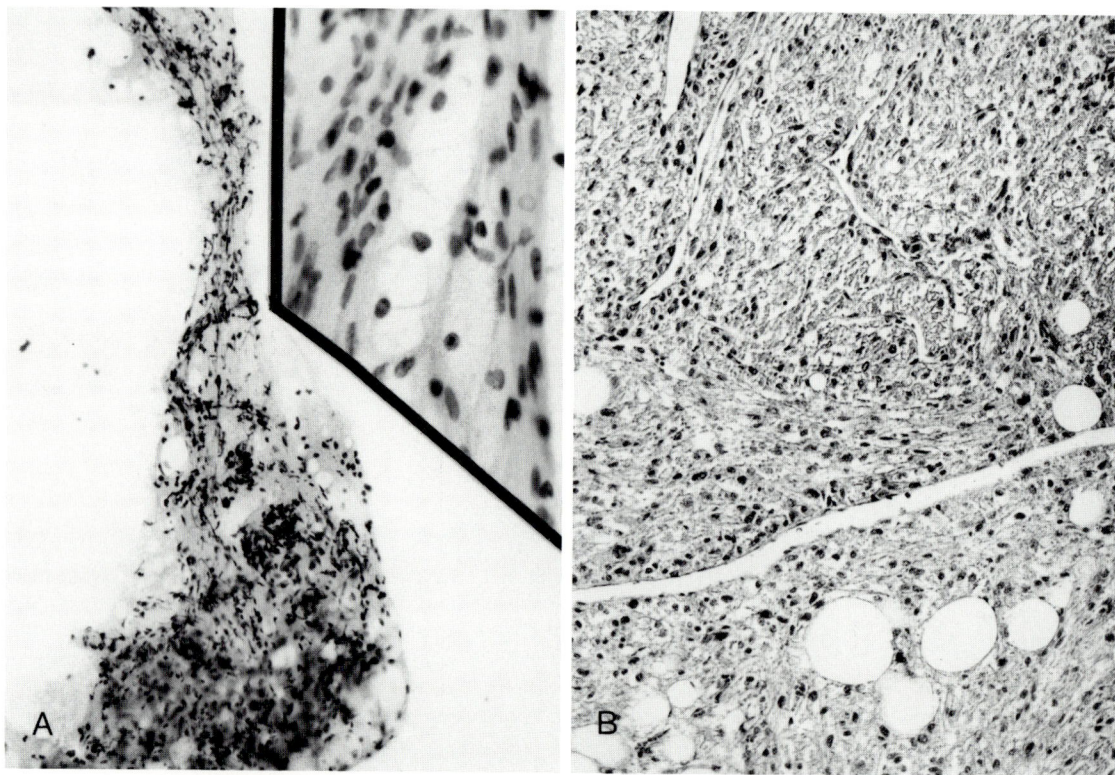

Figure 12.16. Renal angiomyolipoma. **A,** ABC. Note large tissue fragment consisting of spindle cells and fat cells. *Inset* shows the details of the smooth muscle cells and fat cells. ×125; *inset,* ×310. **B,** Histologic section of angiomyolipoma. Note randomly oriented smooth muscle fibers with interspersed adipose cells. Vascular channels are scattered among the smooth muscle fibers and fat. ×125. (Reproduced with permission. Suen KC. Guides to clinical aspiration biopsy. Retroperitoneum and intestine. New York: Igaku Shoin, 1987.)

Diagnostic Pitfalls. Atypical reactive epithelial cells and histiocytes from renal cysts have been mistaken for cells derived from renal cell carcinomas (see "Diagnostic Pitfalls" under "Renal Cell Carcinoma").[23,51] Eisenkraft et al.[52] reported a case of benign solitary multilocular cyst treated by radical nephrectomy because of

the false-positive cytology, although excretory urography, angiography, ultrasonography, and CT scan all suggested a cyst. Koss et al.[51] cautioned that, as a general rule, the diagnosis of cancer should not be established in cyst fluid except on the basis of massive cytologic evidence.

References

1. Kristensen JK, Bartels E, Jorgensen HE. Percutaneous renal biopsy under the guidance of ultrasound. Scand J Urol Nephrol 1974;8:223–226.
2. Zajicek J. Aspiration biopsy cytology, Part 2. Cytology of infradiaphragmatic organs. Basel: S Karger, 1979:1–37.
3. Juul J, Torp-Pedersen S, Gronvall S, et al. Ultrasonically guided fine needle aspiration biopsy of renal masses. J Urol 1985;133:579–581.
4. Orell SR, Langlois SLP, Marshall VR. Fine needle aspiration cytology in the diagnosis of solid renal and adrenal masses. Scand J Urol Nephrol 1985;19:211–216.
5. Pilotti S, Rilke DF, Alasio L, Garbagnati F. The role of fine needle aspiration in the assessment of renal masses. Acta Cytol 1988;32:1–10.
6. Linsk JA, Franzen S. Aspiration cytology of metastatic hypernephroma. Acta Cytol 1984;28:250–260.
7. Nguyen GK. Fine needle aspiration biopsy cytology of metastatic renal cell carcinoma. Acta Cytol 1988;32:409–414.
8. Jeans WD, Penry JB, Roylance J. Renal puncture. Clin Radiol 1972;23:298–311.
9. Lindblom K. Percutaneous puncture of renal cysts and tumors. Acta Radiol 1946;27:66–72.
10. Kristensen JK, Holm HH, Rasmussen SN, Barlebo H. Ultrasonically guided percutaneous puncture of renal masses. Scand J Urol Nephrol Suppl 1972;6:49–56.
11. Gibbons RP, Bush WH, Burnett LL. Needle tract seeding following aspiration of renal cell carcinoma. J Urol 1977;118:865–867.
12. von Schreeb T, Arner G, Skovsted G, Wilstad N. Renal adenocarcinoma: Is there a risk of spreading tumour cells in diagnostic puncture? Scand J Urol Nephrol 1967;1:270–276.
13. Teplick SK, Haskin PK. Imaging modalities. In Kline TS. Handbook of fine needle aspiration biopsy cytology, 2nd ed. New York: Churchill Livingstone, 1988:32.
14. Nosher JL, Amorosa JK, Leiman S, Plafker J. Fine needle aspiration of the kidney and adrenal gland. J Urol 1982;128:895–899.
15. Suen KC. Guides to clinical aspiration biopsy. Retroperitoneum and intestine. New York: Igaku Shoin, 1987:131–163.
16. Bennington JL, Beckwith JB. Tumors of the kidney, renal pelvis and ureter. Atlas of tumor pathology, 2nd Series, Fascicle 12. Washington D.C.: Armed Forces Institute of Pathology, 1975:93–199.
17. Javadpour N. Cancer of the kidney. New York: Thieme-Stratton, 1984:1–13.
18. Duggan MA, Forestell CF, Hanley DA. Adrenal metastases of renal cell carcinoma 19 years after nephrectomy. Fine needle aspiration cytology of a case. Acta Cytol 1987;31:512–516.
19. Skinner D, Colvin R, Vermillion C, Pfister R, Leadbetter W. Diagnosis and management of renal cell carcinoma, a clinical and pathologic study of 309 cases. Cancer 1971;28:1165–1177.
20. Fuhrman SA, Lasky LC, Limas C. Prognostic significance of morphologic parameters in renal cell carcinoma. Am J Surg Pathol 1982;6:655–663.
21. Nguyen GK. Percutaneous fine-needle aspiration biopsy cytology of the kidney and adrenal. Pathol Annu 22:163–191.
22. Helm CW, Burwood RJ, Harrison NW, Melcher DH. Aspiration cytology of solid renal tumors. Br J Urol 193;55:249–253.
23. Plowden KM, Erozen YS, Frost JK. Cellular atypias associated with
benign lesions of the kidney as seen in fine needle aspirates. Acta Cytol 1984;28:648.
24. Yu GSM. Immunocytochemistry and electron microscopy. In Suen KC. Guides to clinical aspiration biopsy. Retroperitoneum and intestine. New York: Igaku Shoin, 1987:197.
25. Tolamo TS, Shonnard JW. Small renal adenocarcinoma with metastases. J Urol 1980;124:132–134.
26. Cass AS. Large renal adenoma. J Urol 1980;124:281–282.
27. Mostofi FK, Davis CJ. Pathology of urologic cancer. In Javadpour N. Principles and management of urologic cancer, 2nd ed. Baltimore: Williams & Wilkins, 1983:65.
28. Bennington JL. Cancer of the kidney—etiology, epidemiology, and pathology. Cancer 1973;32:1017–1029.
29. Lohr E, Leder LD. Renal and adrenal tumors, 2nd ed. Berlin: Springer-Verlag, 1987:27.
30. Bray G, Pendergrass TW, Schaller RT Jr, Kiviat N, Beckwith JB. Preoperative chemotherapy in the treatment of Wilms' tumor diagnosed with the aid of fine needle aspiration biopsy. Am J Pediatr Hematol Oncol 1986;8:75–78.
30a. Quijano G, Drut R. Cytologic characteristics of Wilms' tumors in fine needle aspirates. A study of ten cases. Acta Cytol 1989;33:263–266.
31. Drut R. Neuron-specific enolase-positive rosettes in nephroblastoma: A possible diagnostic pitfall in aspiration cytology. Diag Cytopathol 1987;3:74–76.
32. Williams CB, Mitchell JP. Carcinoma of the ureter—a review of 54 cases. Br J Urol 1973;45:377–387.
33. Farrow GM, Harrison EG Jr, Utz DC, RaMine WH. Sarcomas and sarcomatoid and mixed malignant tumors of the kidney in adults. Cancer 1968;22:545–550.
34. Petersen RO. Urologic pathology. Philadelphia: JB Lippincott, 1986:134–136.
35. Yu GSM, Rendler S, Herskowitz A, Molnar JJ. Renal oncocytoma. Cancer 1980;45:1010–1018.
36. Dickersin GR, Colvin RB. Pathology of renal tumors. In Skinner DG, Lieskovsky G. Diagnosis and management of genitourinary cancer. Philadelphia: WB Saunders, 1988:118–149.
37. Lieber MM, Tomera KM, Farrow GM. Renal oncocytoma. J Urol 1981;125:481–485.
38. Lieber MM. Renal oncocytoma. In Javadpour N. Cancer of the kidney. New York: Thieme-Stratton, 1984:139–148.
39. Barnes CA, Beckman EN. Renal oncocytoma and its congeners. Am J Clin Pathol 1983;79:312–318.
40. Rodriquez CA, Buskop A, Johnson J, et al. Renal oncocytoma: Preoperative diagnosis by aspiration biopsy. Acta Cytol 1980;24:355–359.
41. Alanen KA, Tyrkko JES, Nurmi MJ. Aspiration biopsy cytology of oncocytoma. Acta Cytol 1985;29:859–862.
42. Nguyen GK, Amy RW, Tsang S. Fine needle aspiration biopsy cytology of renal oncocytoma. Acta Cytol 1985;29:33–36.
43. Lingeman JE, Donohue JP, Madura JA, Selks F. Angiomyolipoma: Emerging concepts in management. Urology 1982;20:566–570.
44. Nguyen GK. Aspiration biopsy cytology of renal angiomyolipoma. Acta Cytol 1984;28:261–264.
45. Glenthoj A, Partoft S. Ultrasound-guided percutaneous aspiration of renal angiomyolipoma. Acta Cytol 1984;28:265–268.

46. Barrilero AE. Renal angiomyolipoma: A study of 13 cases. J Urol 1977;117:547–552.

47. Hajdu SI, Foote FW. Angiomyolipoma of the kidney. Report of 27 cases and review of the literature. J Urol 1969;102:396–401.

48. Letourneau JG, Elyaderani MK: Percutaneous biopsy of kidneys and adrenals and drainage of nephric and perinephric fluid collections. In Letourneau JG, Elyaderani MK, Castaneda-Zuniga WR. Percutaneous biopsy, aspiration and drainage. Chicago: Year Book, 1987:79–103.

49. Pollack HW, Banner MP, Arger PH, Peters J, Mulhern CB, Coleman BG. The accuracy of gray-scale renal ultrasonography in differentiating cystic neoplasms from benign cysts. Radiology 1982;143:741–745.

50. Steg A. Does percutaneous puncture still have a role to play in the diagnosis of renal tumors? In Kuss R, Murphy GP, Khoury S, Karr JP. Renal tumors. New York: Alan R Liss, 1981:417–423.

51. Koss LG, Woyke S, Olszewski W. Aspiration biopsy. Cytologic interpretation and histologic bases. New York: Igaku Shoin, 1984:384–408.

52. Eisenkraft S, Englander L, Wolfe RM, Huben RP, Pontes JE. Multilocular cyst of the kidney. A case report. J Surg Oncol 1984;27:45–47.

13

Adrenal

Although the adrenal gland is an anatomic entity, the cortex and medulla differ from one another in their embryonic development, morphology, and function. The cortex develops from the mesoderm on the posterior wall near the urogenital ridge. The medulla is populated by cells originating from the neural crest. These primitive cells mature in the adrenal medulla to become either pheochromocytes or ganglion cells.

Functionally, the outer zone (zona glomerulosa) of the adrenal cortex synthesizes mineralocorticoids, which are responsible for conservation of salt and water and excretion of potassium. The two inner zones (zona fasciculata and zona reticularis) function as one unit and synthesize glucocorticoids and androgens. The adrenal medulla produces epinephrine and norepinephrine.

Based on their structural and functional characteristics, two principal groups of adrenal neoplasms are recognized: *(a)* those arising from the cortex, i.e., cortical adenoma and cortical carcinoma, and *(b)* those arising from the medulla, i.e., pheochromocytoma, neuroblastoma, ganglioneuroblastoma, and ganglioneuroma.

Other less frequently encountered adrenal tumors and tumor-like lesions include myelolipoma,[1,2] primary melanoma, neurofibroma,[3] cysts, tuberculoma,[4] and fungal pseudotumor.[5,5a,5b]

NORMAL CYTOLOGY

Cells of normal adrenal cortex **(Fig. 13.1)**, arranged in small monolayered sheets or in slender cords, are uniform, polygonal cells, with round vesicular nuclei and single small nucleoli. The cytoplasm is either vacuolated or eosinophilic. The vacuolated (clear) cells, derived principally from the zona fasciculata, show diffuse, honeycomb-type cytoplasmic vacuoles and reflect lipid storage. The cytoplasm is fragile, and as a result there are many stripped nuclei and fine lipid droplets in the smear background. The eosinophilic cells, chiefly derived from the zona reticularis, are smaller and compact; the cytoplasm is finely granular, with fewer stored steroids.

Cells from the adrenal medulla **(Fig. 13.2)** are more pleomorphic. They are generally polygonal, with abundant basophilic granular cytoplasm. The nuclei are round and many are eccentrically placed. The chromatin is coarsely granular. Nucleoli are usually conspicuous.

TUMORS OF THE ADRENAL CORTEX
Adrenocortical Adenoma

Cortical adenomas are small, fairly well-circumscribed tumors, 2–4 cm in diameter, and generally weigh less than 100 grams. In general, functioning cortical adenomas make their presence known clinically by producing adrenocortical hormones; nonfunctioning adenomas have rarely been diagnosed during life, despite being found in 2–8% of the autopsy population.[6] However, with increasing usage of ultrasound and computed tomography, more and more nonfunctioning adenomas are being detected during life.

Aspiration Cytology[7,8]

Aspirates from cortical adenomas are moderately cellular, with cells arranged in monolayer sheets or cords in a lipid-rich background. The neoplastic cells resemble the normal cortical cells but may be slightly larger **(Fig. 13.3)**. Varying proportions of large vacuolated cells and compact eosinophilic cells are found. Variation of nuclear size is common **(Fig. 13.4)** but nuclear atypia is minimal or absent. Nucleoli may be small or conspicuous. In a few cases, however, there may be focal cellular polymorphism, with giant cells.

Diagnostic Pitfalls. Neoplastic cells from highly differentiated adenomas closely resemble normal cortical cells; whereas neoplastic cells from pleomorphic adenomas mimic cells of cortical carcinoma. In the first instance, the diagnosis of a benign tumor is made on the basis of the CT or ultrasound finding of an adrenal mass and the observation of benign-appearing cortical cells on FNAB. It is imperative to verify the location of the aspiration needle by computed tomography to ensure its correct placement within the mass. Without this verification by an experienced radiologist, recovered cells, which are assumed to be derived from an adenoma, may in fact have come from the normal part of the cortex.

In the second instance, if the cellular pleomorphism is pronounced, cortical carcinoma must be considered. Usually, other features of cortical carcinoma are also present, such as tumor necrosis, mitoses, and large tumor size (see below).

Adrenocortical Carcinoma

Adrenocortical carcinoma is an uncommon neoplasm, comprising only 0.02–0.04% of all cancers.[9] The majority of cortical carcinomas are functioning, causing Cushing's syndrome or virilization.[10] The typical clinical findings are as follows: a relatively young patient (the mean age for females is 36.6 years and for males, 48 years), a large abdominal mass, weight loss, and various systemic constitutional symptoms. Diagnosis is facilitated by various biochemical tests of urine and serum adrenocortical hormones and metabolites.

Grossly, the tumor size aids in predicting the clinical behavior of the tumor. Schteingart et al.[11] stated that all tumors larger than 7 cm in their series were malignant and that all tumors less than 4 cm were benign. Microscopically, the tumors are composed of vacuolated and eosinophilic cells in varying proportions. The cells tend to be pleomorphic and mitotically active. In some cases, however, the cells are fairly well-differentiated, resembling those seen in cortical

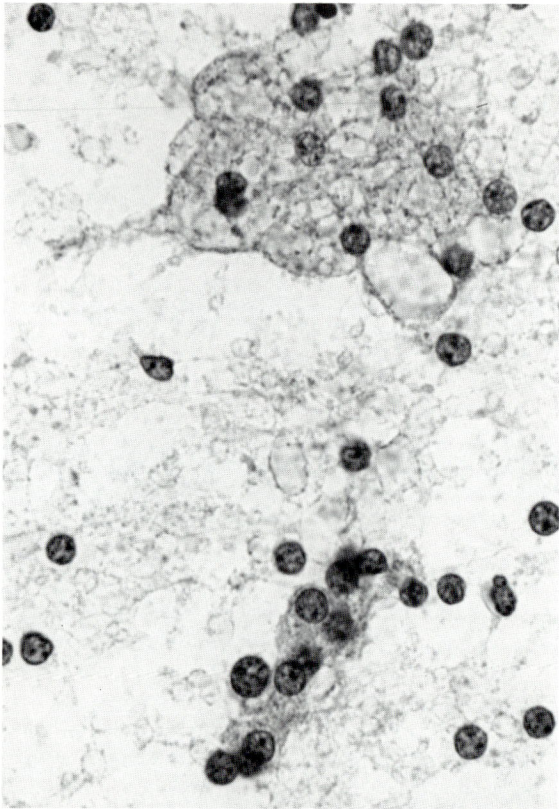

Figure 13.1. Normal adrenal cortex, ABC. Note large vacuolated cells and a small group of compact eosinophilic cells *(bottom half)*. Also note a few stripped nuclei in the background. ×500.

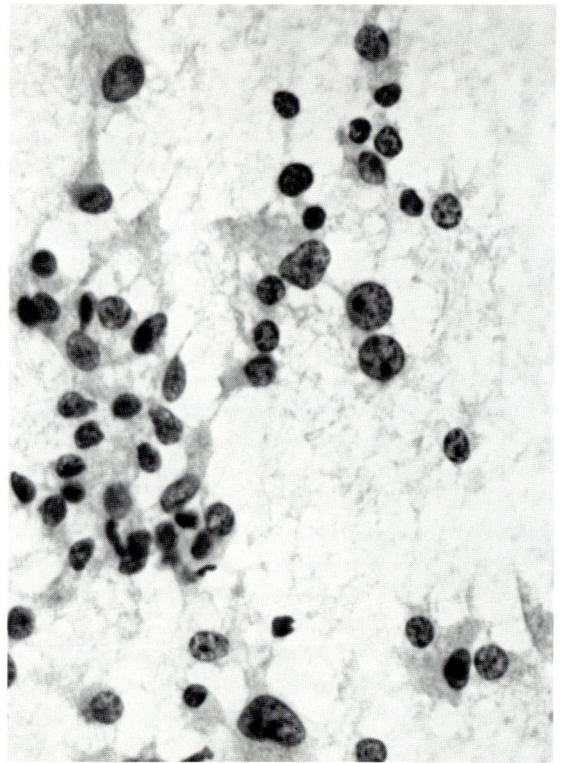

Figure 13.2. Normal adrenal medulla, imprint smear from a surgical specimen. Medullary cells have abundant granular cytoplasm and some cells have prominent nucleoli. Note variability of nuclear size. ×500.

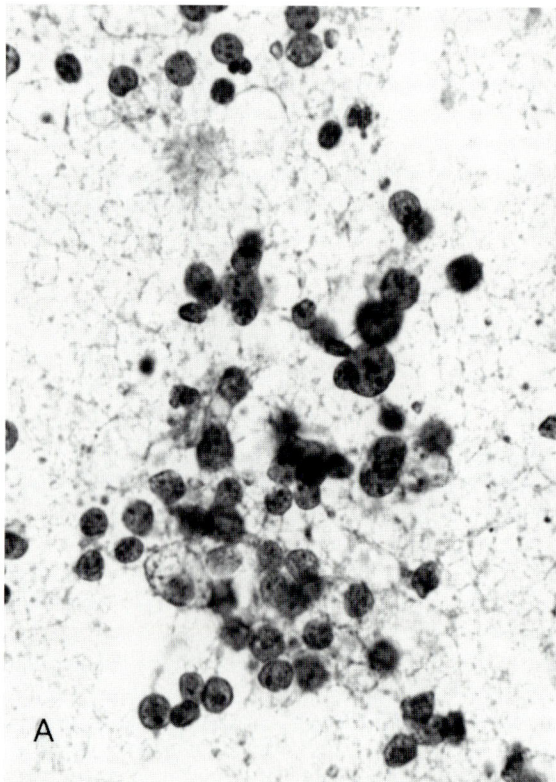

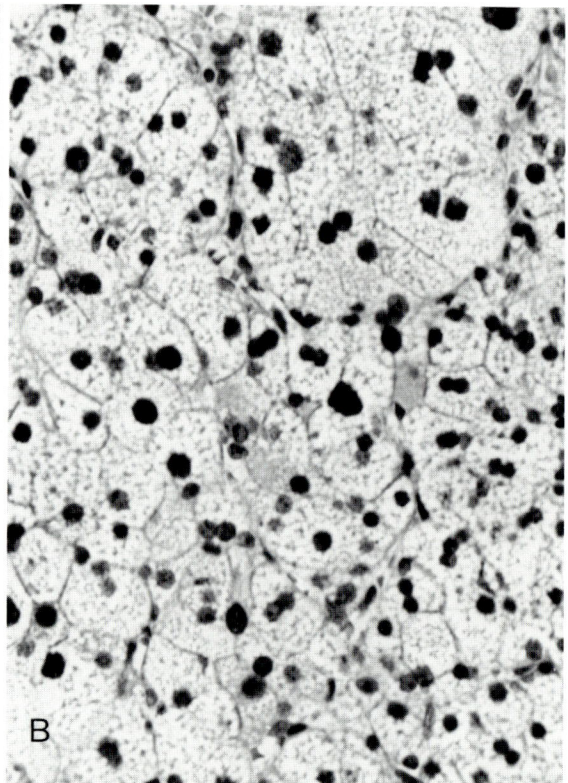

Figure 13.3. Cortical adenoma. **A,** ABC. Note vacuolated cells and lipid droplets in the background. ×500. **B,** Histology of adenoma. Note honeycomb-type cytoplasmic vacuoles. ×310.

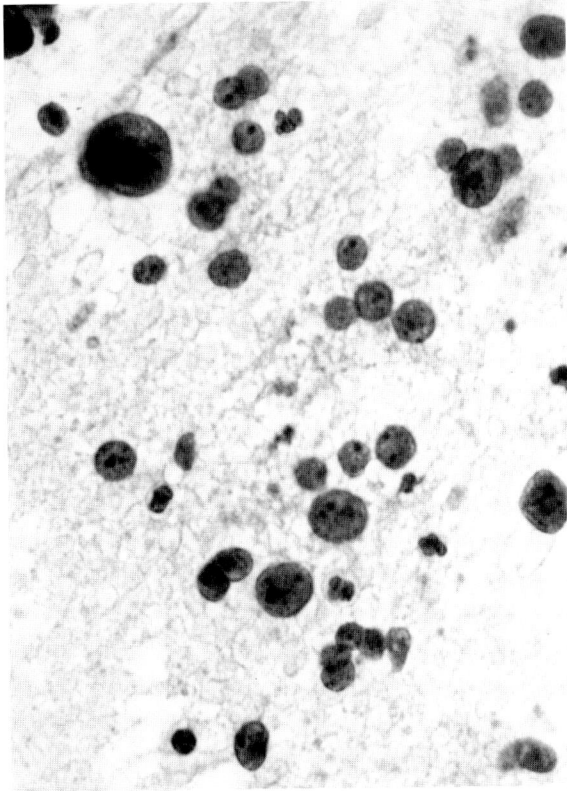

Figure 13.4.

Figure 13.4. Cortical adenoma, ABC. Note many bare nuclei and marked variability of nuclear size. ×500.

Figure 13.5. Cortical carcinoma. **A,** ABC. These cells are cytologically malignant. Both vacuolated cells and granular eosinophilic cells can be seen. ×500. **B,** Histologic section of the resected cortical carcinoma showing obviously malignant cells. Both clear and eosinophilic cells are present. ×310.

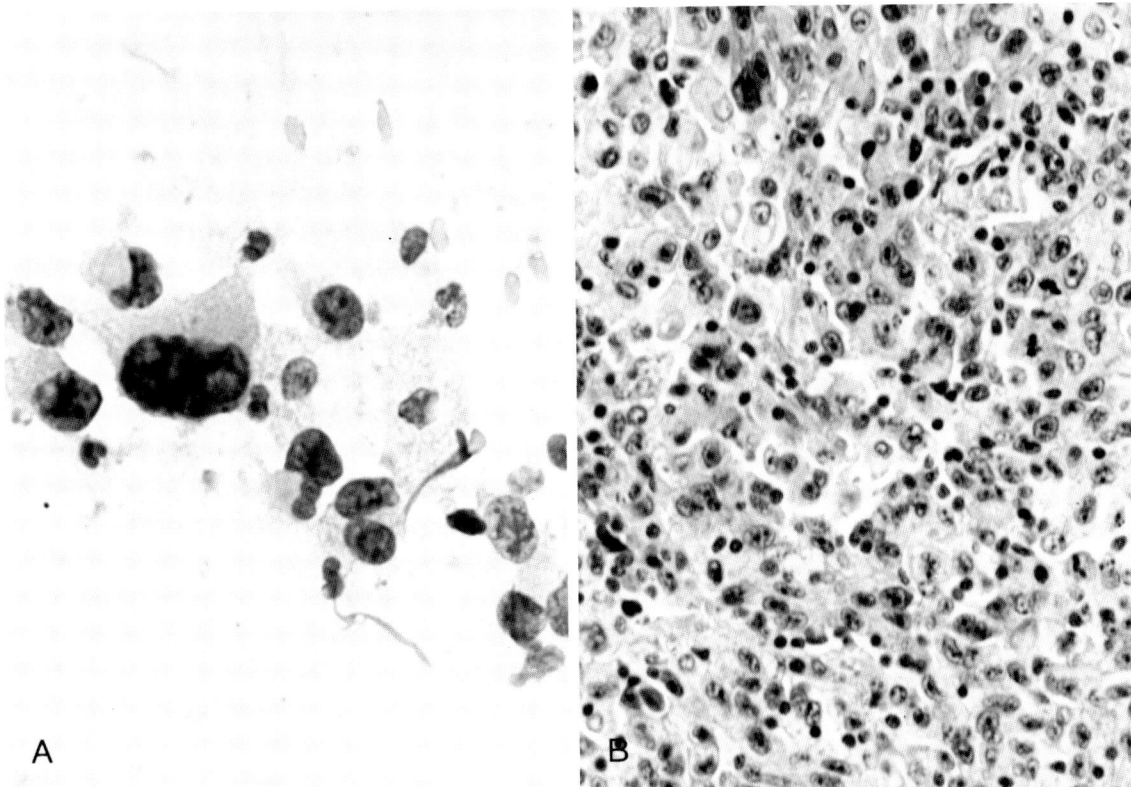

A

B

Figure 13.5.

adenomas. Moreover, focal well-differentiated areas may be seen in an otherwise pleomorphic carcinoma.

Aspiration Cytology[7,8,12–14]

The aspirates are rich in tumor cells, most of which are lying singly because of loss of cell cohesion. Both vacuolated cells and eosinophilic cells are encountered. In two of the four cases in our file the eosinophilic cells predominated and in one case they were present almost to the exclusion of the vacuolated cells. The tumor cells (Fig. 13.5) had pleomorphic nuclei, with irregular coarse chromatin and prominent nucleoli. Numerous mitoses were evident. Our file contains one case of well-differentiated cortical carcinoma. The aspirate (Fig. 13.6) showed more differentiated, lipid-containing cells, which were surprisingly small. The nuclear atypia was subtle, but there were many mitoses and a considerable amount of necrosis.

Diagnostic Pitfalls. The correlation between the histologic appearance and clinical behavior of adrenocortical neoplasms is not entirely accurate, unless the tumor shows capsular or blood vessel invasion, in which case the definitive diagnosis of carcinoma can be made. Bulky tumors (>100 grams) are more likely malignant, although a few appear to behave as simple adenomas.[15] On fine needle aspiration cytology, the following features are usually considered as probable indicators of malignancy: (a) cellular and nuclear pleomorphism, (b) loss of cellular cohesiveness, (c) numerous mitoses, and (d) areas of necrosis.[7] Unfortunately, none of these features by itself is diagnostic of malignancy, because each can be found to some degree in adenomas.[16] In general, although benign tumors can have pleomorphic cellular features, these are more pronounced in carcinomas.

It may be difficult to distinguish poorly differentiated carcinoma of the adrenal cortex from carcinomas metastatic to the adrenal gland. Clinical and laboratory correlation is crucial. Ultrastructural study of the cells of the aspirate may provide valuable information;[16a] cytoplasmic lipid droplets, prominent smooth endoplasmic reticulum, and elongated mitochondria with shelf-like cristae characterize cells of the adrenal cortex (Fig. 13.7). Similarly, differentiation between renal cell carcinoma and adrenocortical carcinoma may cause problems on FNAB because they have many morphologic features in common. Renal cell carcinoma tends to have more clear cells, whereas adrenal carcinoma tends to have pleomorphic eosinophilic cells. The presence of papillae and/or tubules suggests the diagnosis of renal cell carcinoma. Immunoperoxidase staining of the tumors is also helpful in arriving at the correct diagnosis (see ''Renal Cell Carcinoma'' in Chapter 12).

Problems of the Incidentally Discovered Adrenal Masses

The increasing use of modern imaging techniques for metastatic workup in cancer patients has led to the discovery of many incidental small adrenal masses.[17–19] As the nature of the adrenal mass may influence the staging, prognosis, and treatment of the cancer, it is necessary to obtain as definitive a diagnosis as possible. In this situation, the differential diagnosis is between metastatic tumor and primary adrenal tumor. Fine needle aspiration biopsy under ultrasound or CT guidance is ideally suited to assessing such a lesion.[20] An aspirate of a metastatic tumor shows malignant cells that may reveal their tissue origin; an aspirate of an adrenocortical tumor shows adrenocortical cells, and a pheochromocytoma shows neoplastic pheochromocytes (see below). A primary adrenal tumor, whether benign or malignant, should be surgically removed if it produces hormones in sufficient quantity to cause symptoms. In the case of a nonfunctioning, asymptomatic, primary adrenal tumor, it is highly

unlikely that a cytologically diagnosed, asymptomatic cortical adenoma may, in fact, represent a small, incidental cortical carcinoma.[15] The incidence of adrenocortical carcinoma is extremely low (0.02–0.04% of all cancers) and small incidental carcinomas must be even rarer (carcinomas, in general, measure more than 4 cm).[11] On review of the recent literature, O'Leary and Ooi[20a] found 71 cases of incidental adrenal tumors that were treated surgically, and none proved to be adrenocortical carcinoma. Hence, these authors recommend a conservative approach to management of these lesions.

TUMORS OF THE ADRENAL MEDULLA
Pheochromocytoma

Pheochromocytoma is a rare neoplasm, which belongs to the family of neuroendocrine tumors. The majority of pheochromocytomas arise in the adrenal medulla, but extraadrenal pheochromocytomas (paragangliomas) can develop in the organs of Zuckerkandl and the paraganglionic system. About 5–10% of the tumors are familial and may coexist with medullary thyroid carcinoma and parathyroid hyperplasia.[21] Pheochromocytomas produce catecholamines and hence hypertension. Clinically, fewer than 50% of the patients have the typical, paroxysmal hypertensive episodes, and 14% have atypical signs or an absence of signs.[22,23] When a clinical diagnosis of pheochromocytoma is made, it can be substantiated by measuring increased quantities of catecholamines or their metabolites (e.g., vanillylmandelic acid) in the patient's urine or serum. FNAB becomes superfluous in these cases. In the literature, FNAB has been performed in tumors in which the diagnosis of pheochromocytoma was not suspected.[7,23–26] Aspiration of a catecholamine-producing tumor is not without risk: a case of fatality following the procedure has been reported.[22] Hence, clinical expertise for emergency treatment of catecholamine storm should be available.

Histologically, the cells of pheochromocytoma resemble the mature pheochromocytes of the normal medulla.[16] Although generally polygonal in configuration, the tumor cells are sometimes fusiform or multinucleated. They are arranged in alveolar groupings or trabeculae in close association with thin-walled vessels or sinuses. About 10% of the tumors are malignant but in the absence of metastasis no histologic features exist that can be used to separate the benign from the malignant.

Aspiration Cytology

The aspirates are cellular and often contain much blood due to tumor vascularity. The cells are arranged in small loose alveolar groups or are lying singly. The ABC has a pleomorphic appearance because of the great variability in cell size and shape.[27] Three main types of tumor cells are identified: polygonal cells (55%), pleomorphic cells (43%), and spindle cells (2%).[28] The relatively uniform, polygonal cells have round, vesicular nuclei, some of which are eccentrically situated. The cytoplasm is moderate in amount and foamy or finely granular. The cell borders are not always distinctively recognizable. The polygonal cells may be small or large in size. The small cells are reminiscent of carcinoid cells (Fig. 13.8). The larger cells, especially when they contain conspicuous nucleoli and abundant cytoplasm, are reminiscent of ganglion cells (Fig. 13.9). The pleomorphic giant cells (Fig. 13.10) show hyperchromatic nuclei with chromatin smudging; nuclei may be multiple and nucleoli are prominent. The cytoplasm is homogenous and eosinophilic. It should be noted that these pleomorphic giant cells have no association with clinical malignancy. The spindle cells (Fig. 13.11) are the least common and show fusiform nuclei and pale eosinophilic cytoplasm with ill-defined borders.

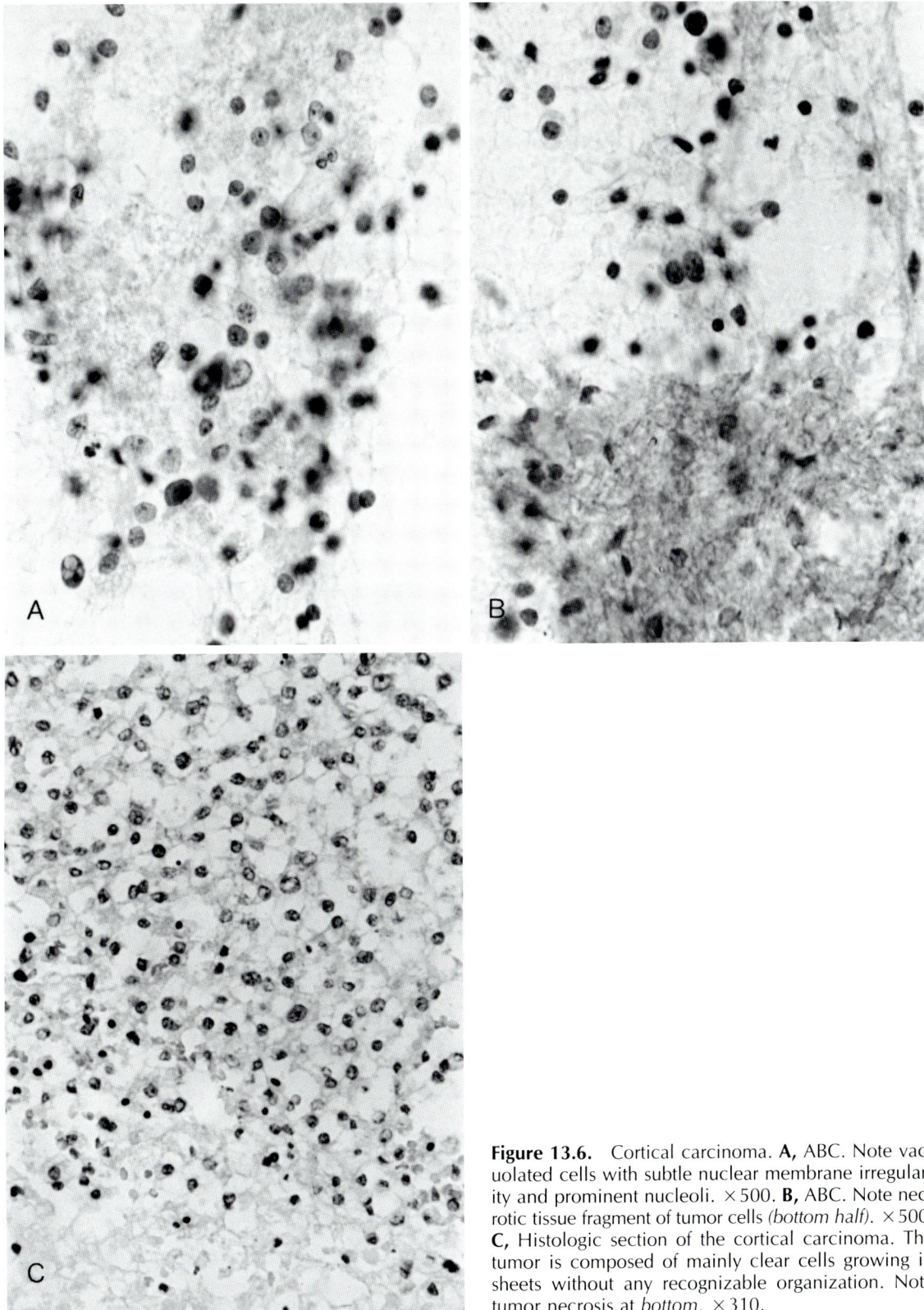

Figure 13.6. Cortical carcinoma. **A,** ABC. Note vacuolated cells with subtle nuclear membrane irregularity and prominent nucleoli. ×500. **B,** ABC. Note necrotic tissue fragment of tumor cells *(bottom half).* ×500. **C,** Histologic section of the cortical carcinoma. The tumor is composed of mainly clear cells growing in sheets without any recognizable organization. Note tumor necrosis at *bottom.* ×310.

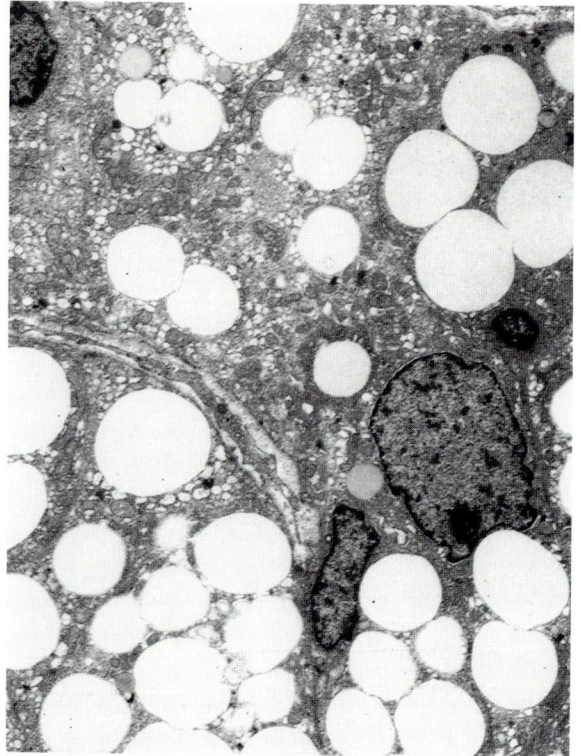

Figure 13.7.   Ultrastructure of cortical carcinoma, cell block. Note abundant cytoplasmic lipid globules, prominent smooth endoplasmic reticulum, and mitochrondria. These features are characteristic of steroid hormone-producing cells. Uranyl acetate and lead citrate preparation, ×3680.

Figure 13.8.   Pheochromocytoma. **A,** ABC. Note rather uniform, small, polygonal cells in alveolar arrangement. ×310. **B,** Tissue section. Note morphologic resemblance to carcinoid tumor. ×310.

Figure 13.7.

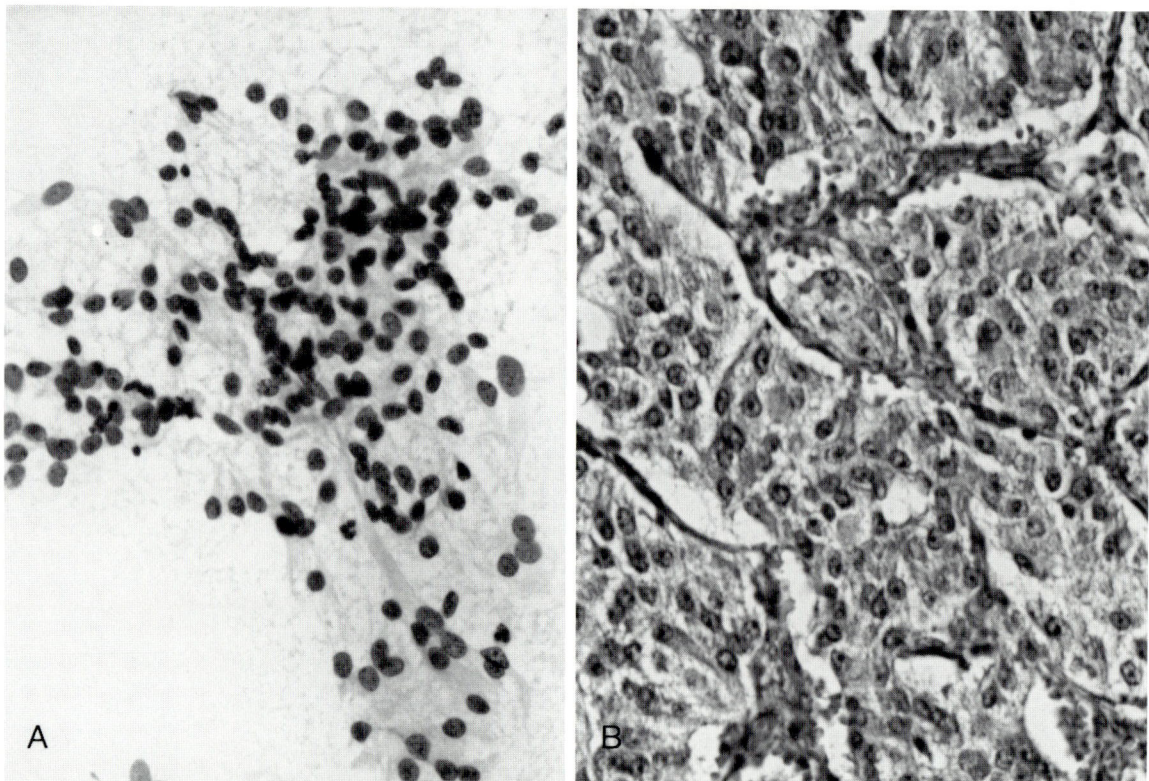

Figure 13.8.

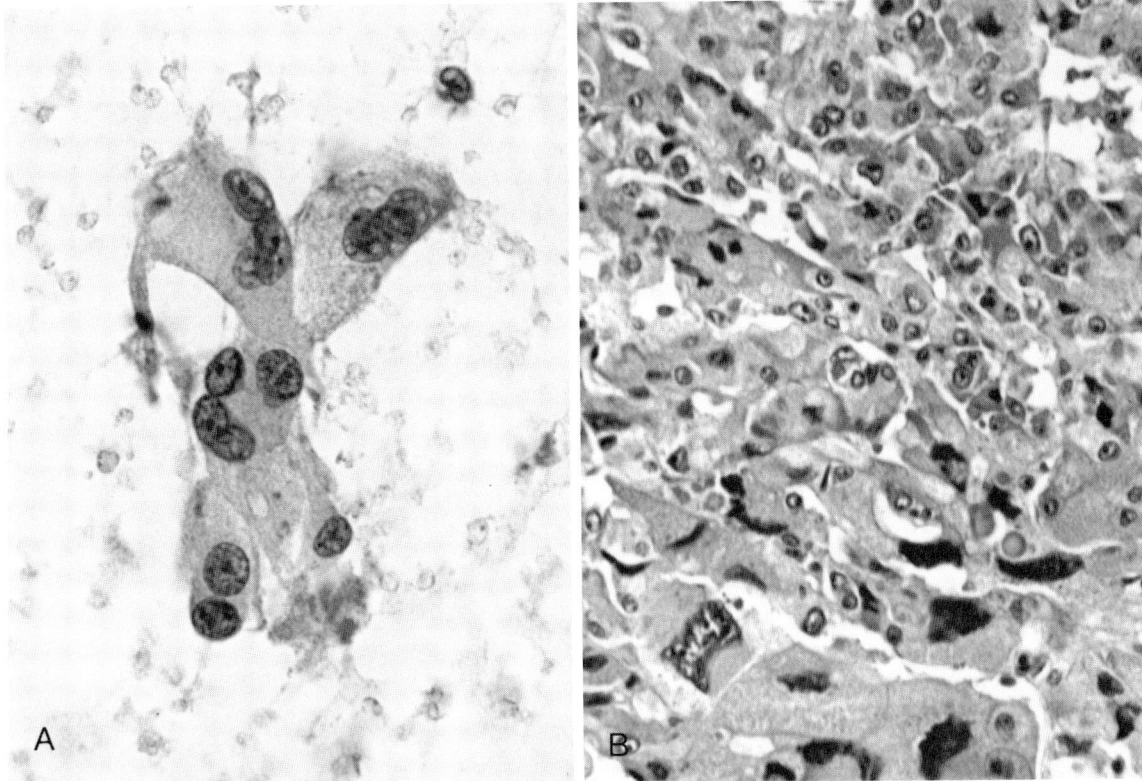

Figure 13.9.   Pheochromocytoma. **A,** ABC. Note large polygonal cells with abundant granular or foamy cytoplasm and prominent nucleoli. ×500. **B,** Tissue section. Note large eosinophilic polygonal cells and many bizarre giant cells *(bottom).* ×310.

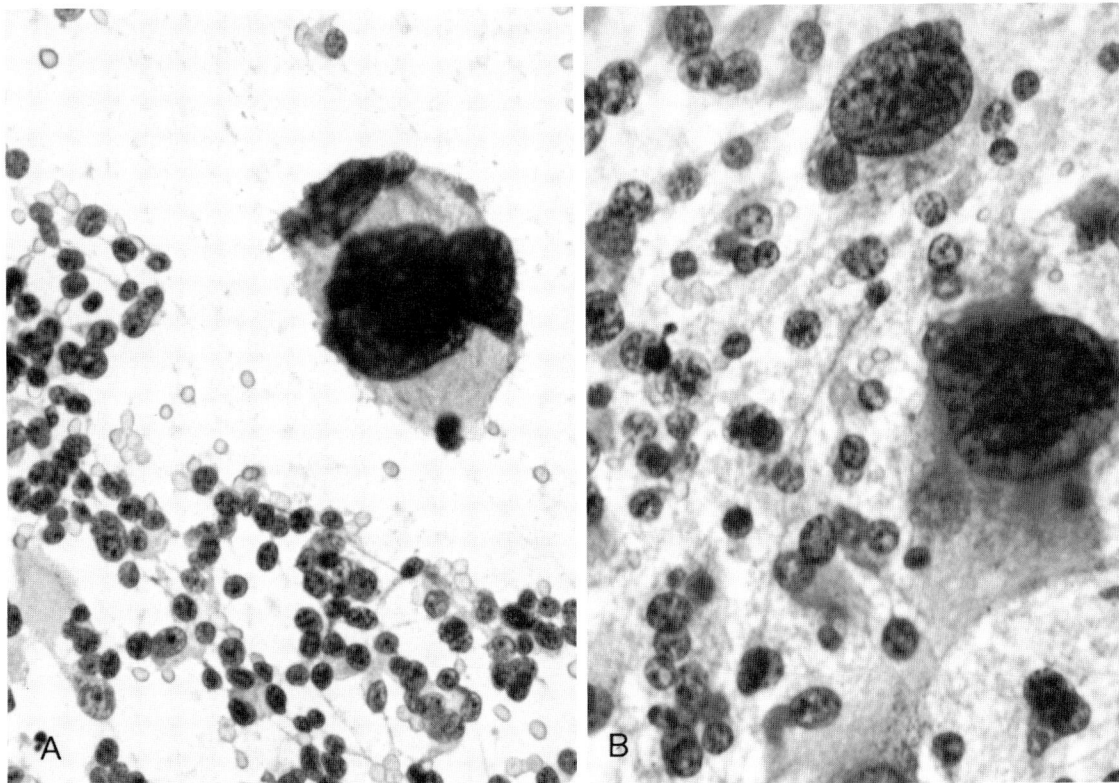

Figure 13.10.   Pheochromocytoma, ABC. **A** and **B,** Note admixture of carcinoid-like cells and bizarre giant cells. **A,** ×310; **B,** ×500.

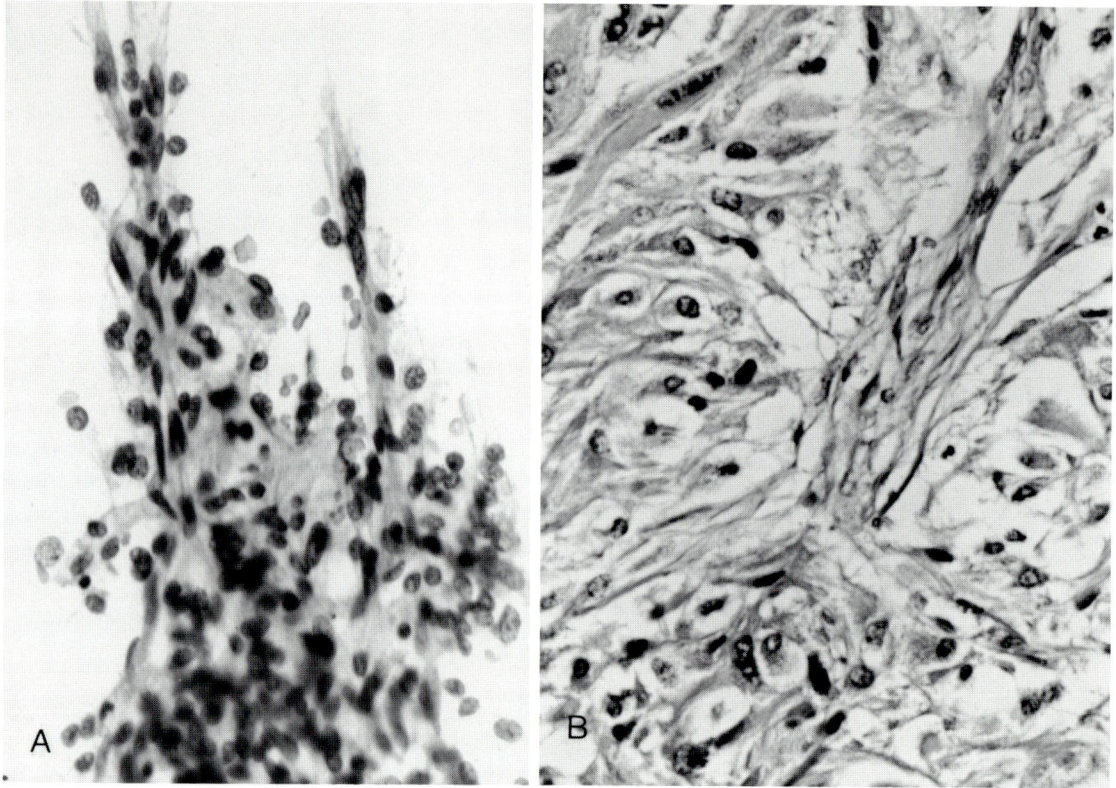

Figure 13.11.

Figure 13.11. Pheochromocytoma. **A,** ABC. Note spindle cells with eosinophilic cytoplasm. This aspirate was reported as "suspicious for sarcoma." ×310. **B,** Tissue section. Note spindle cells. ×310.

Figure 13.12. Ultrastructure of pheochromocytoma, needle aspirate. Note characteristic membrane-bound, dense-core neurosecretory granules. Uranyl acetate and lead citrate preparation. ×26,000.

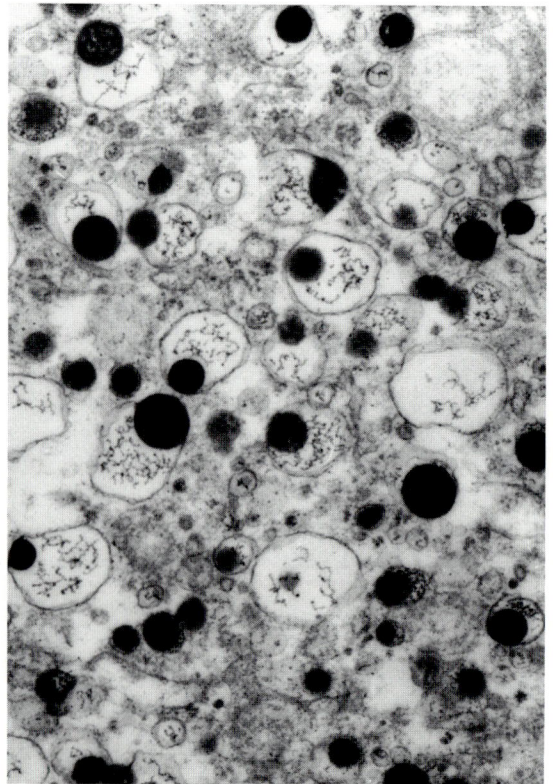

Figure 13.12.

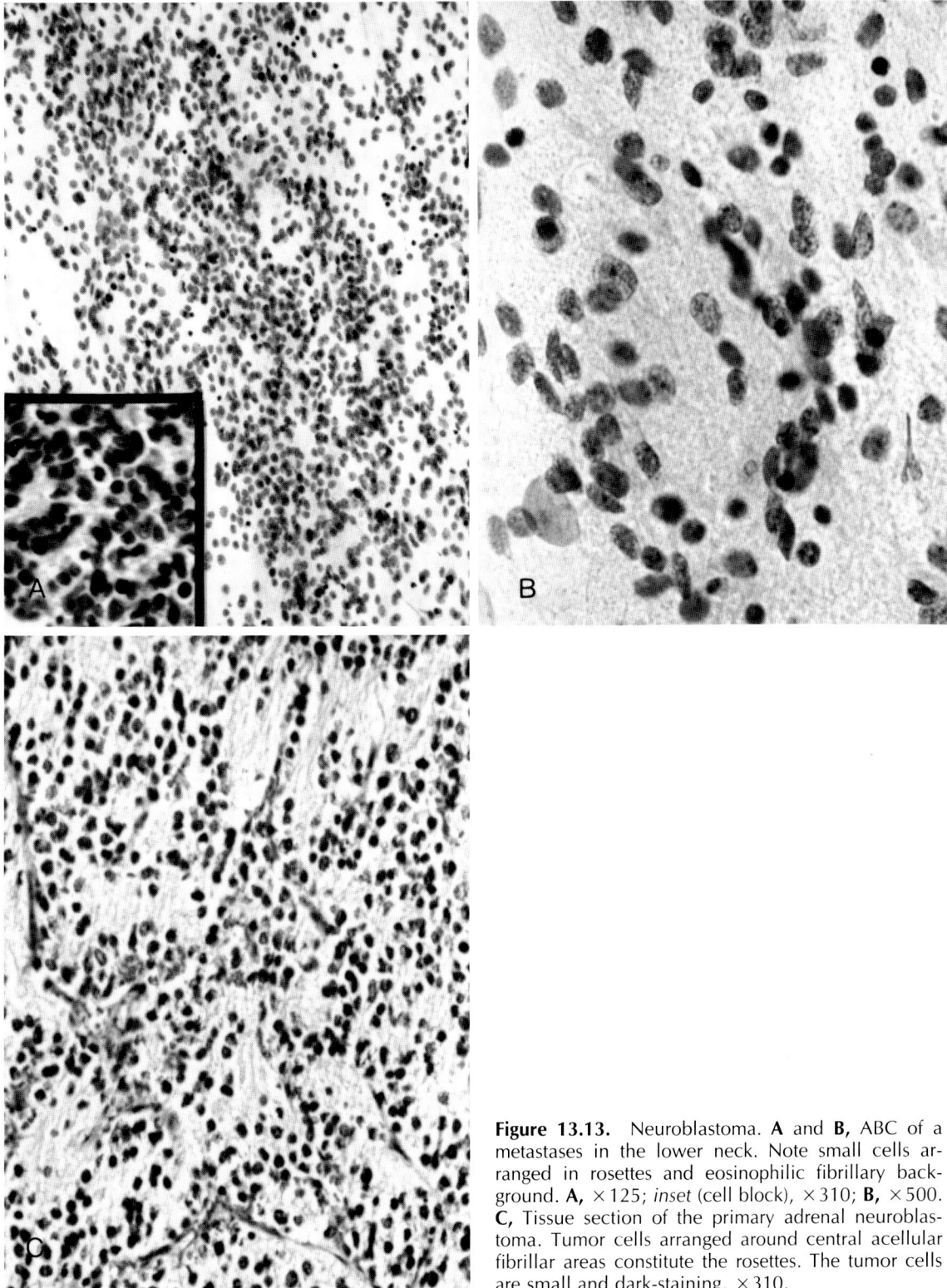

Figure 13.13. Neuroblastoma. **A** and **B,** ABC of a metastases in the lower neck. Note small cells arranged in rosettes and eosinophilic fibrillary background. **A,** ×125; *inset* (cell block), ×310; **B,** ×500. **C,** Tissue section of the primary adrenal neuroblastoma. Tumor cells arranged around central acellular fibrillar areas constitute the rosettes. The tumor cells are small and dark-staining. ×310.

Diagnostic Pitfalls. Pheochromocytoma is a rare tumor. When the cytopathologist encounters his or her first FNAB case, it is not uncommon to make an erroneous diagnosis of sarcoma or giant cell malignancy because of cellular polymorphism.[7,24,25] The following characteristics are helpful in the diagnosis. *(a)* In aspirates obtained from pheochromocytomas, even though the pleomorphic giant cells may immediately catch one's attention, the uniform polygonal cells, singly or in small clusters, are almost always present if sought. The latter are the prototype cells seen in all neuroendocrine tumors. *(b)* Despite marked cellular pleomorphism, mitoses are not abundant. When mitoses are easily found, a tumor other than pheochromocytoma should be suspected.[29]

It is occasionally difficult to determine whether an adrenal tumor is a cortical carcinoma or pheochromocytoma. The absence of cytoplasmic lipid vacuoles and the absence of mitoses favor pheochromocytoma. If adequate aspirated material is available for electron microscopic studies, the diagnosis is easy. Typical membrane-bound, dense-core, neurosecretory granules, averaging 270 nm in size, are found in pheochromocytoma cells **(Fig. 13.12)**.

Neuroblastoma

Neuroblastomas are primarily seen in infants and children less than 4 years of age. In accordance with their origin from neural crest, neuroblastomas may arise in many locations. Most are found in the adrenal medulla; some arise in the ganglionic tissue of the retroperitoneum. About 18% of neuroblastomas arise above the diaphragm in the chest or neck. In approximately 12% of cases, the primary site cannot be determined.[30] Seventy percent of patients evidence metastases at the initial presentation.[31] Spontaneous regression or maturation to ganglioneuroma has been reported in occasional cases.

Histologically, neuroblastomas exhibit a diffuse growth of rather uniform small cells, typically arranged in groups of small morula-like structures. In about one-third of cases, well-formed rosettes can be identified.

Aspiration Cytology[32–36]

The smears are cell-rich. The tumor cells **(Fig. 13.13)** are small and oval, with hyperchromatic nuclei, finely stippled chromatin, and scanty cytoplasm. The nuclear membranes show occasional lobulation. Each nucleus contains one or two round, small, but occasionally conspicuous, nucleoli. The cells are arranged in loose clusters. The well-known rosette formation can be recognized in 50% of our cases. These are formed by radial arrangement of cells around a space containing delicate eosinophilic neurofibrils. Similar fibrillary material creating a streaming effect is also seen in the smear background. These features are readily appreciated in the more differentiated tumors.

Diagnostic Pitfalls. Neuroblastomas present the pathologist with the diagnostic problem of the small cell tumor of childhood, in which such neoplasms as Wilms' tumor, Ewing's sarcoma, rhabdomyosarcoma, and malignant lymphoma must be considered in the differential diagnosis (the ABC of these tumors has already been discussed elsewhere in this book). The observation of rosettes and eosinophilic neurofibrils aids in correct diagnosis. Even in their absence, the presence of small round cells on FNAB, coupled with

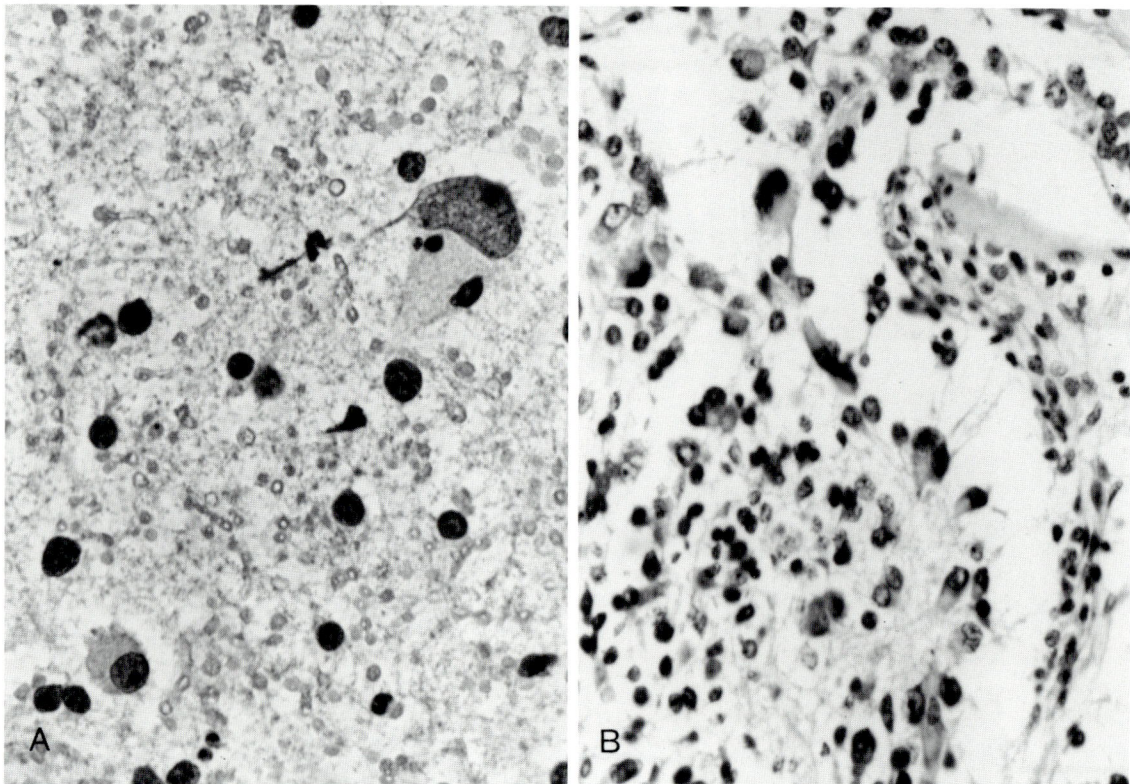

Figure 13.14. Ganglioneuroblastoma in retroperitoneum. **A,** ABC. Note small neuroblasts and large ganglion cells with nucleoli and ample eosinophilic cytoplasm. ×500. **B,** Histology of the resected tumor showing admixture of neuroblasts and ganglion cells. ×310.

laboratory evidence of secretion of catecholamines or its metabolites, is diagnostic of neuroblastoma.

Ganglioneuroblastoma

While neuroblastomas are primitive neoplasms, ganglioneuroblastomas are partly differentiated neuroblastomas. The biologic behavior of these uncommon neoplasms is reported to be intermediate between neuroblastomas and ganglioneuromas. Ganglioneuroblastomas are most commonly found in the mediastinum and retroperitoneum, and only uncommonly found within the adrenal. Aspirates obtained from these tumors **(Fig. 13.14)** show all stages of neuroblastic maturation with variable mixtures of immature neuroblasts and variably mature ganglion cells. The ganglion cells are large cells with eccentric nuclei, prominent nucleoli, and ample eosinophilic cytoplasm.

Ganglioneuroma

Ganglioneuromas represent the benign form of the clinical spectrum and, unlike neuroblastomas, they occur most commonly in adults. The sites of predilection are the mediastinum and retroperitoneum, and only occasionally they originate in the adrenal gland. Small immature neuroblasts should not be present in the tumor. Aspirates show admixture of ganglion cells and spindle cells with serpentine nuclei. See Chapter 8, ''Mediastinum,'' for the cytologic discussion of this tumor.

References

1. DeBlois G, DeMay RM. Adrenal myelolipoma diagnosis by computed-tomography guided fine needle aspiration. Cancer 1985;55:848–850.
2. Pinto MM. Fine needle aspiration of myelolipoma of the adrenal gland. Acta Cytol 1985;29:863–866.
3. Page DL, DeLellis RA, Hough AJ. Tumors of the adrenal. Atlas of tumor pathology, 2nd Series, Fascicle 23. Washington, D.C.: Armed Forces Institute of Pathology, 1986:261.
4. Yee ACN, Gopinath N, Ho CS, Tao LC. Fine needle aspiration biopsy of adrenal tuberculosis. J Can Assoc Radiol 1986;37:287–289.
5. Heaston DK, Handel DB, Ashton PR, Korobkin M. Narrow gauge needle aspiration of solid adrenal masses. AJR 1982;138:1143–1148.
5a. Anderson CJ, Pitts WC, Weiss LM. Disseminated histoplasmosis diagnosed by fine needle aspiration biopsy of the adrenal gland. A case report. Acta Cytol 1989;33:337–340.
5b. Valente PT, Calafati SA. Diagnosis of disseminated histoplasmosis by fine needle aspiration of the adrenal gland. Acta Cytol 1989;33:341–343.
6. Sommers SC. Adrenal glands. In Kissane JM. Anderson's pathology, Vol. 2, 8th ed. St. Louis: CV Mosby, 1985:1442.
7. Suen KC. Guides to clinical aspiration biopsy. Retroperitoneum and intestine. New York: Igaku Shoin, 1987:165–189.
8. Katz RL, Patel S, Mackay B, Zornoza J. Fine needle aspiration cytology of the adrenal gland. Acta Cytol 1984;28:269–282.
9. Sipio JC, Rohner TJ, Drago JR. Adrenal cortical carcinoma. J Surg Oncol 1986;31:52–55.
10. Warner NE. Pathology of the adrenal gland. In Skinner DG, Lieskovsky G. Diagnosis and management of genitourinary cancer. Philadelphia: WB Saunders, 1988:199.
11. Schteingart DE, Oberman HA, Friedman BA, Conn JW. Adrenal cortical neoplasms producing Cushing's syndrome. Cancer 1968;22:1005–1013.
12. Cochand-Priollet B, Jacquenod P, Warnet A, Ferrand J, Galian A. Adrenal cortical carcinoma: A case diagnosed by fine needle aspiration cytology. Acta Cytol 1988;32:128–130.
13. Zornoza J, Ordonez N, Bernardino ME, Cohen MA. Percutaneous biopsy of adrenal tumors. Urology 1981;18:413–416.
14. Levin NP. Fine needle aspiration and histology of adrenal cortical carcinoma. A case report. Acta Cytol 1981;25:421–424.
15. Symington T. The adrenal cortex. In Bloodworth JMB. Endocrine pathology: General and surgical, 2nd ed. Baltimore: Williams & Wilkins, 1982:457–462.
16. Benda JA. Adrenal neoplasms: Pathologic features. In Culp DA, Loening SA. Genitourinary oncology. Philadelphia: Lea & Febiger, 1985:497–509.

16a. Yazdi HM, Dardick I. What is the value of electron microscopy in fine-needle aspiration biopsy? Diagn Cytopathol 1988;4:177–182.
17. Copeland PM. The incidentally discovered adrenal mass. Ann Intern Med 1983;98:940–945.
18. Mitnick JS, Bosniak MA, Megibow Aj, Naidich DP. Non-functioning adrenal adenomas discovered incidentally on computed tomography. Radiology 1983;148:495–499.
19. Katz RL, Shirkhoda A. Diagnostic approach to incidental adrenal nodules in the cancer patient. Cancer 1985;55:1995–2000.
20. Gross BH, Goldberg HI, Moss AA, Harter LP. CT demonstration and guided aspiration of unusual adrenal metastases. J Comput Assist Tomogr 1983;7:98–101.
20a. O'Leary TJ, Ooi TC. The adrenal incidentaloma. Can J Surg 1986;29:296–298.
21. Steiner AL, Goodman AD, Powers SR. Study of a kindred with pheochromocytoma, medullary thyroid carcinoma, hyperparathyroidism and Cushing's syndrome: Multiple endocrine neoplasia, type II. Medicine 1968;47:371–409.
22. McCorkell SJ, Niles NL. Fine-needle aspiration of catecholamine-producing adrenal masses: A possibly fatal mistake. AJR;145:113–114.
23. Casola G, Nicolet V, vanSonnenberg E, Withers C, Bretagnolle M, Saba RM, Bret PM. Unsuspected pheochromocytoma: Risk of blood-pressure alterations during percutaneous adrenal biopsy. Radiology 1986;159:733–735.
24. Nguyen GK. Cytopathologic aspects of adrenal pheochromocytoma in a fine needle aspiration biopsy. A case report. Acta Cytol 1982;26:354–358.
25. Moussouris HF, Koss LG, Rosenblatt R, Kutcher R. Thin needle aspiration biopsy of abdominal organs. In Koss LG, Coleman DV. Advances in clinical cytology, Vol 2. New York: Masson Publishing, 1984:226–228.
26. Montali G, Solbiati L, Bossi MC, De Pra L, Di Donna A, Ravetto C. Sonographically guided fine-needle aspiration biopsy of adrenal masses. AJR 1984;143:1081–1084.
27. Gonzalez-Campora R, Otal-Salaverri C, Panea-Flores P, Lerma-Puertas E, Galera-Davidson H. Fine needle aspiration cytology of paraganglionic tumors. Acta Cytol 1988;32:386–390.
28. Leder LD, Richter HJ. Pathology of renal and adrenal neoplasms. In Lohr E, Leder LD. Renal and adrenal tumors, 2nd ed. Berlin: Springer-Verlag, 1987:1–68.
29. Sherwin RP. The adrenal medulla, paraganglia and related tissues. In Bloodworth JMB. Endocrine pathology. Baltimore: Williams & Wilkins, 1968:256–315.
30. Stamler FW. Pediatric genitourinary neoplasms. Pathologic features. In Culp DA, Loening SA. Genitourinary oncology. Philadelphia: Lea & Febiger, 1985:530–545.

31. Koop CE, Schnaufer L. The management of abdominal neuroblastoma. Cancer 1975;35:905–909.

32. Silverman JF, Dabbs DJ, Ganick DJ, Holbrook CT, Geisinger KR. Fine needle aspiration cytology of neuroblastoma, including peripheral neuroectodermal tumor, with immunocytochemical and ultrastructural confirmation. Acta Cytol 1988;32:367–376.

33. Akhtar M, Ashraf A, Sabbah RS, Mohamed B, Sakey K, Nash EJ. Aspiration cytology of neuroblastoma: Light and electron microscopic correlations. Cancer 1986;57:797–803.

34. Miller TR, Bottles K, Abele JS, Beckstead JH. Neuroblastoma diagnosed by fine needle aspiration biopsy. Acta Cytol 1985;29:461–468.

35. Head DR, Kennedy PS, Goyette RE. Metastatic neuroblastoma in bone marrow aspirate smears. Am J Clin Pathol 1979;72:1008–1011.

36. Farr GH, Hajdu SI. Exfoliative cytology of metastatic neuroblastoma. Acta Cytol 1972;16:203–206.

14

Prostate and Testis

THE PROSTATE

Fine needle aspiration biopsy of the prostate is becoming a well-accepted diagnostic procedure in both Europe and North America.[1-9a] The aspiration is traditionally performed transrectally. A special needle guide may or may not be used, depending on the aspirator's personal preference. **Figure 14.1** depicts the needle guide, devised by Franzen and associates.[10] It consists of a metal tube, slightly curved to conform to the contour of the palpating index finger. The distal end is funnel-shaped, thereby permitting easy entrance of the needle. Near the proximal end of the guide is a steering ring through which the tip of the gloved index finger is fitted. An adjustable metal plate midway along the guide serves to stabilize the instrument by resting on the operator's palm. The metal steering ring is secured on the index finger by a finger cot and the finger is then inserted into the rectum. When the suspicious area of the prostate is palpated, the fine needle is introduced through the guide to the lesion. Although the Franzen needle guide is widely used, Kline et al.[3-6] were able to show also that the accuracy of the aspiration technique is independent of the use of specially designed equipment. Kline and her colleagues use the simple, 90–mm, 18– or 20–gauge spinal needle and disposable syringe for the procedure. In recent years, at our institution and at many others[11-13] direct sonography of the prostate gland is obtained with a real time linear-array transrectal probe, and any suspected abnormal nodule can be more accurately aspirated perineally under continuous ultrasonic monitoring.

Diagnostic Accuracy

The sensitivity of FNAB to diagnose prostatic cancer varies considerably from series to series, ranging from 68 to 99%, depending largely on the experience of the aspirator and the cytopathologist.[5,13a] The clinical usefulness of FNAB can be evaluated by comparing it with the conventional core biopsy method. Chodak et al.[8] studied 62 cases in which both aspiration and core biopsies were performed. The sensitivity of FNAB in diagnosing cancer was 98% (45 of 46 biopsies) compared to 81% (37 of 46) for the core biopsy method. There is a definite learning curve as shown by Lin et al.,[14] who reported a false-negative rate of 27%; many of the unsatisfactory results occurred due to changeover of residents. False-positive diagnoses are largely caused by misinterpretation of chronic prostatitis (see below).[15-17] Epstein[16] diagnosed the first eight cases of prostatitis as malignant. Faul and Shmiedt[17] reported that 20% of their first 170 aspirates of chronic prostatitis were interpreted as suspicious. Other sources of false-positive reports include ductal dysplasia, contamination (e.g., seminal vesicle cells), and therapy-in-

duced alterations.[6] With experience, the false-positive rate can be greatly reduced.

Benign Prostatic Hyperplasia

Benign prostatic hyperplasia (BPH) is a common condition afflicting men over 50 years of age. In all likelihood, it results from the hormonal imbalance between estrogen and testosterone. The prostate gland shows diffuse or focal nodular enlargement, and the patient may have urinary symptoms, such as frequency, hematuria, weak stream, and urinary retention. Microscopically, the nodules are composed of closely packed, hyperplastic glands with tall, often papillary epithelium (**Fig. 14.2**). Stromal hyperplasia and interstitial inflammation are also common.

Aspiration Cytology

The ABC reveals a variable cellularity, depending on whether the glandular or the stromal areas are sampled. Generally, the aspirates are hypocellular, which is an important feature of benignity. The glandular epithelium often appears as large monolayered sheets of 50 or more cells (**Fig. 14.3**). Less frequently, multilayered tissue fragments and small acini are also present. Discrete cells are uncommon. The glandular epithelial cells are uniform, polygonal or columnar in shape, with distinct cell borders, producing a honeycomb pattern (**Fig. 14.4**). The cells have a moderate amount of lacy cytoplasm. The nuclei are vesicular, oval or round, with finely granular chromatin and small nucleoli. At the periphery of the cell groups are a few elongated or triangular-shaped basal, or reserve, cells.[18]

Other cell types may also be seen, such as stromal, squamous, and inflammatory cells and epithelial cells from the rectal mucosa and seminal vesicles. Stromal cells (**Fig. 14.5**) appear as spindle cells lying singly or in small groups of 3 or 4 cells. Squamous cells may originate from the anal mucosa or from squamous metaplasia, induced by estrogen therapy, infarction, or prostatitis. Epithelial cells of the seminal vesicles (**Fig. 14.6**) may show large, hyperchromatic nuclei with prominent nucleoli. These cells may be mistaken for carcinoma cells by the unwary.[18a] The former, however, have finely granular chromatin, smooth nuclear membranes, and ample cytoplasm with abundant brown lipofuscin granules. Rectal mucosal cells can be distinguished by their tall columnar shape, cytoplasmic vacuolation, and nuclear palisading. Corpora amylacea (concretions) are round hyaline bodies, which measure 100–200 μm in diameter and show laminations and smooth borders (**Fig. 14.7**). Their significance is unknown. They can be seen in both benign conditions and in carcinomas.

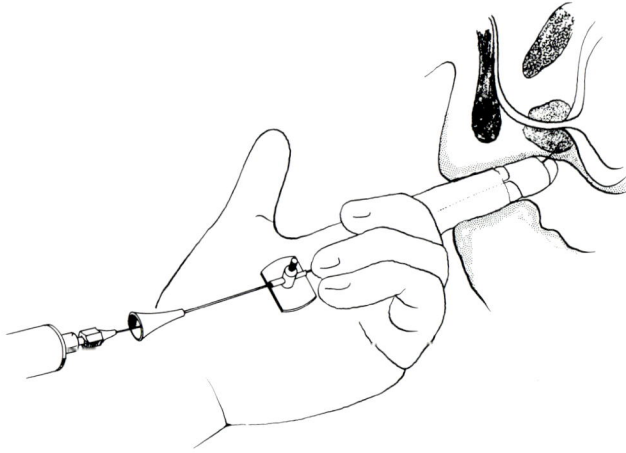

Figure 14.1.

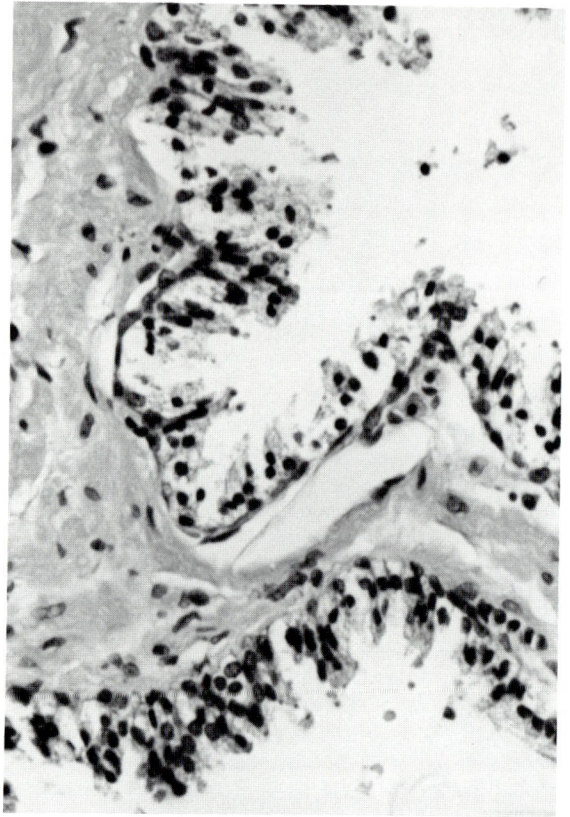

Figure 14.2.

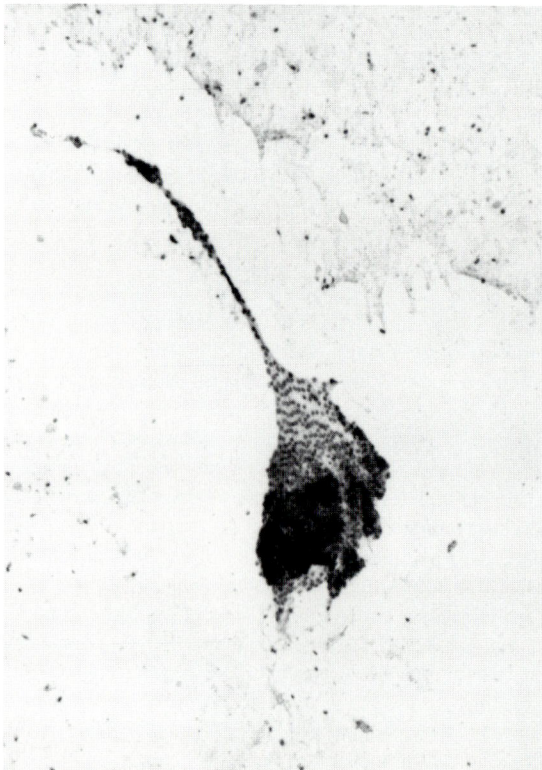

Figure 14.3.

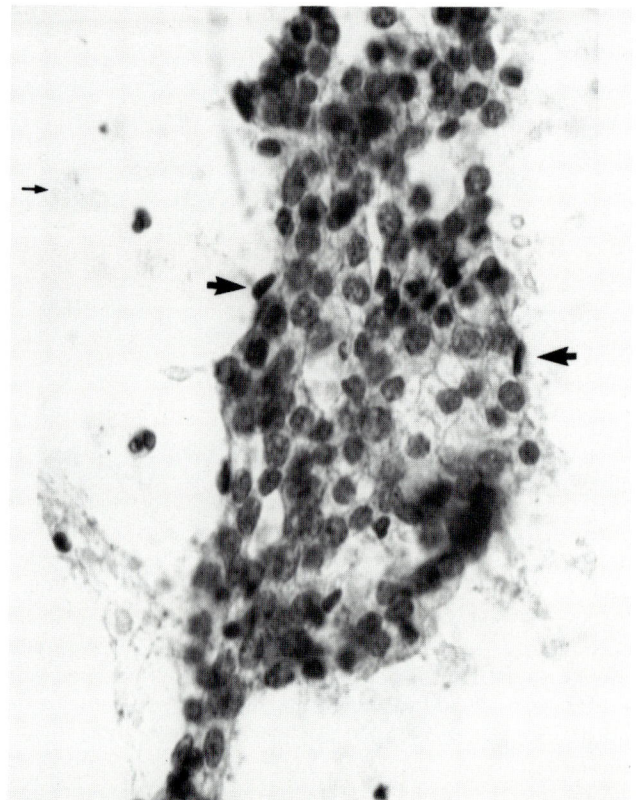

Figure 14.4.

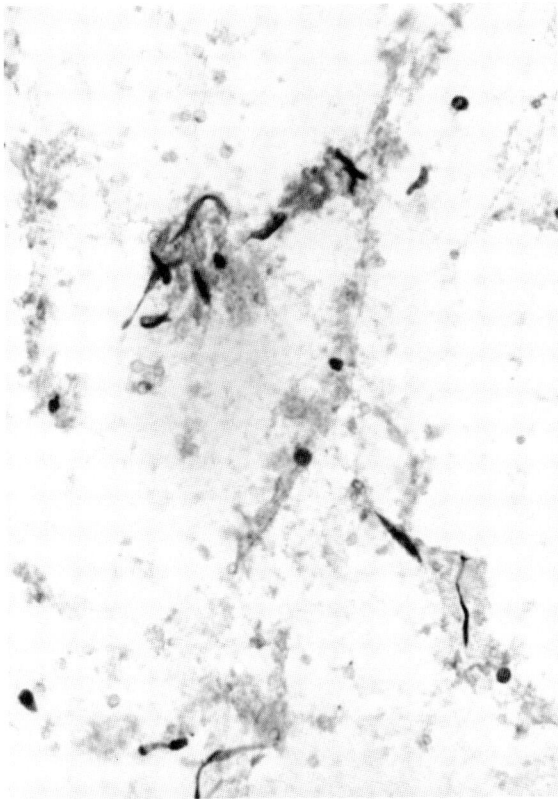

Figure 14.5. Benign prostatic hyperplasia, ABC. Note spindle-shaped stromal cells. ×310.

Diagnostic Pitfalls. Interpretation of aspirates from BPH would include the differential diagnosis of normal prostatic epithelium on one hand and well-differentiated adenocarcinoma on the other. Kline[6] cautioned that the epithelial cells from BPH cannot be distinguished from those of the normal prostate. The question then arises as to what constitutes an adequate or satisfactory specimen. She considers a specimen procured by an experienced operator to be ade-

quate with as few as four to six epithelial cell groups per slide. However, this same aspirate, obtained by a novice, would be interpreted as "unsatisfactory; insufficient cells for diagnosis." In other words, a negative report is only meaningful in the hands of a skillful team.

In the differential diagnosis of BPH and carcinoma, the number of cells comprising each cell group may provide a useful clue.

Figure 14.1. The Franzen apparatus for transrectal aspiration biopsy of the prostate (see text). The needle guide is mounted on the aspirator's left index finger and rests on the thenar of the palm. The plunger of the syringe is retracted by the right hand.

Figure 14.2. Histology of benign prostatic hyperplasia. Note dilated glands, lined by hyperplastic columnar epithelium forming small papillary tufts. ×310.

Figure 14.3. Benign prostatic hyperplasia, ABC. The smear is relatively hypocellular. A large tissue fragment is seen at the center. Note cobblestone arrangement of the cells. ×80.

Figure 14.4. Benign prostatic hyperplasia, ABC. Note uniform cells with regular round nuclei, well-defined cell borders, and a honeycomb or mosaic pattern. Also note flattened, spindle-shaped reserve or myoepithelial cells (arrows) at the periphery. ×500.

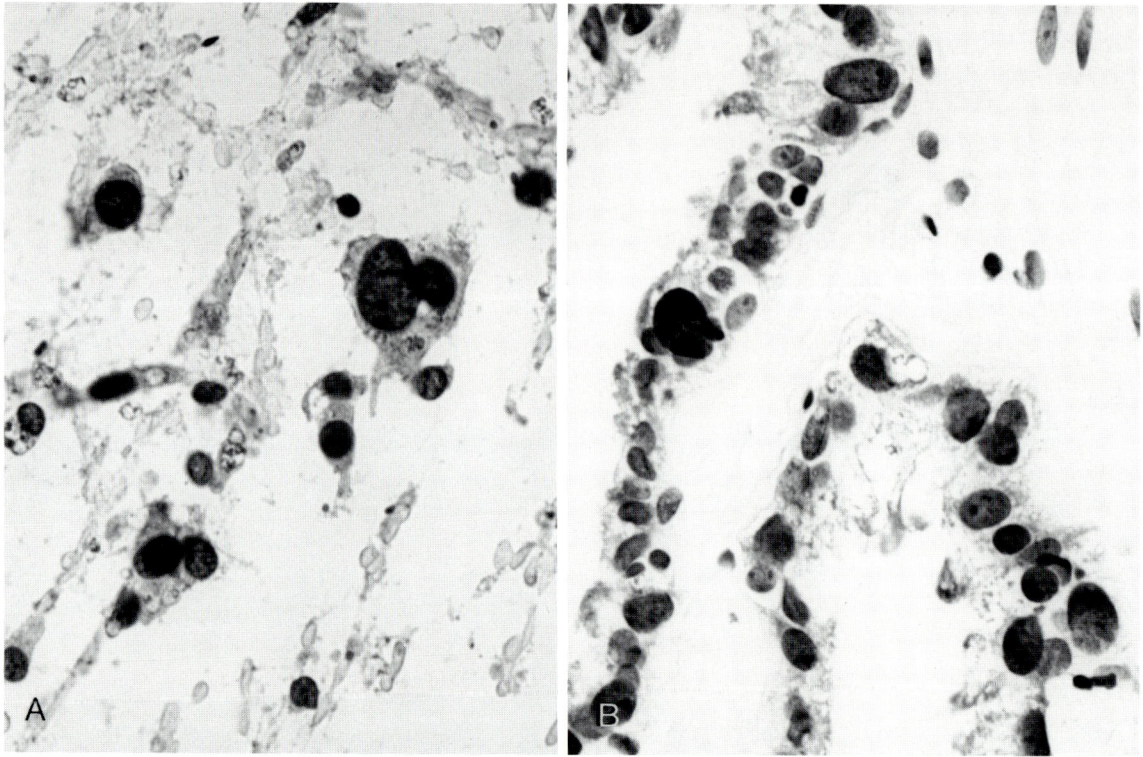

Figure 14.6.

Figure 14.6. Epithelial cells of the seminal vesicle. **A,** ABC. Note hyperchromatic cells with considerable anisonucleosis. Many intra- and extracellular lipofuscin granules can be seen. ×500. **B,** Histologic section of seminal vesicle. Note pleomorphism of the epithelial lining cells. ×500.

Figure 14.7. Corpus amylaceum. Note concentric laminations. ×310.

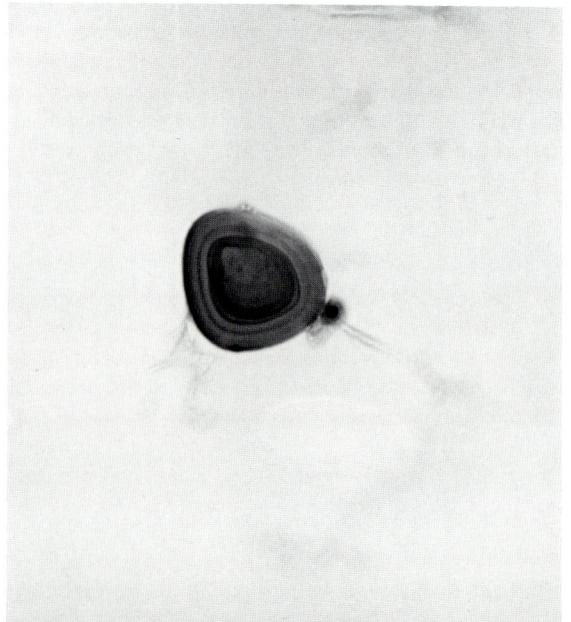

Figure 14.7.

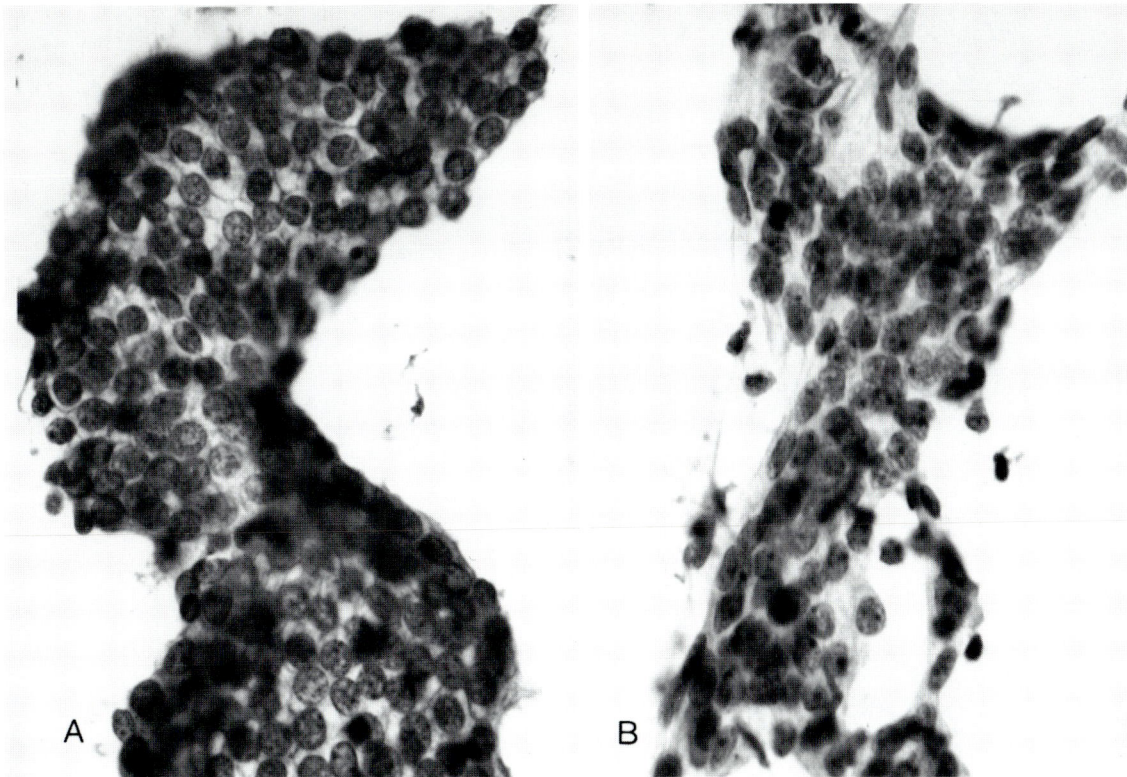

Figure 14.8.   Contrast ABC. **A,** Benign prostatic hyperplasia, tissue fragment. Note cellular uniformity, and smooth outer border of the tissue fragment. ×500. **B,** Well-differentiated adenocarcinoma of the prostate, tissue fragment. Note nuclear overlapping, indistinct cytoplasmic membranes and loss of smoothness at edge of tissue fragment. ×500.

Groups of 50–200 cells are usually derived from benign prostatic hyperplasia. Microacinous groups of 3–10 cells are "suspect,"[3] although acinar arrangement is by no means synonymous with carcinoma.[16] When one examines carefully the spatial relationship of the cells comprising the cell groups, one will find that in BPH the cells are located equidistant from each other with retention of polarity **(Fig. 14.8A)**. This contrasts with the malignant cell groups in which the nuclei are overlapping and randomly arranged, with a loss of polarity **(Fig. 14.8B)**. Epstein[16] further pointed out that benign tissue fragments have smooth outer borders formed by orderly polarized cells, whereas the smoothness is lost in carcinomatous tissue fragments. For further discussion, see "Adenocarcinoma."

Prostatitis

Acute prostatitis is usually caused by bacterial infections, and the diagnosis is made on clinical features, such as fever, dysuria, and a tender, swollen prostate gland. FNAB is not necessary for diagnosis. In fact, it is contraindicated because of the risk of sepsis.

Chronic prostatitis may be caused by bacteria, but frequently no bacteria are identified. Chronic prostatic inflammation, particularly the granulomatous variant, may present on digital rectal examination an indurated prostate that simulates carcinoma.[19]

Aspiration Cytology

The ABC of chronic prostatitis **(Fig. 14.9)** is generally cell-rich and polymorphic. In the background are lymphocytes, histiocytes, and neutrophils. The ductal epithelial cells are plentiful, appearing in monolayered sheets as well as in clumps. Because of the inflammation and edema, the cells appear to be dyshesive. There are cellular and nuclei enlargement, hyperchromasia, anisonucleosis, and distinct nucleoli of small to medium size. Such atypical epithelial changes, representing an injury-repair response, are not specific for any one type of prostatitis, but they are most severe in granulomatous prostatitis.[15,18] Although chronic granulomatous prostatitis may be caused by fungi or acid-fast organisms, in the majority of cases the causative factor remains elusive.

Diagnostic Pitfalls.   The hypercellularity and epithelial atypia seen in chronic prostatitis may mimic well-differentiated adenocarcinoma. In the former, the nuclear membranes usually are regular and large eosinophilic nucleoli are rare.[6] Kline[3] advised that the diagnosis of carcinoma in the presence of inflammation must be based only on well-preserved cells showing all major criteria of malignancy (see below). In doubtful cases and to avoid a falsely positive cancer diagnosis, aspiration should be repeated about 6–12 weeks after appropriate treatment for prostatitis.[15]

Adenocarcinoma

Adenocarcinoma of the prostate is the second most common malignancy in American men, accounting for 99,000 new cases and some 28,000 deaths each year.[20] There are no known risk factors. It is rare under age 40 years, and it does not occur in the absence of testes.

Among other factors, the grade of a prostatic carcinoma is considered a valuable prognostic factor. Currently two grading sys-

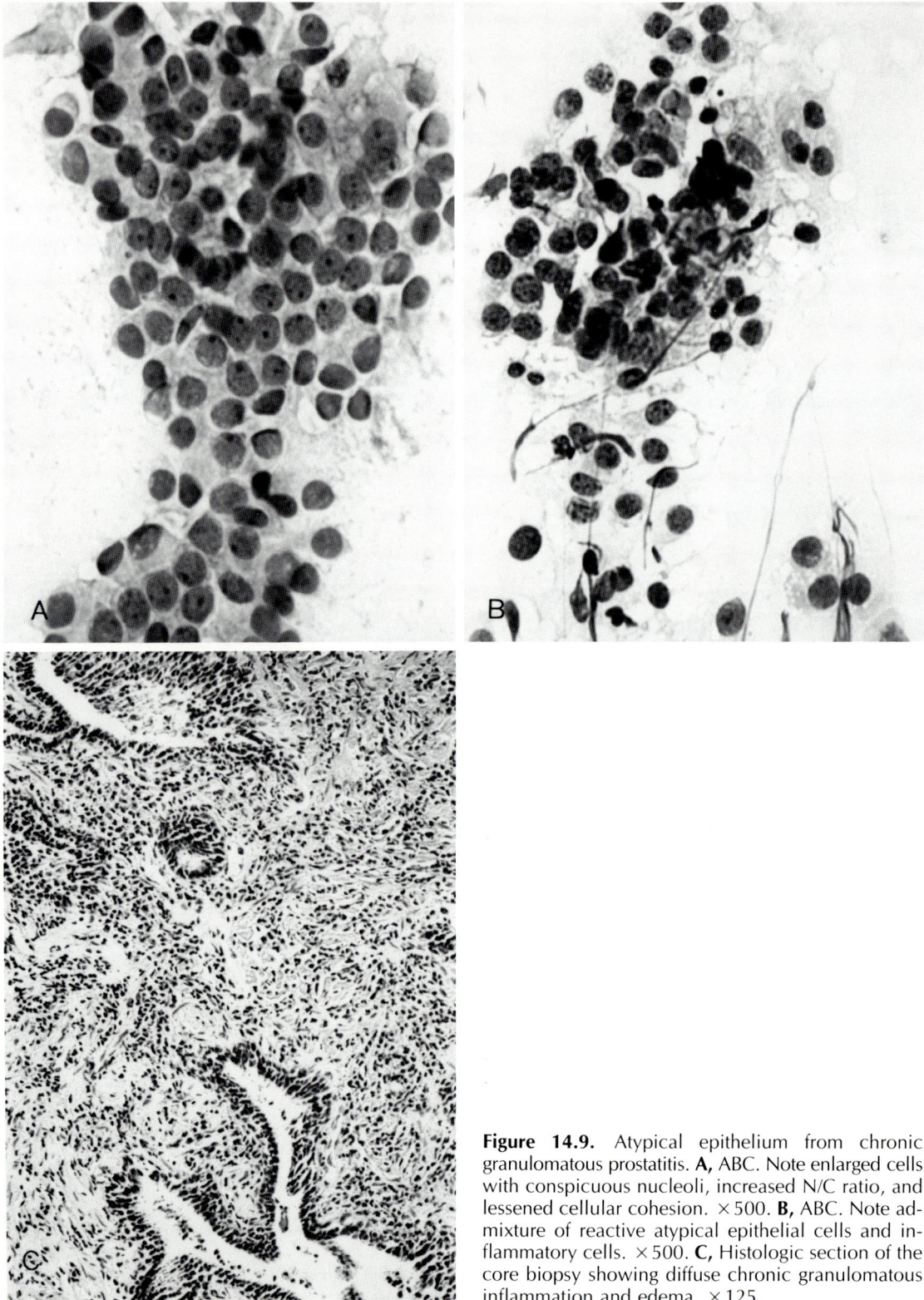

Figure 14.9. Atypical epithelium from chronic granulomatous prostatitis. **A,** ABC. Note enlarged cells with conspicuous nucleoli, increased N/C ratio, and lessened cellular cohesion. ×500. **B,** ABC. Note admixture of reactive atypical epithelial cells and inflammatory cells. ×500. **C,** Histologic section of the core biopsy showing diffuse chronic granulomatous inflammation and edema. ×125.

tems are widely used: one proposed by Gleason and Mellinger and the other by Mostofi. Gleason and Mellinger[21] use a system that recognizes a primary and a secondary histologic pattern of the tumor and also takes into consideration the clinical stage. Mostofi's system,[22,23] which divides prostatic adenocarcinomas into well-differentiated, moderately differentiated, and poorly differentiated, is simpler to use in FNAB. The histology of well-differentiated adenocarcinomas (**Fig. 14.10**) resembles the appearance of normal glands. Only slight nuclear anaplasia is apparent, but there is architectural crowding of the acini and glands, which are occupied by a single, monotonous population of cells without the myoepithelial cells. Moderately differentiated carcinomas (**Fig. 14.11**) show irregularly shaped glands and acini, and the tumor cells exhibit definitely more nuclear atypia. A poorly differentiated carcinoma (**Fig. 14.12**) is suggested by a predominant solid growth pattern and marked cellular pleomorphism. Cytologic grading based on FNAB material has been advocated by various workers, particularly those from Scandinavia, and their results show high correlation with histologic sections.[2,9,24]

Aspiration Cytology

Kline and Kannan[5] have published a set of major and minor cytologic criteria for diagnosing prostatic adenocarcinomas. The major criteria of malignancy include hypercellularity, dyshesion, anisonucleosis, nuclear membrane irregularity, and macronucleoli. The minor criteria are microacini, polarity loss with crowding and piling of nuclei, cell enlargement, and indistinct cell borders. A diagnosis of carcinoma is made with four major criteria or high cellularity plus two major and two minor criteria. A "suspicious" diagnosis is made with a cell-rich aspirate and two or three minor criteria.[4]

Tables 14.1 and **14.2** tabulate the cytologic features of benign and malignant prostatic FNAB specimens, compiled from several articles and text.[3–7,13a,16] Cytologic diagnosis of poorly differentiated adenocarcinomas (**Fig. 14.13**) presents no difficulty because many or all of the major criteria are present. The cell clusters show marked cellular dyshesion. The more poorly differentiated the tumor is, the more numerous are the isolated cells. Chromatin is clumped; nuclear membranes are irregular; macronucleoli are present. Aspirates from

TABLE 14.2. Cytologic Categories of Prostatic Adenocarcinoma

Aspiration Cytology	Well-differentiated	Moderately Differentiated	Poorly Differentiated
Cell sheets	Many and large	Some	Few or none
Microacini	Common	Some	Few
Dissociated cells	Few	Some	Many
Cell cohesion	Fair	Lessened	Poor

moderately differentiated carcinomas (**Fig. 14.14**) consist of dyshesive cell clusters as well as some isolated cells. The major criteria of malignancy are also readily apparent. Diagnosis of well-differentiated carcinoma, on the other hand, may be difficult because in some cases the major criteria of malignancy are absent and interpretation is heavily based on the minor criteria. The aspirates show cohesive aggregates as well as smaller cell groups with irregular or scalloped borders (**Fig. 14.15**). Within the groups, the cells are haphazardly arranged with a loss of nuclear polarity. Microacini, composed of 5–10 relatively uniform cells forming circles or crescents, are often seen (**Figs. 14.16** and **14.17**).

Diagnostic Pitfalls. False-negative diagnoses are mostly attributable to well-differentiated adenocarcinomas because of their cytologic resemblance to benign prostatic hyperplasia. When only atypical or suspicious-appearing cells are obtained, a repeat aspirate from another area of the lesion may yield cells with more obviously malignant features. Additionally, the sensitivity of detecting well-differentiated carcinomas may be improved by paying attention to the minor criteria set out by Kline and associates.[4,5] Not infrequently, the smears also contain a few sheets of normal glandular cells lying side by side with the malignant cells. Comparative study will facilitate the diagnosis, as the differences are readily apparent (see **Fig. 1.7**). More recently, Ostrzega et al.[25] suggested that using immunoperoxidase technique to identify prostatic basal cells can aid in differentiating benign and malignant cell sheets in prostatic aspirates.

False-positive diagnoses may result from misinterpretation of

TABLE 14.1. Benign versus Atypical versus Malignant Prostatic Epithelium, ABC

Cytology	Benign Epithelium	Atypical Epithelium	Malignant Epithelium
Cellularity[a]	Variable	Rich	Rich
Cell group	Large monolayered sheets with honeycomb appearance	Large sheets, and clusters	Small and large sheets, clusters, microacini, and dispersed cells
Cell dyshesion[a]	Nil	Slight to moderate	Moderate to marked
Nuclear membrane irregularity[a]	Nil	Nil	Present
Anisonucleosis[a]	Nil	Slight	Slight to marked
Nucleoli[a]	Small	Small to large	Large
Nuclear chromatin	Uniform distribution	Uniform distribution	Frequently irregular with clumping and clearing
Nuclear polarity	Well-maintained	More or less maintained	Disturbed cell crowding and nuclear overlapping
Cell enlargement	Not observed	Observed	Observed
Cytoplasmic border	Distinct	Indistinct	Indistinct
Inflammatory cells	Absent	Often present	Absent

[a]Major criteria, according to Kline and Kannan.[5]

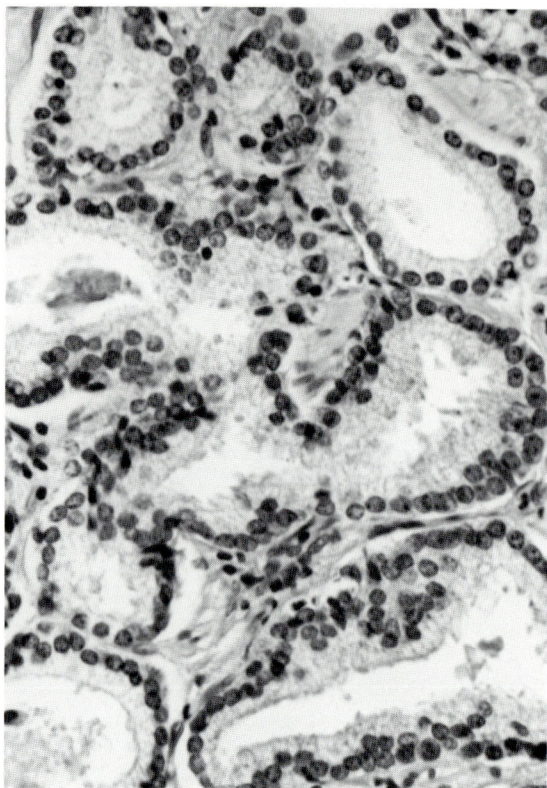

Figure 14.10.

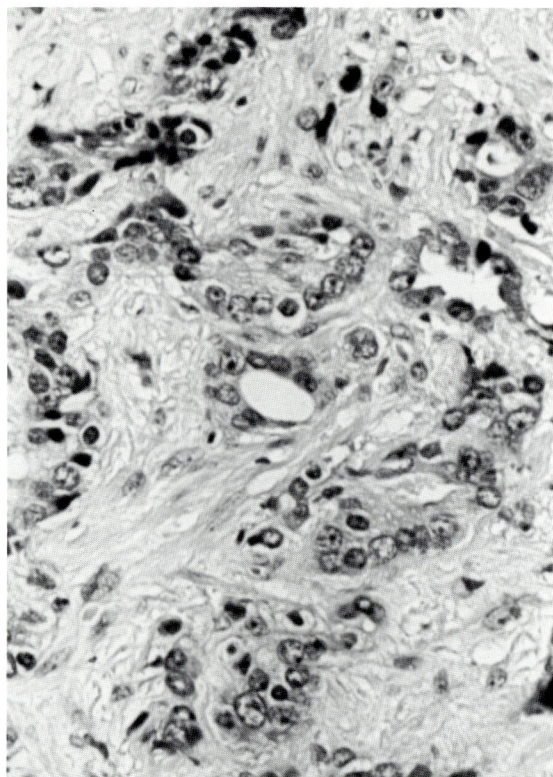

Figure 14.11.

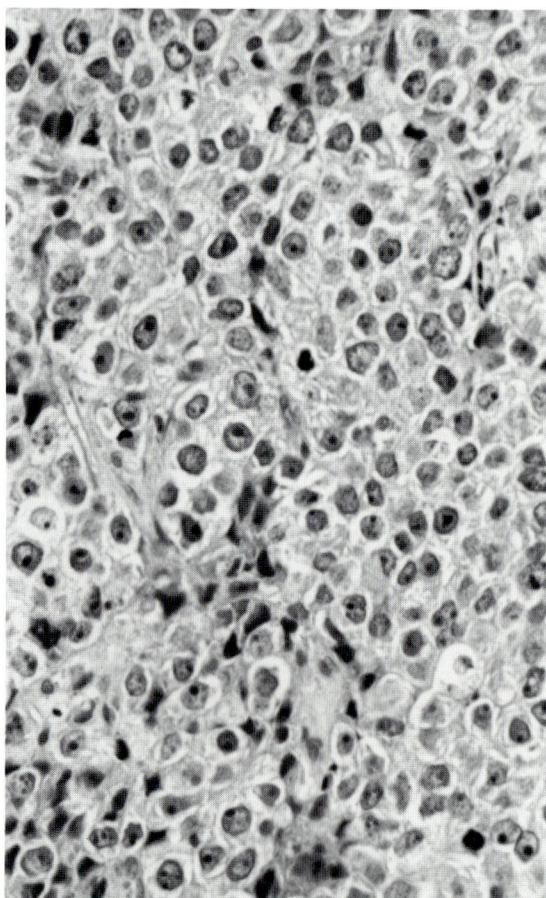

Figure 14.12.

Figure 14.10. Histology of well-differentiated prostatic adeno-carcinoma. ×310.

Figure 14.11. Histology of moderately differentiated prostatic adenocarcinoma. ×310.

Figure 14.12. Histology of poorly differentiated prostatic ad-enocarcinoma. ×310.

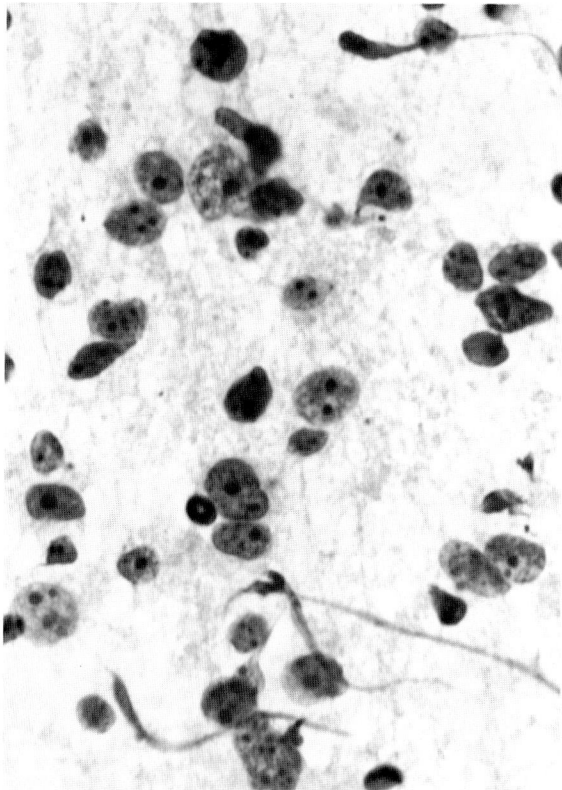

Figure 14.13. Poorly differentiated prostatic adenocarcinoma, ABC. Note complete loss of cellular cohesion, pleomorphic nuclei and macronucleoli. ×500.

Figure 14.13.

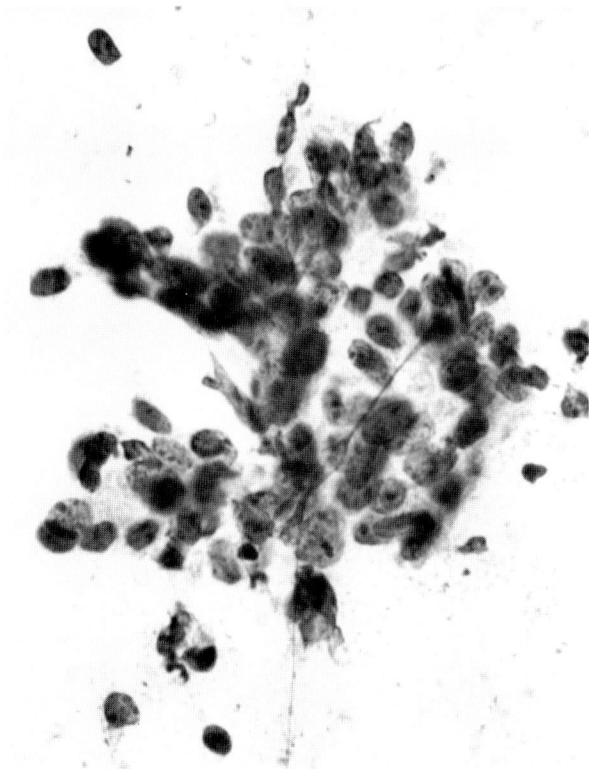

Figure 14.14. Moderately differentiated prostatic adenocarcinoma, ABC. Note imperfect gland formation and marked overlapping of nuclei. ×500.

Figure 14.14.

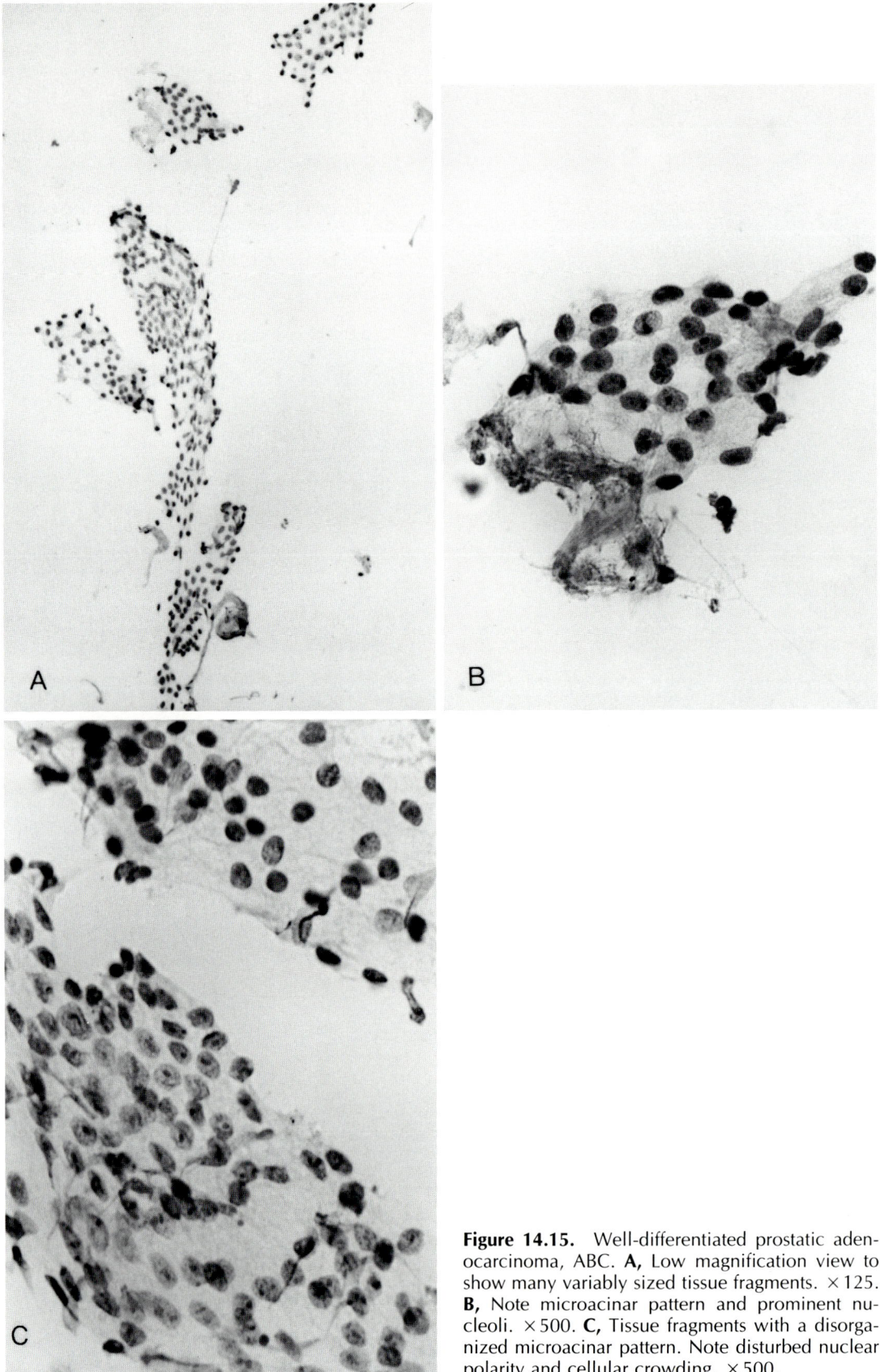

Figure 14.15. Well-differentiated prostatic adenocarcinoma, ABC. **A,** Low magnification view to show many variably sized tissue fragments. ×125. **B,** Note microacinar pattern and prominent nucleoli. ×500. **C,** Tissue fragments with a disorganized microacinar pattern. Note disturbed nuclear polarity and cellular crowding. ×500.

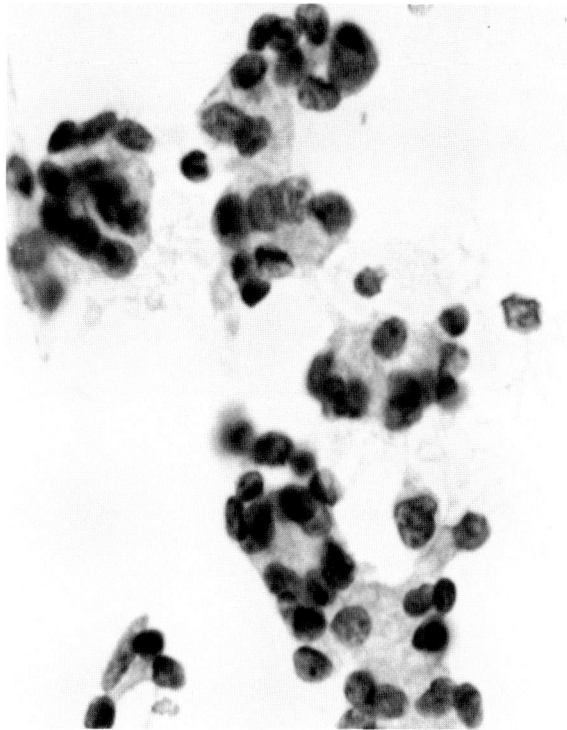

Figure 14.16. Well-differentiated prostatic adenocarcinoma, ABC. Note individual microacinar units. ×500.

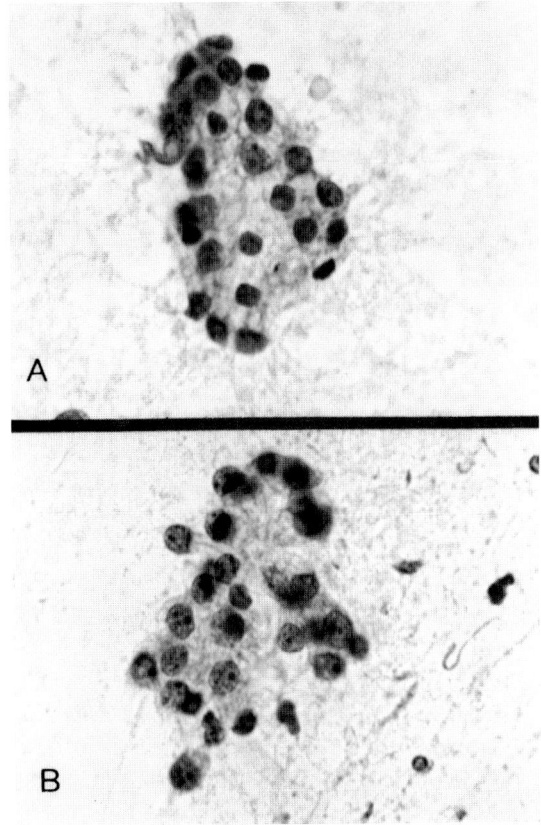

Figure 14.17. Contrast ABC. **A,** Microacinus from benign prostatic hyperplasia. Cells are equidistant from each other. ×500. **B,** Microacinus from well-differentiated prostatic adenocarcinoma. Note nuclear piling and prominent nucleoli. ×500.

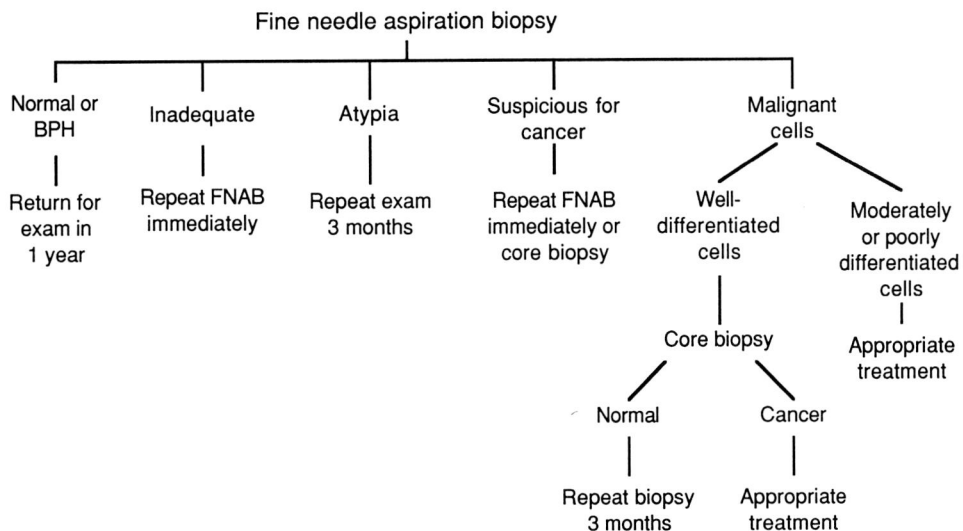

Figure 14.18. Flow diagram for use of fine needle aspiration biopsy of the prostate. (From Chodak GW, Steinberg GD, Bibbo M, Wied G, Straus FS III, Vogelzang NJ, Schoenberg HW. The role of transrectal aspiration biopsy in the diagnosis of prostatic cancer. J Urol 135:299–302, © by Williams & Wilkins, 1986.)

cells derived from the seminal vesicles, chronic prostatitis, or ductal dysplasia.[3,18a,26] The marked atypia seen in these benign conditions are generally focal. Chodak and associates[8] do not render the diagnosis of cancer unless more than half of the slide shows malignant cells, and they would repeat the aspiration for those cases with a smaller number of malignant or highly atypical cells. A ''positive'' cytologic report of moderately or poorly differentiated carcinoma is equivalent to tissue diagnosis;[6] on the other hand, if well-differentiated carcinoma is diagnosed, it is suggested that a core biopsy be performed to avoid the possibility that benign or atypical hyperplasia may be confused with well-differentiated cancer (**Fig. 14.18**).[8]

It is worth noting that Greenebaum[27] recently described the presence of megakaryocytes (due to accidental penetration of the needle into the ischium) and ganglion cells in needle aspirate specimens of the prostate. The megakaryocytes mimic anaplastic carcinoma, and the ganglion cells, well-differentiated adenocarcinoma. The author pointed out that the paucity of ''atypical'' cells and the sparsity or absence of prostatic epithelium in the aspirates were clues to the cytologist that the findings represented contaminants rather than a prostatic cancer.

THE TESTIS

Although testicular tumors account for only 1% of all malignant neoplasms in males, they are the most common malignant tumors of men between the ages of 25 to 29 years.[28] Ninety-five percent of the testicular neoplasms are of germ cell origin; the other 5% arise mainly from Leydig or Sertoli cells. In Scandivania, FNAB has been used successfully in the diagnosis of primary testicular tumors with no significant risk of tumor spread.[29] The technique is also used in evaluating spermatogenesis in cases of infertility.[30] However, at most medical centers in North America, including our own, FNAB is mainly used for diagnosing metastases of testicular tumors.[30a] Experience with FNAB of testicular tumors is limited and diagnostic accuracy has not yet been determined.

Germ Cell Tumors

Germ cell tumors are a group of neoplasms derived from the primitive germinal epithelium. Typically, they arise in the testes and ovaries, although occasional tumors may develop in extragonadal sites along the midline of the body, such as the mediastinum, retroperitoneum, sacrococcygeal region, and pineal body. In a few of our cases, the testicular tumor first presented with metastatic disease while the primary tumor remained occult, and it behooves the cytopathologist to recognize the morphologic characteristics of these neoplasms on FNAB. Kapila et al.[31] reported that the appearances of germ cell tumors are sufficiently characteristic to make specific cytologic diagnosis possible, particularly when augmented with immunocytochemical stains. **Table 14.3** lists the histologic types of germ cell tumors. One should also remember that it is not uncommon to have more than one histologic type present in a particular tumor.

Seminoma

Seminoma is the most common germ cell tumor in males, comprising from 35 to 70% of the primary tumors of the testis.[32] The identical tumor arising in the ovary is called dysgerminoma and is less common. The ABC of seminomas (**Fig. 14.19**) shows large, uniform, round or polyhedral cells that resemble the primitive germinal epithelial cells. The large, round nuclei are centrally located and hyperchromatic, with one or two macronucleoli. The cytoplasm is moderate in amount, clear or granular, and the cytoplasmic borders are distinct. The cells are generally dispersed singly in the smear.

TABLE 14.3.   Histologic Types of Germ Cell Tumors

Seminoma (dysgerminoma)
Embryonal carcinoma
  Adult type
  Infantile type (yolk sac tumor)
Choriocarcinoma
Teratoma
  Mature
  Immature
Mixed germ cell tumor (specify each component)

Diagnostic Pitfalls. The undifferentiated round cells of seminoma with prominent nucleoli must be differentiated from other malignant round cells showing prominent nucleoli, such as those derived from melanoma, large cell lymphoma and hepatocellular carcinoma. In malignant melanoma, many cells have eccentric nuclei (plasmacytoid appearance) with prominent nucleoli, and cytoplasmic pigment granules are frequently seen. Often spindle-shaped cells are present (see Chapter 4, under ''Malignant Melanoma''). In large cell lymphoma, the cells are less uniform, and nuclear cleaving is an important diagnostic feature. The cells are stained positively for leukocyte common antigen with immunocytochemical techniques. Hepatocellular carcinoma consists of polygonal cells with eosinophilic granular cytoplasm, and the characteristic trabecular or adenomatoid pattern of cellular arrangement may be present (see Chapter 9).

Embryonal Carcinoma

Embryonal carcinoma is a highly malignant neoplasm and comprises about 20% of all testicular tumors.[32] Histologically, the tumor resembles an anaplastic adenocarcinoma. The ABC (**Fig. 14.20**) shows large malignant cells with irregular, round or oval nuclei and prominent eosinophilic nucleoli. Unlike seminoma cells, the cytoplasmic borders of the embryonal carcinoma cells are indistinct, resulting in formation of many syncytial cell sheets. Some cells also group like adenocarcinomas, producing abortive glands or papillary structures.

Diagnostic Pitfalls. Cells of embryonal carcinoma may be mistaken for adenocarcinoma. In general, adenocarcinomas of a comparable glandular differentiation will show a lesser degree of nuclear pleomorphism. The possibility of embryonal carcinoma should be considered if the papilloglandular clusters are composed of cells showing pleomorphic nuclei with irregular macronucleoli, especially when the aspirate is obtained from a young adult.

Yolk Sac Tumor

Yolk sac tumor (infantile embryonal carcinoma, endodermal sinus tumor) is now recognized as a separate entity, although in the old literature it was grouped together with the embryonal carcinoma.[33] The morphologic appearance closely resembles embryonal carcinoma, except that the cells tend to be smaller and less pleomorphic (**Fig. 14.21**). The nuclei appear regular and round with prominent nucleoli.[31] The tumor exhibits various architectural patterns: anastomosing reticular network, glandular and papillary structures, solid cell sheets, cystic spaces, and the so-called endodermal sinuses, i.e., glomeruloid structures composed of a mesodermal core with a central capillary and an outer layer of cells with an epithelial appearance. Round, pink-staining, PAS-positive, diastase-resistant globules can sometimes be found in the cytoplasm of the tumor cells as well as extracellularly. These globules have been shown by immunocytochemical techniques to contain α-fetoprotein (AFP) and α_1-

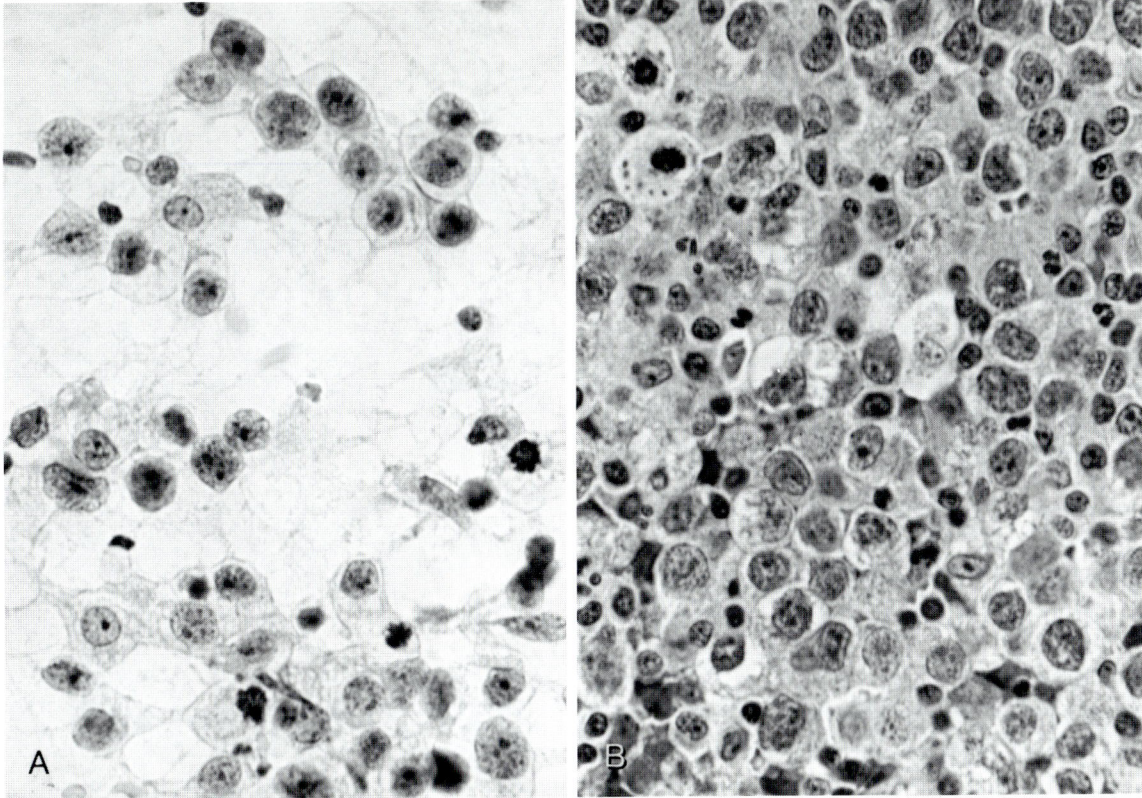

Figure 14.19.   Seminoma presenting first as massive lymphade-nopathy in the retroperitoneum. **A,** ABC. Note dyshesive, rather uniform cells with large round nuclei, large nucleoli, and distinct cell membranes. ×500. **B,** Histology of the primary testicular seminoma. Note uniformity of the neoplastic cells with distinct cell borders. ×310.

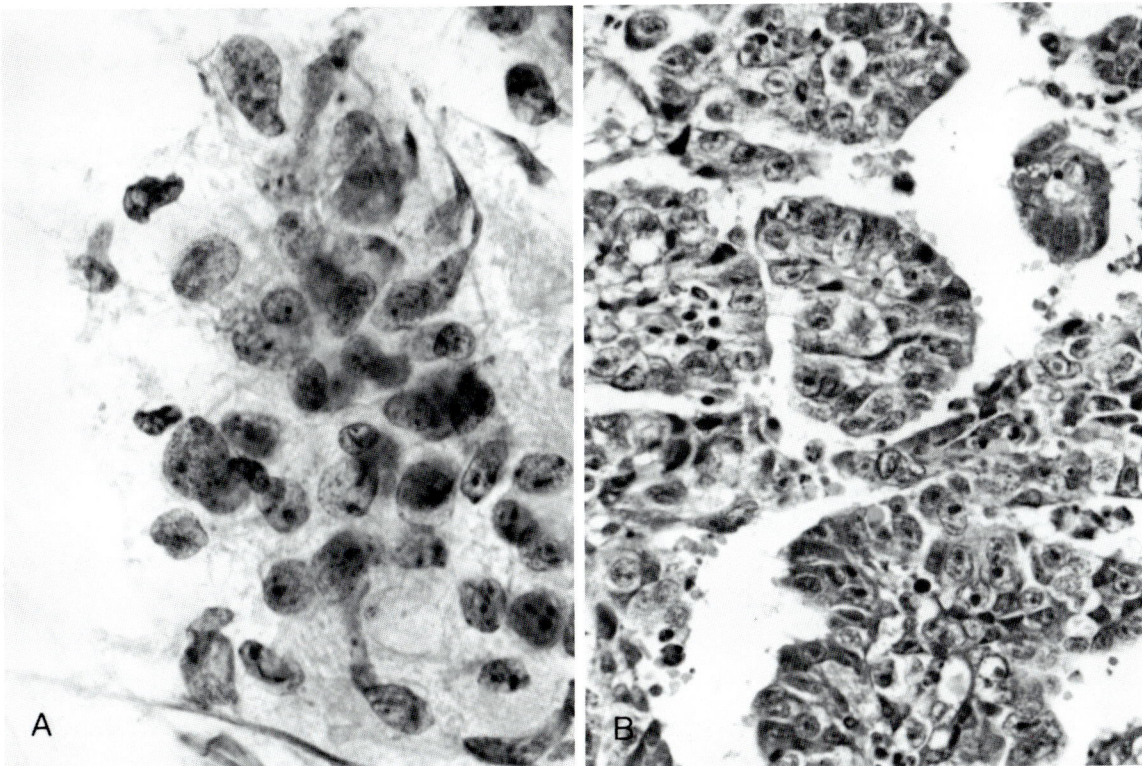

Figure 14.20.   Metastatic embryonal carcinoma originating from a testicular teratoma. **A,** ABC. The neoplastic cells are arranged in epithelial groups resembling adenocarcinoma. Note irregu-larly shaped nuclei, multiple prominent nucleoli, and indistinct cell membranes resulting in syncytium. ×500. **B,** Histologic sec-tion showing embryonal carcinoma with a papillo-glandular growth pattern. ×310.

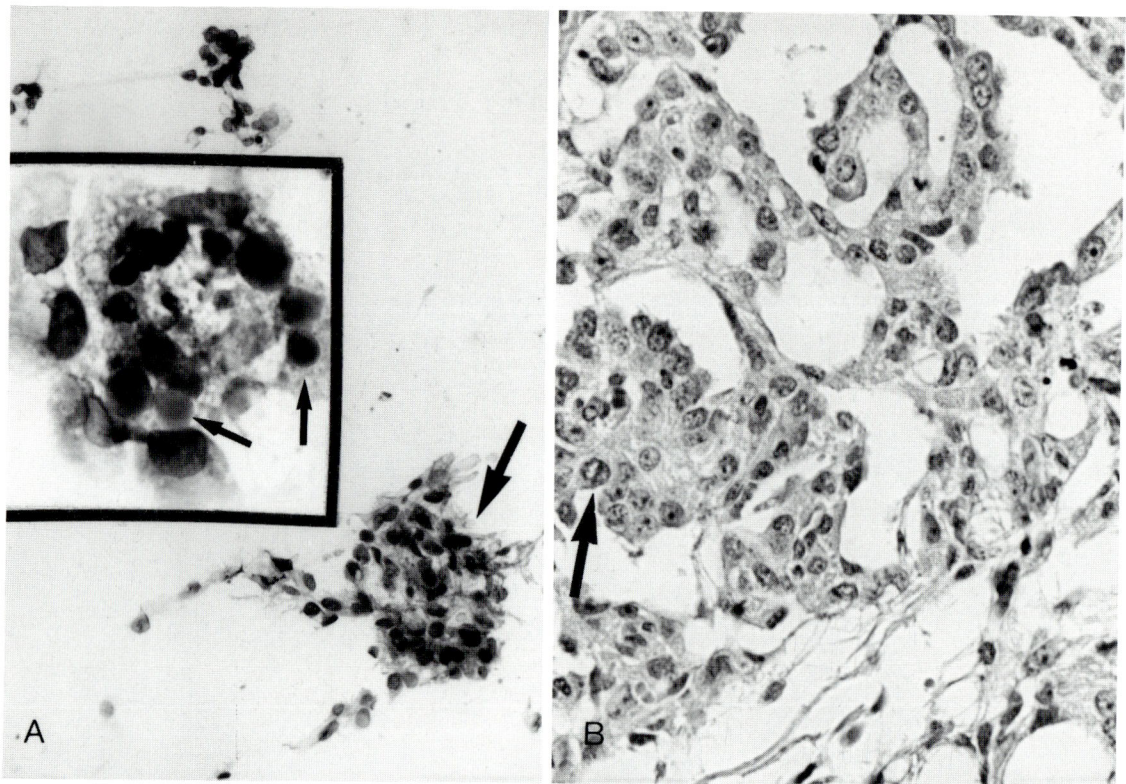

Figure 14.21.   Metastatic yolk sac tumor in retroperitoneum. **A,** ABC. Tumor cells are smaller and more uniform than those of embryonal carcinoma. *Thick arrow* indicates a cell cluster resembling a glomeruloid structure. *Inset* shows numerous eosi-nophilic globules *(thin arrows)*, which contain α-fetoproteins. ×125; *inset,* ×500. **B,** Histologic section of yolk sac tumor. Note relatively uniform cells with prominent nucleoli, a reticular growth pattern, and a glomeruloid structure *(arrow).* ×310.

antitrypsin. Very often, patients with yolk sac tumors also have elevated levels of AFP in their sera.

Choriocarcinoma

Choriocarcinoma is the most malignant of germ cell tumors. Serum and urine levels of human chorionic gonadotropins (HCG) are elevated. In order to make the diagnosis in the aspirate, two types of cells must be present—the syncytiotrophoblast and the cytotrophoblast **(Fig. 14.22)**. Syncytiotrophoblast cells are large bizarre multinucleated cells with abundant ground-glass-type, eosinophilic cytoplasm, which can be occasionally vacuolated. Cytotrophoblast cells are large, cuboidal cells with a single dark nucleus and clear cytoplasm. Ishizuka et al.[34] have emphasized large nucleoli as one of the striking features. Since the tumor almost always contains extensive hemorrhage, the smear backgound is typically bloody.

Diagnostic Pitfalls.   Hudson[35] cautioned the possibility of confusing choriocarcinoma cells with cells derived from giant cell anaplastic carcinoma or keratinizing squamous cell carcinoma. In choriocarcinomas, the highly hemorrhagic smear background is characteristic, and immunostaining for HCG will show a positive reaction in the tumor cells **(Fig. 14.22C)**.

Teratoma

Teratomas are complex neoplasms composed of tissues derived from two or more germ cell layers. The component tissues can be histologically mature or immature. The mature (''adult'') teratomas are commonly cystic and the cyst walls are lined by mature keratinizing squamous epithelium, with other mature tissues in the walls such as sebaceous glands, intestinal and respiratory epithelia, adipose tissue, bone, and cartilage (see Chapter 8, ''Mediastinum''). Mature teratomas occurring in young children and in women are benign and do not metastasize. Conversely, in adult males even the most mature teratomas may metastasize and cause death.

Immature teratomas are malignant neoplasms characterized by the presence of a mixture of mature (adult) and embryonal tissues in varying proportions. The predominant component is usually neural tissue, including glial elements as well as neuroepithelium forming tubules and rosettes **(Fig. 14.23)**. In a detailed study of 58 cases of immature teratomas of the ovary, Norris et al.[36] have shown that the malignant potential is directly proportional to the quantities of immature tissues and to the degree of immaturity.

Malignant elements from other germ cell tumors, such as embryonal carcinoma or choriocarcinoma, may be present in a teratoma (teratocarcinoma), and the presence of these elements should be specified in the diagnosis.

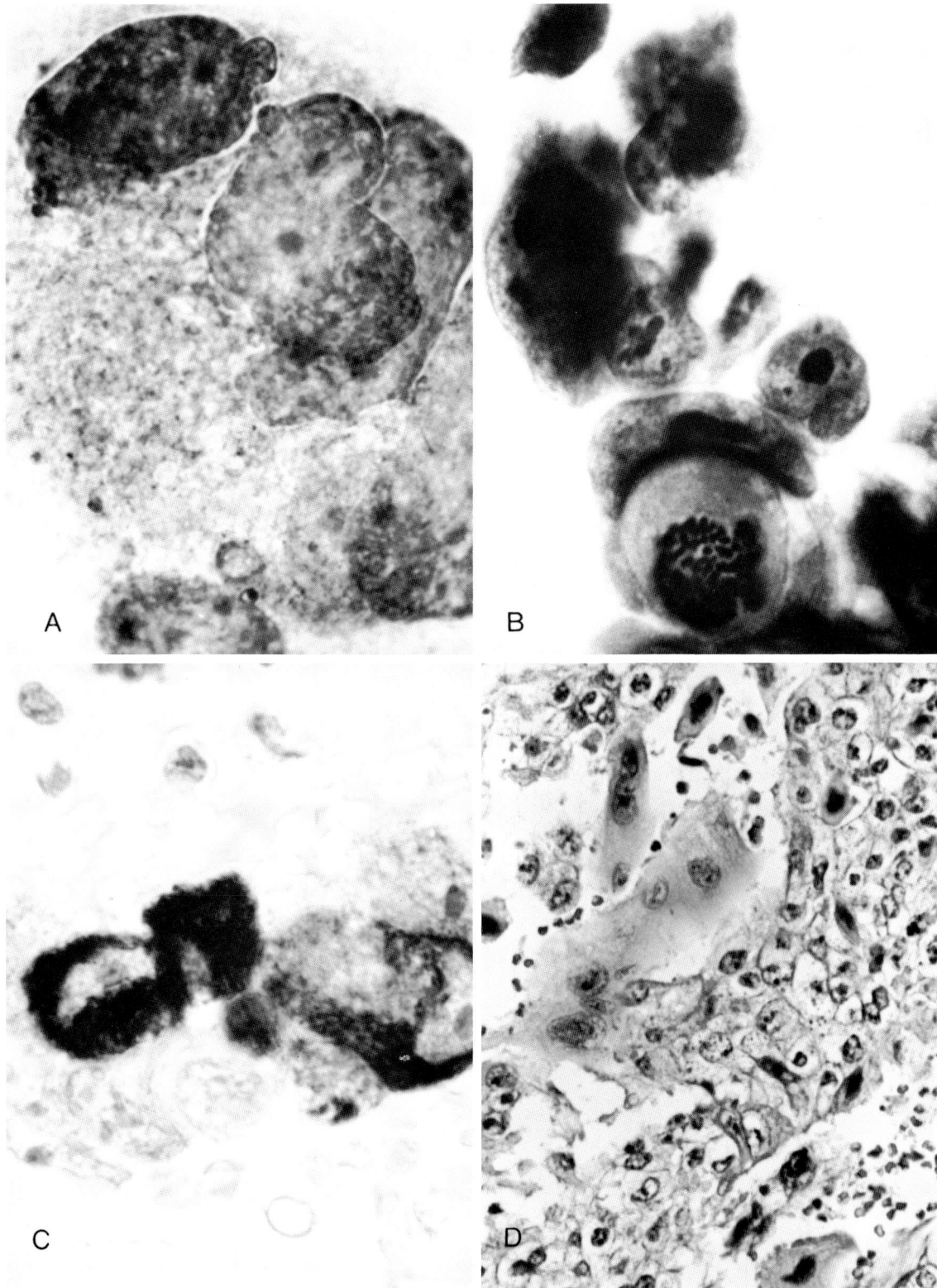

Figure 14.22. Choriocarcinoma, primary in the retroperitoneum, ABC. **A,** Malignant syncytiotrophoblast cell showing multinucleation, marked nuclear pleomorphism, and ground-glass cytoplasm. ×1000. **B,** Malignant cytotrophoblast cells with macronucleoli and an atypical mitosis. ×1000. **C,** Cluster of tumor cells showing strong cytoplasmic staining for β-HCG. Avidin-biotin peroxidase technique. ×1000. (**A–C:** Courtesy of Dr. N. Jetha, Shaughnessy Hospital, Vancouver, Canada.) **D,** Histology of choriocarcinoma (not the same case) to illustrate the characteristic admixture of cytotrophoblast cells and syncytiotrophoblast cells. ×310.

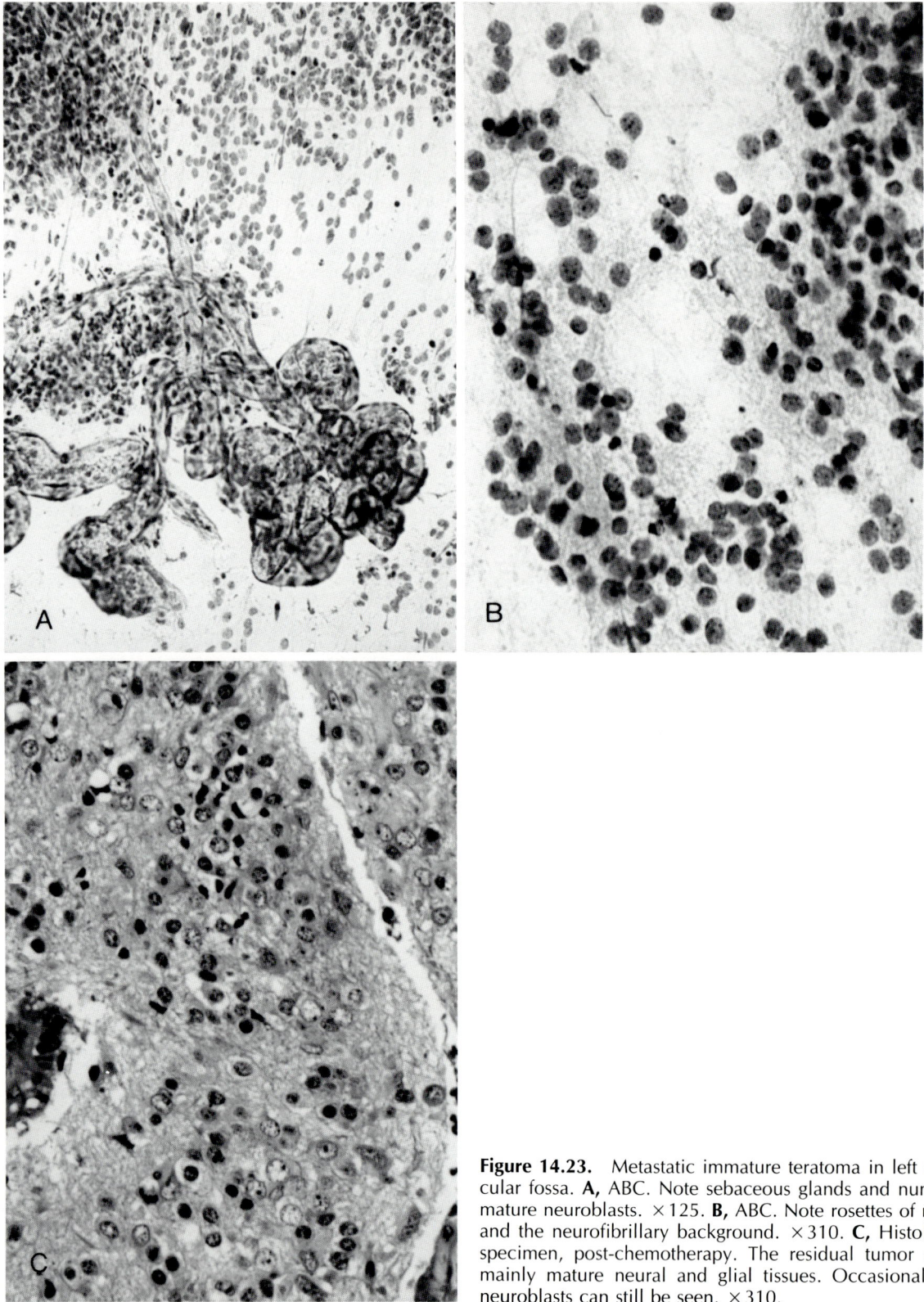

Figure 14.23. Metastatic immature teratoma in left supraclavicular fossa. **A,** ABC. Note sebaceous glands and numerous immature neuroblasts. ×125. **B,** ABC. Note rosettes of neuroblasts and the neurofibrillary background. ×310. **C,** Histology of the specimen, post-chemotherapy. The residual tumor consists of mainly mature neural and glial tissues. Occasional immature neuroblasts can still be seen. ×310.

References

1. Willems JS, Lowhagen T. Transrectal fine needle aspiration biopsy for cytologic diagnosis and grading of prostatic carcinoma. Prostate 1981;2:381–395.
2. Esposti PL. Cytologic malignancy grading of prostatic carcinoma by transrectal aspiration biopsy. A five-year follow-up study of 469 hormone-treated patients. Scand J Urol Nephrol 1971;5:199–209.
3. Kline TS. Guides to clinical aspiration biopsy. Prostate. New York: Igaku Shoin, 1985.
4. Kline TS, Kohler FP, Kelsey DM. Aspiration biopsy cytology (ABC). Its use in diagnosis of lesions of the prostate gland. Arch Pathol Lab Med 1982;106:136–139
5. Kline TS, Kannan V. Prostatic aspirates. A cytomorphologic analysis with emphasis on well-differentiated carcinoma. Diagn Cytopathol 1985;1:13–17.
6. Kline TS. Handbook of fine needle aspiration biopsy cytology, 2nd ed. New York: Churchill Livingstone, 1988:365–392.
7. Linsk JA, Axilrod HD, Solyn R, Delaverdac C. Transrectal cytologic aspiration in the diagnosis of prostatic carcinoma. J Urol 1972;108:455–459.
8. Chodak GW, Steinberg GD, Bibbo M, Wied G, Straus FS II, Vogelzang NJ, Schoenberg HW. The role of transrectal aspiration biopsy in the diagnosis of prostatic cancer. J Urol 1986;135:299–302.
9. Carter HB, Riehle RA Jr, Koizumi JH, Amberson J, Vaughan ED Jr. Fine needle aspiration of the abnormal prostate: A cytohistological correlation. J Urol 1986;135:294–298.
9a. Casey JH, Silenieks AI. Fine-needle aspiration cytology of prostate: Experience in a nonacademic practice. Semin Diagn Pathol 1988;5:294–300.
10. Franzen S, Giertz G, Zajicek J. Cytological diagnosis of prostatic tumors by transrectal aspiration biopsy: A preliminary report. Br J Urol 1960;32:193–196.
11. Rifkin MD, Kurtz AB, Goldberg BB. Sonographically guided transperineal prostatic biopsy. Preliminary experience with a longitudinal linear-array transducer. AJR 1983;140:745–747.
12. Spirnak JP, Resnick MI. Transrectal ultrasonography. Urology 1984;23:461–467.
13. Cooner WH. Ultrasound in prostatic cancer. JAMA 1988;259:1015.
13a. Bentley EM, Mallery WR, Mueller JJ, Anderson MC, Schott AW, Flegel G, Still R. Fine needle aspiration of the prostate gland in the community hospital. A predictive value analysis. Acta Cytol 1988;32:499–503.
14. Lin BPC, Davies WEL, Harmata PA. Prostatic aspiration biopsy. Pathology 1979;11:607–614.
15. Maksem JA, Johenning PW, Park CH, Galang CF. Prostatitis and aspiration biopsy of the prostatic gland. Cytopathology Check Sample C88–1. Chicago: American Society of Clinical Pathologists, 1988.
16. Epstein NA. Prostatic biopsy. A morphologic correlation of aspiration cytology with needle biopsy histology. Cancer 1976;38;2078–2087.
17. Faul P, Shmiedt E. Cytologic aspects of diseases of the prostate. Int Urol Nephrol 1973;5:297–310.
18. Koss LG, Woyke S, Olszerwsky W. Aspiration biopsy. Cytologic interpretation and histologic bases. Tokyo: Igaku Shoin, 1984:223–249.
18a. Droese M, Voeth C. Cytologic features of seminal vesicle epithelium in aspiration biopsy smears of the prostate. Acta Cytol 1976;20:120–125.
19. Kelalis PP, Greene LF, Harrison EG Jr. Granulomatous prostatitis. A mimic of carcinoma of the prostate. JAMA 1965;191:111–113.
20. Silverberg E, Lubera JA. Cancer statistics, 1988. CA 1988;38:5–22.
21. Gleason DF, Mellinger GT, The Veteran's Administration Cooperative Urological Research Group. Prediction of prognosis for prostatic adenocarcinoma by combined histologic grading and clinical staging. J Urol 1974;111:58–64.
22. Mostofi FK. Problems of grading carcinoma of prostate. Semin Oncol 1976;3:161–169.
23. Mostofi FK. Grading of prostatic carcinoma. Cancer Treat Rep (Part 1) 1975;59;111–117.
24. Zajicek J. Aspiration biopsy cytology, Part 2. Cytology of infradiaphragmatic organs. Basel: S Karger, 1979:129–166.
25. Ostrzega N, Cheng L, Layfield LJ. Keratin immunoreactivity in fine-needle aspiration of the prostate: An aid in the differentiation of benign epithelium from well-differentiated adenocarcinoma. Diagn Cytopathol 1988;4:38–41.
26. De Gaetani CF, Trentini GP. Atypical hyperplasia of the prostate. A pitfall in the cytologic diagnosis of carcinoma. Acta Cytol 1978;22:483–486.
27. Greenebaum E. Megakaryocytes and ganglion cells mimicking cancer in fine needle aspiration of the prostate. Acta Cytol 1988;32:504–508.
28. Rosai J. Ackerman's surgical pathology, 6th ed. St. Louis: CV Mosby, 1981:876.
29. Zajicek J. Aspiration biopsy cytology, Part 2. Cytology of infradiaphragmatic organs. Basel: S Karger, 1979:104–128.
30. Persson PS, Ahren C, Obrant KO. Aspiration biopsy smear of testis in azoospermia: Cytological versus histological examination. Scand J Urol Nephrol 1971;5:22–26.
30a. Glant MD, Wall RW, Clark SA, Roth L. Cytopathology of germ-cell neoplasms metastatic to lymph nodes: Diagnosis by fine needle aspiration. Acta Cytol 1988;32:762.
31. Kapila K, Hajdu SI, Whitmore WF, Golbey RB, Beattie EJ. Cytologic diagnosis of metastatic germ cell tumors. Acta Cytol 1983;27:245–251.
32. Mostofi FK, Price EB Jr. Tumors of the male genital system. Atlas of tumor pathology, 2nd Series, Fascicle 8. Washington, D.C.: Armed Forces Instiue of Pathology, 1973.
33. Dixon FJ, Moore RA. Tumors of the male sex organs. Atlas of tumor pathology, Fascicles 31b and 32. Washington D.C.: Armed Forces Institute of Pathology, 1952:48–104.
34. Ishizuka Y, Oota K, Masubuchi K. Practical cytodiagnosis. Toyko: Igaku Shoin, 1972:112;157.
35. Hudson EA. Sputum cytology of metastatic choriocarcinoma: A case report. Acta Cytol 1981;25:29–32.
36. Norris HI, Zirkin HJ, Benson WL. Immature (malignant) teratoma of the ovary. A clinical and pathologic study of 58 cases. Cancer 1976;37:2359–2372.

15

Female Genital Organs

Fine needle aspiration biopsy does not play a key role in the primary diagnosis of many common gynecologic cancers. For example, carcinomas of the vagina, vulva, and cervix are accessible to direct inspection and punch biopsy. Endometrial cancers are diagnosable by uterine curettage. Although Scandinavian workers[1,2] have advocated FNAB of ovarian tumors, this usage has remained controversial in North America because of the potential risk of causing intraperitoneal tumor dissemination.[3,4] On the other hand, simple, thin-walled cysts of paratubal, paraovarian, or ovarian origin and endometriotic cysts can be aspirated and evacuated by needle aspiration, especially at laparoscopic examination.[5,6] Most of the medical centers in North America follow the suggestions proposed by Geier and Strecker[7] and use FNAB for: *(a)* recurrence and metastasis of previously diagnosed gynecologic tumors, *(b)* patients too frail for laparotomy, and *(c)* benign ovarian cysts. Pelvic lesions can be aspirated transvaginally or transrectally, using the Franzen's apparatus as in prostatic aspirations.[1,2,7–9] Bulky masses can be aspirated transabdominally. Sepsis has been reported following transrectal biopsy of ovarian tumors.[7]

Diagnostic Accuracy

In general, the diagnostic accuracy of FNAB of ovarian tumors has been reported to be 90–95%.[1] "Unsatisfactory" specimens have been reported in 2–11% of the aspirates studied.[1,7,10] Kjellgren and Angstrom[11] were able to suggest or diagnose 94% of 116 malignant intrapelvic tumors by FNAB. Of 113 benign conditions, six were suspected to contain malignant cells and four were diagnosed as malignant tumors. Therefore, the cytologic false-positive rate was 3.3%, or 8.8% if suspected diagnoses were included. Sevin et al.[8] reported a reliability of 96.4% in distinguishing between malignant and benign conditions, and a 97.9% specificity. Geier and Strecker[7] correctly interpreted 91% of the satisfactory smears from the malignant tumors and all of the aspirates from the benign tumors.

THE OVARIES
Benign Cystic Lesions

The "chocolate" endometriotic cyst occurs chiefly in young women and is the most common nonneoplastic indication for fine needle aspiration biopsy. Kjellgren and Angstrom[11] studied 48 cases, 69% of which showed decomposed blood, siderophages, and degenerate epithelial cells. According to these workers, this cytologic picture is typical, even if not pathognomonic, for endometriosis. Twelve percent of the cases were unsatisfactory, containing only fresh blood and mesothelial cells. There were no false-positive diagnoses of malignancy. The endometrial epithelial cells **(Fig. 15.1)** are small, with a scant amount of cytoplasm, and tend to occur in two-dimensional aggregates. The nuclei are uniform, with coarsely granular chromatin and smooth nuclear membranes. The nucleoli are not prominent and there is little or no anisonucleosis. The endometrial cells can be distinguished from colonic epithelial cells, which are tall columnar cells with vesicular nuclei and abundant cytoplasm.[9]

A variety of thin-walled cysts are also targets for FNAB. These include simple epithelial inclusion cysts, paraovarian cysts, and some cystadenomas. The cysts contain clear fluid and a variable number of macrophages. In addition, scant degenerated epithelial cells may be identified. These epithelial cells are usually cytologically nondescript, thus precluding precise classification of the cysts.[11]

Sex Cord-Stromal Tumors

Sex cord-stromal tumors, also referred to by the alternate name of gonadal stromal tumors, share a common characteristic: they have the capability of producing hormones and account for a large proportion of functioning ovarian tumors. The most common members of this group are the thecomas and the granulosa cell tumors. The thecomas are benign ovarian neoplasms and are generally not the targets for FNAB. The aspirates are cell-poor because of the fibrotic tumor matrix and show a few benign spindle cells. Most of our experience and the reports from the literature have been concerned with recurrences of granulosa cell tumors.

Granulosa cell tumor is a malignant member of the sex cord-stromal tumors. It has a low malignant potential and is well known for its late recurrence. Distant metastases are uncommon. Some of the recurrences can be quite bulky and most are in the pelvis and lower abdomen, providing easy targets for fine needle aspiration biopsy.[12–14] We have encountered three such cases. Histologically, these tumors contain not only granulosa cells but also variable numbers of spindle cells, reminiscent of theca cells and fibroblasts.

Aspiration Cytology of Granulosa Cell Tumor

Cell Morphology. Two types of cells are seen: the granulosa cells, which are the predominant cell type, and the spindle cells. The granulosa cells **(Fig. 15.2)** are small and relatively uniform, oval to low columnar, and have vesicular nuclei with small single nucleoli. Nuclei with longitudinal grooves may be seen in about 10–20% of the granulosa cells. The spindle cells are the theca or stromal cells, having elongated or fusiform, bland nuclei and pale eosinophilic cytoplasm. These cells are not present in large numbers and may be easily overlooked.

Cellular Pattern. Aspirates from granulosa cell tumors yield abundant cellular material with a clean background. The cells are arranged singly or in compact groups. Others form pseudorosette structures **(Fig. 15.3)**. By focusing at various levels, a central clear

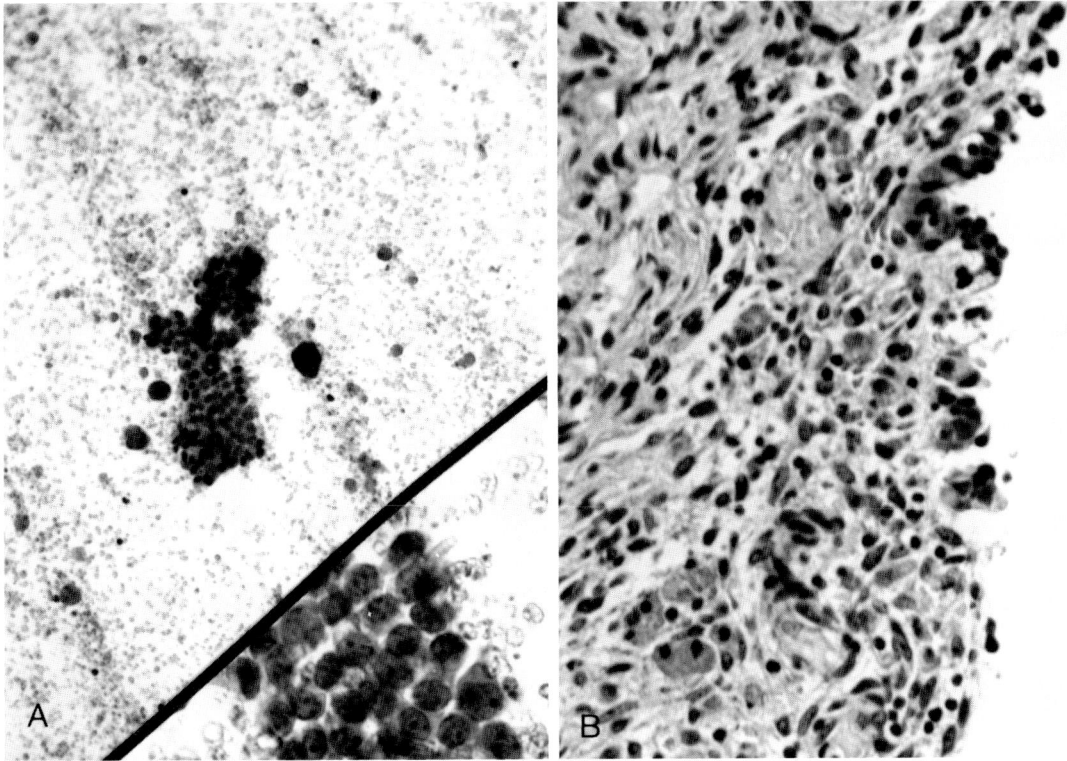

Figure 15.1.

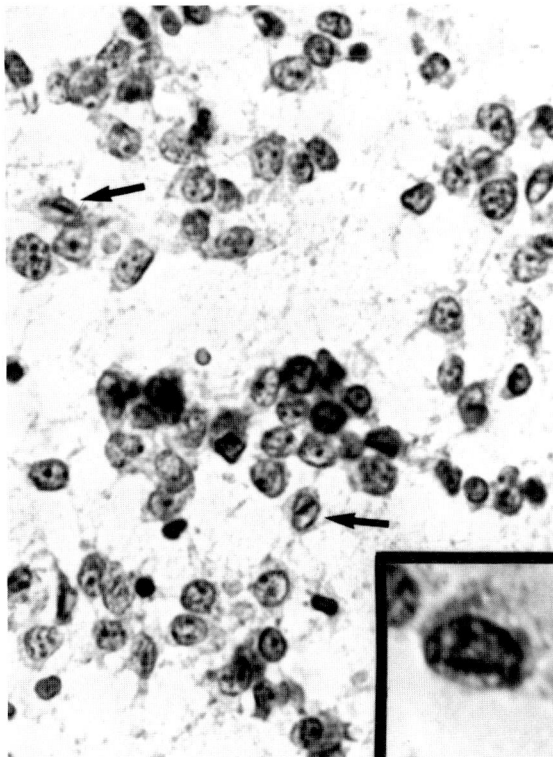

Figure 15.2.

Figure 15.1. Chocolate endometriotic cyst. **A,** ABC. Note abundant decomposed blood, hemosiderin-laden macrophages and a monolayered sheet of endometrial epithelial cells. *Inset* shows endometrial epithelial cells in orderly honeycomb arrangement. ×125; *inset,* ×500. **B,** Histology of an endometriotic cyst. The cyst is incompletely lined by a layer of endometrial epithelial cells. Numerous hemosiderin-laden macrophages are seen in the cyst wall. ×310.

Figure 15.2. Granulosa cell tumor, ABC. Note pale vesicular nuclei and longitudinal nuclear grooves *(arrows* and *inset).* ×500; *inset,* ×1250.

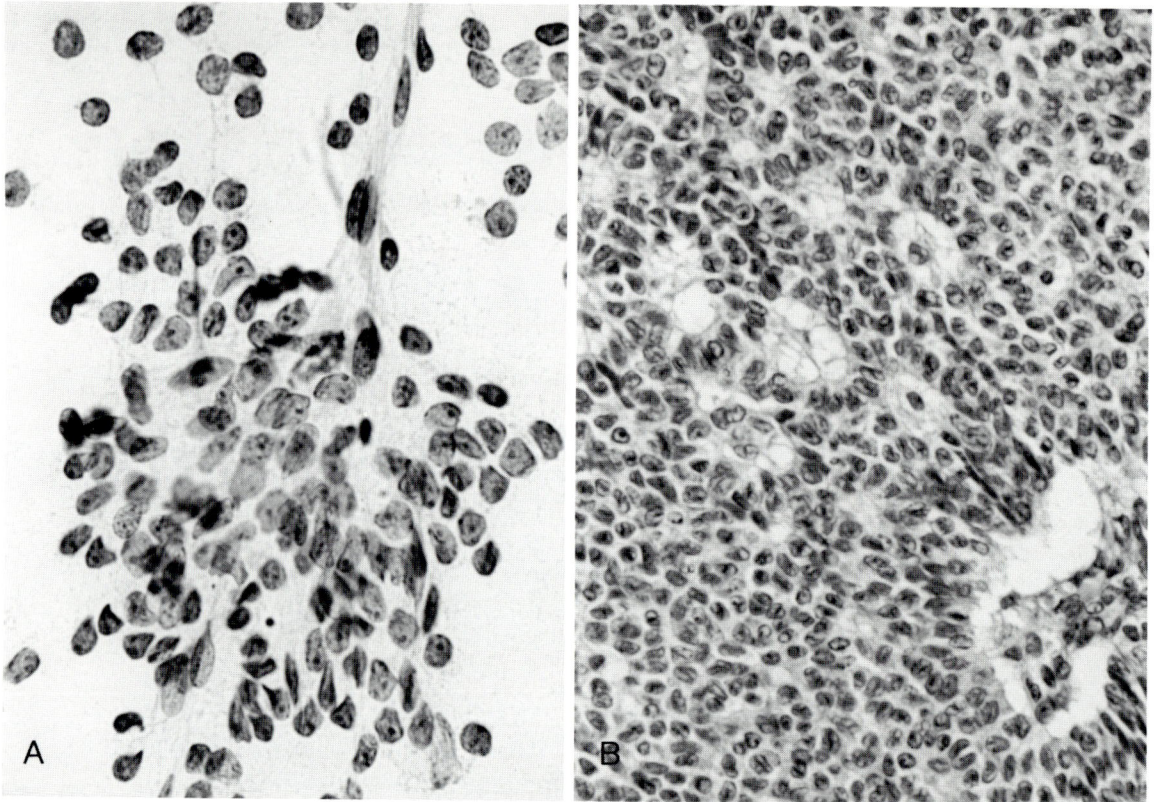

Figure 15.3.   Granulosa cell tumor. **A,** ABC. Note pseudorosette arrangement of tumor cells, corresponding to Call-Exner bodies. The theca cells are represented by the spindle cells. ×500. **B,**

Histologic section of granulosa cell tumor showing solid growth pattern as well as formation of Call-Exner bodies. ×310.

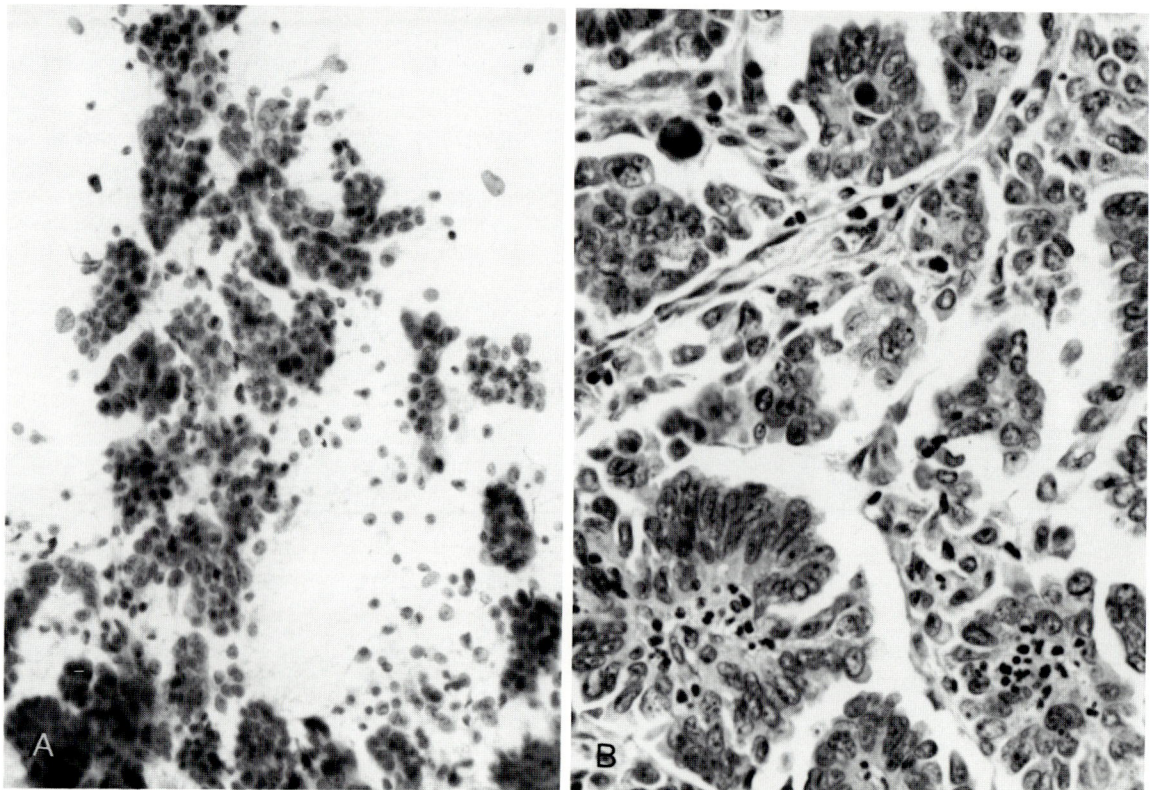

Figure 15.4.   Serous adenocarcinoma of the ovary. **A,** ABC. Note typical branching papillary pattern. ×125. **B,** Histology of the papillary serous adenocarcinoma. ×310.

or pale eosinophilic area may be seen in such pseudorosettes, which correspond to the Call-Exner bodies seen in histologic sections.

Diagnostic Pitfalls. In a patient with a previously known granulosa cell tumor, the cytologic diagnosis is fairly apparent. However, some of these tumors may recur two to three decades after the removal of the primary tumor, and diagnostic problems may arise if the clinical history does not include this information.

Although the longitudinal nuclear groove is characteristic of granulosa cell tumor, it is by no means specific. Grooved nuclei can be seen in reactive mesothelial cells, cleaved lymphocytes, Brenner tumor, and papillary thyroid carcinoma.

Common neoplasms that may be mistaken for granulosa cell tumors are carcinoid tumor, undifferentiated carcinoma, and large cell lymphoma.[15] Cells of carcinoid tumor generally show slightly more cytoplasm, which is finely granulated. The nuclei are uniformly round and lack indentations or grooves. The acini of carcinoid tumors are more sharply outlined than the Call-Exner bodies. An undifferentiated carcinoma may simulate a diffuse granulosa cell tumor. The nuclei of undifferentiated carcinoma are hyperchromatic, usually of unequal size and shape, whereas those of granulosa cell tumor are typically pale, fairly uniform in size and shape, and often grooved. Malignant lymphomas are distinguished by a dispersed cell pattern. No psuedorosetes or other organoid structures are formed. Immunoperoxidase staining of lymphocytes for leukocyte common antigen is positive.

Adenocarcinomas

In contrast to testicular neoplasms, the vast majority of which are germ cell in origin, 80–90% of ovarian malignancies are of epithelial origin (adenocarcinomas). Ovarian adenocarcinomas are divided into the following histologic subtypes: serous, mucinous, endometrioid, clear cell, and undifferentiated. Although past literature has suggested otherwise, it is now apparent that these different histologic subtypes behave similarly, stage for stage and grade for grade. In the past, a better prognosis was affixed to the mucinous and endometrioid subtypes, but prognosis is now recognized to be more closely related to the fact that these tumors are more often better differentiated (hence of lower grade) and found in earlier stages.[16] Ovarian adenocarcinoma is notorious for its tendency to spread on peritoneal surfaces not only in the pelvis but throughout the peritoneum. Metastases in the pelvis and abdomen are readily subjected to FNAB, with or without radiologic guidance.

Aspiration Cytology

The cytologic diagnosis of adenocarcinomas of the ovary generally poses no problems. The tumor cells exhibit the usual cytologic criteria of malignancy, such as abnormal chromatin pattern, irregular nuclear membranes, and enlarged nucleoli. The N/C ratio is high.

The ABC of serous adenocarcinomas **(Fig. 15.4)** typically show acino-papillary structures. Psammoma bodies, frequently surrounded by tumor cells, may be seen **(Fig. 15.5)**. The tumor cells are low columnar or oval, with scant homogenous amphophilic cytoplasm. In endometrioid carcinomas **(Fig. 15.6)**, tumor cells show glandular and, less frequently, papillary arrangements, resembling those from endometrial carcinoma. Compared with serous carcinoma, endometrioid carcinoma has larger cells with frequently prominent nucleoli and eosinophilic cytoplasm.[9] The aspirates from mucinous adenocarcinomas **(Fig. 15.7)** consist of large cells in glandular clusters and cell balls. A variable number of the cells contain cytoplasmic mucin vacuoles, which can be demonstrated by mucicarmine stain on air-dried smears. Malignant cells from clear cell carcinomas **(Fig. 15.8)** exhibit the lowest N/C ratio of all adenocarcinomas due to their large

cytoplasmic volume. The nuclei are round and contain a single prominent nucleoli. For the most part, the cytoplasm is pale, granular, and eosinophilic. Some cells exhibit cytoplasmic vacuoles of various sizes, and these cells correspond to the clear cells seen in histologic sections. In our experience, cytoplasmic clearing is generally more striking in histologic sections than in aspirates, due to paraffin processing.

Diagnostic Pitfalls. Although it is relatively easy to recognize the tumors as adenocarcinomas, the pathologist may not be able to classify them as to correct type. Unless psammoma bodies and papillary structures are seen, differentiation between the serous and the endometrioid type is difficult or impossible.[11] Moreover, it is important to remember that psammoma bodies by themselves are not diagnostic of ovarian carcinoma since they can be found in benign conditions, such as mesothelial proliferations and cystadenomas.

Metastatic colonic carcinomas to the ovary may morphologically simulate mucinous, serous, and endometrioid adenocarcinomas of the ovary. The clear cell variant of ovarian carcinoma may be confused with clear cell carcinomas from other sites, the most common of which is renal cell carcinoma. The cytologic picture of some undifferentiated ovarian carcinomas may mimic a lymphoma or sarcoma. A team approach to diagnosis cannot be overemphasized. At our institutions, most of the gynecologic aspirations are done on recurrent or metastatic lesions. The knowledge of the type of primary cancer and the availability of previous histologic slides for review facilitate ABC interpretation.

Germ Cell Tumors

Compared with epithelial cancers, germ cell tumors of the ovary are infrequent. For a description of the cytology of this group of tumors, see Chapter 14, ''Testis.''

THE UTERUS AND CERVIX
Adenocarcinomas

Recurrent cervical and uterine cancers in the vaginal vault, in the parametria, or elsewhere in the pelvis can be aspirated transvaginally or transrectally. The ABC of endometrial adenocarcinomas is similar to the endometrioid type of ovarian adenocarcinoma described previously and will not be repeated. The most common glandular cervical cancer is the adenocarcinoma of the endocervical columnar cell type. Histologically, it varies from well-differentiated to poorly differentiated, the most common variety being moderately differentiated with interbranching glands.[17] The ABC of endocervical adenocarcinomas shows columnar tumor cells, in which the cytologic criteria of adenocarcinoma **(Fig. 15.9)** are readily apparent. The tumor cells resemble, to a variable extent, normal endocervical cells; the cytoplasm is often the secretory type with fine vacuolation. The cells are arranged in a papillo-glandular pattern. Cytologic distinction from endometrial and colonic adenocarcinomas may not be feasible without clinical data.

Clear cell adenocarcinomas, morphologically identical to those arising in the ovary, can also be primary in the vagina, cervix, or endometrium. Clear cell carcinoma of the vagina or cervix occurs typically in young females with exposure to diethylstilbestrol administered to mothers during pregnancy.[18] In contrast, clear cell carcinomas arising in the ovary or endometrium occur sporadically in older women.

Squamous Cell Carcinoma

The common sites of origin of squamous cell carcinomas are the cervix, vagina, and vulva. The cytologic features of the keratin-

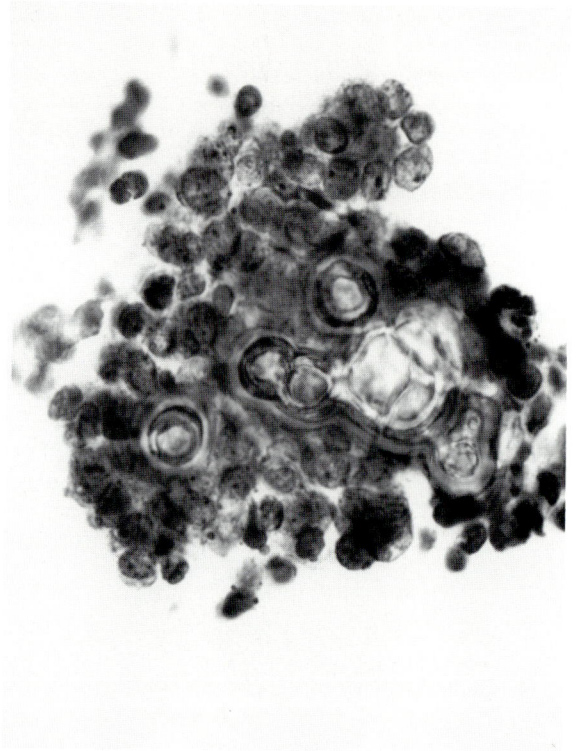

Figure 15.5.   Serous adenocarcinoma of the ovary, ABC. Note psammoma bodies surrounded by tumor cells. ×500.

Figure 15.6.   Endometrioid adenocarcinoma of the ovary. **A,** ABC. Thick tissue fragment with a microglandular pattern. Note oval to somewhat elongated nuclei. ×500; *inset,* ×125. **B,** Histology of endometrioid adenocarcinoma showing gland formations. ×310.

Figure 15.5.

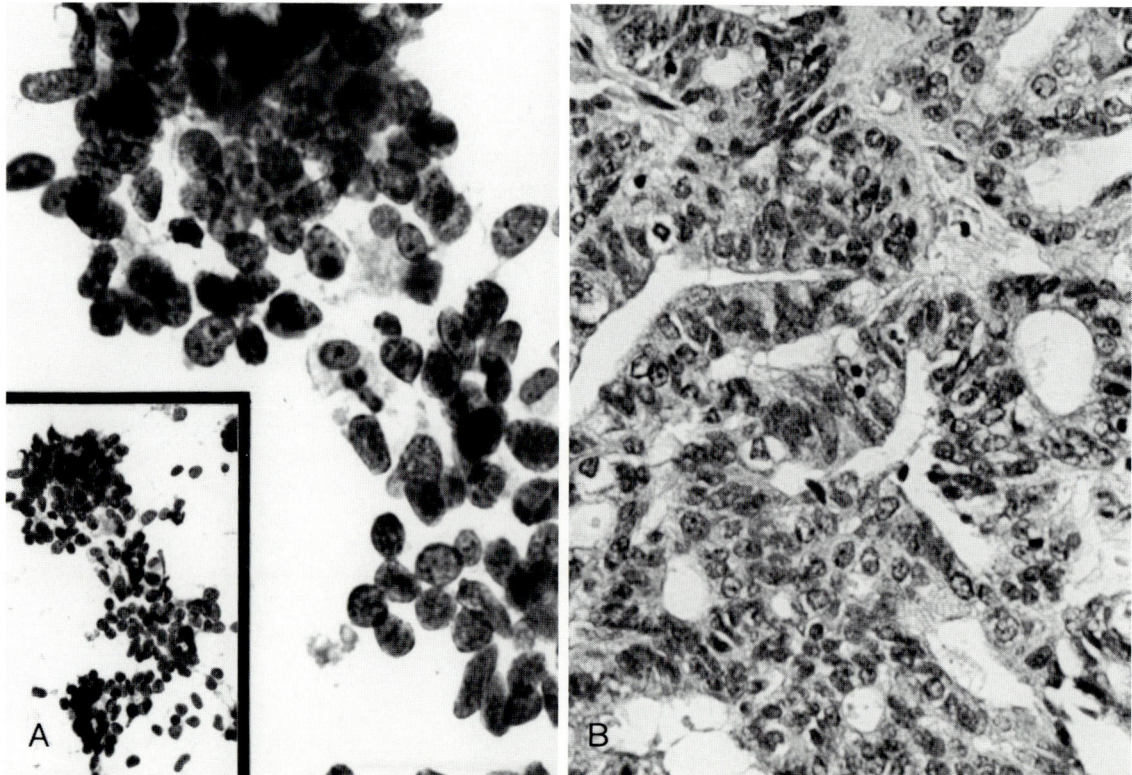

Figure 15.6.

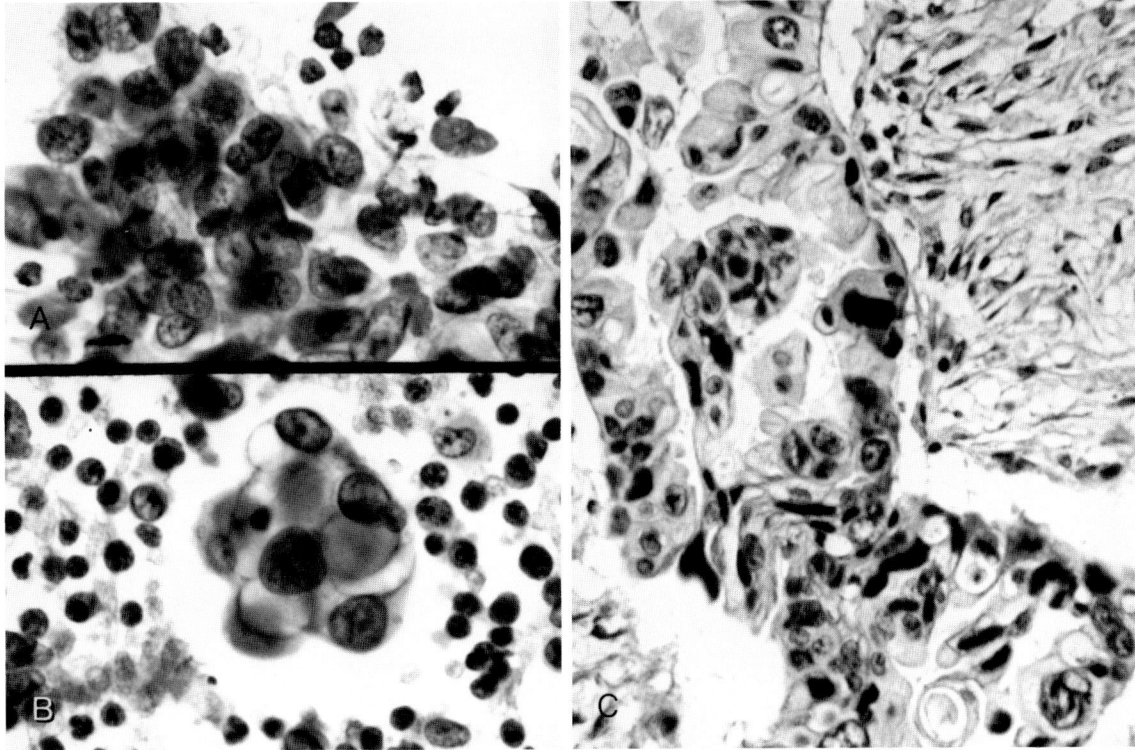

Figure 15.7.

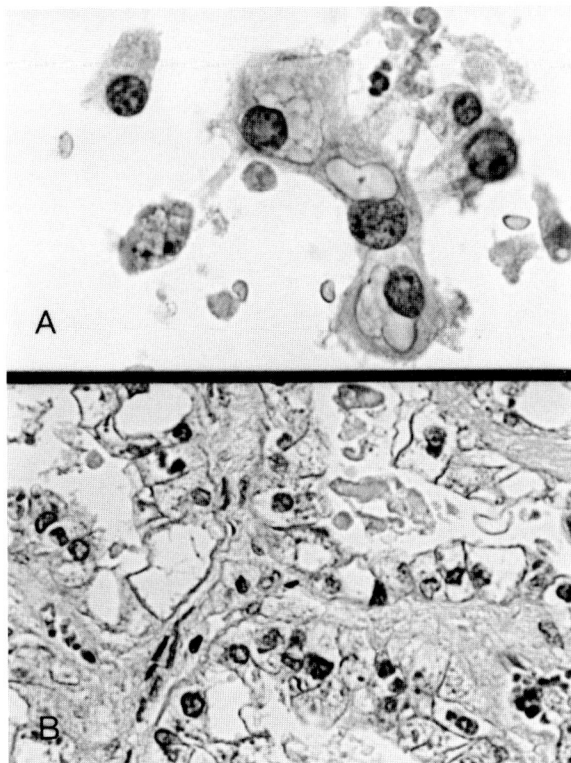

Figure 15.7. Mucinous adenocarcinoma of the ovary. **A** and **B,** ABC. Note clusters of malignant glandular cells. Tumor cells in **B,** show cytoplasmic mucin vacuoles. **A,** ×500; **B,** ×500. **C,** Histology of mucinous adenocarcinoma showing malignant mucinous cells. ×310.

Figure 15.8. Clear cell carcinoma of the ovary. **A,** ABC. Note vacuolated cytoplasm. ×500. **B,** Histologic section showing the clear cells forming tubules. ×310.

Figure 15.8.

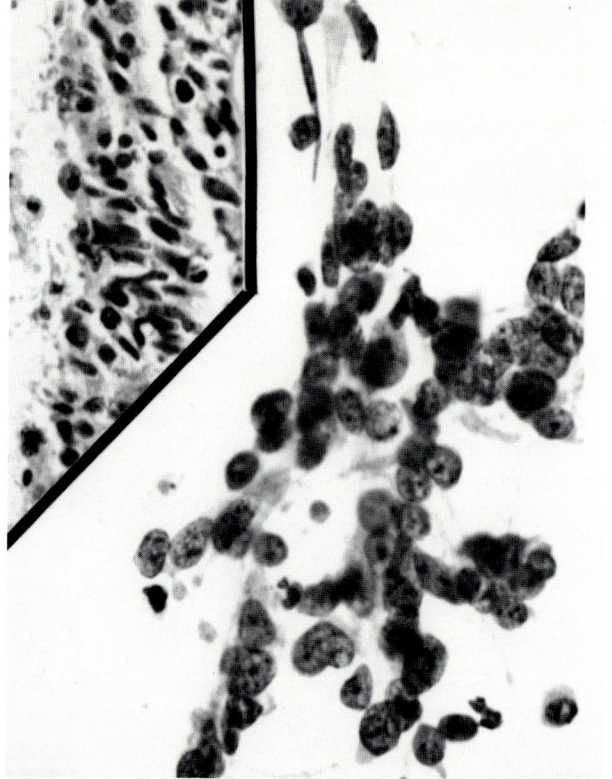

Figure 15.9.   Moderately differentiated endocervical adenocarcinoma, ABC. Note glandular cells with prominent nucleoli. *Inset* shows the histology of the original biopsy featuring columnar cells reminiscent of endocervical cells. ×500; *inset,* ×310.

Figure 15.10.   Nonkeratinizing squamous cell carcinoma of the cervix. **A,** ABC. A syncytial cell aggregate with irregular border. ×310. **B,** Histology of the squamous cell carcinoma. A sheet of malignant squamous cells showing morphologic similarity to the sheet seen in the aspirate. ×310.

Figure 15.9.

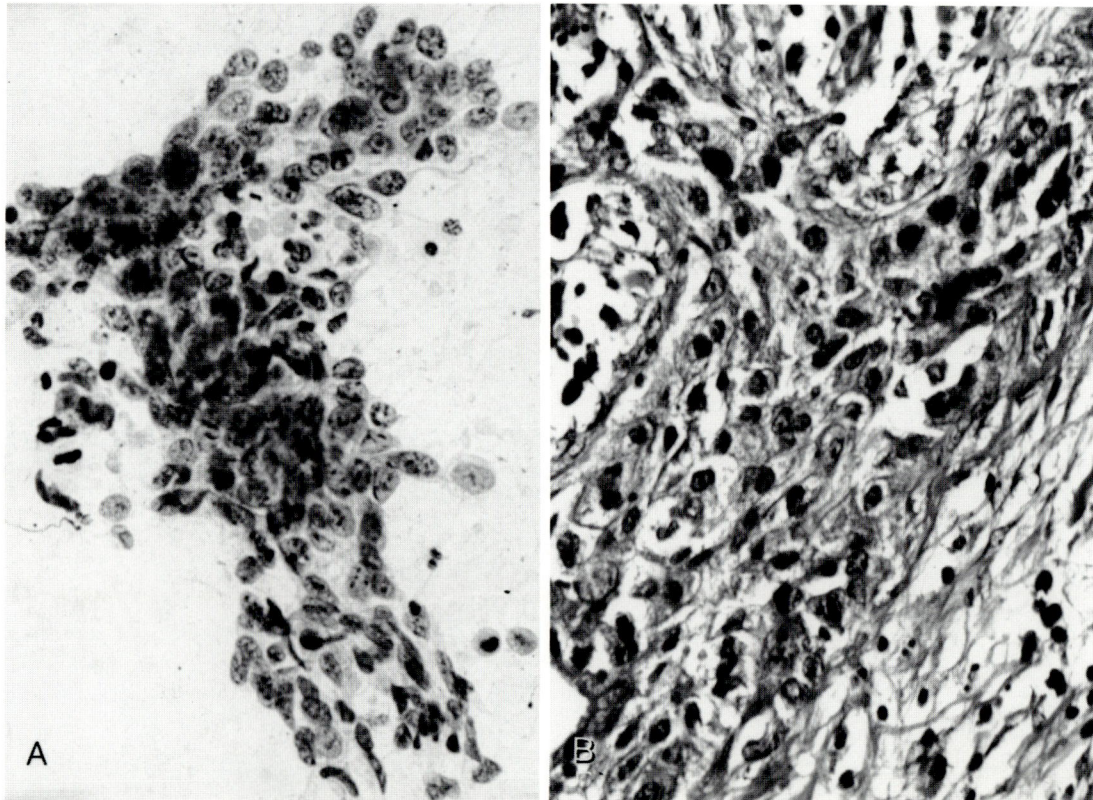

Figure 15.10.

izing squamous cell carinomas of the female genital tract and of the other sites are similar and need not be repeated here (see Chapter 7). The aspirates from poorly differentiated, nonkeratinizing squamous cell carcinoma (Fig. 15.10) consist of tumor cells appearing in large aggregates, as opposed to isolated cells in well-differentiated, keratinizing squamous carcinomas. The cell aggregates, unlike glandular tissue fragments, have irregular borders, with cells jutting out from the periphery. The nonkeratinizing squamous cells are relatively uniform in size and smaller than their keratinizing counterparts. The N/C ratio is high. The homogenous, dense cytoplasm and central nuclei contrast with the finely vacuolated cytoplasm and eccentric nuclei of adenocarcinoma.

Sarcomas

Uterine sarcomas are bulky tumors that occur most frequently in the elderly. Because of their large size, primary and recurrent sarcomas can often be readily aspirated transabdominally.[19] Leiomyosarcomas are the most frequent and constitute about 40% of uterine sarcomas. The ABC shows many tissue fragments composed of spindle cells arranged in fascicles (Fig. 15.11). The nuclei are cigar-shaped and hyperchromatic. The chromatin is coarse and irregularly distributed. The nuclear membranes are thickened. The cytoplasm is generally abundant, granular or fibrillary. In well-differentiated leiomyosarcomas, nuclear atypia is less obvious, and it may be difficult to differentiate them from cellular leiomyomas. The presence of mitoses is in favor of leiomyosarcoma.

Malignant mixed mesodermal tumors (malignant mixed müllerian tumors) are diagnosable cytologically.[20-22] The presence of an epithelial component, coupled with elongated mesenchymal cells or sarcoma cells, is the clue to correct diagnosis (Fig. 15.12). The epithelial component is usually an adenocarcinoma. The stromal component most often consists of fibrosarcoma-like cells, and in the heterologous variant, striated muscle, osteoid, and cartilage may be present.

Endometrial stromal sarcoma is relatively uncommon in the experience of any one laboratory. The tumor is composed entirely of cells reminiscent of endometrial stromal cells (Fig. 15.13). The neoplasmic cells are small and relatively uniform, lying singly or arranged in small clusters. The nuclei are short spindle or oval. The chromatin is finely granular, with a somewhat irregular distribution, and there are 1-2 small nucleoli. Cytoplasm is minimal, basophilic, and ill-defined. Mitotic figures are seen readily in high-grade tumors but are few in low-grade tumors.[23]

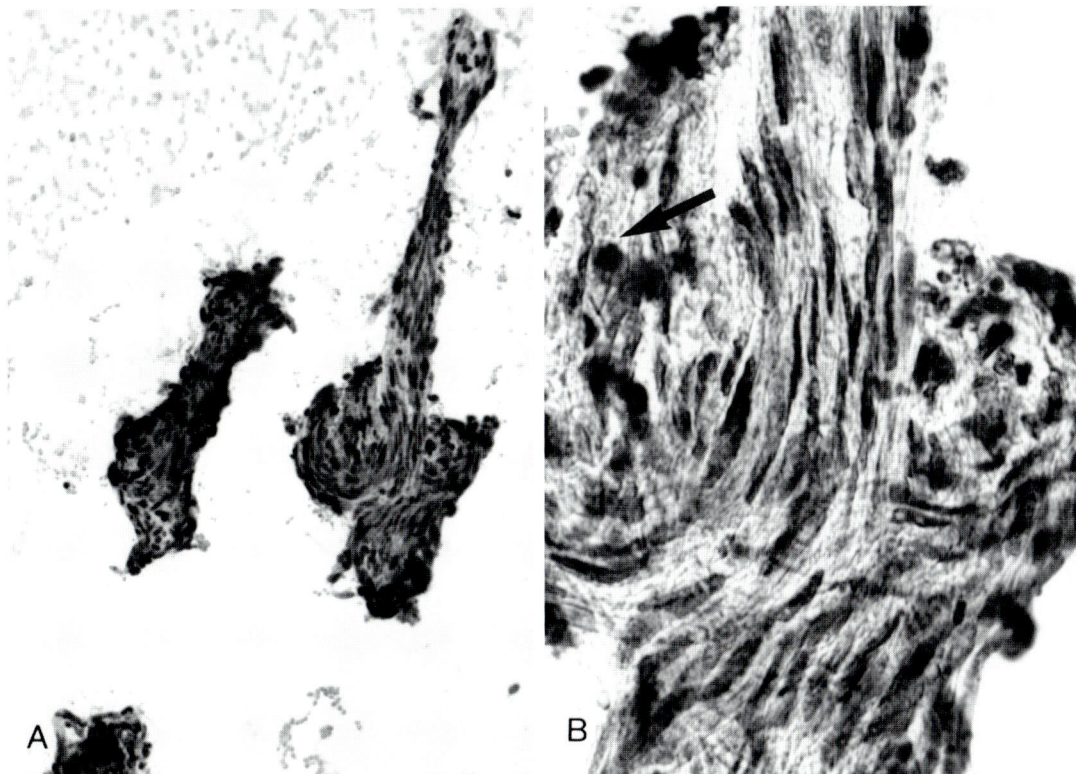

Figure 15.11.   Uterine leiomyosarcoma, ABC. **A,** Note tissue fragments composed of spindle cells in parallel arrangement. ×125. **B,** Note irregularly distributed chromatin and irregular nuclear membranes. *Arrow* indicates a mitosis. ×500.

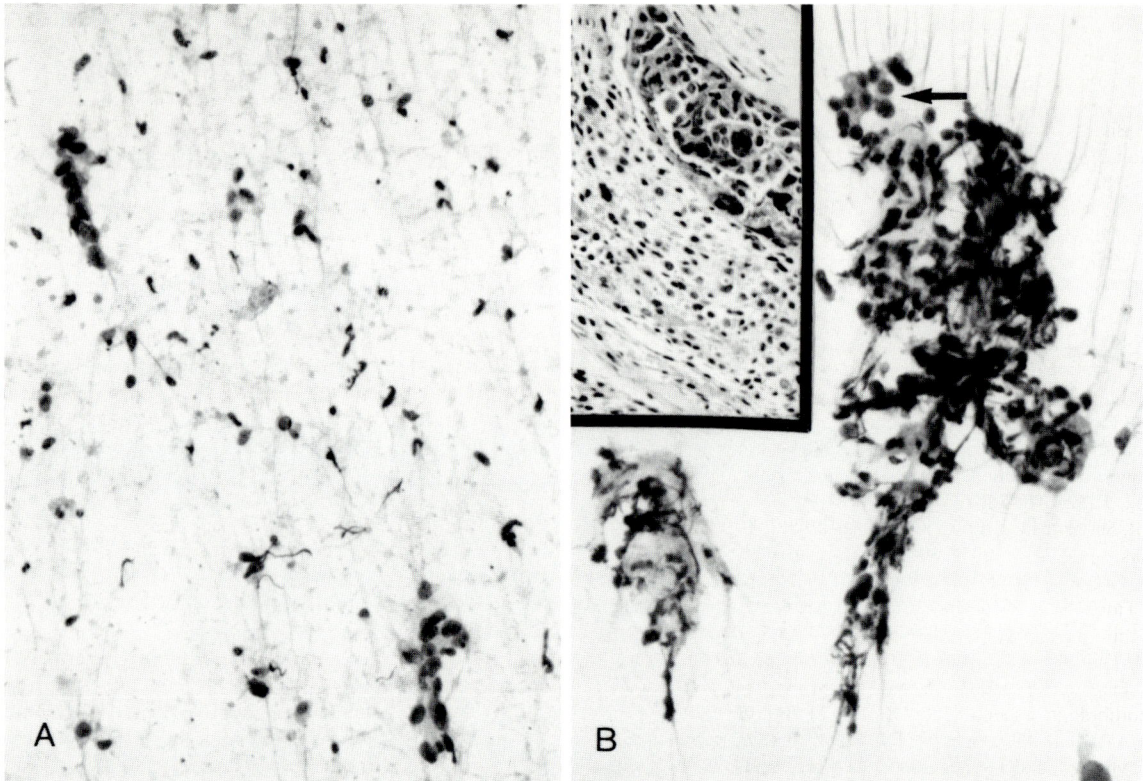

Figure 15.12.   Mixed mesodermal tumor, ABC. **A,** Note two cohesive strips of columnar epithelial cells and many scattered spindle cells. ×160. **B,** Note fragments of malignant spindle cells with a small cluster of epithelial cells *(arrow). Inset,* Histologic section showing a focus of adenocarcinoma surrounded by spindle sarcoma cells. ×210; *inset,* ×125.

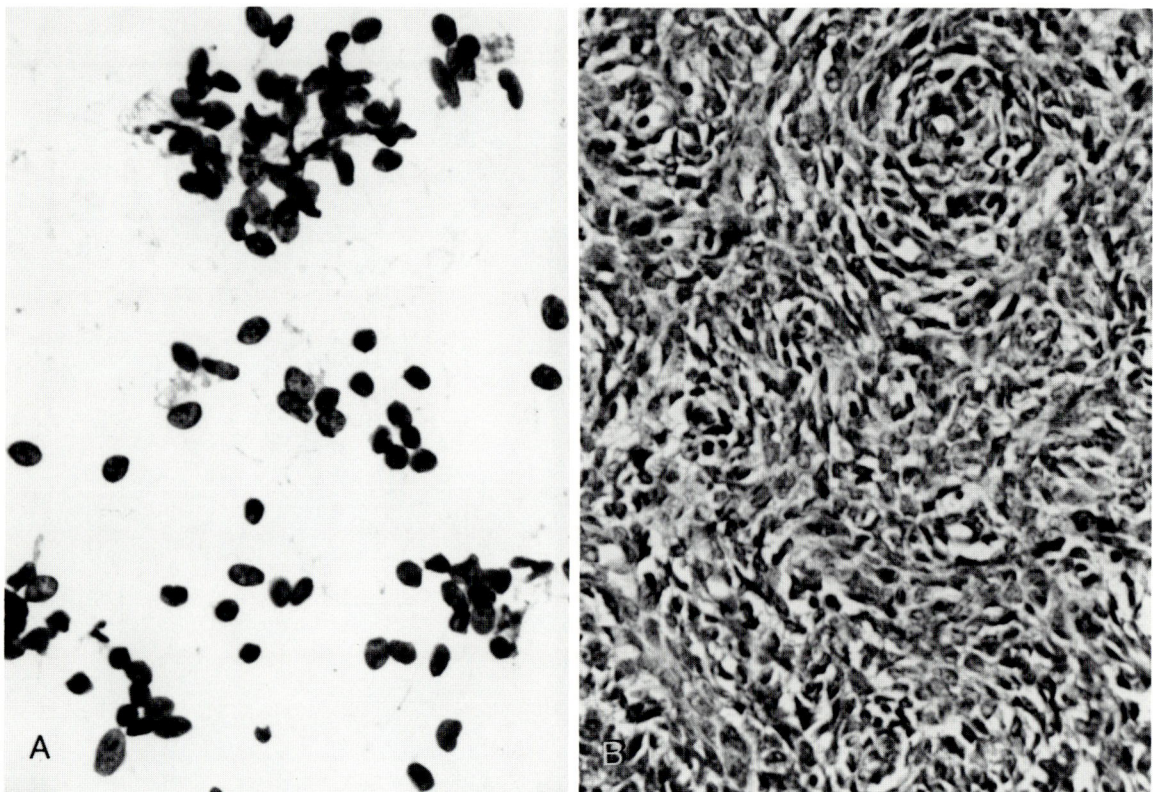

Figure 15.13.   Endometrial stromal sarcoma, recurrent in the pelvis. **A,** The aspirate is composed of loose clusters of plump spindle cells with hyperchromatic nuclei. ×500. **B,** Histologic section of the recurrent, low-grade endometrial stromal sarcoma showing densely packed stromal cells. ×310.

References

1. Kjellgren O, Angstrom T. Transvaginal and transrectal aspiration in diagnosis and classification of ovarian tumors. In Zajicek J. Aspiration biopsy cytology, Part 2. Cytology of infradiaphragmatic organs. Basel: S Karger, 1979:80–103.

2. Kjellgren O, Angstrom T, Bergman F, Wiklund DE. Fine needle aspiration biopsy in diagnosis and classification of ovarian carcinoma. Cancer 1971;28:967–976.

3. Hajdu SI, Melamed MR. Limitations of aspiration cytology in the diagnosis of primary neoplasms. Acta Cytol 1984;28:337–345.

4. Christopherson WW. Cytologic detection and diagnosis of cancer: Its contributions and limitations. Cancer 1983;51:1201–1208.

5. Rioux JE. Operative laparoscopy. J Reprod Med 1973;10:249–255.

6. Kovacic J, Rainer S, Levicnik A. Aspiration cytology of normal structures and non-neoplastic cysts of the ovary. In Blaustein A. Pathology of the female genital tract, 2nd ed. New York: Springer-Verlag, 1982:716–740.

7. Geier GR, Strecker JR. Aspiration cytology and E$_2$ content in ovarian tumors. Acta Cytol 1981;25:400–406.

8. Sevin B, Greening SE, Nadji M, Ng ABP, Averette HE, Nordqvist SRB. Fine needle aspiration cytology in gynecologic oncology. I. Clinical aspects. Acta Cytol 1979;23:277–281.

9. Nadji M, Greening SE, Sevin B, Averette HE, Nordqvist SRB, Ng ABP. Fine needle aspiration cytology in gynecologic oncology. II. Morphologic aspects. Acta Cytol 1979;380:380–388.

10. Moriarty AT, Glant MD, Stehman FB. The role of fine needle aspiration cytology in the management of gynecologic malignancies. Acta Cytol 1986;30:59–64.

11. Kjellgren O, Angstrom T. Aspiration biopsy cytology of ovarian tumors. In Blaustein A. Pathology of the female genital tract, 2nd ed. New York: Springer-Verlag, 1982:741–751.

12. Fidler WJ. Recurrent granulosa-cell tumor: Aspiration cytology findings. Acta Cytol 1982;26:688–690.

13. Ehya H, Lang WR. Cytology of granulosa cell tumor of the ovary. Am J Clin Pathol 1986;85:402–405.

14. Stamp GWH, Krausz T. Fine needle aspiration cytology of a recurrent juvenile granulosa cell tumor. Acta Cytol 1988;32:533–539.

15. Brenda JA, Zaleski S. Fine needle aspiration cytologic features of hepatic metastasis of granulosa cell tumor of the ovary. Differential Diagnosis. Acta Cytol 1988;32:527–532.

16. Clarke-Pearson DL, Creasman WT. Ovarian cancer. In Moossa AR, Robson MC, Schimpff SC. Comprehensive textbook of oncology. Baltimore: Williams & Wilkins, 1986:845.

17. Ferenczy A, Winkler B. Carcinoma and metastatic tumors of the cervix. In Kurman RJ. Blaustein's pathology of the female genital tract, 3rd ed. New York: Springer-Verlag, 1987:218–256.

18. Sedlis A, Robboy SJ. Diseases of the vagina. In Kurman RJ. Blaustein's pathology of the female genital tract, 3rd ed. New York: Springer-Verlag, 1987:121–127.

19. Massoni EA, Hajdu SI. Cytology of primary and metastatic uterine sarcomas. Acta Cytol 1984;28:93–100.

20. Suen KC. Guides to clinical aspiration biopsy. Intestine and retroperitoneum. New York: Igaku Shoin, 1987:89–91.

21. Nguyen GK, Berendt RC. Aspiration biopsy cytology of metastatic endometrial stromal sarcoma and extragenital mixed mesodermal tumor. Diagn Cytopathol 1986;2:256–260.

22. Silverman JF, Gardner J, Larkin EW, Finley JL, Norris HT. Ascitic fluid cytology in a case of metastatic malignant mixed mesodermal tumor of the ovary. Acta Cytol 1986;30:173–176.

23. Morimoto N, Ozawa M, Kato Y, Kuramoto H. Diagnostic value of mitotic activity in endometrial stromal sarcoma. Acta Cytol 1982;26:696–698.

16

Diagnostic Immunocytochemistry

Immunocytochemistry is the identification of a tissue constituent in situ according to its antigenic constitution by means of a specific antigen-antibody reaction tagged by a visible label. The advantage of immunocytochemistry over histochemical stains and electron microscopy is its increased specificity. The immunoperoxidase methodology, using antibodies tagged with horseradish peroxidase, is the most widely used today. The sites of peroxidase localization are demonstrated by addition of hydrogen peroxide and a chromogen; the interaction results in the formation of a colored precipitate that can be seen with an ordinary light microscope. Among the many immunoperoxidase staining procedures, the two most commonly used are the peroxidase-antiperoxidase and the avidin-biotin techniques. For technical details of various immunoperoxidase procedures, interested readers are referred to specialized publications.[1-5] Commercial kits containing antisera needed for routine diagnostic work are now readily available and have made results reliable and reproducible in the hands of conscientious technologists.

Clinical Applications

The principal applications of immunocytochemistry to diagnostic cytology are briefly summarized as follows:

(a) Immunocytochemical techniques enhance considerably our ability to diagnose and classify tumors, especially poorly differentiated tumors whose origins cannot be determined solely with the use of routine stains or special cytochemical stains. With immunochemical staining techniques, antibodies directed against tissue-specific antigens can be used to differentiate tumors as epithelial, lymphoid, neural, or mesenchymal.[6-10a] In some instances a very specific diagnosis can be made when a cell-specific substance is identified, such as demonstration of calcitonin in medullary thyroid carcinomas,[11] myoglobin in rhabdomyoblastic tumors, and prostate-specific antigen in prostatic adenocarcinomas.[12,13] Similarly, functional classification of pancreatic endocrine tumors based on the specific polypeptides they produce are now possible.[14]

(b) Immunocytochemistry can aid in distinguishing between reactive lymphoid hyperplasia and malignant lymphoma. In reactive conditions the B-lymphocyte population exhibits polyclonality, expressing both κ and λ light chains; conversely, a monoclonal B-cell population is consistent with malignant lymphoma.[8] Although there are cases of B-cell lymphoma that produce both κ and λ chains, such an event is rare.

Moreover, a number of lymphocyte antibodies capable of detecting specific subsets of lymphocytes are now available and aid in more precise characterization of individual lymphomas.[15]

(c) Small groups of metastatic cancer cells can be demonstrated immunocytologically in bone marrow, lymph nodes, and serous fluids at a time when the cell groups are too small or too few to be detected by conventional light microscopy.[16-20]

(d) Some markers may provide prognostic information. In breast cancer, the expression of carcinoembryonic antigen (CEA) appears to correlate with the presence of lymph node metastases.[21] Similarly, CEA-positive carcinoid tumors of the lung have been shown to behave more aggressively than their CEA-negative counterparts.[22]

(e) Through the use of immunostains, infectious agents such as hepatitis B virus, herpes simplex virus, and human papilloma virus can be readily diagnosed.[23,24]

Tumor Markers

In diagnostic immunocytochemistry, the term *tumor marker* is used to designate those substances that are stored or secreted by the tumor cells and which can be demonstrated immunochemically in

TABLE 16.1. Some Common Markers Used for Immunocytologic Diagnosis of Tumors

Marker	Diagnostic Implications
Cytokeratin[6,7,25]	Epithelial tumors, mesothelioma
Epithelial membrane antigen (EMA)[26]	Epithelial tumors, mesothelioma (some lymphomas rarely)
Vimentin[7,25,27]	Mesenchymal tumors (some carcinomas)
Leukocyte common antigen[28,29]	White cell series
Lymphocyte subsets[15]	Typing of lymphoma
α-Fetoprotein[30]	Yolk sac tumor, hepatocellular carcinoma
Carcinoembryonic antigen (CEA)[16]	Many adenocarcinomas (mesothelial cells generally negative)
Desmin[7,25,27]	Muscle tumors
Neuron-specific enolase[31]	Neuroendocrine tumors, neuroblastoma, Wilms' tumor, melanoma
Hormones (e.g., calcitonin, thyroglobulin, gastrin, human chorionic gonadotropin)[13,14,30]	Endocrine tumors
Myoglobin[32]	Rhabdomyoblastic tumors
Prostate-specific antigen[11]	Prostatic carcinoma
Prostatic acid phosphatase[12]	Prostatic carcinoma
S100 protein[33]	Nerves, Schwann cells, chondrocytes, melanocytes, Langerhans' cells, APUD cells

TABLE 16.2. Coexpression of Cytokeratin/Vimentin

1. Epithelial neoplasms: renal cell carcinoma, some papillary thyroid carcinomas, some adenocarcinomas of the endometrium, ovary, and lung, adenoid cystic carcinoma, pleomorphic adenoma of salivary gland
2. Sarcomas: synovial sarcoma, epithelioid sarcoma
3. Other neoplasms: mesothelioma, thymoma, Wilms' tumor, chordoma

tissue sections, smears, or cell suspensions. **Table 16.1** is a brief list of tumor markers commonly used in diagnostic pathology.[6,7,11–16,25–33] It should be noted that many tumor markers are not absolutely specific. Familiarity with the immunocytologic profiles of various tumors is crucial in the correct interpretation of the results. Using a combination of carefully selected antibodies, one can usually arrive at a correct diagnosis when other information, such as clinical and conventional morphologic data, is also taken into consideration. For example, an anaplastic melanoma may cause diagnostic confusion with poorly differentiated carcinoma and lymphoma. Despite a lack of specificity for S100 protein for melanoma, the presence of this antigen supports such a diagnosis, if concomitant evaluation of cytokeratin and leukocyte common antigen are negative. Another commonly encountered problem is the demonstration in some carcinomas of vimentin, which is generally regarded as a marker for mesenchymal tumors. Thus, antivimentin antibody should not be used alone in the evaluation of mesenchymal tumors. In a proper clinical context, a mesencyhmal tumor is implicated if vimentin is positive and cytokeratin is negative. Coexpression of both cytokeratin and vimentin suggest other possibilities **(Table 16.2)**.[34–36]

Specimen Preparations

Immunoperoxidase techniques can be effectively applied to direct cell smears, cytocentrifuge preparations (Cytospins), and cell blocks. The direct smears or cytocentrifuge smears are fixed in high-quality acetone for 8–10 minutes, prior to immunostaining. It is important not to underfix or overfix the smears. A too long fixation time may destroy the antigen. Many cell membrane antigens (particularly those of hematopoietic cells) are readily destroyed by any fixative and are best demonstrated in air-dried cytologic samples. Material for cell block should be placed in B5 or Bouin's fixative, and then embedded in paraffin or resin.

We do not perform immunoperoxidase studies indiscriminately. We make a decision only after light microscopic examination of the specimen. If immunoperoxidase studies are indicated and cell block preparation is not available, we prefer cytocentrifuge smears to direct smears. The cytocentrifuge technique (we use Cytospin II, Shandon Instruments, Sewickley, PA) has many advantages, such as

low background staining with minimal interference from tissue fluid, good preservation of cellular morphology, and ease of preparing multiple smears from the cytocentrifuge material, thus enabling one to perform a panel of immunostains.[37] The slides should be removed from the cytocentrifuge as soon as it stops, so that cells may air dry as quickly as possible. If cells take too long to dry, poor cytologic detail may result. The slides are then fixed in cold (4 °C), high-quality acetone for about 8–10 minutes and stored in a refrigerator until they are stained.

Precautions and Pitfalls

In immunocytologic studies, meticulous attention to procedural detail and caution in interpretation are as necessary as in any other laboratory methodology.

(a) When evaluating a new antiserum, it is important to use a positive tissue on which to determine the optimal dilution that gives the strongest staining of the antigen with minimal background staining. If the dilution is too low, strong background activity may interfere with interpretation; if the dilution is too high, the specific antigen may not stain.

(b) Appropriate negative and positive controls must be run with each sample. A negative control slide is prepared by replacing the primary antiserum with nonimmune normal serum from the same species, or by staining a known negative smear. For positive control, a slide prepared from a known positive source should be fixed and stained in a manner identical to that of the unknown slides being studied. It is always necessary to include a known positive slide or else negative results cannot be assessed.

(c) A negative result by itself does not exclude any diagnosis. A number of factors may give rise to negative results, such as suboptimal specimen fixation, improper technique, or use of unsuitable antibodies or antibodies that are excessively diluted.

(d) False-positive results may arise from artifacts—crushed tissue, dead cells, and debris that may stain nonspecifically. In a sample containing a mixed cell population, care must be taken to distinguish neoplastic cells from nonneoplastic cells.

(e) One should be aware of the fact that many of these antibodies are still under investigation and their alleged specificities may be based on preliminary studies. The cytopathologist should limit the use of immunostains in one of the two clearly defined situations: to narrow a differential diagnosis and to support a diagnosis. In the final analysis, immunocytochemical evaluation must be subjugated to the assessment of routinely stained cytomorphology.

(f) When evaluating difficult diagnostic problems, a panel of carefully selected antibodies, rather than a single antibody, should be used.

References

1. Sternberger LA. Immunocytochemistry, 2nd ed. New York: John Wiley & Sons, 1979.
2. DeLellis RA, Sternberger LA, Mann RB, Banks PM, Nakane PK. Immunoperoxidase technics in diagnostic pathology. Report of a workshop sponsored by the National Cancer Institute. Am J Clin Pathol 1979;71:483–488.
3. Bourne JA. Handbook of immunoperoxidase staining methods. Santa Barbara: Dako Corp., 1983.
4. Falini B, Taylor CR. New developments in immunoperoxidase techniques and their application. Arch Pathol Lab Med 1983;107:105–117.
5. Nadji M, Morales AR. Immunoperoxidase: Part I. The technique and its pitfalls. Lab Med 1983;14:767–771.
6. Domagala W, Lubinski J, Weber K, Osborn M. Intermediate filament typing of tumor cells in fine needle aspirates by means of monoclonal antibodies. Acta Cytol 1986;30:214–224.
7. Gown AM, Vogel AM. Monoclonal antibodies to human intermediate filament proteins. III. Analysis of tumors. Am J Clin Pathol 1985;84:413–424.
8. Levitt S, Cheng L, DuPuis MH, Layfield LJ: Fine needle aspiration diagnosis of malignant lymphoma with confirmation by immunoperoxidase staining. Acta Cytol 1985;29:895–902.

9. Nadji M. The potential value of immunoperoxidase techniques in diagnostic cytology. Acta Cytol 1980;24:442–447.

10. Chess Q, Hajdu SI. The role of immunoperoxidase staining in diagnostic cytology. Acta Cytol 1986;30:1–7.

10a. Keshgegian AA. ABCs of immunocytochemistry. In Kline TS. Handbook of fine needle aspiration biopsy cytology, 2nd ed. New York: Churchill Livingstone, 1988:419–431.

11. DeLellis RA, Rule AH, Spiler I, et al. Calcitonin and carcinoembryonic antigen as tumor markers in medullary thyroid carcinoma. Am J Clin Pathol 1978;70:587–594.

12. Keshgegian AA. Immunocytochemistry. In Kline TS. Guides to clinical aspiration biopsy. Prostate. New York: Igaku Shoin, 1985:115–125.

13. Keshgegian AA, Kline TS. Immunoperoxidase demonstration of prostatic acid phophatase in aspiration biopsy cytology (ABC). Am J Clin Pathol 1984;82:586–589.

14. Mukai K, Greider MH, Grotting JC, Rosai J. Retrospective study of 77 pancreatic endocrine tumors using the immunoperoxidase method. Am J Surg Pathol 1982;6:387–399.

15. Martin SE, Zhang HZ, Magyarosy E, et al. Immunologic methods in cytology: Definitive diagnosis of non-Hodgkin's lymphoma using immunologic markers to T- and B-cells. Am J Clin Pathol 1984;82:666–673.

16. Watts AE, Said JW. Specific tumor markers in diagnostic cytology. Immunoperoxidase studies of carcinoembryonic antigen, lysozyme and other tissue antigens in effusions, washes and aspirates. Acta Cytol 1983;27:408–416.

17. Ghosh AK, Mason DY, Spriggs AI. Immunocytochemical staining with monoclonal antibodies in cytologically "negative" serous effusions from patients with malignant disease. J Clin Pathol 1983;36:1150–1153.

18. Ghosh AK, Hatton C, O'Connor N, et al. Detection of metastatic tumor cells in routine bone marrow smears by immuno-alkaline phosphatase labelling with monoclonal antibodies. Br J Haematol 1985;61:21–30.

19. Menard S, Rike F, Torre GD, et al. Sensitivity enhancement of the cytologic detection of cancer cells in effusions by monoclonal antibodies. Am J Clin Pathol 1985;83:571–576.

20. Redding WH, Monaghan P, Imrie SF, et al. Detection of micrometastases in patients with primary breast cancer. Lancet 2:1271–1274, 1983.

21. Shousha S, Lyssiotis T, Godfrey VM, Scheuer PJ. Carcinoembryonic antigen in breast cancer tissue: A useful prognostic indicator. Br Med J 1979;1:777–779.

22. Bishopric GA, Ordonez NG. Carcinoembryonic antigen in primary carcinoid tumors of the lung. Cancer 1986;58:1316–1320.

23. Bedrossian UK, de Arce EAL, Bedrossian CWM. Immunoperoxidase method to detect herpes simplex virus in cytologic specimens. Lab Med 1984;15;673–676.

24. Ulich T, Thorne C, Cheng L, Lewin KJ, Gitnick GL. Chronic active hepatitis of hepatitis B and non-A, non-B etiology: Immunoperoxidase staining of hepatitis B surface antigen in a series of 66 needle biopsies. Am J Surg Pathol 1982;6:33–39.

25. Osborn M, Weber K. Tumor diagnosis by intermediate filament typing: A novel tool for surgical pathology. Lab Invest 1983;48:372–394.

26. Pinkus GS, Kurtin PJ. Epithelial membrane antigen—A diagnostic discriminant in surgical pathology. Immunohistochemical profile in epithelial, mesenchymal, and hematopoietic neoplasms using paraffin section and monoclonal antibodies. Hum Pathol 1985;16:929–940.

27. Altmannsberger M, Dirk T, Osborn M, Weber K. Immunohistochemistry of cytoskeletal filaments in the diagnosis of soft tissue tumors. Semin Diagn Pathol 3:306–316, 1986.

28. Kurtin PJ, Pinkus GS. Leukocyte common antigen—A diagnostic discriminant between hematopoietic and nonhematopoietic neoplasms in paraffin sections using monoclonal antibodies: Correlation with immunologic studies and ultrastructural localization. Hum Pathol 1985;16:353–364.

29. Warnke RA, Gatter KC, Falini B, et al. Diagnosis of human lymphoma with monoclonal antileukocyte antibodies. N Engl J Med 309:1275–1281, 1983.

30. Kurman RJ, Scardino PT, McIntire KR, Waldmann TA, Javadpour N. Cellular localization of alpha-fetoprotein and human chorionic gonadotropin in germ cell tumors of the testis using an indirect immunoperoxidase technique. Cancer 1977;40:2136–2151.

31. Dhillon AP, Rode J, Leathem A. Neuron-specific enolase: An aid to the diagnosis of melanoma and neuroblastoma. Histopathology 1982;6:81–92.

32. Corson JM, Pinkus GS. Intracellular myoglobin—A specific marker for skeletal muscle differentiation in soft tissue sarcomas. Am J Pathol 1981;103:384–389.

33. Kahn HJ, Marks A, Thom H, Baumal R. Role of antibody to S100 protein in diagnostic pathology. Am J Clin Pathol 1983;79:341–347.

34. Gould VE. The coexpression of distinct class of intermediate filaments in human neoplasms. Arch Pathol Lab Med 1985;109:984–985.

35. Miettinen M, Franssila K, Lehto VP, et al. Expression of intermediate filament protein in thyroid gland and thyroid tumors. Lab Invest 1984;50:262–270.

36. Holthoeffer H, Miettinen A, Paasivuo et al. Cellular origin and differentiation of renal carcinomas. Lab Invest 1983;49:317–326.

37. Yu GSM. Immunocytochemistry and electron microscopy. In Suen KC. Guides to clinical aspiration biopsy. Retroperitoneum and intestine. New York: Igaku Shoin, 1987:191–206.

Index

(Page numbers in italics refer to illustrations)